Multiplanar CT
of the Spine

Multiplanar CT
of the Spine

Stephen L. G. Rothman, M.D.
William V. Glenn, Jr., M.D.
Medical Science Center
Multi-Planar Diagnostic Imaging, Inc.
Torrance, California

with 990 illustrations, 16 in full-color

University Park Press · Baltimore

University Park Press
International Publishers in Medicine and Allied Health
300 North Charles Street
Baltimore, Maryland 21201

Copyright © 1985 by University Park Press

Sponsoring Editor: Larry W. Carter
Director of Production: Berta Steiner
Cover and text design by: Caliber Design Planning, Inc.
Typeset by: Waldman Graphics, Inc.
Manufactured in the United States by Halliday Lithograph

Cover illustrations: Failed L4-5 interbody fusion. **A:** Prone axial
view. **B:** Sagittal view. **C:** Coronal view, with the curve defined
on the sagittal plane parallel to the spinal canal.

Illustration sequence: A B
                              C

Library of Congress Cataloging in Publication Data

Main entry under title:
Multiplanar CT of the spine.
    Includes index.
    1. Spine—Radiography. 2. Tomography. 3. Spine—
Diseases—Diagnosis. I. Rothman, Stephen L. G.,
1942–   II. Glenn, William V. [DNLM: 1. Spine—
radiography. 2. Tomography, X-Ray Computed. WE 725 M961]
RD533.M85 1984   616.7′3′07572   84-17344
ISBN 0-8391-1910-0

This book is dedicated to our parents
Anita and Jerry Rothman
Doris and Dr. William V. Glenn, Sr.

Contents

Preface

A few years ago a radiologist, a computer graphics engineer, a talented computer programmer, and a systems analyst asked a group of back surgeons, "If you were devising a CT examination of the spine, with no regard to what the manufacturers provide, what would you ask for?"

From that session and other meetings with similar surgical groups emerged a unique method of performing CT examinations of the spine. In essence, the examination includes (1) life-size imaging, (2) a complete series of axial, sagittal, and coronal images, and (3) a film organization comparable to myelography and therefore understandable by spine physicians.

This volume is unique among major CT books. It represents a single, unified approach to spine CT based on the experience gained from the analysis of 14,000 spine examinations by a single scientific group. We do not approach spine CT as an ancillary examination among a group of radiographic studies because we firmly believe that a complete CT examination provides all the radiographic information necessary to treat the majority of spine disorders. Our first premise is that the well-performed and well-interpreted CT scan precludes a myelogram in most cases.

This book includes discussion on how we perform CT of the spine and how to analyze the CT spine examination so as to derive from it all available information. We emphasize a suggested lumbar scanning procedure and the concomitant film organization and reporting form (including an anatomic grading system for various components of the lumbar spine), and a logical film-reading sequence.

The authors of this book have a unique experience. They have been involved with the development and/or clinical testing of five versions of multiplanar reformation from four CT manufacturers on three generations of body scanners. All but one of these multiplanar capabilities have been

of the interactive type, which involves the radiologist spending much time at the console.

The approach described herein requires no computer expertise and no sitting at the console. The radiologist works only from the film, the medium with which he is most comfortable. The objective is, simply, efficiency. Efficiency is also the reason for using precisely the same scanning technique and film organization for all cases. The result is that the radiologist is freed from any interaction at the physician's console and from any need for monitoring the scanning of individual spine cases. The radiologist has been returned once again to the viewbox or alternator, where he usually spends his day.

For the CT scanning facility faced with rapidly increasing demands for spine CT, already saturated schedules must somehow make room for what may eventually become the largest patient category in "body" scanning. One solution is to limit severely the number of CT spine examinations; another is to find ways whereby the busy facility can stretch to accommodate this fastest growing demand segment in diagnostic CT. The latter solution requires a real effort to optimize the efficiency of each component of the CT spine diagnostic process: scanner, computer, technologist's time, use of film, reading efficiency of the radiologists, and last but perhaps most important the confidence with which the resulting films are understood by the referring physician.

Optimal CT spine diagnosis is not achieved simply by locating a CT scanner that can make high-resolution transverse images. The challenge is to provide easily understood image data that can be efficiently transferred to film and thoroughly understood by the viewer. Variables that impact acceptance include the number of films per study, information content per film and per image, easy location of position in a series of similar pictures, and finally adequate visual cues for correlating the correct image with the correct interspace. Whether the referring physician chooses a CT scan or a myelographic examination, he should be able to go to the patient's film jacket and place either set of films on the viewbox with equal ease and equal understanding regarding the primary findings. A CT spine case becomes tedious when treated as a lengthy series of individual pictures rather than as a coherent unit or sequence of carefully registered and cross-referenced images.

The implications of increased use of CT in spine-related diagnoses are not all positive. A concern often expressed by spine surgeons is that CT's elucidation of numerous surgically tempting abnormalities may increase inappropriate surgery on clinically silent bone spurs, laminar thickening, disc/anulus bulging, facet hypertrophy, or foraminal encroachment. To avoid surgery inspired by pictures, CT's morphologic details must be presented to the surgeon in a standardized format that is thorough, easily understood, and not conducive to misinterpretation. The surgeon himself must confidently understand the CT images in order to make precise correlations with patient history,

neurologic examination, and other diagnostic information.

It is our contention that the ultimate role of spine CT and the extent of its utilization will be determined by referring orthopedic surgeons, neurosurgeons, and neurologists—they are the physicians who currently order myelograms. If myelography for spinal stenosis and disc disease is to be largely supplanted by noninvasive CT, these are the referring specialists who first must be made to feel comfortable and competent with CT. Ideally, they will be taught to understand CT examinations to the degree that they now understand myelographic studies.

Although the exact film formats described herein are produced only by the use of specialized computer software not yet available to every institution in the United States, the clinical approach is generic in that if enough time, energy, and resources are made available to perform a *complete* examination of the spine adequate reformations can be produced using the programs provided by the CT manufacturers.

Our major objective is to show CT of the spine for what it can be: the single most important diagnostic tool for the evaluation of spinal disorders.

Acknowledgments

Gratitude is expressed to the overworked and harried technical staff at MPDI—Nadim Sawaya, Richard Amador, Jack Estrada, Mary Kay Catterall, Carolyn Leonard, and Venita Smith—for their herculean efforts in the preparation of the illustrations for this book. Special thanks to Larry Carter for his constant encouragement, editorial expertise, and original decision to make this book happen. Special thanks also to Berta Steiner for the superb layout and attention to production detail.

While there were many talented people who contributed to the realization of this book, recognition of Jerry Lindley is of particular importance. She spent hundreds of hours reviewing, typing, and editing the manuscript, always questioning how best to express ideas. Jerry finished her arduous task before revealing how ill she really was. She moved ''home'' within weeks in order to enjoy each new day with her parents and family in Tulsa. Her days were limited for reasons that medical school teaches us all too vividly. Jerry was thrilled to see the final page proofs of the entire book on August 31, 1984. She died three days later on September 2. Those of us who were close will miss her many talents, tireless energy, and her friendship. We are deeply touched and most grateful for the courage it took to push ''her book'' to completion.

Contributors

Perry E. Camp, M.D.
Medical Director
Whitman Institute of Neuro Science
Walla Walla, Washington

William V. Glenn, Jr., M.D.
Chairman, MPDI Medical Science Center
Torrance, California

Ronald L. Kaufman, M.D.
Assistant Professor of Medicine—Rheumatology
USC School of Medicine
Los Angeles, California and
Associate Medical Director
Rancho Los Amigos Hospital
Downey, California

Charles W. Kerber, M.D.
MPDI Medical Science Center
Torrance, California

Wolfgang Rauschning, M.D.
Senior Visiting Scientist
Researcher Director
Foundation for Advanced Medical Display Technology
Torrance, California and
Associate Professor
Department of Orthopedic Surgery
Uppsala University
Sweden and
Visiting Associate Professor
Department of Radiological Science
UCLA School of Medicine
Los Angeles, California

Michael L. Rhodes, Ph.D.
Director of Computer Science
MPDI Medical Science Center
Torrance, California

Stephen L. G. Rothman, M.D.
Director of Medical Science
MPDI Medical Science Center
Torrance, California

Leon L. Wiltse, M.D.
Staff, Long Beach Memorial Hospital
Long Beach, California and
Honorary Clinical Professor of Orthopedic Surgery
University of California, Irvine
Irvine, California

Foreword

Before the discovery of x-rays by Roentgen in 1895, physicians and surgeons were extremely frustrated because of the lack of a method to appropriately examine the spine and the nervous structures that were contained within it, and which sprang from it. At that time there were no really trained neurologists or neurosurgeons, but the inability to properly examine the spine did not improve very much following the development of these two specialties of medicine and surgery.

Frustration continued for several decades, even after the discovery of x-rays, for in spite of the fact that it was possible to get frontal, lateral and oblique radiographs of the spine, this examination was helpful only in a small percentage of cases. Following the serendipitous description of myelography by Sicard and Forestier in 1922, it was hoped that, at last, a good and "complete" method of examination had been devised. However, the lack of a good contrast medium for myelography, which lasted two decades until the development of Pantopaque, hampered the widespread use of myelography.

The cause of sciatica was not understood until after the first description of herniation of the intervertebral discs by Mixter and Barr in 1934. Once the diseases of the intervertebral disc became part of medical knowledge, the indications for myelography increased greatly, and after Pantopaque was introduced into the market, the number of myelographic examinations increased precipitously. Myelography, then, became the most commonly performed examination procedure of the spine aside from plain film examination. Myelography, however, is invasive and, when performed with Pantopaque, it often led to some undesirable minor and sometimes severe complications in patients who are sensitive to this contrast medium. Even the more recently developed water-soluble contrast media have some undesirable effects on sensitive patients.

Thus, the development of computed tomography of the spine was indeed a most welcome refinement, occurring several years after the discovery of CT, and long after it had been successfully applied to the diagnosis and management of diseases of the brain.

The two main authors of this book, Drs. Rothman and Glenn, the latter a true pioneer in spinal computed tomography, have accumulated a tremendous experience and have analyzed probably the largest number of spinal CT with multiplanar reconstruction of any group in the United States. However, in this work, they have not limited themselves to demonstrating anatomy and pathology via computed tomography with axial, sagittal and coronal reconstructions, but have included an exquisite demonstration of the anatomy as shown in cross-sections. The color and black and white reproductions presented here by Rauschning are a most welcome complement to a book dealing with cross-sectional diagnosis by computed tomography. The chapter "Planning and Performing Spine Surgery with CT/MPR" by Camp and Kerber is also a welcome addition to a radiologic imaging book.

An interesting aspect of this work is the almost complete lack of any contrast media myelographic examination in the illustrations. I believe that this represents a trend and that with the passage of time, myelography will be utilized less frequently. The next book of this type will be one combining computed tomography with multiplanar reconstruction and magnetic resonance imaging of the spine and intraspinal structures. Further reduction in myelography can be expected.

I believe that the authors have succeeded in compiling a book representing the state-of-the-art in CT diagnosis of the spine.

Juan M. Taveras, M.D.
Massachusetts General Hospital
Boston, Massachusetts

Foreword

Few would argue that one of the greatest advances in medical diagnosis of all times has been that of computerized axial tomography. In a few short years CT has advanced from an experimental idea to a remarkably sophisticated system available to virtually everyone living in the world's developed countries.

This book is written especially for the radiologist, the neurosurgeon and the orthopaedic surgeon, but anyone who treats spinal disease will be benefited. It is unique in that it is a detailed treatise on the spine from a perspective of radiologists who specialize in CT. The authors bring together most of the current knowledge of the spine as it relates to CT and present it in a succinct fashion.

The illustrations are of excellent quality and are nearly all original.

The authors have made an effort to correlate what is seen on the CT image with actual pathology. Some correlation with symptoms is also made.

This book differs from any previously published work in that it is the work of a single group, rather than a compilation of several chapters written by many different authors. Because of this it is more integrated and is without the inevitable overlaps, repetitions and omissions that occur when many authors are involved.

Probably no other diagnostic modality is burdened with more difficulty in transferring to the mind of the surgeon that which is in the mind of the radiologist who reads the CT image. In this book the authors address this problem and present in detail their method of organizing the image material supplied by the computer into something understandable to the treating physician. After all, it is he who must use that information in the treatment of the patient.

One of the criticisms often leveled against CT has been that it shows too much and that there is difficulty distinguishing the incidental from the truly significant. This of course will remain a problem, but the system of grading lesions from 1 to 5 presented here does help a great deal.

For all these reasons this treatise becomes a valuable contribution and forms a basis for understanding the minutiae of normal and abnormal CT findings in the spine. The presentation makes this knowledge more readily available to the surgeon and helps him to decide if surgery is necessary and if so the type and extent of that surgery.

Leon L. Wiltse, M.D.
Long Beach, California

Foreword

Diagnostic imaging of the spinal column, spinal cord, and spinal roots has changed so much even in the career of one neurosurgeon that it is difficult to remember the former concerns and problems concerning x-ray studies of the spinal column. Presently, the problem is evaluating the information obtained from diagnostic imaging. The commonest complaint in spinal disorders is local and/or radicular pain, and most complaints are related to some activity—required, disliked, enjoyed or compensatory. This relationship of a subjective complaint to a specific activity that is often a gain-producing symptom requires objective measurements to diagnose and treat effectively. Despite an older clinician's concern, diagnostic imaging increasingly has become the foundation upon which diagnosis and therapy are based.

The images being produced are of such apparent anatomical quality that clinicians may accept information that has not been diagnostically verified. Such information often suggests new diagnoses which may or may not contribute to the symptoms, or to any symptom-producing disease state.

In conditions such as trauma and tumors of the spine, the problems are different. The images both confirm the diagnoses and accurately define the position and extent of bony displacement or tumors. Frequently, the quality is such that the images may not require contrast, or may require such small amounts of contrast material that the contrast is poorly visualized or not visualized with conventional x-rays. The clinician must be aware that such exams are often more limited than standard myelography and that, as with any imaging technique, this value is relative to the accuracy of the localization.

Recently, the most commonly used imaging technique has been high resolution x-ray computerized tomography (CT). This book summarizes the experiences of practicing clinicians with this technique, places in perspective the various methods used to improve the information obtained from CT, and, where possible, relates the experiences of treatment. It provides guidelines to clarify the use of CT in the diagnosis and treatment of spinal conditions, since it allows the physician treating these disorders to evaluate the available techniques of CT scanning as they relate to the disease entities being considered, to understand some of the techniques' limitations as well as advantages, and, hopefully, at least from my point of view, to determine the place of the obtained information in the diagnosis and treatment of spinal disorders. The necessity of such a presentation should be apparent to all. Perhaps this book and its successors will hasten the time when the problems and limitations of diagnostic imaging of the spine will be clarified, and the value of such imaging defined.

William Collins, M.D.
Chief, Department of Neurosurgery
Yale University, School of Medicine

Multiplanar CT
of the Spine

Scanning Technique for Lumbar Spine Computerized Tomography

1

There is no standardized technique for the performance of a computerized tomographic (CT) evaluation of the spine. The basic principles stated here allow the reader to devise the best method for his own scanner and clinical practice.

Methodology of Spine CT

CT of the spine is approached in a variety of ways. The process selected is affected by a combination of available CT system options and the personal preferences of the radiologist and referring physicians. A partial list of the approaches currently used includes:

1. *Axial scans; nontilted gantry; interspaces only.* This is the least complete examination. A portion of each vertebra is omitted from the study, and axial scans are not parallel to the discs. Limited reformation is possible, but anatomic areas are so small they are of limited value (Fig. 1.1A).
2. *Axial scans; nontilted gantry; contiguous or overlapped scans covering vertebral-body segments and interspaces.* This technique is common. Axial scans are generally performed using high milliamperagesettings in an attempt to optimize low contrast resolution. Proponents of this technique believe that they can, with experience, correctly compensate mentally for the distortion pro-

duced by axial scans traversing disc spaces obliquely (Figs. 1.1B, C).
3. *Axial scans; tilted gantry; interspaces only.*This commonly performed technique optimizes the axial scans for evaluation of the disc spaces by using high milliamperage. It has the advantage of reducing geometric angular distortion of the disc, but by its very nature it skips a portion of each vertebral segment (Fig. 1.1D).
4. *Axial scans; tilted gantry; contiguous or overlapped scans covering vertebral-body segments and interspaces.* This technique is an expansion of the previous system. Its tilted-axial scans include an entire vertebral segment. The plane of the scan parallels each interspace, but the entire vertebral body is covered by at least one slice (Fig. 1.1E). This is a more complete examination than that in (3), but it has a minor drawback in that the overlapped angled scans tend to radiate the same anatomy on the posterior portion of the patient, thereby raising the absorbed dose to the center of the low back.
5. *Sparse multiplanar; two or three sagittal and coronal images; used either routinely or when extra effort is needed to clarify a finding.*Two variations of this technique are commonly advocated. One variation uses a series of parallel 5-mm-thick axial slices, and the other uses a series of parallel overlapped 5-mm-thick axial slices. The proponents of this method use the scanner's internal reconstruction algorithms to produce sagittal and

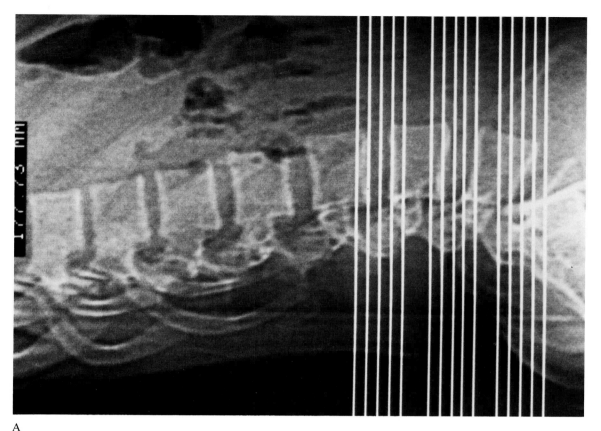

A

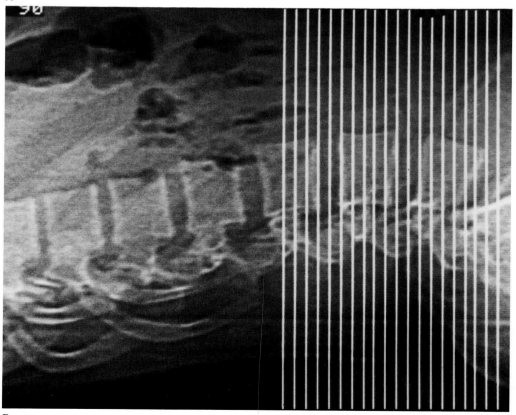

B

FIGURE 1.1 Methods of spine CT. **A.** Digital ScoutView showing axial disc-space technique; non-tilted gantry. **B.** Digital ScoutView; continuous 5–mm axial scans; non-tilted gantry. **C.** Digital Scoutview; overlapping continuous 5–mm axial scans; nontilted gantry. **D.** Digital ScoutView; angled gantry; interspaces only. (*Figure continued* on page 4.)

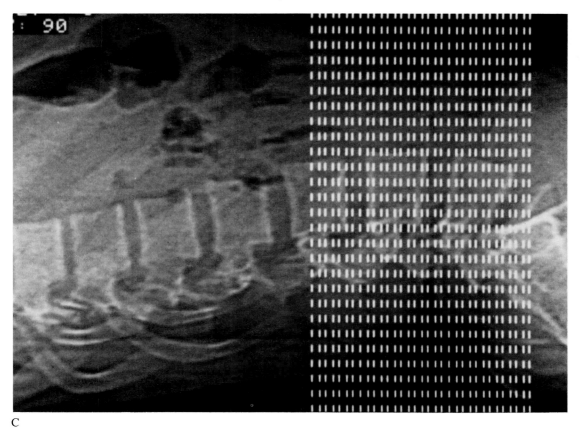

C

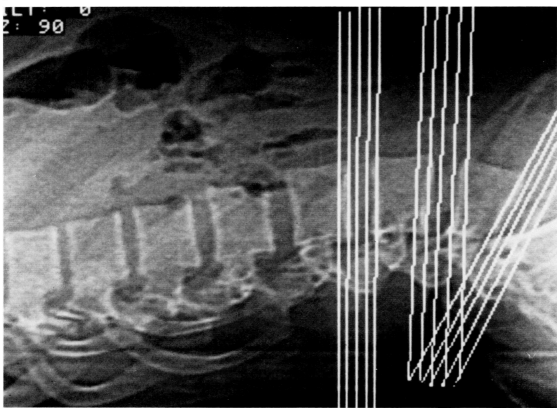

D

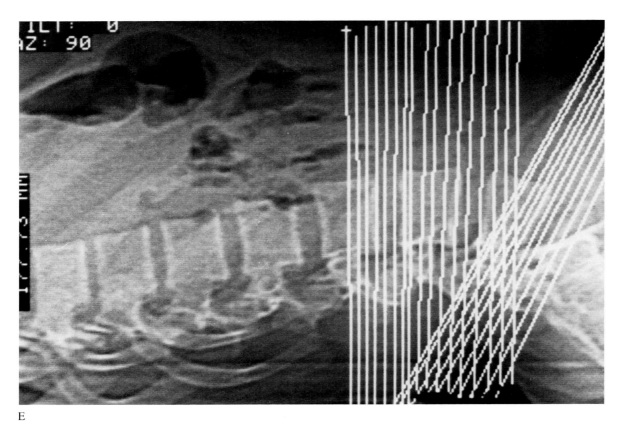

E

FIGURE 1.1 (*cont'd*)   Methods of spine CT. **E.** Digital ScoutView; angled gantry; interspaces and vertebral bodies.

coronal images at selected planes on selected cases. This method is becoming most widely used as reformation algorithms become more user-friendly (Fig. 1.2). This method is somewhat limited because the reformations are made at random planes, presumably where the pathology is most likely to occur. In most cases, this suf-

fices. However, because by its very nature the examination is incomplete, unsuspected pathology that is not present on the randomly selected reformation is missed.

6. *Detailed multiplanar; complete set of sagittal and coronal images, reformatted from thin overlapping scans.* This technique, advocated by the authors, is called the

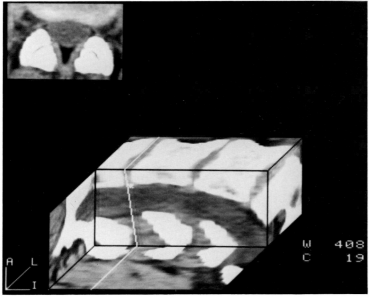

A

FIGURE 1.2   Multiplanar reformations using intrinsic scanner programs. **A.** Siemens Somatom. **B.** Technicare 2010. **C.** Picker 1200. (*Figure continued* on page 6.)

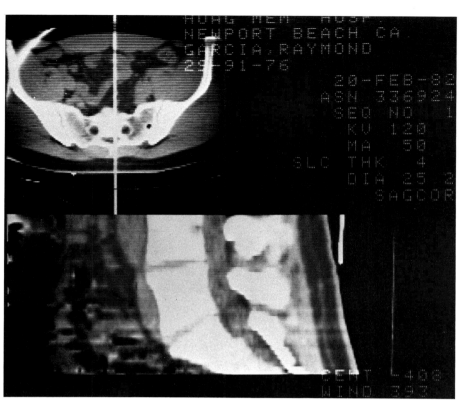

B

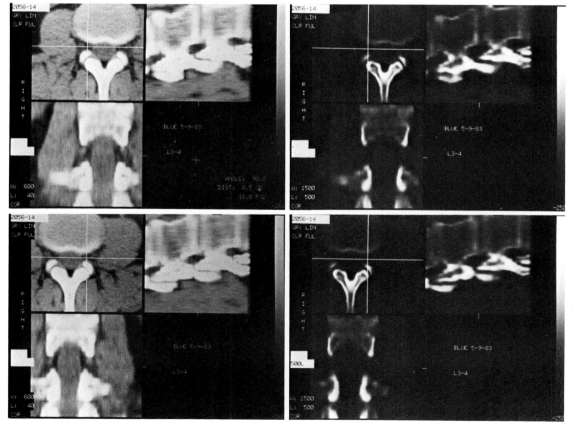

C

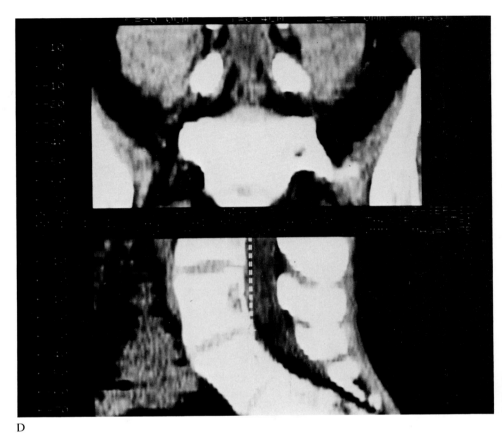

D

FIGURE 1.2 (*cont'd*) Multiplanar reformations using intrinsic scanner programs **D.** GE 9800.

CT/MPR method. The complete series of thin sagittal reformations preclude the necessity for tilting the gantry because there is no geometric distortion of the disc space on the sagittal view. We believe that we can actually reduce the per-slice milliamperage on the axial scans because the total information content of the three parallel

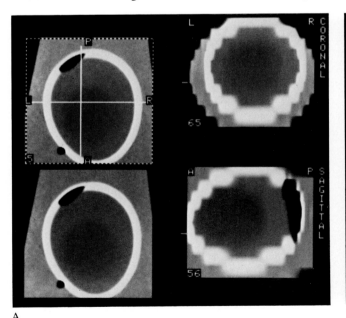

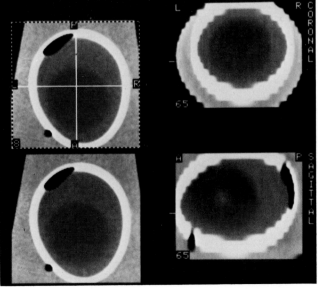

A   B

FIGURE 1.3 CT reformations from axial scans of varying slice thicknesses. Scans were performed on an egg embedded in gelatin. **A.** 5–mm slices every 5 mm. **B.** 5–mm slices every 3 mm. **C.** 1.5–mm slices every 1.5 mm. **D.** 1.5–mm slices every 1 mm.

views more than compensates for the subtle increase in contrast resolution gained by high-milliamperage techniques. We always use the thin overlapping slice technique. We believe that the Z-axis resolution offered by using contiguous 3-mm slices when available, or overlapped 5-mm scans when necessary, produces reformations with quality sufficiently higher than those produced from parallel 5-mm slices (Fig. 1.3).

Patient Preparation and Positioning

Patient cooperation and comfort are essential for high-quality spine CT. The examination is explained to the patient, who is given an honest estimate of the actual scanning time in order to prepare for a potentially lengthy period in the gantry. If necessary, the patient voids before lying on the table so that no patient motion occurs during the examination.

As a general rule, patients are scanned supine with the knees flexed over a pillow and a rigid plastic scoop (Fig. 1.4). Flexing the knees reduces the lumbar lordosis, thereby reducing the back pain that frequently occurs in the extended supine position. It also rotates the L5–S1 disc space into a more perpendicular plane, thereby reducing the obliquity of the scanning angle.

On occasion, when patients cannot lie supine because of either severe pain or a recent spinal operation, it is necessary to perform the CT scan with the patient prone. It is important to realize that respiration causes significant motion of the vertebral column in the prone position. Each

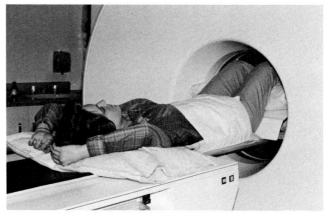

FIGURE 1.4 Patient in position for lumbar spine CT examination, with knees flexed and as comfortable as possible.

exposure is made in the same portion of the respiratory cycle, either at the end of deep inspiration or at the end of expiration. Respiration causes no significant spinal motion in most patients in the supine position.

Patients may be placed into the scanner either head first or feet first, depending on scanner design. The CT scanning system needs information on how the patient is positioned so that the left and right markers are annotated correctly on the final film. The patient is centered in the gantry, and whenever possible a ScoutView (General Electric Company, Milwaukee, Wisconsin) or a digital radiograph is performed in at least the lateral projection. It is frequently helpful to produce the digital radiograph in both

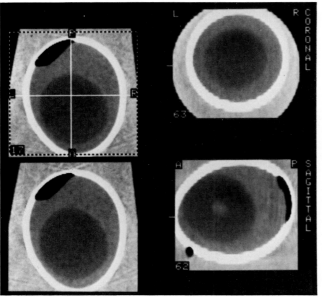

C

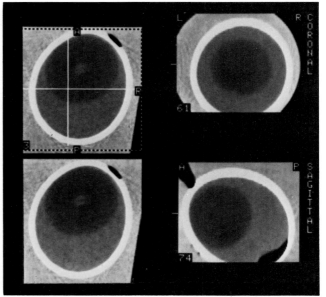

D

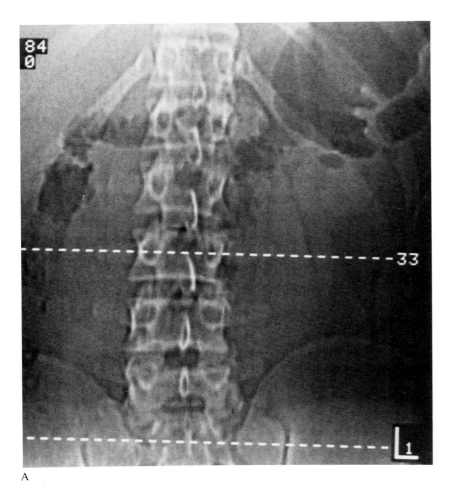

A

FIGURE 1.5 AP (**A**) and lateral ScoutView (**B**) indicating the limits of the patient to be scanned for a routine three-level spine series and tilted-axial surveys above the area of reconstruction.

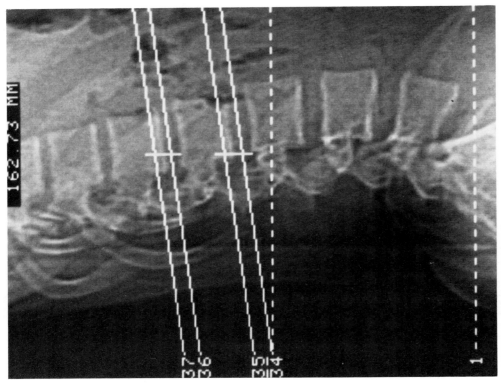

B

lateral and frontal projections. This frontal radiograph is useful for counting the number of vertebral segments, and it prevents mislabeling of transitional vertebrae. Digital radiography is the key to successful spine CT because it allows very precise localization of the slice level (Fig. 1.5).

Size of Scan Field

Typically, when studying the abdomen or the pelvis, whole-body scanners reconstruct a circle with a diameter of approximately 42 cm. This allows visualization of the entire circumference of the body on the viewing monitor. The pixel size is usually in the range of 1.5 × 1.5 mm. Standard head scanning programs reconstruct a circle approximately 10 cm in diameter and have a pixel size of approximately 1 × 1 mm.

When studying the spine, it is useful to reduce the circle of reconstruction to an area smaller than that used for the standard "body" technique. This has two advantages and one disadvantage. Reducing the size of the circle of reconstruction produces a concomitant decrease in the pixel size, thereby producing scans of higher spatial resolution. These scans are also magnified so that only the reduced circle of reconstruction fills the viewing monitor. Typically, spine scans are produced on "head-size" scanning programs with reconstruction circles in the range of 20–25 cm. For 320 × 320 image matrices, pixel sizes are as small as 0.7 mm. The disadvantage is that a portion of the patient is outside the circle of reconstruction, and it is therefore conceivable that pathology outside the spine could be missed. With most CT systems it is possible to scan the patient with a scanning circle wide enough to include all of the necessary anatomy but to reconstruct only those anatomic areas of interest. This is called "target reconstruction." It prevents some of the artifact caused by having a portion of the patient outside the circle of reconstruction and allows the scan to be displayed using small pixels. This is the technique that we use routinely (Fig. 1.6).

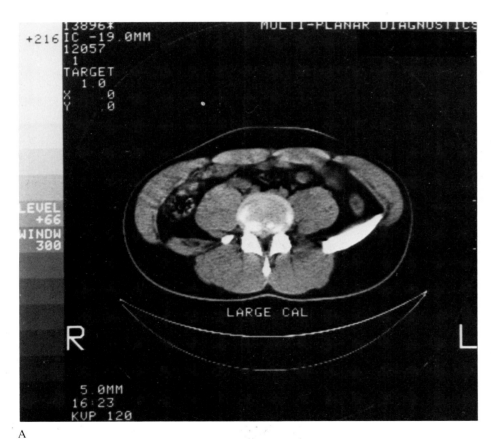

A

FIGURE 1.6   Axial spine scans produced on a GE 8800 scanner. **A.** Large-body calibration file, 42 cm. (*Figure continued* on pages 10–12.)

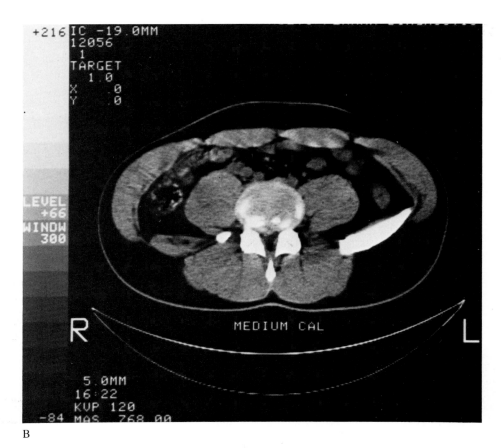

B

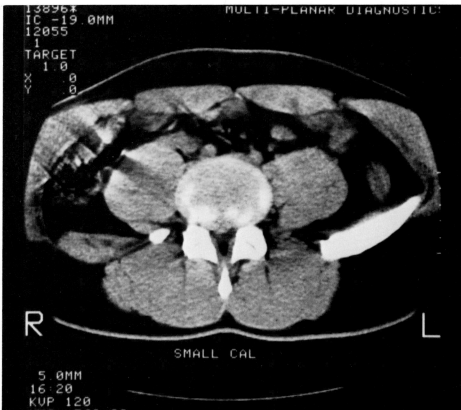

C

FIGURE 1.6 (*cont'd*) Axial spine scans produced on a GE 8800 scanner. **B.** Medium-body calibration file, 35 cm. **C.** Head calibration file, 25 cm. **D–F.** Previous scans viewed at the same magnification using the "target" reconstruction algorithm. (*Figure continued on page 12.*)

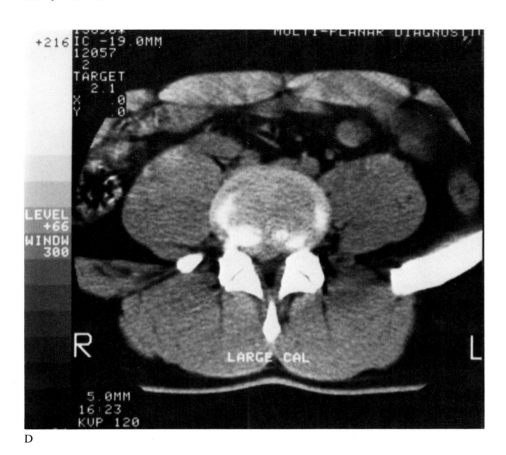

D

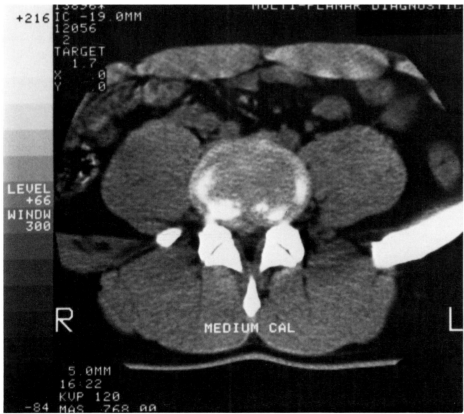

E

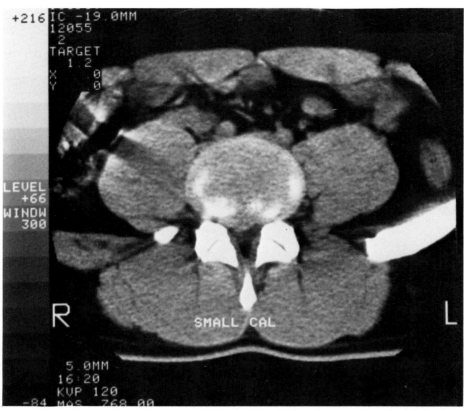

F

FIGURE 1.6 (*cont'd*)   Axial spine scans produced on a GE 8800 scanner. **D–F.** Previous scans viewed at the same magnification using the "target" reconstruction algorithm.

Slice Thickness

Most CT manufacturers offer variability of slice thickness. It is possible to scan the spine using very thin (1.5 mm), moderately thin (3–5 mm), or standard slices (10 mm) slices. Examples of each of these three distinct slice thicknesses for the same lumbar level in the same patient are shown in Figure 1.7. It is rarely advisable to scan using thick slices, because of the partial-volume effect. Slices of 10 mm almost always include disc and vertebral bodies averaged on the same slice.

Theoretically, it is advisable to scan with very thin slices (1.5 mm) for maximal reduction of the volume effect; however, this technique has a major drawback. In order to achieve images with the low signal/noise ratio needed for differentiating disc material from intraspinal contents it would be necessary to raise the milliamperage dramatically. Halving the slice thickness would require doubling the dose; therefore reducing the slice thickness to 1.5 mm would require more than five times the milliamperage to achieve an image of the same quality. It is therefore advisable to scan lumbar spines using slices of intermediate thickness.

Slices 5 mm thick reduce the volume averaging to within tolerable levels while not requiring milliamperage settings to be so high that tube cooling becomes a major problem. If sagittal/coronal reformatting is to be done, these 5 mm thick slices are taken every 3 mm with a 2-mm overlap. This has the virtue of maintaining the quality of the individual slices while providing excellent spatial resolution in the reformatted coronal and sagittal planes (Fig. 1.8).

Some scanners allow 3-mm slices, which seems a logical compromise. This provides better geometric resolution than do 5-mm slices and is likely to allow sufficient contrast resolution even in the lower lumbar spine. For scanner units of this type (e.g., GE 9800), it is appropriate to scan the patients using a series of nonoverlapped, contiguous 3-mm slices for reformation.

Advantages and Limitations of Gantry Angulation

When reformations are not to be performed, the plane of the CT scans is parallel to the disc in order to keep artifacts to a minimum. Angled CT slices may traverse a bony vertebral end-plate and a portion of the soft-tissue disc or anulus. The posterior soft-tissue shadow of a normal anulus

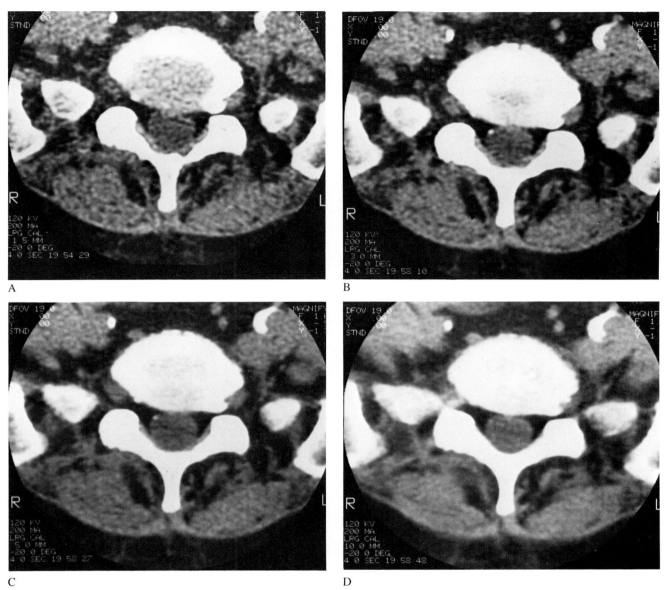

FIGURE 1.7 Axial scans at the same level, performed on a GE 9800 scanner. **A.** 1.5 mm slice thickness. **B.** 3 mm slice thickness. **C.** 5 mm slice thickness. **D.** 10 mm slice thickness.

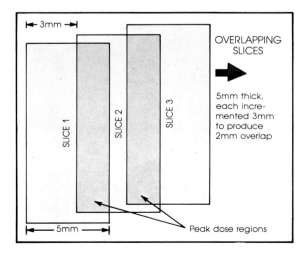

FIGURE 1.8 Slice thickness and overlap for the high-detail CT/MPR portion of the study.

may thus be mistaken for herniated or bulging disc. To reduce this artifact, the scanner is tilted such that each intervertebral disc space comes to lie parallel to the plane of the scan. This may require redisplaying digital radiographs several times during the examination and retilting the gantry between each disc space. The L5–S1 interspace may be impossible to position properly, however, as in the case of patients with a deep lumbar lordosis. Should this occur, placing the patient prone may straighten the L5–S1 interspace somewhat.

Multiplanar reformation eliminates the necessity for tilting the gantry because the amount of anulus bulge or disc herniation can be measured accurately on the sagittally reconstructed images. Advanced multiplanar capabilities can simulate a tilted gantry by producing tilted-axial images through reformation techniques, which are not limited mechanically by gantry architecture (gantry tilt of more than 20° in either direction is uncommon).

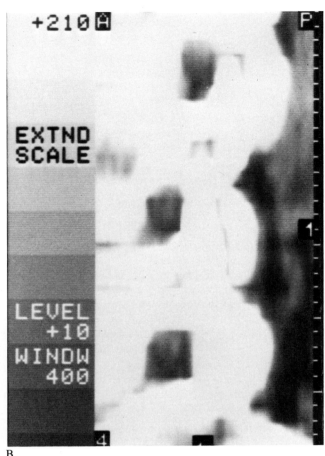

B

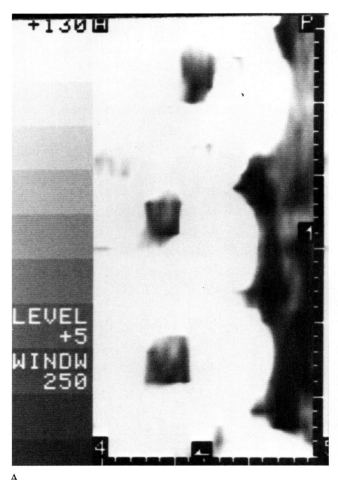

A

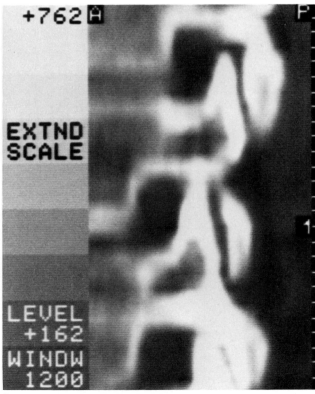

C

FIGURE 1.9 Effect of windowing and linear measurement. A series of sagittal reformations, all photographed with different mean and window settings but with the same geometric magnification. Note the difference in the size of the neural foramina. **A.** Window 250. **B.** Window 400. **C.** Window 1200.

Multiplanar Reformation of Axial Spine Scans

It is the opinion of the authors, based on 14,000 CT spine examinations, that sagittal and coronal reformation of axial CT data is an indispensable part of the study. Just as a lateral chest radiograph is an essential portion of the evaluation of the chest, so too is the sagittally reformatted image an essential portion of the evaluation of spine disease.

As mentioned earlier, when limited to 5 mm thick axial scans, it is critical to overlap the axial slices when a multiplanar reconstruction of spine data is desired. Taking 5 mm thick slices every 3 mm delivers statistics that are adequate for differentiating disc from spinal contents. In addition, resolution along the Z axis for reconstructed sagittal and coronal images is fine enough to show anatomy without "staircase" or "blocky" artifacts.

Nearly all scanners currently available feature some type of reformatting program capable of creating adequate sagittal and coronal images. Although the details of operation vary among manufacturers, the concept is the same. A region-of-interest "box" encompassing the entire spinal canal is superimposed on the axial scans. The reformatting programs then "dissect" this box of pixels out of each of the axial images, thereby creating a rectangular data block. Images are then produced, at the direction of the technologist, by reorganizing the data block into a series of parallel sagittal, coronal, or oblique slices.

Additional Data Manipulation

Linear and Area Measurements

Most CT reconstruction programs contain algorithms for producing linear and area measurements. Accurate measurements of canal diameter and surface area are possible, although they require added physician or technologist interaction with the computer. These measurements are most important if the multiformat camera images are not life-size.

It is important to note that the window width and level affect the accuracy of any linear or area measurements (Fig. 1.9). When bony structures are viewed with narrow viewing windows the edges appear expanded, and consequently the inner diameter of a long ring is smaller than when measured with a very wide window. Standardization then becomes very important. Accurate measurement of the diameter of the spinal canal depends on the angle of the slice. Oblique scanning angles result in images with reduced diameter or area of the neural ring. As a rule, it is easier to accurately measure the diameter of each spinal segment on sagittally reformatted images. This allows the assessment of stenosis when it occurs between the posterior portion of one vertebral body and the anterior face of the lamina of an adjacent vertebra (Fig. 1.10).

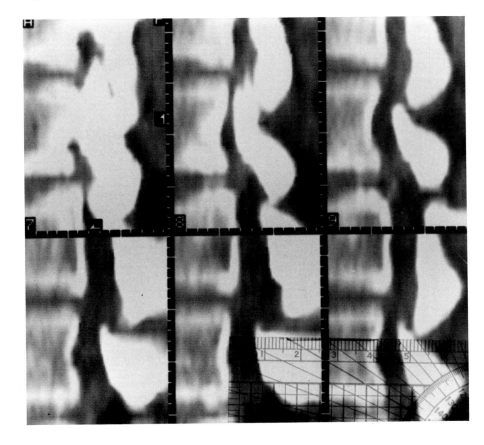

FIGURE 1.10 Accurate measurement of canal size on life-size sagittal reformations.

Mineral Content Measurements

Although it is probable that a more accurate measurement of bone-mineral physiology can be obtained by scanning cortical and medullary bone of the forearm,[1] it has been suggested that vertebral body bone-mineral assay is a useful procedure. The details of the methodology can be found in the works of Genant et al.[2] He and his co-workers developed a simple phantom for standardization of bone mineral on CT spine scans. As experience is gained using these physiological techniques, they will add an additional dimension to the evaluation of the spine.

High-Resolution Bone-Detail CT

Most scanners provide special high-resolution "sharpening" filters capable of producing very high resolution images of bony anatomy.

When spine scanning is performed for the evaluation of a bony lesion, the technique of the examination must be modified accordingly. Once the lesion has been identified and localized to a specific segment, a special sequence of scans designed to produce images of maximal high-contrast resolution (bone detail) is initiated. Slice thickness is reduced to the minimum—typically 1.5 mm. The algorithm is altered to reduce the pixel size to limits of the individual machine—typically 3–4 mm. The convolution filter is modified so that smoothing is reduced to a minimum or eliminated by the use of sharpening filters. If possible, the x-ray attenuation sampling rate is increased, which further improves geometric resolution.

It must be recalled that the modifications just described dramatically reduce the statistical quality of the actual CT measurements. The signal/noise ratio is reduced by each of the modifications. Because of this, there is marked diminution in low-contrast resolution, hence soft-tissue detail is reduced. Because bone anatomy is a series of parallel, very high density trabeculae with low-density fat and marrow interposed, the inherent contrast of the tissue is high. We therefore benefit from improving the geometric resolution of the system without serious image degradation caused by a low signal-to-noise ratio (Fig. 1.11).

Types of Lumbar Examinations

Three distinct lumbar spine examinations are routinely ordered by referring physicians (Fig. 1.12). Each type of examination has a high-detail portion for the vertebral bodies and interspaces of primary interest and a survey portion for additional interspaces. The high-detail, or CT/MPR, portion of each examination requires a closely spaced series of parallel overlapping images obtained with no gantry tilting. The survey portion of each examination is limited to just the interspaces and is performed by obtaining one or two axial slices at 5-mm intervals with the gantry tilted to the angulation of the interspace.

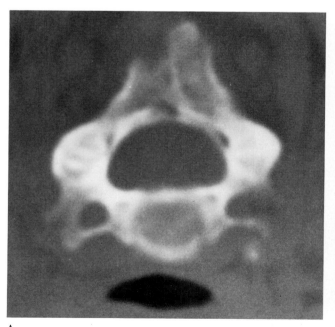 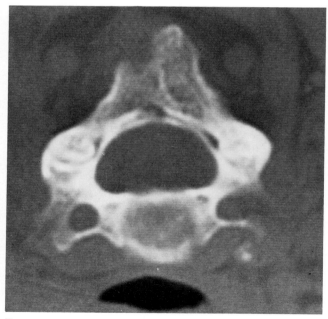

A   B

FIGURE 1.11   Variations in convolution filters for bone and soft tissue. **A.** Axial scan, 5 mm thick slice, soft-tissue optimization. **B.** Axial scan, 5–mm-thick slice, bone optimization. **C.** Axial scan, 1.5 mm thick slice, soft-tissue optimization. **D.** Axial scan, 1.5–mm-thick slice, bone optimization.

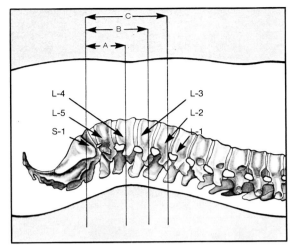

FIGURE 1.12 Types of CT/MPR lumbar studies (reformation area only). (A) Limited examination: two disc spaces reformatted, three spaces tilted-axial slices. (B) Standard examination: three disc spaces reformatted, two spaces tilted-axial slices. (C) Extended examination: four disc spaces reformatted, one space tilted-axial slices.

A limited study covers the region from upper S1 through the midbody of L4. This normally requires 1–24 slices for the CT/MPR portion and an additional 3–6 slices for the remaining upper three lumbar interspaces, which are surveyed. A standard study covers from the midbody of S1 to the midbody of L3 with 25–34 slices and an additional 4–6 slices for survey images through the upper two lumbar interspaces. An extended study covers from upper S1 to the midbody of L2 with 4–45 slices plus an additional 1–2 tilted survey images for the L1–2 interspace.

Suggested Lumbar Procedure

The first step, as outlined earlier, is to place the patient in the scanner feet first with knees supported in a flexed position. It is important that the patient is positioned within the scanning aperture so that the spine is in the center of the scanning field, with the sagittal and coronal planes of the spine parallel with the table.

The iliac crest represents a good landmark to an anteroposterior and lateral ScoutView. The next step is to set beginning and ending locations for the scans in the study; the lateral ScoutView is used for this purpose. The first slice location is through the midbody of S1. The last slice location in a standard three-level lumbar examination is placed at the lower margin of the L3 pedicle. The reason for starting at S1 is that if patients move between axial scans (thereby creating motion artifact on reformatted coronal and sagittal images) they usually do it late in the study because of impatience, pain, or both. Because most lumbar abnormalities are either at L4–5 or L5–S1, it compromises the overall examination accuracy least when motion occurs late in the examination at the L3–4 interspace level, where the frequency of abnormality is considerably less (Fig. 1.13).

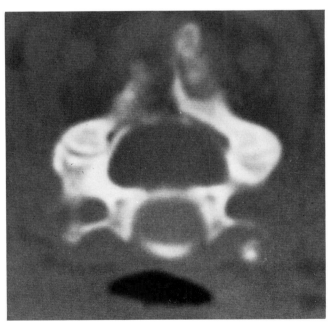

C

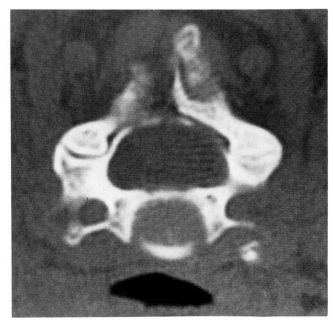

D

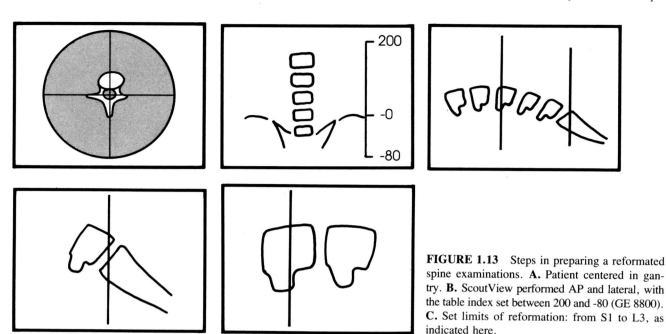

FIGURE 1.13 Steps in preparing a reformated spine examinations. **A.** Patient centered in gantry. **B.** ScoutView performed AP and lateral, with the table index set between 200 and -80 (GE 8800). **C.** Set limits of reformation: from S1 to L3, as indicated here.

Dose and Scan-Time Considerations

The overlapping sequence of 5 mm thick axial images taken every 3 mm produces a 2-mm area of overlap, which corresponds to the peak dose regions. The recommended dose and technique factors are illustrated in Figure 1.14. For a medium-size adult with a waistline measurement of 32–37 inches, the recommended technique is 480 mA, with peak entry skin dose of 5.4 rads resulting from the overlapped image sequence. By following procedures recommended in Figure 1.14, an average patient mix allows 45-min scheduling intervals without undue stress. Tube cooling time lengthens extended studies for large patients to 1 hr.

The rather low milliamperage settings reflected in Figure 1.14 represent a deliberate attempt to run the scanner at well below manufacturer-recommended tube settings. There are three reasons for this: (1) the tube cooling intervals are minimized. By avoiding the higher milliamperage settings, the tube anode rotates at lower revolutions per minute, thereby, hopefully, maximizing tube life. (2) Every attempt is made to minimize patient exposure. (3) The alternative sets of coronally and sagittally reformatted images compensate to some degree for the slightly reduced axial image quality from the lower milliamperage settings. In other words, this methodology can sacrifice some dose and some image quality because the reformatted image planes offer other, additional chances of picking up subtle abnormalities.

References

1. Orphanoudakis SC, Jensen PS, Rauschkolb EN, et al: Bone mineral analysis using single-energy computed tomography. Invest Radiol 14:122–130, 1979
2. Genant HK, Cann CE: Spinal osteoporosis: advanced assessment using quantitative computed tomography. In Genant HK (ed): Spine Update 1984. Radiology Research and Education Foundation, University of California Printing Department, San Francisco, 1983, pp. 331–343

PATIENT TYPE	WAIST (INCHES)	TUBE mA	NO. VIEWS	TOTAL mAS	PEAK ENTRY SKIN DOSE (RADS)
Large Adult	38-44	320	576	614	7.3
Medium Adult	32-37	250	576	480	5.4
Small Adult	26-31	200	576	384	4.1
Child	N/A	320	288	307	2.1
Infant	N/A	250	288	240	1.6

FIGURE 1.14   Suggested technique factors for GE 8800 scanner.

Film Organization and Case Reporting

2

It is important for the final CT images to be photographed and presented to the radiologist and referring physician in an easily understood format. The CT examination should be displayed in a manner that allows easy correlation with routine spine films and myelography. An attempt is made to condense the axial examination onto the fewest possible films without unduly reducing the image size. Reducing the amount of film "juggling" required to organize the stack of axial images is helpful to the radiologist reading the films and to his surgical colleagues in the operating room. This can be accomplished by magnifying the area of interest and removing extraneous anatomy from the final film image. When this is done, it is prudent to include at least some of the full axial scans in order to eliminate the possibility of missing significant nonspinal lesions causing back pain. It is also desirable to produce films that are photographed for both bone and soft-tissue detail. The goal of the filming format is to allow the radiologist to interpret all facets of the study without the necessity of using the scanner console to manipulate the images.

Complete Case on Six Large Films

Like other multiplanar software packages, CT/MPR requires a region-of-interest "box" to be set around the spine, as in Figure 2.1. The box creates a rectangular three-dimensional block of data through all the carefully registered, overlapped axial slices. Digital picture elements, or pixels, within this block are used to calculate picture elements in order to form the coronal and sagittal sequences of images. Two key processing steps precede the formation of sagittal and coronal images. First, the supine image data is rotated 180 degrees to present spinal anatomy in a surgical, or prone, orientation (Fig. 2.2). Second, all of the axial picture data are expanded so that the axial, coronal, and sagittal sequences of images are perfectly life-size when photographed in 4-on-1 format with the GE CT camera. The axial image sequences produced by CT/MPR processing are then condensed into groups of four or six so that they can be photographed efficiently. One such composite image is illustrated in Figure 2.3. Note that appended to the right side

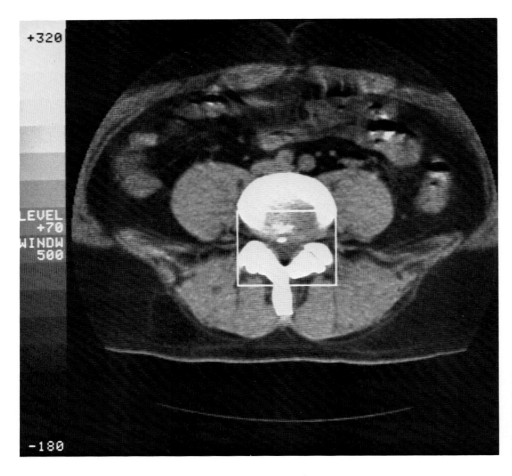

FIGURE 2.1 Region of interest. A region-of-interest box is placed around the spinal canal on the highest, lowest, and middle slices of a stacked series of axial scans.

of the composite views are anterioposterior and lateral digital radiographs. Superimposed on these digital images are the number and the position of the attached axial scans. This aids in localization and identification of the axial images.

The first two films in our series contain all of the axial images in composite groupings of six axial slices. Each composite grouping represents one button push on the camera and one storage file or picture file with the scanner's computer system. The 42 axial images in this four-level example study require only seven photographic exposures.

The reformation algorithm computes a complete set of equally spaced sagittal images, beginning from the left side of the reconstruction box (Fig. 2.4). These individual sagittal views are then organized into groups by the computer and sequentially numbered for efficient photography. The distance (in millimeters) between the sagittal images is identical to the motion of the table between axial slices (Fig. 2.5).

The final step in the reformation is to use the sagittal scan data to compute coronal planes (Fig. 2.6). The coronal scans are numbered sequentially and displayed from posterior to anterior in groups of two. Each pair is photographed by a single button push (Fig. 2.7). The axial, sag-

ittal, and coronal views generally require four films when photographed life-size.

The lumbar spinal canal is actually a curved structure, sweeping backward, producing a variable lumbar lordosis. Planar coronal reformations therefore produce reformatted planes where vertebral body and neural canal are projected on the same image. It may require multiple coronal scans to display the desired curved surface. It was therefore decided to produce a special type of coronal view that would follow the curve of the posterior border of the vertebral bodies. To achieve this, the usual series of axial scans is reformatted in the sagittal plane, and a selected sagittal reference slice is chosen. The technologist selects points along the posterior edge of the spinal canal. The reformation algorithm then computes a complex polynomial that describes the curve drawn on the screen, and the computer creates a series of parallel curves around the calculated curve. Images of each of these curvilinear planes are then produced. By this method one can ''straighten'' the lumbar lordosis so that on one single curved coronal reformation all of the exiting nerve roots can be seen simultaneously and compared (Fig. 2.8). The authors have performed several thousand examinations using this technique and believe it to be superior to the usual planar coronals in most lumbar

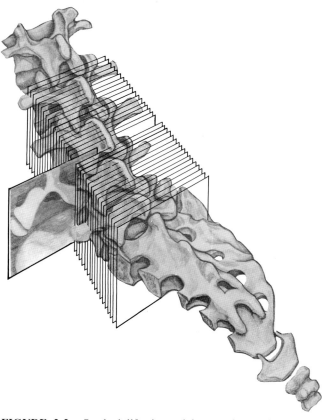

FIGURE 2.2 Stacked life-size axial scans in surgical orientation.

cases. We have recently chosen to eliminate planar coronals entirely and substitute these curved views in our standard examination. Many examples of these views are presented throughout this text.

As in any radiographic procedure, one should produce images along planes perpendicular to the axis of the anatomic area of interest. Therefore oblique reformations may be of importance in selective cases. The cervical neural foramina are small structures that are angled forward and downward and are ideally visualized by performing reformations perpendicular to their bony axes (Fig. 2.9). In the authors' clinical experience oblique reformations are rarely of use in lumbar CT scanning. The lumbar foramina are sagittally oriented and are well seen on the sagittal views. Theoretically, the planar surfaces of the articular facets would be best studied in oblique views. In actual practice, these views add little new clinical information.

Detailed Localization Strategy

To facilitate localization of anatomic structures on the composite images, a series of parallel tick marks is included. Tick marks located along the top or bottom of an axial image localize the position of the sagittal images, counting

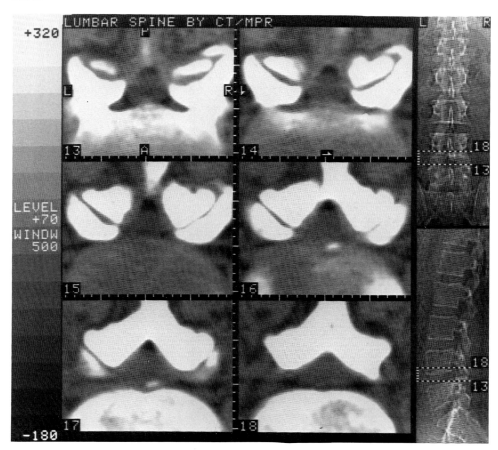

FIGURE 2.3 Composite axial grouping. Six sequential axial scans and two digital Scout-Views are presented as one TV-screen image and photographed with a single push of the camera button. Tick marks positioned along the edges of the images are used for localization.

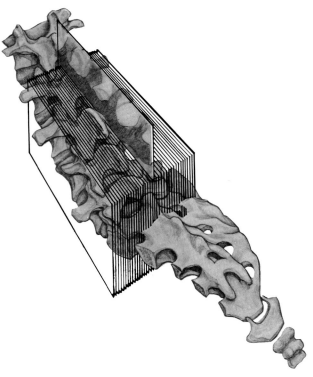

from left to right. Tick marks located along the side of an axial image represent the position of the coronal images, counting from posterior to anterior. Every fifth tick mark is large. The interval between any two tick marks is automatically determined by the couch increments specified at the time the original axial data were obtained. These intervals are 3 mm for lumbar spine cases. The same life-size CT/MPR processing adjusts to 1.5 mm for cervical spine work. As an exercise, look at the annular calcification in axial scan No. 16 in Figure 2.10A. Count across the bottom tick marks. The calcification is aligned with the 11th tick mark from the left and therefore should be found on sagittal view No. 11. Look now at the composite sagittal scans in Figure 2.10B. The calcification is seen as expected on sagittal scan No. 11. Count the tick marks along the side of the scan. You will see that the calcification aligns with the 16th tick mark, representing axial scan No. 16. By counting the bottom tick marks on the sagittal view, we would expect to find the calcification on coronal scan No. 10, the 10th tick mark from the back. Observe coronal scan No. 10 in Figure 2.10C; the calcification is at the level of axial scan No. 16.

FIGURE 2.4 Sequential life-size sagittal reformations in surgical orientation.

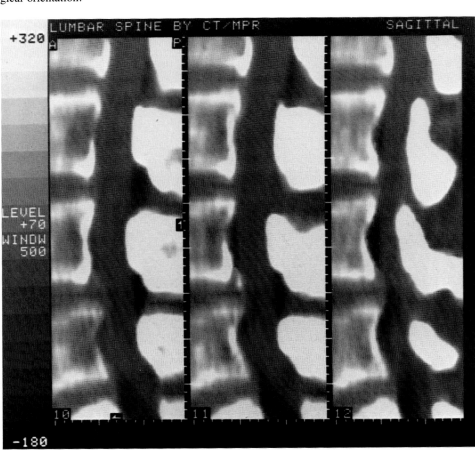

FIGURE 2.5 Composite sagittal grouping. Three sequential sagittal views, with localizor tick marks, are presented as a single TV-screen image and photographed with a single push of the camera button. Images are numbered, with the left-most structures on the left.

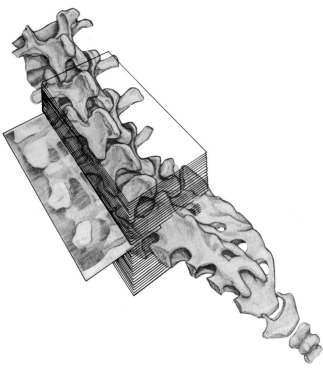

It is very easy to work from a specific spot on a given image of one sequence to the corresponding spot on a single image within either of the other two image sequences. The tick marks represent a static film equivalent to the blinking-dot localizer, which is an interactive function on the viewing console.

It is important to create a series of bone-windowed views for evaluation of the spinal canal, facets, and neural foramina. We have chosen to photograph these bone images using the 12-on-1 format in order to conserve film. Measurements are always made on the life-size pictures.

One final sequence of images is included to ensure proper evaluation of the retroperitoneal and paravertebral spaces. This includes a composite of whole-body axial images that are reduced in size by 75% (Fig. 2.11).

The total number of 14 × 17 inch films per case depends on the extent of the study (limited, standard, or extended) and the filming format (4-on-1 or 12-on-1). A standard study requires five or six films with the 4-on-1 format and two or three films with the 12-on-1 format. The 12-on-1 approach conserves film but does not maintain the life-size attribute inherent in the 4-on-1 format.

FIGURE 2.6 Sequential coronally reformatted images displayed in surgical orientation.

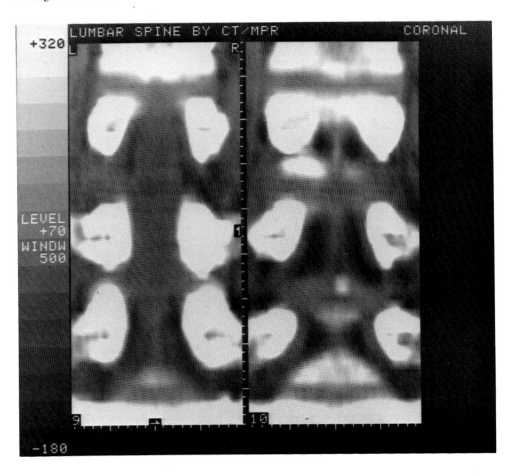

FIGURE 2.7 Composite coronal grouping. Two sequentially numbered coronal images are displayed from back to front in surgical orientation. Localizor tick marks are present along the bottom and the side.

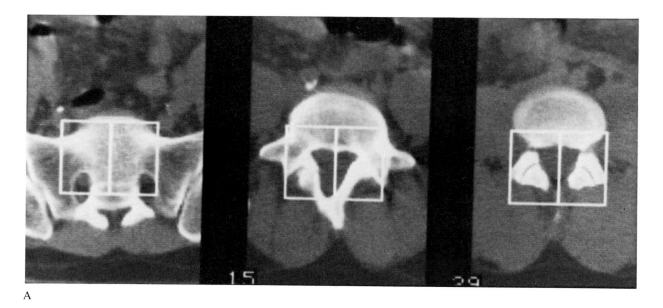

A

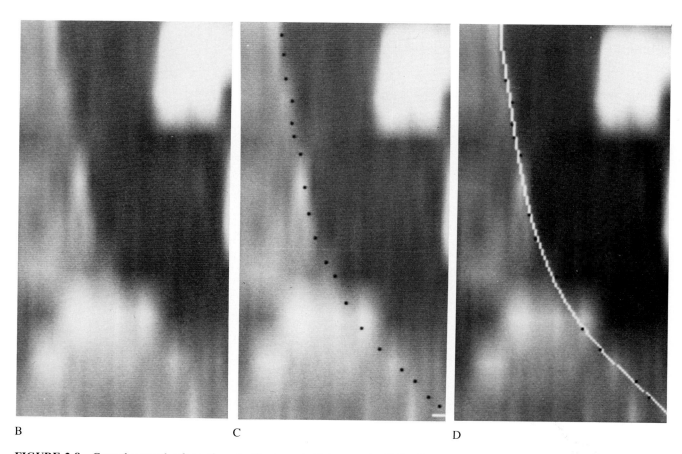

B   C   D

FIGURE 2.8   Curved coronal reformation. **A.** The lowest, highest, and middle slices of a stack of axial scans are displayed. The midsagittal plane is marked. **B.** A crude sagittal reconstruction is produced by reconstructing every third axial pixel. **C.** The technologist traces the plane of the posterior border of the vertebral bodies by placing dots on the screen. **D.** The computer generates a curve corresponding to the chosen dots. **E.** The computer then generates a series of parallel curves and curved coronal scans corresponding to each of the computed curves.

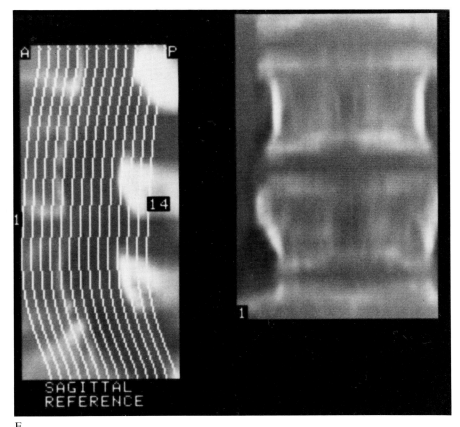

E

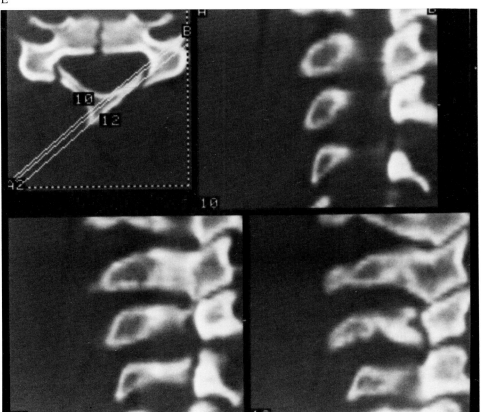

FIGURE 2.9 Oblique reconstruction format. An axial slice is used as a reference. From this slice, the axis of the oblique plane is set by the technologist. The computer then produces images along the path of the requested axis and perpendicular to it. These oblique slices are annotated on a reference axial image for correct localization.

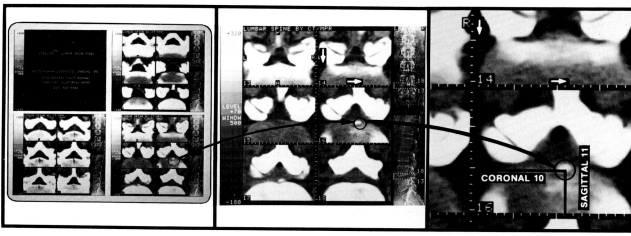
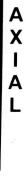

A

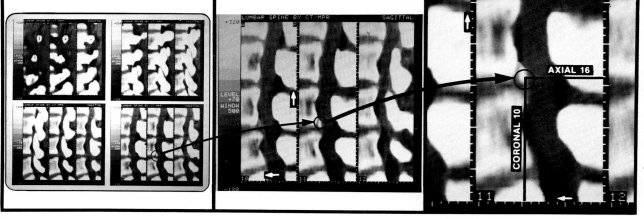
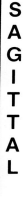

B

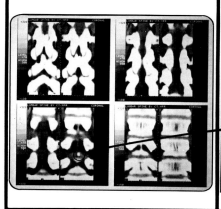
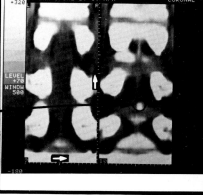
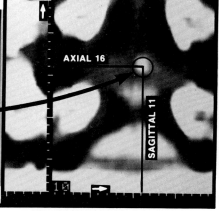
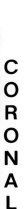

C

FIGURE 2.10   Axial life-size composite film. **A.** One 14 × 17 inch sheet of film contains three composite axial groupings. Close-up of the lower right-hand corner demonstrates a calcification in the anulus on axial slice No. 16. Note on the enlarged view of this slice that by projecting the calcification on the tick marks one is able to identify on which coronal and which sagittal views the calcification should appear. **B.** One 14 × 17 inch sheet of film with four composite sagittal groupings. On the close-up of the right lower quadrant one notes the calcification on sagittal view No. 11. On the enlargement of sagittal view No. 11 the calcification projects to the 16th tick mark from the bottom and the 10th tick mark from the back. **C.** One 14 × 17 inch sheet of film with four composite coronal views on the magnified view. The calcification is seen where predicted on coronal view No. 10.

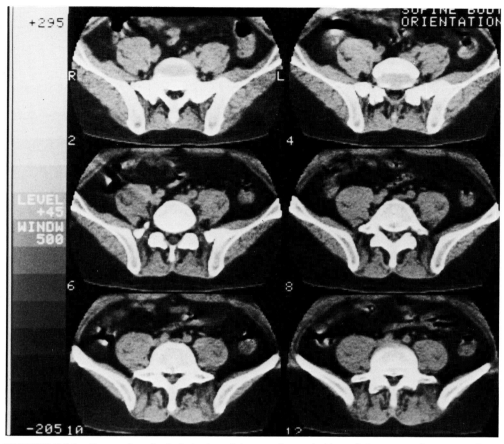

FIGURE 2.11 Composite of whole-body axial scans for evaluation of the retroperitoneum and paravertebral spaces. Note that only every second slice is photographed. This is adequate, as there is a 2–mm overlap on each slice.

Sample Reporting Form

The current lumbar CT reporting form (Fig. 2.12) conforms to the prone surgical orientation of the CT/MPR format. The top half is for summarizing the objective findings, and the bottom half is for supporting details, which include graded findings at each lumbar level, specification of key images showing the major abnormalities, and miscellaneous notations. The graded findings are organized so that each lumbar level is represented by a horizontal row of blanks. Each column of blanks indicates a specific structure (e.g., left facet) at the various lumbar levels. The columns are organized so that left-sided structures are on the left side of the form and right-sided structures are on the right side of the form. Left-sided structures are also on the left side of the films. This conforms with the prone axial image orientation favored by referring surgeons. This left/right orientation is maintained within the three columns that constitute the "trijoint complex" and "central canal."

Along the edges of the reporting form are perforations for tractor-fed computer printers. This allows continuous-

form printing of the lumbar CT reports once the summary (top half of report) and the supporting details (bottom half) have been entered at computer terminals (CRTs) by the medical transcribers. The summaries are dictated. The graded findings for specific structures are penciled in on xeroxed copies of the form.

The reporting form need not be computer-printed. For 1 year, before our computer-based reporting and retrieval system were established, this form was completed by the transcriber at a typewriter in the conventional manner.

The advantages of a computer-based reporting system are several. First, the continuous-form printing provides the opportunity to generate several original reports, thus eliminating either a xeroxing step or the separation of a multicarboned single report. Moreover, each physician receiving a CT report gets an original. A second advantage is CRT recall of reports for handling telephone inquiries. In addition to speed, the prompt display of a report on the CRT allows the telephone inquiry to be handled during the original phone call rather than requiring a second call after the film jacket and report have been retrieved from the film file.

SEE REVERSE SIDE FOR FILM ORGANIZATION AND EXAMPLES ILLUSTRATING 1-5 GRADING SYSTEM

Graded Findings and Abbreviations:

1 = Normal (1MM)	**4** = Moderate (5MM)	**VC** = Vacuum Change
2 = Slight (2MM)	**5** = Severe (>6MM)	**OR** = Osteophytic Ridging
3 = Mild (3MM)	**★** = Soft Tissue	**PD** = Pars Defects

FH = Flavum Hypertrophy	**Sp** = Spur	**IJ** = Irregular Joint
LAM = Laminectomy	**F** = Fused	**DN** = Degenerative Narrowing
HL = Hemilaminectomy	**NF** = Not Fused	**SL** = Sub Lux

	TRI-JOINT COMPLEX			CANAL				OTHER	
	LEFT FORAMEN	LEFT FACET	DISC/ ANNULUS	RIGHT FACET	LT. LAT. RECESS	CENTRAL	RT. LAT. RECESS	RIGHT FORAMEN	
L1-L2	___	___	___	___	___	___	___	___	___ L1-L2
L2-L3	___	___	___	___	___	___	___	___	___ L2-L3
L3-L4	___	___	___	___	___	___	___	___	___ L3-L4
L4-L5	___	___	___	___	___	___	___	___	___ L4-L5
L5-S1	___	___	___	___	___	___	___	___	___ L5-S1
	___	___	___	___	___	___	___	___	

Miscellaneous Findings

Lumbar Segments _____ Transitional Segment _____

Residual Pantopaque: _____ Few Drops; _____ Several CC's

Radiologist

_____

(Typed Name)

_____

(Signature)

Key Images

	Lifesize		Non-Lifesize
Axial	_____	Bone Density Axial	_____
Sagittal	_____	Bone Density Sagittal	_____
Coronal	_____	Bone Density Coronal	_____
Other	_____	Reduced Full Field Supine Images	_____

ALL EXAMS SUPERVISED AND INTERPRETED BY: PROFESSIONAL SCANNING MEDICAL GROUP, INC., TORRANCE, CA

FIGURE 2.12 CT reporting form; front.

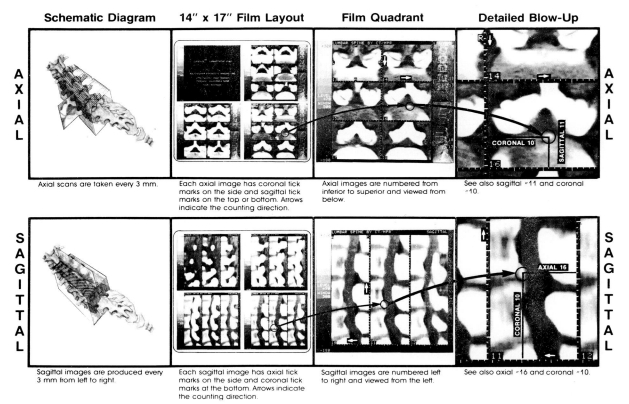

Schematic Diagram	14" x 17" Film Layout	Film Quadrant	Detailed Blow-Up
A X I A L — Axial scans are taken every 3 mm.	Each axial image has coronal tick marks on the side and sagittal tick marks on the top or bottom. Arrows indicate the counting direction.	Axial images are numbered from inferior to superior and viewed from below.	See also sagittal #11 and coronal #10. — **A X I A L**
S A G I T T A L — Sagittal images are produced every 3 mm from left to right.	Each sagittal image has axial tick marks on the bottom and coronal tick marks at the bottom. Arrows indicate the counting direction.	Sagittal images are numbered left to right and viewed from the left.	See also axial #16 and coronal #10. — **S A G I T T A L**

FIGURE 2.13 CT reporting form; reverse.

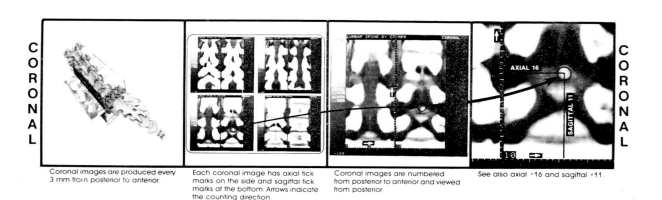

Coronal images are produced every 3 mm from posterior to anterior.

Each coronal image has axial tick marks on the side and sagittal tick marks at the bottom. Arrows indicate the counting direction.

Coronal images are numbered from posterior to anterior and viewed from posterior.

See also axial #16 and sagittal #11.

GRADING SYSTEM EXAMPLES

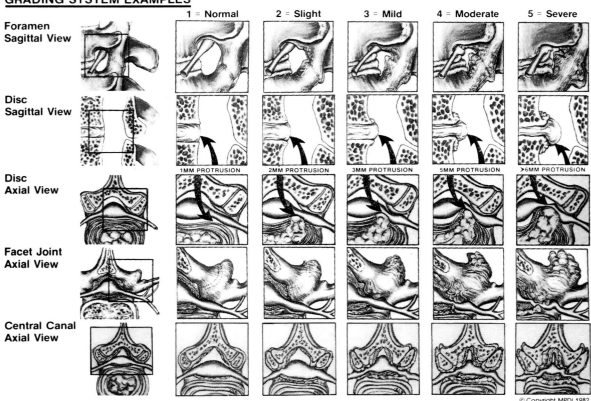

© Copyright MPDI 1982

FIGURE 2.13 (*cont'd*)

A third benefit is easier transcribing in that mailing addresses for the referring physician need not be typed in full for the report and again for the mailing labels. A directory of referring physicians' correct names and addresses in the computer allows these lines to be inserted automatically into the report or on mailing labels simply by triggering an alphabetic search of the physician directory. Only the first few letters of the physician's last name are required for this search. A fourth benefit is integration of reporting with other computer-based functions, e.g., billing and scheduling. Patient and referring physician information can be entered once and yet serve many functions. A fifth advantage of the computer-based reports is case retrieval. Because of the 1–5 grading system, the data base can be searched for groups of patients fulfilling specific criteria.

The reverse side of the lumbar reporting form is also divided into top and bottom halves (Fig. 2.13). The top half summarizes the organizational details of axial, sagittal, and coronal sequences of images and the interrelationships inherent in this film format for localization purposes. The top half is simply a visual summary of the details given in this chapter. The bottom half of the reverse side shows the grading system used for key components of the lumbar spine. This is discussed in the following section.

1–5 Grading System with Anatomic Drawings

The first horizontal row of diagrams in Figure 2.13 represents foramina as seen in the sagittal view. Briefly, using the drawings as visual guidelines for the 1–5 grading system, foraminal evaluations focus on the nerve root and to what extent there might be either a bony or a soft-tissue entrapment. The sagittal view is optimal because it demonstrates not only the foraminal opening but also the nerve root itself. The nerve root is located in the anterior superior quadrant of the foramen. Inferior end-plate spurring encroaches on the anterior inferior aspect of the foramen.

The most common abnormal soft tissue within a foramen is lateral anulus or disc material, swollen nerve root, or scarring from prior surgery. These are sometimes difficult to distinguish. Suffice it to say that abnormal soft tissue which fills a normal-size foramen can represent nerve root entrapment in the absence of bony stenosis.

The second and third rows in Figure 2.13 represent the sagittal and axial views of disc protrusion. When a bulge is detected, its protrusion is measured on the life-size films in both the axial and the sagittal views. The measured soft-tissue bulge is graded according to the scale on the form. For example, a 3-mm protrusion is a mild (grade 3) disc; a 5-mm protrusion is a moderate (grade 4) disc; protrusions exceeding 6 mm are classified as severe. The grading system is applied to focal disc herniations, which are usually lateral diffuse circumferential disc/anulus bulging or osteophytic spurring from sclerosis of the opposing end-plates. What is assessed is the amount of protrusion into the anterior aspect of the central canal. The amount of protrusion is graded as such and does not take into account the proportional extent to which the cross-sectional area of the central canal is compromised. Obviously, a grade 4 moderate disc/anulus protrusion has greater significance in a congenitally small spinal canal than in a very large spinal canal.

The fourth row in Figure 2.13 illustrates the progressive stages of facet-joint abnormality that the 1–5 grading system attempts to quantify subjectively. Key observations include overall size of the articular processes and the presence of any associated periarticular spurs, particularly anteriorly where such spurs can easily compromise a nerve root in either the lateral recess or the foramen. Appropriate abbreviations for irregular joint (IJ), degenerative narrowing (DN), subluxation (SL), vacuum change (VC), fusion (F), or spurring (Sp) augment the grading system in order to reflect various types of degenerative change within or about the facet joint. The grading system per se is basically an estimate of overall size of the combined articular processes and their associated spurs.

The bottom row in Figure 2.13 illustrates the various shapes and sizes of the central canal and its lateral recesses, corresponding to the grading system. What is attempted is to quantify subjectively the cross-sectional area that remains for the dural sac and nerve roots. Encroachment can be bony or soft tissue in nature; use of the grading system does not distinguish between these possibilities. The causes for a reduced cross-sectional area can come from any direction.

When possible, a comment is made regarding the anticipated myelographic defect (ventral, posterior, lateral, etc.) that lumbar myelography would likely demonstrate.

Suggested Reading Sequence

The order in which a radiologist or a referring physician evaluates x-ray films largely depends on the order in which films are placed on viewboxes and the sequence of structures to be evaluated on individual films. To avoid the confusion associated with unnecessary shuffling of films, the order of films in x-ray jackets for film files and in mailing envelopes to referring physicians is controlled very carefully. The order is always as follows:

Life-size
1. Axial composites
2. Sagittal composites
3. Coronal composites

Nonlife-size
4. Bone-density axial composites
5. Bone-density sagittal composites
6. Bone-density coronal composites
7. Reduced full-field supine images
7. Survey images of upper lumbar interspaces

The first step in analyzing a lumbar CT case is to label the appropriate interspace levels on all three views and determine whether there are four, five, or six lumbar segments. The sagittal images are then viewed in order to grade the left and right foramina, in that order. The posterior margins of each interspace are scanned to determine the presence of an anterior extradural defect. Measurements of these protrusions can then be made on both the sagittal and the axial views; these measurements are correlated with a specific rating for each interspace in the disc/anulus column. Pertinent abbreviations, e.g., OR (osteophytic ridging), VC (vacuum change), or Sp (spur), are included. The axial scans are evaluated. The lateral recesses and the facet anatomy are quantitated and described.

The coronal composite images are generally of less use than either the axial or sagittal views. Coronal images are surveyed for soft-tissue densities at the interspace levels, which might help lateralize a disc protrusion or establish a relationship between a bulging/herniated lateral disc and a traversing nerve root.

The next step is to review bone-density axial composite views in order to grade the articular processes and any manifestation of degenerative change, e.g., periarticular erosions, joint space irregularity, or facet-joint spurring.

The bone-density sagittal and coronal views tend to be of little use in soft-tissue abnormalities, e.g., disc herniations. They are extremely important, however, in as-

NAME _____

AGE _____ DATE _____

1. What was your chief complaint when you visited your doctor?

_____

2. Describe your pain (i.e., burning, sharp, etc.).

_____

3. Does the pain go down your arm or leg? _____. In the back or front? _____

Left, right or both? _____

4. Does anything make it worse (i.e., Standing, sitting, lying down, etc.)

_____

5. What do you think caused the problem?

_____

6. When you awake in the morning is your pain better or worse?

_____

7. Do you have any numbness? _____. Where? _____

_____

8. Do you have any weakness? _____. Where? _____

9. Have you had any bowel or bladder changes?

Describe _____

_____

10. Have you had spine surgery? _____

When? _____

What was done? _____

_____

11. Do you have any other medical conditions?

_____

_____

12. Describe your general health.

_____

_____

_____

PLEASE SHADE IN THE AREAS WHICH HURT

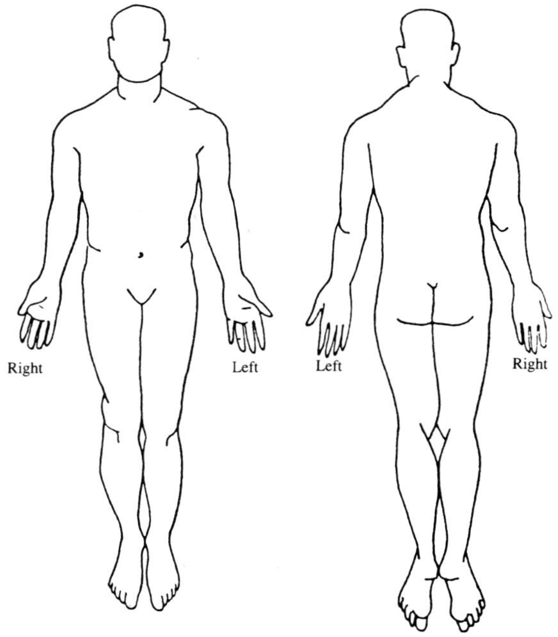

Right   Left   Left   Right

FIGURE 2.14 Patient questionnaire.

sessing bony changes (lytic/blastic abnormalities), spurs, and solidity or continuity of fusion bone.

The reduced full-field supine images are reviewed for any abnormalities outside the immediate vicinity of the spine. It is surprising how often an unsuspected but significant abnormality is seen on these "minified" full-field images. Not infrequently, a far lateral disc/anulus bulge or herniation or a somewhat subtle soft-tissue interface between a bulging disc and other soft-tissue contents of the spinal canal is more easily evaluated on these minified images.

Finally, the last film contains the upper lumbar survey images at L1–2 and L2–3. Appropriate structures are graded. As each film is reviewed, key images that best demonstrate the abnormalities are specified. It is helpful to make notations, place arrows, and record measurements on these key images for use by the referring physician who receives the films or by the surgeon in the operating room.

Once the various spine components at each level have been graded, the final summary can be dictated quickly. Use of the grading system not only helps to organize summary statements but also provides the supporting details. If at any time during review of a case there is an interruption, it is always easy to go back and resume filling in the bottom half of the form. Without a reporting form, a distracting phone call often requires reevaluating the entire case point by point.

Patient Questionnaire

It is very important to have an adequate clinical history available when interpreting lumbar spine CT. Minor ana-tomic abnormalities are often found on the side opposite the clinical complaints or at a level seemingly inconsistent with the presenting symptom complex. Unfortunately, our clinical colleagues are often vague in their requests. The single most common request for scanning is "rule out disc herniation," with no indication for side or level. To some extent we can improve on our histories by educating surgeons to ask more specific questions, which obviously will ensure more correct and insightful diagnoses.

The patient questionnaire shown in Figure 2.14, designed by Dr. C. Kerber, is completed by our patients while they sit in the waiting room before scanning. This allows them to ask the receptionist to explain anything that seems vague and aids in obtaining clinically useful information. The questionnaire was designed to allow the patients to express, in their own words, the nature, character, location, and when possible the cause of the pain. Patients are also asked to draw in the pattern of discomfort. This combination is very useful in differentiating those patients with clearly defined clinical syndromes from those whose back pain may be related more to their legal status than to the status of their discs.

We *always* interpret the scan *before* reviewing this questionnaire so that observations are made and quantitated objectively, without bias. The questionnaire is then reviewed and an attempt made to correlate the objective findings with the history. When there is good correlation, this is so stated in the dictated case summary. If correlation is weak or nonexistent, this too is indicated. Many patients have minor anatomic abnormalities. It is crucial to indicate whenever possible which of these may bear clinical relevance.

Detailed Sectional Anatomy of the Spine

3

Wolfgang Rauschning

Morphologic studies on the human spine constitute a special challenge because of the spine's complex topographic anatomy and the intimate relationship between the supporting skeleton and the contiguous soft tissues (muscles, discs, joint capsules) as well as the neurovascular contents of the spinal canal and intervertebral foramina. The improving resolution and multiplanar image reformatting capabilities of modern CT scanners call for accurate anatomic reference material. Such anatomic images should be available without distortion, in natural colors, and in considerable detail. The images should present the anatomy in the correct axial, sagittal, and coronal planes and should also be sufficiently closely spaced so as to follow the thin cuts of modern CT scanners.

This chapter details one of several recent attempts to correlate gross anatomy with the images depicted by high-resolution CT. The methods of specimen preparation, sectioning, and photographing have been documented elsewhere.[1,2]

Overall Spinal Morphology

The terminology used in this chapter follows the glossary prepared by the Committee on the Spine, American Academy of Orthopaedic Surgeons (Document 675-80). The two exceptions are our use of ''spinous process'' instead of ''spine'' and ''spinal canal'' instead of ''vertebral canal.''

The spinal column is a curved structure with the major curves visible in the sagittal plane: the cervical (lordotic), thoracic (kyphotic), and lumbar (lordotic) curves. Angulation is also present between the fifth lumbar vertebra and the posteriorly convex sacrum.

The spine normally comprises 24 vertebrae (7 cervical, 12 thoracic, and 5 lumbar), the sacrum, and the coccyx. The vertebrae are connected to each other by the intervertebral discs, facet joints, and ligaments. The spine is surrounded by thick layers of paraspinal muscles and has a richly anastomosing arterial supply and venous drainage. The bony spinal canal contains the spinal cord with its meningeal envelopes. Thirty-one pairs of spinal nerves arise from the spinal cord. The first cervical pair emerges between the occiput and the atlas and the eighth pair emerges below the seventh cervical vertebra. Caudal to the first thoracic segment the spinal nerves are numbered according to the upper vertebra at any given interspace (i.e., T2 roots and L3 roots at the T2–3 and L3–4 interspaces, respectively).

Vertebrae

Except for the atlas (C1), typical vertebrae consist of both anterior and posterior elements. The anterior elements include the vertebral bodies, intervertebral discs, and longitudinal ligaments. The posterior elements are, collectively, the pedicles, the laminae, and the articular processes, transverse processes, and spinous processes, with intervening joint capsules and ligaments.

The bodies are cylindrical blocks of cancellous bone covered by a thin layer of cortical bone except at the endplates. The cross-sectional shape and dimensions vary greatly, increasing in size in the craniocaudal direction. The cancellous bone of the cervical spine has a fine texture, but toward the lumbar spine the bone texture becomes considerably coarser. The vertebrae contain the most voluminous amount of hematopoietic red marrow in the body. That fact

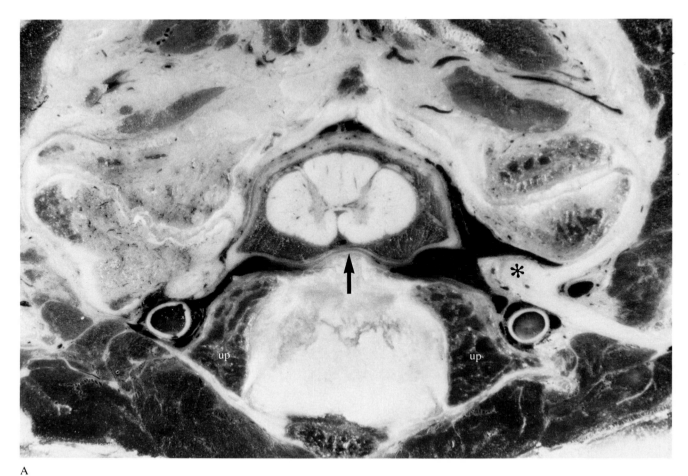

A

FIGURE 3.1 Axial sections from the C2–3 disc into the atlas. (All axial sections in this chapter are viewed from below and oriented in the prone position.) **A.** Severe degenerative arthritis of the left C2–3 facet joint. Degeneration and central bulge of the disc (*arrow*). The right C3 dorsal root ganglion is seen immediately posterior to the vertebral artery (*asterisk*); the ventral and dorsal roots are branching from this ganglion. The uncinate processes (*up*) are oriented in the sagittal plane. **B,C.** The vertebral arteries run through angle-shaped canals in the axis. **D,E.** Note the close relationship of the vertebral arteries to the atlantoaxial joints. The epidural space is occupied by wide venous sinuses, which are continuous with the foraminal venous plexus and venous sinuses surrounding the vertebral artery. The ligamentum flavum is seen only in the C2–3 interspace (*arrowheads* in **D** and **E**). **F,G.** The lower portion of the dens is seen in **F**; **G** shows the upper segment of the odontoid process and the transverse ligament. **H.** Close-up of **G**. Axial section through the spinal canal at the level of the transverse ligament of the atlas (*tl*). A true synovial joint is seen between the cartilage-covered posterior circumference of the dens (*d*) and the transverse ligament. Loose areolar tissue intermingled with veins occupies the space lateral to the odontoid process. Thin septa of fibrous tissue and fat subdivide the epidural venous sinuses. The dorsal and ventral preganglionic nerve roots form from a greater number of small rootlets. They are separated as they pierce the thecal sac. The gray and white matter can be clearly distinguished in the spinal cord. (*Figure continued* on pages 35–38.)

seems to underscore the early optimism regarding a significant future role for magnetic resonance imaging (MRI) in the spine, i.e., physiological evaluation of marrow. For morphologic bone detail, CT will probably remain superior.

Small vascular foramina pierce the cortex of the vertebral bodies. The flat or slightly concave, nearly parallel end plates consist of dense cancellous bone to which the hyaline cartilage endplate is firmly attached. On dried vertebral specimens a prominent circular ridge of cortical bone derived from the united anular apophysis surrounds this spongy central portion of the vertebral endplate. Thin CT scans parallel to the endplate often show the annular apophysis. The vertebral bodies are usually wider at the endplates and have a waist-shaped narrowing of their inter-

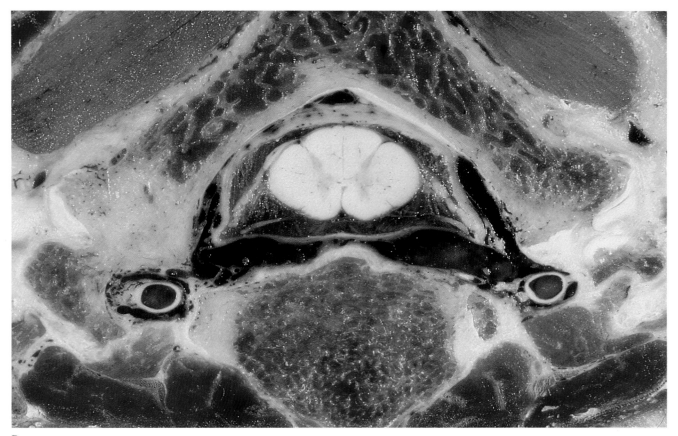

B

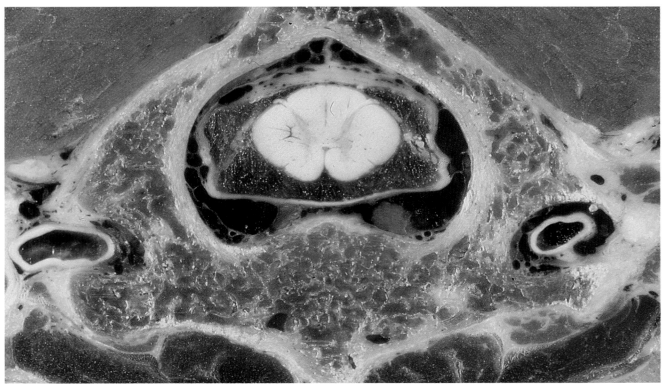

C

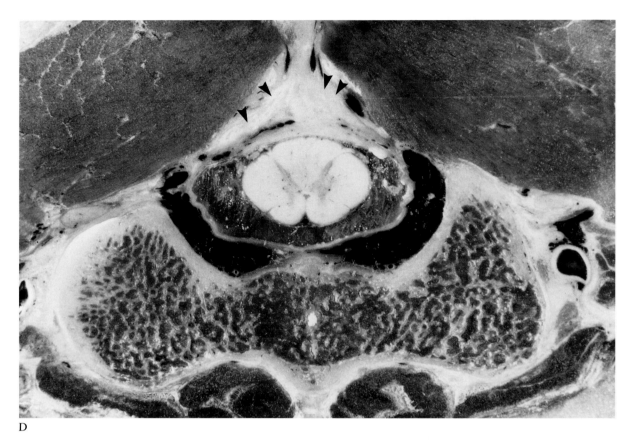

D

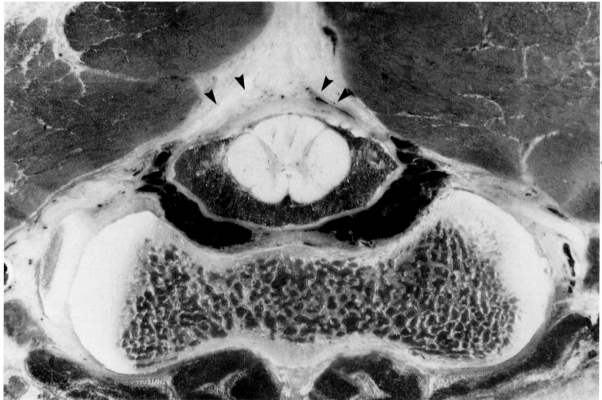

E

FIGURE 3.1 (*cont'd*)

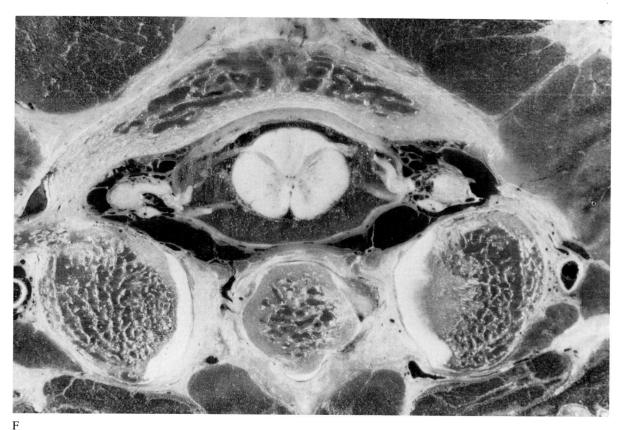

F

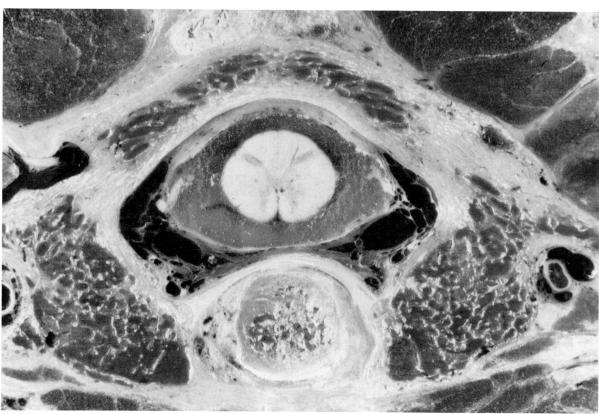

G

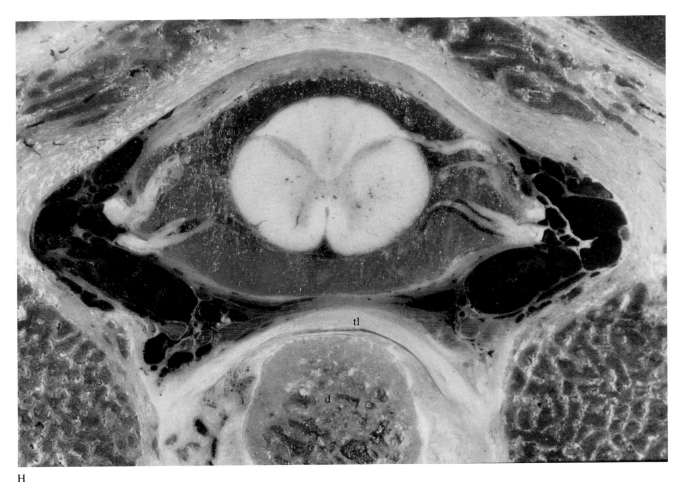

H

FIGURE 3.1 (*cont'd*)   See legend page 34.

mediate portion. The posterior surface is flat or slightly concave and is pierced by veins draining through large vascular foramina.

3.1.2 Intervertebral Discs

Refer to Figures 3.1–3.9.

In the healthy spine intervertebral discs protrude slightly beyond the edges of the adjacent vertebra. This is because they have a slightly larger circumferential dimension than the contiguous vertebral end-plates. The intervertebral discs are elastic, biconvex, or wedge-shaped, and functionally they bulge somewhat into the spinal canal during extension. Their contribution to the total length of the vertebral column is 20–25% in both the cervical and thoracic regions and 30–35% in the lumbar region. The nucleus pulposus is situated in the central and posterior portion of the discs. It is a gelatinous, pulpy substance derived from the notochord. The peripheral part of the disc is composed of concentrically oriented layers of fibrocartilaginous tissue intermingled with strong collagenous strands running obliquely at different angles. This peripheral portion is known as anulus

fibrosus. Its fibrous strands are anchored into the annular apophysis and also attach to the vertebral body beyond the end-plate by blending with the periosteum (Sharpey's fibers) and the longitudinal ligaments.

Anterior Longitudinal Ligament

Refer to Figure 3.9.

The anterior longitudinal ligament is a flat fibrous band located along the anterior surface of the vertebral column. It consists of deep unisegmental and superficial plurisegmental layers. The ligament originates at the base of the skull as a thin band. As it descends, it rapidly increases in width, covering most of the anterior surface of the cervical vertebrae. In the thoracic spine it becomes narrower. In the lumbar spine, however, the anterior longitudinal ligament again increases considerably in width and thickness. It is attached to the bodies of the vertebrae by loose areolar tissue and partially fills in their anterior concavities. At the discs the ligament becomes broader and is inseparably interwoven with the fibers of the anulus fibrosus.

Posterior Longitudinal Ligament

Refer to Figures 3.4, 3.8, and 3.9.

The posterior longitudinal ligament is a flat fibrous band that also has a deep localized unisegmental layer of strands and a more superficial layer extending over several disc levels. It runs from the foramen magnum along the posterior surface of the vertebral bodies and intervertebral discs and forms a narrow band behind the vertebral bodies. The ligament bridges the central concavity of the posterior surface of the vertebral body in a bowstring fashion from one disc to another. Not infrequently, longitudinal ridges of dense bone project beneath the ligament. The posterior longitudinal ligament becomes thinner, wider, and less distinct at the disc levels, where it blends with the obliquely oriented fibers of the anulus fibrosus.

Vertebral Arch

Refer to Figures 3.1, 3.4, 3.5, and 3.8–3.10.

A pair of pedicles emerge at the upper lateral posterior aspect of the vertebral bodies. The level at which the pedicles arise from the vertebral bodies, as well as their length, thickness, and direction, determine to a considerable degree the size and configuration of the bony boundaries of the spinal canal and the neuroforamina. Pairs of articular processes with cartilage-covered articular facets project cranially and caudally from the pedicles, forming the zygoapophyseal or facet joints. Together with the intervertebral disc at the same level and the intervening ligaments, these facet joints represent the motion-segment unit between two vertebrae. The facet joints are innervated by medial branches of the dorsal rami of the spinal nerves. Posteriorly, the angulated or curved flat laminae close the vertebral (neural) arch.

The lateral transverse processes and the posterior spinous processes mainly constitute lever arms and, as such, serve as attachment sites for tendons, ligaments, and muscles. The posterior bony elements are composed of thick cortical bone with only minimal amounts of red marrow and cancellous bone. Several ligaments act as passive restraints of spinal mobility. They are the supraspinous ligaments, the interspinous ligaments, and the ligamenta flava. Like the facet-joint capsules, they are elastic to facilitate the segmental spinal mobility. The supraspinous ligament runs over the tips of the spinous processes, forming thick fibroelastic strands, which also project laterally and merge into the coarse thoracolumbar fascia. The interspinous ligament is continuous with the heavy nuchal ligament in the cervical spine. It is considerably thinner, with a loose arrangement of obliquely crossing fibers, between which may be holes and defects.

Ligamentum Flavum

Refer to Figures 3.1, and 3.4–3.10.

The ligamentum flavum is an arcade of yellow elastic tissue between the arches of the vertebrae. In the cervical spine it is very thin, but it gradually increases in thickness in the thoracic spine and becomes thickest (4–5 mm) in the lower lumbar spine. When the posterior wall of the spinal canal is viewed from the front there is only a narrow band of cortical bone of the lamina exposed. The ligamentum flavum has a wide attachment to the anteroinferior border of the lamina above and a small area of insertion to the upper rim of the lamina below. This typical insertion of the ligamentum flavum allows the upper and lower portions of a lamina to be distinguished on axial CT scans as well as on gross anatomic sections, because the lower border of a lamina always has a thick layer of ligamentum flavum at its anterior margin; at the upper border of the lamina below, the ligamentum flavum predominantly attaches posteriorly to the upper rim of the lamina. Except for the lower lumbar and upper cervical spine, the ligamentum flavum is not visible from behind, because of the overlapping of the spinous processes. The ligamentum flavum extends laterally and blends with the thick medial and superior portions of the facet-joint capsules; laterally and inferiorly the joint capsules are thinner.

Spinal Canal

Refer to Figures 3.1, 3.4, and 3.9.

The spinal canal is delimited anteriorly by the posterior surface of the vertebral bodies and the intervertebral discs, laterally by the pedicles and the facet joints, and posteriorly by the ligamentum flavum and the neural arch. In the thoracic and the upper cervical spine the canal has a round shape in cross section, whereas in the lower cervical and the lower lumbar spine it is triangular or half-moon in shape. The spinal canal can be divided into a central portion, housing the thecal sac, and the extradural soft tissues anterior and posterior to the dura. The extradural spaces extending anterolaterally from the border of the dura to the medial border of the intervertebral foramen are called lateral recesses. These recesses contain, primarily, the spinal nerve roots in the periradicular dural sheath; because of this, the recesses are also referred to as the radicular canals or root canals.

Thecal Sac and Spinal Cord

Refer to Figures 3.1, 3.2, and 3.4–3.12.

The spinal cord is continuous with the medulla oblongata at the level of the foramen magnum. It tapers to form the conus medullaris and terminates between the first and second lumbar vertebrae. The cord is elliptical in the cervical region, with a greater transverse than anteropos-

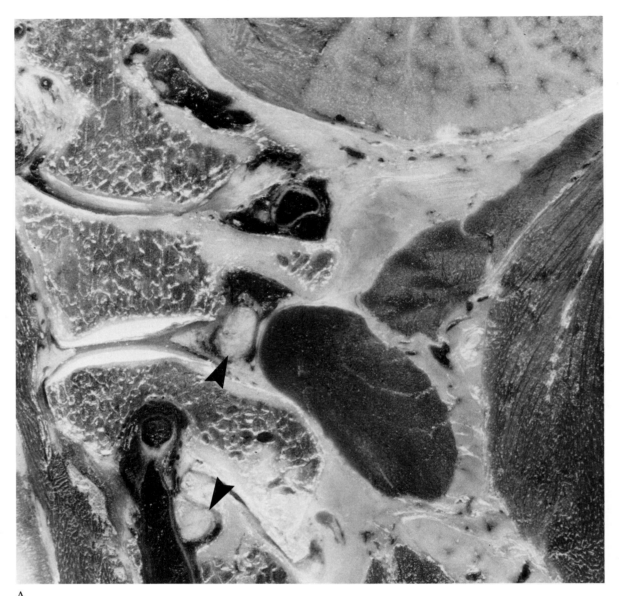

A

FIGURE 3.2 Sagittal sections through the upper cervical spine (occiput through C3). The left occipitoatlantal, atlantoaxial, and C2–3 facet joints are shown in **A** and **B**. Note that the thick dorsal root ganglia of the second and third cervical nerves are surrounded by venous sinuses. **C** shows that ''the thick dorsal root ganglia of the second and third cervical nerves are surrounded by venous sinuses.'' (*Figure continued* on pages 41–43.)

terior (AP) diameter, and round in the thoracic region. The diameter of the spinal cord varies considerably among subjects at identical levels. The spinal cord expands between the C4 and T2 levels of the vertebral column and again between T10 and T12. At these levels the large nervous plexuses passing to the upper and lower extremities emerge.

The lateral cord diameter is approximately 13 mm at the cervical thickening and 8 mm at the lower thoracic levels. The thinnest portions of the cord are at the upper and mid-thoracic levels, where it usually measures 7–8 mm and occupies only a small proportion of the spinal canal.

The spinal cord is covered by the pia mater, which

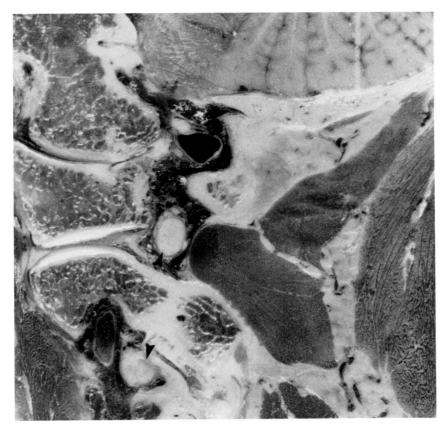

B

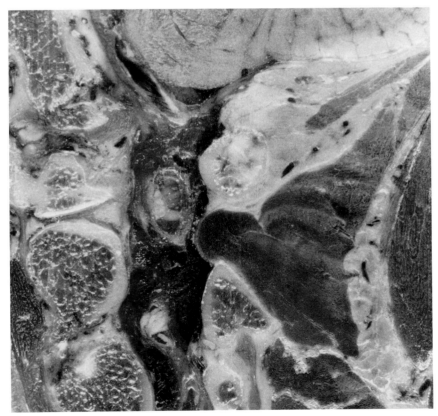

C

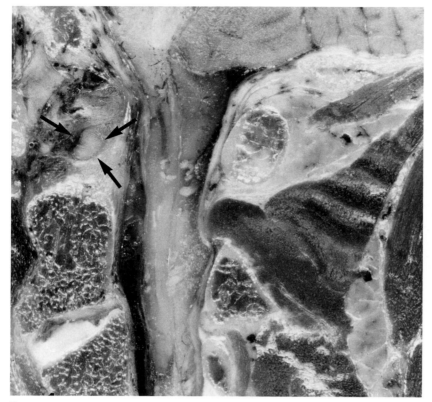

D

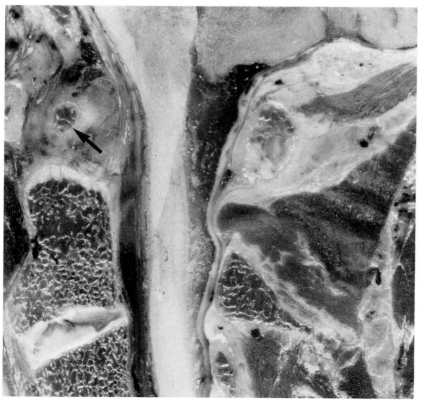

E

FIGURE 3.2 (*cont'd*)   Sagittal sections through the upper cervical spine (occiput through C3). In **D**, the thecal sac is opened, exposing the spinal cord, nerve roots, and dentate ligament. Here the transverse ligament is almost round in cross section (*arrows*). Because of a waist-shaped narrowing in its upper portion, the tip of the odontoid process seems to be separated from the dens in paramedian sections (*open arrow* in **E**). Midline sections (**F** and **G**) show the central canal of the spinal cord, the synovial joints between the anterior arch of the atlas (*asterisk*), the flat transverse ligament (*crossed arrow*) with the odontoid process, and the tectorial membrane (*tm* in **G**).

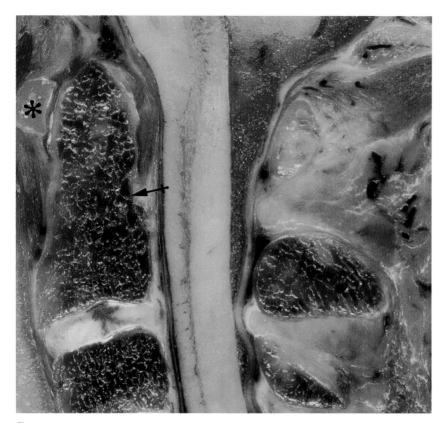

F

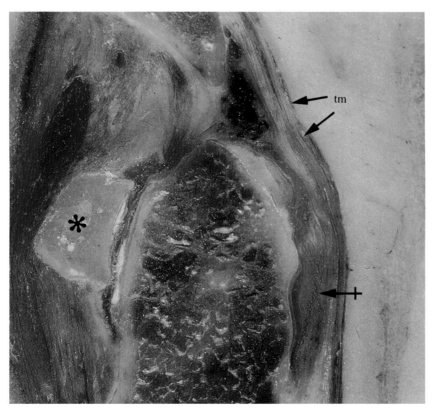

G

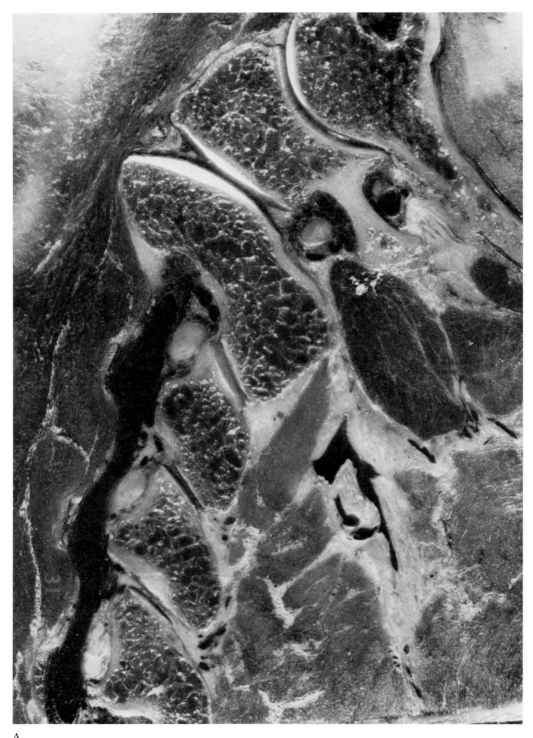

A

FIGURE 3.3 Sagittal section through the articular pillars, from the occiput to C4. **A.** This section shows the typical ball-and-socket configuration of the occipitoatlantal joint. The articular surfaces of the atlantoaxial joint are both convex. The cartilage is thicker centrally than in the peripheral portion of the joint. The subchondral bone contour is almost straight. **B.** Meniscoid synovial tags project into this joint anteriorly and posteriorly. The nerve roots below the level of the axis are accommodated in furrows at the anterior upper aspect of the articular pillars, allowing the vertebral artery to take a straight course. Meniscoid synovial tags are visible in the lateral portion of the facet joints (*arrowheads* in **C**).

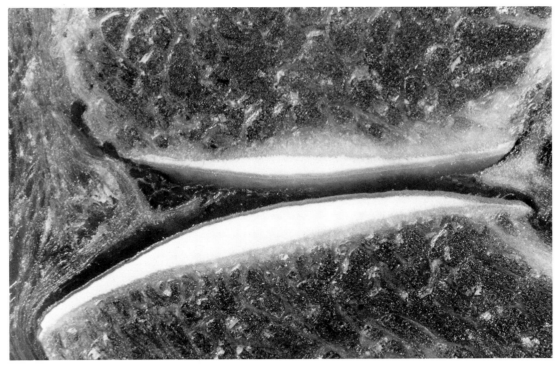

B

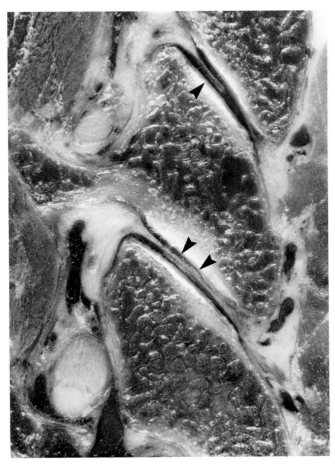

C

laterally merges to form the dentate ligaments. These are suspensory attachments of the cord to the thecal sac. The anterior median fissure is a deep longitudinal groove in the anterior surface of the cord. The dorsal and ventral roots of the cervical and thoracic spinal cord are formed from many dendritic root filaments that emerge from the antero- and posterolateral sulci of the cord. The dorsal rootlets of the cervical spine are considerably thicker than the ventral rootlets. These filaments or rootlets merge stepwise to form the ventral and dorsal roots of the spinal nerves, separated by the dentate ligament.

As a result of the faster longitudinal growth of the vertebral column in relation to the spinal cord, the rootlets and spinal nerve roots run almost horizontally in the upper cervical spine, then take a progressively more oblique, vertical, and anteriorly directed course at lower levels of the cord. The lumbosacral spinal roots arise directly from the cord and surround the conus medullaris by four bundles of nerve roots in the anterolateral and posterolateral compartments of the subarachnoid space. This arrangement results in the typical X-shaped configuration of the lumbosacral roots seen on axial CT scans and anatomic sections through the conus medullaris.

The ventral and the longer dorsal roots converge somewhat anteriorly toward the subpedicular gutter and pierce the thecal sac separately. At these points of exit there are short but separate sleeves of the arachnoid and dura, which merge after a short distance and form between them the interradicular foramen. Within the intervertebral foramen just below the pedicle, one can identify a localized swelling

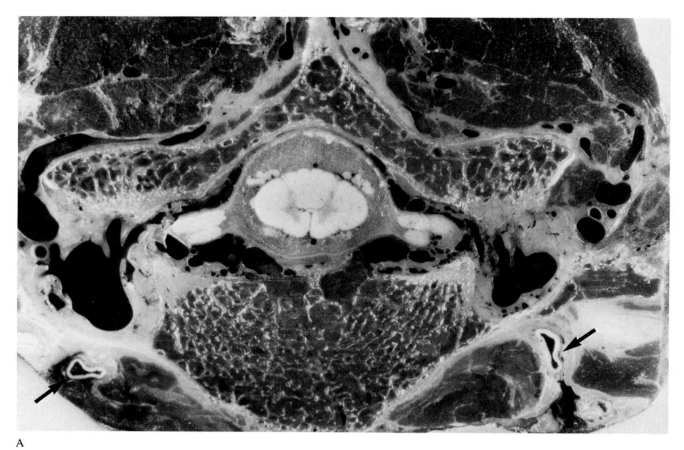

A

FIGURE 3.4   Axial sections through C7, the C6–7 disc, and C6. This specimen had been frozen
in moderate flexion. The resulting distraction of the wedge-shaped articular processes causes considerable widening of the foraminal venous plexuses (**F** and **G**). The posterior margin of the
vertebral bodies and the disc is straight; the lamina and the ligamentum flavum have a circular
curvature (**A–C**). The vertebral artery (*arrows*) runs outside the transverse foramen of C7 (**A–E**).
The artery enters the transverse foramen of C6 (**F** and **G**). The uncinate processes in the lower
cervical spine project from the posterolateral margin of the upper end-plates (*up* in **D** and **E**).
Radiate tears and a small disc herniation are seen in the posterior portion of the anulus (*arrowheads*
in **D** and **E**). Note also the relationship between the dorsal root ganglion (*g*) and the vertebral
artery. (*Figure continued* on pages 47–49.)

of the nerve root; this is the dorsal root ganglion. Distally,
the spinal cord has a thin caudal extension, the filum terminale internum, running together with the nerve roots of
the cauda equina. The thecal sac ends at the midsacral level,
where it dwindles into the thin filum durae matris spinalis
and affixes to the coccyx.

Intervertebral Foramen

Refer to Figures 3.1, 3.2. 3.4, 3.5, and 3.7–3.11.

  The intervertebral or "neural" foramina are actually
osseofibrous tunnels rather than true foramina. They are
continuous with the lateral recesses of the spinal canal. It
is through the foramina that the segmental nerves and vessels emerge. In the cervical region the spinal nerve roots
and their foramina take an obliquely caudal, lateral, and
anterior course. In the thoracic and lumbar regions the intervertebral foramina are directed laterally. The intervertebral
foramina of the cervical and thoracic spine are located behind the lower portion of the body of the vertebra above.
The upper bony wall is formed by the notch at the inferior
and medial margin of the pedicle. In the cervical spine the
floor of the neuroforamen (i.e., the upper rim of the pedicle)
is at the level of the upper end-plate of the vertebra below.
In the thoracic spine the floor of the neuroforamen (pedicle
of the lower vertebra) is above the level of the intervertebral
disc. In the cervical spine the anterior osseous wall of the
neuroforamen is formed by the uncinate process of the lower
vertebra. In the thoracic spine the inferior lateral portion of
the vertebral body delimits the neuroforamen. In the lumbar
spine the intervertebral foramen has an inverted teardrop
configuration, with the wider upper portion under the pedi-

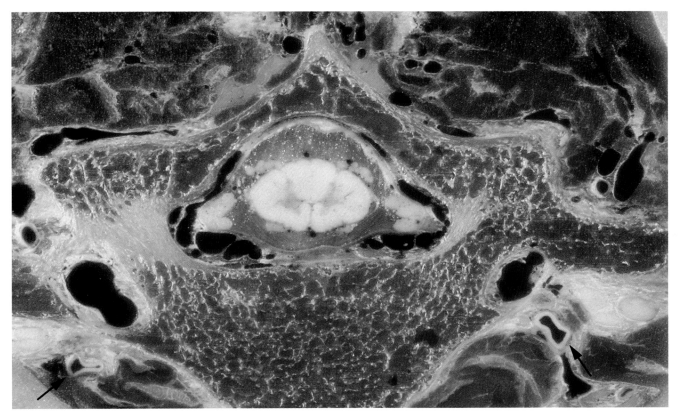

B

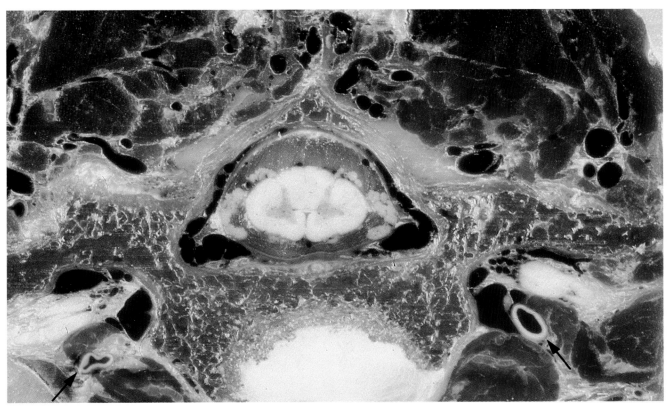

C

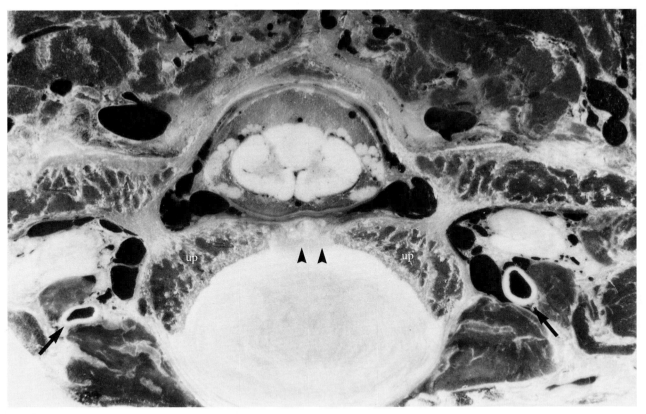

D

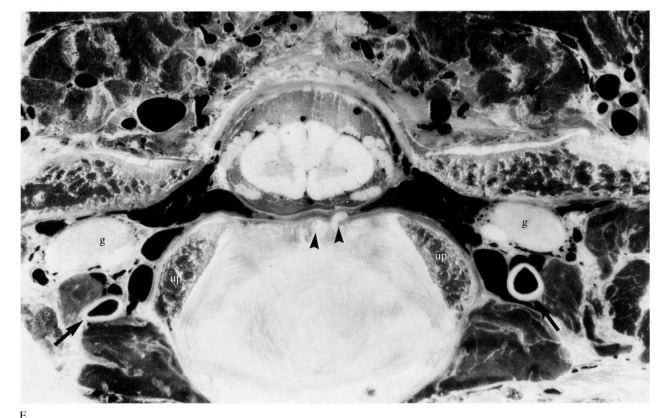

E

FIGURE 3.4 (*cont'd*)   See legend page 46.

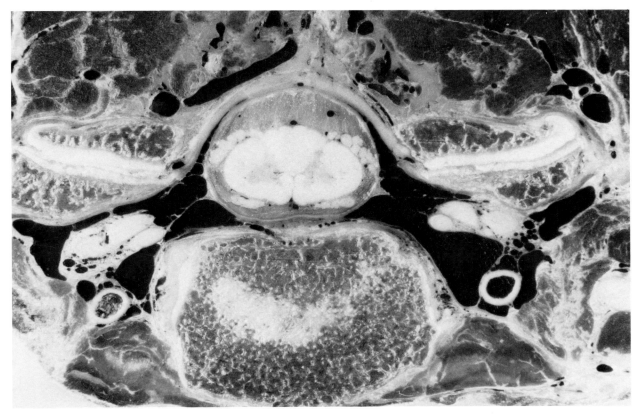

F

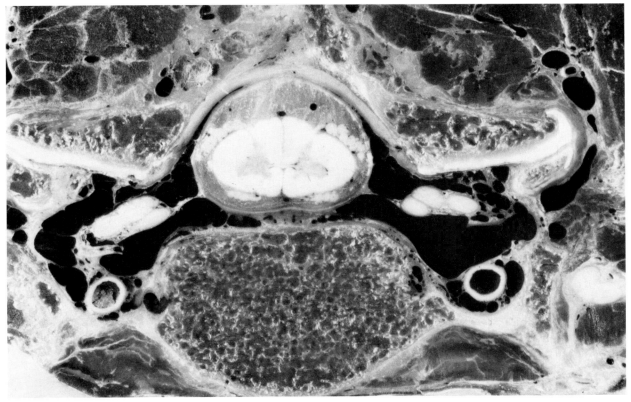

G

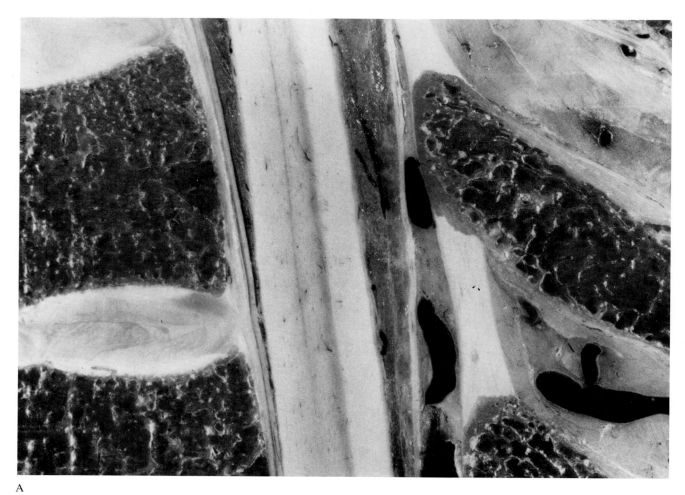

A

FIGURE 3.5 Sagittal sections at the cervicothoracic junction. Note the outlet of the basivertebral vein (*asterisk* in **A** and **B**) as well as a blood vessel traversing the subarachnoid space (*arrowheads* in **B**). The epidural venous plexus increases in volume toward the lateral recess and the neuroforamen. Note the typical insertion of the ligamentum flavum (*lf*) into the anterior aspect of the upper lamina and the upper rim and posterior aspect of the lamina below (**C**). Sections **D–F** show how the nerve roots run close to the pedicle surrounded by venous sinuses. The dentate ligament separates the ventral nerve roots from the dorsal nerve roots (*open arrows* in **C**). The uncovertebral joint is marked by a *crossed arrow* in **G**. (*Figure continued* on pages 51–53.)

cle of the upper vertebra and the narrower lower portion delimited anteriorly by the thick and slightly posteriorly bulging intervertebral disc and posteriorly by the base of the superior articular process, the ligamentum flavum (joint capsule), and the base of the inferior articular process.

The floor of the lumbar intervertebral foramen is below the upper endplate of the lower vertebra because the lumbar vertebral bodies (contrary to the cervical and thoracic vertebrae) have a notch at the upper aspect of the pedicle, the incisura vertebralis superior. All vertebral bodies have a subpedicular notch, the incisura vertebralis inferior. The shape and size of a given intervertebral foramen varies considerably, both from specific movements in different positions and from loading of the spine.

The superior portion of a typical intervertebral foramen contains the sheath of the dura, with the dorsal root ganglion and the ventral spinal root, the spinal branch of the segmental artery, radicular veins, and the recurrent (sinuvertebral) nerve. This particular nerve arises from the dorsal division of the spinal nerve and then reenters the spinal canal to supply the posterior portion of the anulus fibrosus, the posterior longitudinal ligament, and the periosteum of the vertebral body. The inferior portion of the intervertebral foramen contains intervertebral veins and fat tissue. The thoracic spinal nerves are comparatively thin and occupy a far smaller proportion of the foramina than do those in the lumbar spine. They are surrounded by wide venous sinuses and some fat tissue, and are often located

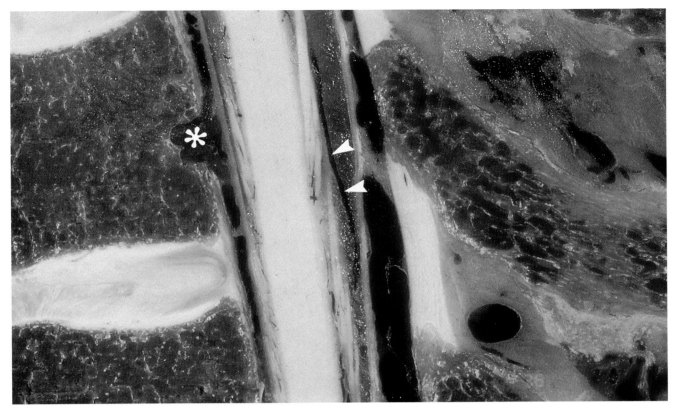

B

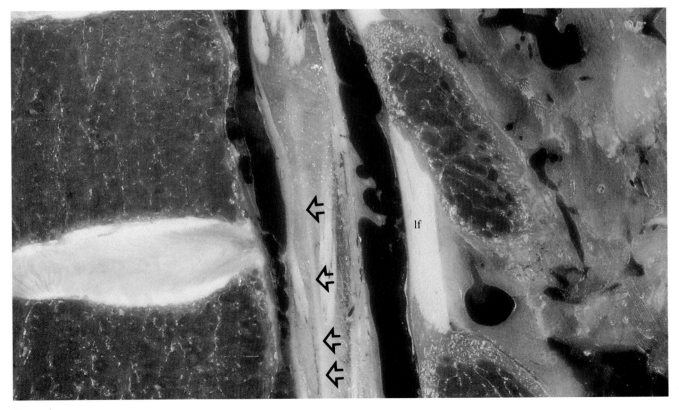

C

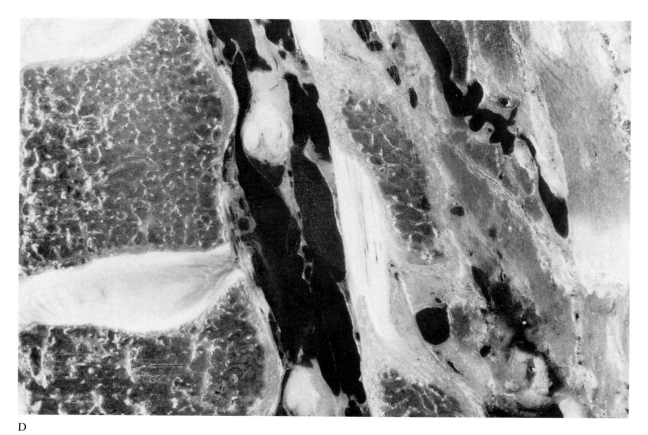

D

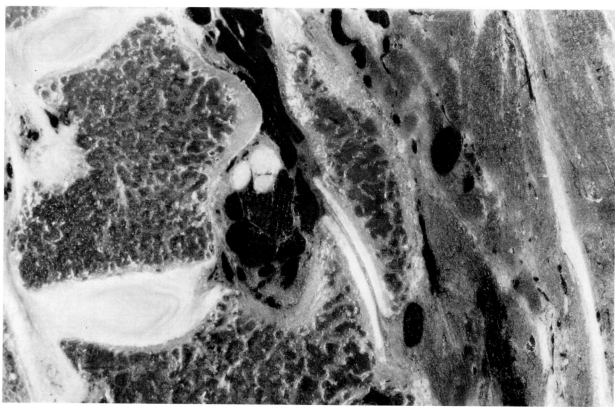

E

FIGURE 3.5 (*cont'd*)   See legend page 50.

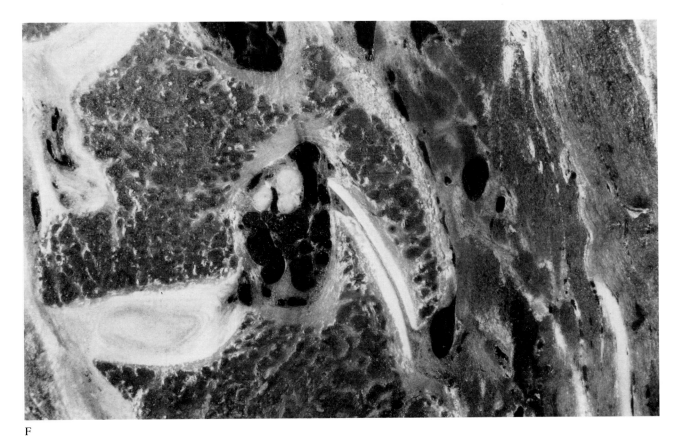

F

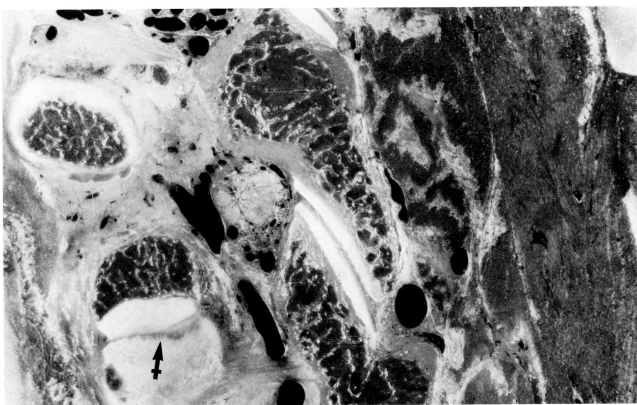

G

well away from the pedicle. By contrast, the lumbar spinal nerve roots are much thicker and occupy a greater portion of the upper neuroforamen, the subpedicular notch.

Arterial Supply of the Spine

The anterior spinal arteries supply the blood to the anterior portions of the spinal cord. The multiple spinal branches take origin from the vertebral arteries (cervical spine), dorsal branches of the intercostal arteries (thoracic spine), dorsal branches of the lumbar arteries (lumbar spine), and dorsal branches of the lateral sacral arteries (sacrum).

The vertebrae and the internal structures of the spinal canal are supplied by the spinal branches of the cervical vertebral arteries and the segmental arteries of the thoracolumbar spine and the sacrum. These arterial branches enter the intervertebral foramen, where they divide into ventral and dorsal medullary arteries, posterior central arteries, and anterior laminar arteries. The medullary arteries follow the corresponding ventral and dorsal nerve roots to the spinal cord. After reaching the cord, these small arteries run in longitudinal grooves on the cord, covered by the pia mater. The posterior central arteries supply the anterior wall of the spinal canal through nutrient foramina beneath the posterior longitudinal ligament. The anterior laminar arteries terminate as a delicate arterial network on the inner surface of the neural arches.

Vertebral Veins

The epidural intraspinal space is predominantly filled with fat and rich venous plexuses. Dorsal and ventral venous plexuses drain the spinal canal and its contents. The latter is in continuity with the basivertebral veins, which traverse the central part of the vertebral body through prominent foramina that are easily identified on CT scans. The basivertebral veins connect the ventral internal veins with the anterior external venous plexuses. In a similar manner, the smaller posterior internal venous plexuses communicate with their external counterparts through the neuroforamen, longitudinal midline spaces between the ligamenta flava, and osseous channels in the laminae and pedicles. The segmental intervertebral veins drain intraspinal blood into the vertebral, intercostal, ascending lumbar, and lateral sacral veins. The spinal veins have no valves, and therefore bidirectional flow may occur.

Regional Characteristics of the Spine

The Craniocervical Junction

Refer to Figures 3.2 and 3.3.

The atlas lacks a vertebral body. It consists of anterior and posterior arches which are fused to a pair of lateral masses containing the facets. The superior facets are con-

cave and articulate with the convex occipital condyles. Inferiorly, the convex articular facets of the atlas articulate with the convex superior facets of the axis. Foramina for the vertebral arteries traverse the laterally projecting transverse processes of C1. The dens, or odontoid process of the axis, is a peglike projection that extends upward behind the anterior arch of C1. It has true synovial articulations with the anterior arch of the atlas and the transverse ligament. The axis and atlas are anchored to the skull base by several layers of strong ligaments. The apical and alar ligaments of the odontoid process are covered by the strong cruciform ligament.

The lateral bands of the cruciform ligament, commonly referred to as the transverse ligament, can usually be demonstrated on axial CT scans. All of these ligaments are covered posteriorly by the broad tectorial membrane, which is an expansion of the anterior layer of the posterior longitudinal ligament. Posteriorly, the occiput and atlas are connected by the thin, wide, elastic posterior atlanto-occipital membrane. The vertebral artery and first cervical nerve pass through this membrane. Anteriorly, the broad atlanto-occipital and atlantoepistrophic ligaments are partially hidden by the anterior longitudinal ligament.

Cervical Spine from C3 to C7

Refer to Figures 3.3–3.5.

The cross-sectional shape of vertebral bodies in the cervical spine is that of a trapezoid. They are about twice as wide from side to side as in the sagittal dimension. Superior and inferior endplates are roughly parallel and slope obliquely downward anteriorly. The discs are slightly wedge-shaped, wider anteriorly than posteriorly. Projecting superiorly from the lateral edges of the superior endplates are paired ridges—the uncinate processes. The uncinate processes of C3 through C5 are oriented in the sagittal plane; those of C6 and C7 are located at the posterolateral border of the endplate. These processes fit into corresponding notches laterally and posterolaterally in the lower endplates of the upper vertebrae. The intervertebral discs abruptly decrease in height toward their lateral and posterolateral border. Oblique clefts in the disc following the medial contour of the uncinate processes (an acquired condition) give the impression of true articulations, commonly referred to as the uncovertebral or von Luschka joints. Osteoarthritic osteophytes arising from these pseudojoints may encroach on the spinal nerve roots and vessels during their long course through the intervertebral foramen.

Whereas the intervertebral or facet joints in the lumbar and thoracic region project behind the vertebral bodies and the pedicles, the cervical facet joints extend laterally and slightly posteriorly to the vertebral bodies. The transverse processes arise anterior to the facet joints. The transverse process is a composite structure derived from a costal anlage anteriorly and a real transverse process posteriorly.

The anterior portion of the transverse process projects laterally and slightly anteriorly from the anterolateral corner of the vertebra. It terminates as a markedly superiorly extending horn-shaped thickening—the anterior tubercle. This tubercle is especially thick and prominent in C6, whereas C7 is devoid of this process.

The pedicle, round or oval in cross section, projects from the upper posterior portion of the vertebra and runs in a lateral and slightly dorsal direction toward the strong articular pillar. Forming a horizontal ridge at the anterior aspect of the pars interarticularis, it is continuous with the transverse process proper. This transverse process takes a more caudad oblique course and terminates as the posterior tubercle lateral and inferior to the tubercle of the rib anlage process. The distal portions of these two processes are connected by a caudally convex bridge of bone, the costotransverse bar, which forms the lateral bony border of the transverse foramen. The deep furrow at the superior aspect of the transverse process carries the spinal nerve and segmental vessels. The dorsal root ganglion is located behind the vertebral artery and is partially accommodated in a shallow, oblique groove in the superior articular process. The transverse foramina, commonly slightly larger on the left than on the right, contain the vertebral artery, surrounded by veins, fat, and sympathetic nerves. As a rule, the transverse foramen of the seventh cervical vertebra contains only vertebral veins. The vertebral artery usually enters the transverse foramen of C6; occasionally it enters at a higher level.

Throughout the cervical region, posteriorly, broad V-shaped laminae emerge from the pedicles and meet in the midline to form short, caudally sloping spinous processes, most of which have bifid tips and deep grooves on their lower surface. Except for the seventh cervical vertebra, the vertebra prominens, the spinous processes are too short to reach the superficial fascia. Their interspinous and supraspinous ligaments have a strong midsagittal elastic prolongation, the ligamentum nuchae.

The cervical spinal canal is wide and has a round configuration cranially and a more triangular one caudally. Epidural fat tissue is sparse, and wide venous plexuses are present in the lateral parts of the canal. These venous channels surround roots and nerves as they leave the intervertebral foramina and form wide sinuses. The lack of large amounts of epidural fat in the cervical canal, in contrast to the lumbar canal, makes it more difficult to differentiate between the soft-tissue structures in the cervical spinal canal on a noncontrast CT scan.

Another typical anatomic feature is the arrangement of muscles in the cervical spine. Posteriorly, a number of short unisegmental muscles (rectus capitis superior minor and major, superior and inferior oblique) insert in the atlas. Distal to the atlas, the multisegmental semispinalis and longissimus cervicis muscles make up the cervical portion of the multifidus. These deep muscles are covered by the thick semispinalis and longissimus capitis as well as the super-

ficial layer of the splenius capitis and the trapezius. Laterally, the three scalenus muscles are attached to tubercles on the tips of cervical transverse processes. Anteriorly, the cervical vertebral column is covered by the longus capitis, the longus colli, and their enveloping fascia.

Thoracic Spine

Refer to Figures 3.6–3.8.

As a reflection of the thoracic kyphosis, the thoracic vertebral bodies are slightly wedge-shaped. The upper thoracic vertebrae are commonly ovoid in cross section, with a larger sagittal than transverse diameter. Through the midthoracic and lower thoracic regions they gradually become larger and broader. The discs which are thin in the upper thoracic spine are thicker at progressively lower levels. The pedicles are long, and the joint facets are oriented in the coronal plane. The upper 10 thoracic vertebrae have caudally angulated laminae. They form overlapping osseous shingles together with the slender, long, obliquely downward-directed spinous processes. Thick, round transverse processes are also characteristic. They run obliquely craniad posteriorly to provide the costotransverse articulations at the level of the intervertebral discs. Each rib articulates with two adjacent vertebral bodies and the intervening disc. These so-called costocentral joints have a thick fibrous capsule—the radiate ligament. Several strong costotransverse ligaments add further support to the rib articulation.

A thin layer of epidural fat and veins surrounds the thecal sac in a relatively even distribution. Large venous sinuses occupy the lateral recesses and intervertebral foramina. The thoracic spinal roots are quite thin. They emerge from the thecal sac, forming short, cone-shaped axillary pouches at the inferomedial border of the pedicles. The nerve-root sheaths of the dura are short. The thin thoracic spinal roots occupy a small proportion of the intervertebral foramen and visualize less well on CT scans than do the thick lumbosacral roots.

Between the ribs, three layers of intercostal muscles (intercostalis externus, internus, and intimus) run in different directions. Anteriorly, the crura of the diaphragm and the large vessels constitute contiguous paraspinal soft tissues. Posteriorly, the various portions of the sacrospinal muscle (erector trunci) are located within the shallow triangular compartment between the spinous processes and the transverse processes of the thoracic spine, the posterior angles of the ribs, and the thoracolumbar fascia. The deepest layer, the multifidus, is covered posteriorly and laterally by the spinalis thoracis, longissimus thoracis, iliocostalis thoracis, and lumborum muscles. The superficial muscles of the thoracic spine form wide and thin muscular plates with mainly obliquely oriented fibers—the serratus posterior inferior, rhomboideus major and minor, latissimus dorsi, and trapezius.

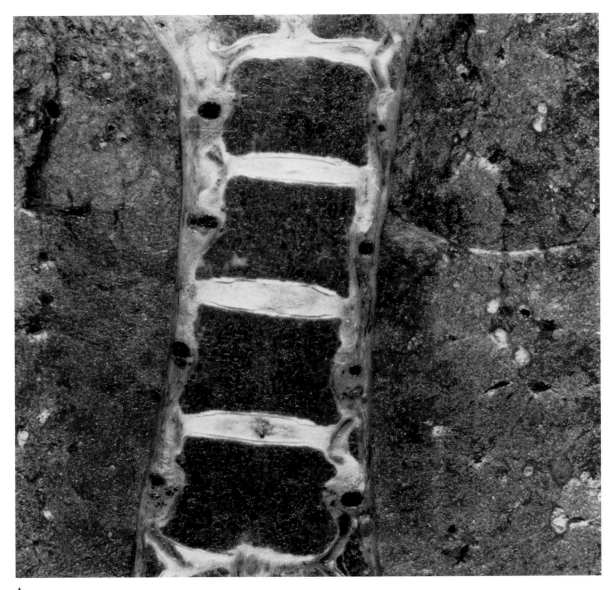

A

FIGURE 3.6 Coronal sections through the midthoracic spine. The intervertebral discs are thin (**A**), and the end-plates of the vertebral bodies are almost parallel. Segmental vessels can be distinguished at the midportion of each vertebra. The spinal canal opens (**B**). Note the wedge-shaped heads of the ribs articulating with cartilaginous facets of the two adjacent vertebral bodies (**B, C** and **D**). They are also attached to the disc (costocentral joints). Posteriorly (**F**), the ribs articulate with the transverse processes (costotransverse joints). The two ligamenta flava join in the midline and are continuous with the interspinous ligament (**E, F** and **G**). (*Figure continued* on pages 57–59.)

Lumbar Spine

Refer to Figures 3.7–3.11.

As a consequence of the great weight load borne by the lumbar spine, the lumbar vertebral bodies are large, round, or elliptical and are wider transversely than in the sagittal plane. The lower lumbar vertebrae are slightly wedge-shaped, accounting in part for the lumbar lordosis. The lumbar intervertebral discs have a similar wedge shape,

adding to the lordosis. This is most pronounced at the L5-S1 level. The lumbar discs are the thickest in the entire vertebral column (10–15 mm). The pedicles of the lumbar vertebrae are short and strong, and the laminae are broad and thick. The lower borders of the laminae terminate at the level of the next lower disc so that a small space exists between adjacent laminae. The spinous processes are heavy and rectangular. The superior articular processes diverge

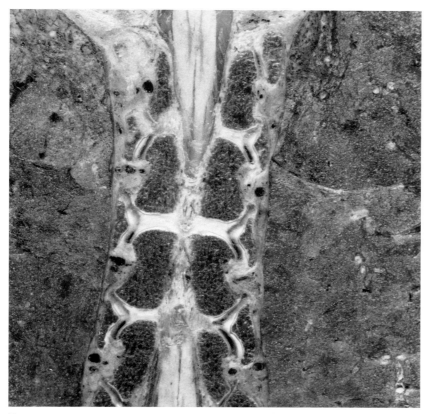

B

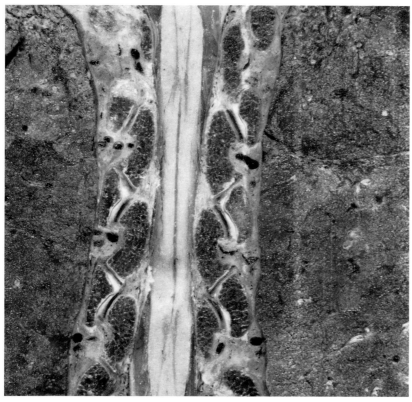

C

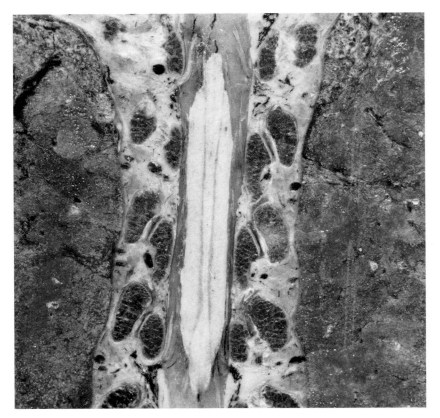

D

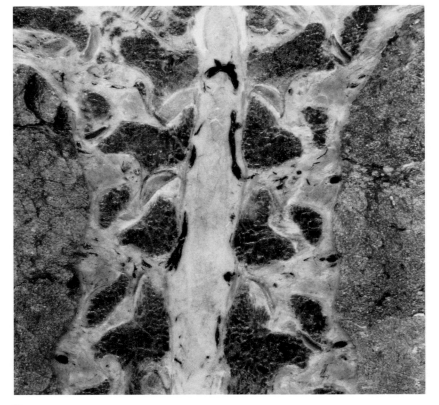

E

FIGURE 3.6 (*cont'd*)   See legend page 56.

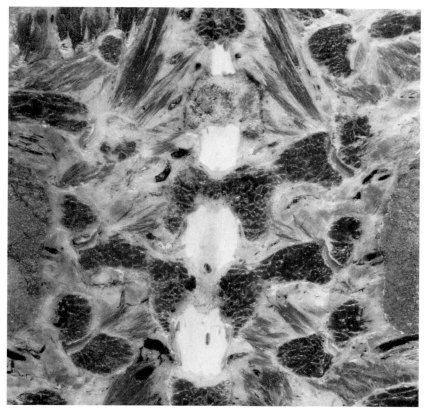

F

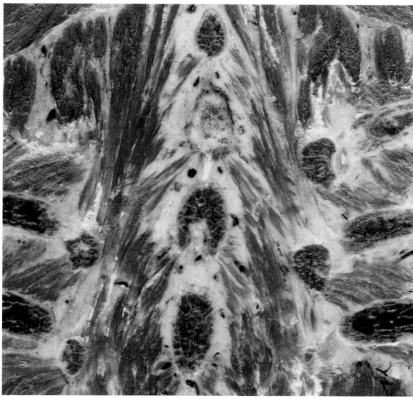

G

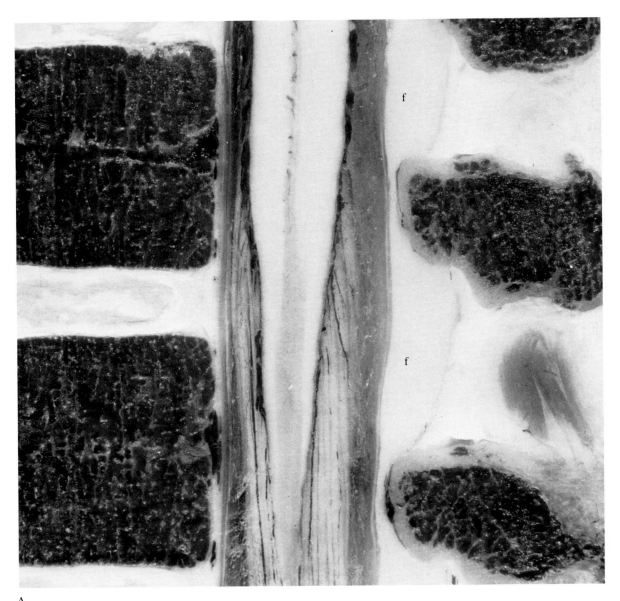

A

FIGURE 3.7 Sagittal sections through the thoracolumbar junction (T12 and L1) and the conus medullaris. The central canal of the spinal cord and the midline longitudinal blood vessels of the cord are demonstrated in (**A**). The outlet of the basivertebral vein is seen in **A–C**. A fat pad (*f*) lies under the ligamentum flavum but does not extend under the lamina. Note the nerve-root bundles of the cauda equina in **B** and **C**. There is an almost abrupt increase in intervertebral disc height from the lower thoracic to the upper lumbar segments (**D**). The longitudinal ventral internal veins interconnect the retrovertebral venous plexuses from one level to the other (*arrowheads* in **E**). The dorsal root ganglia occupy only a minor portion of the intervertebral foramina (**F**). (*Figure continued on pages 61–63.*)

both cranially and dorsally. On axial CT scans the lumbar facet joints frequently assume a biplanar or curvilinear configuration, with the anterior portions oriented toward the coronal plane and the posterior ones oriented more sagittally.

The transverse processes are flattened anteroposteriorly and run slightly dorsally and upward. They represent attachment sites for the intertransverse ligaments, which laterally are continuous with the lumbar aponeurosis. At the base of the transverse processes, short accessory processes project from the dorsal inferior surface. They represent distinct landmarks on axial CT images, as they indicate scans through the lower portion of the pedicles. The transverse processes of the fifth lumbar vertebra are attached to the

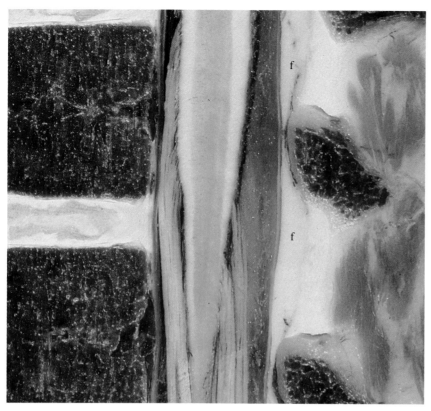

B

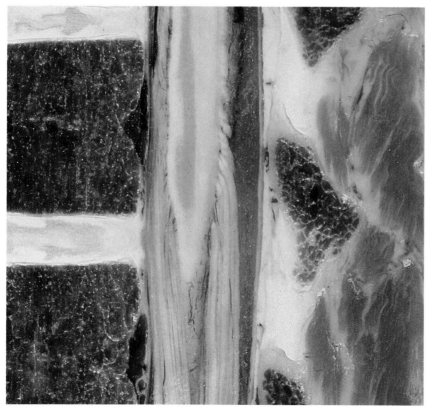

C

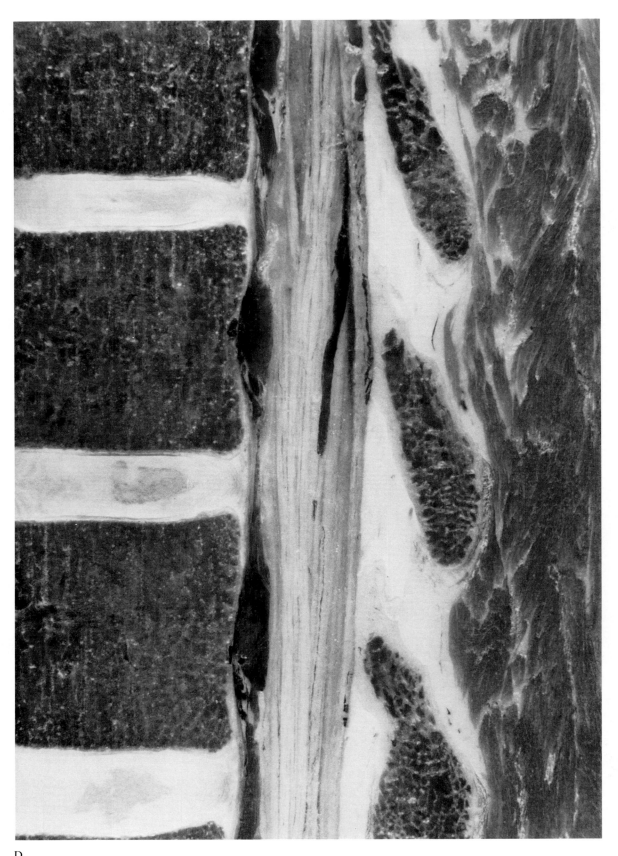

D

FIGURE 3.7 (*cont'd*)   See legend page 60.

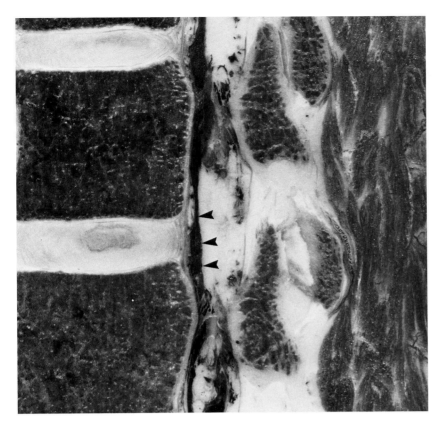

E

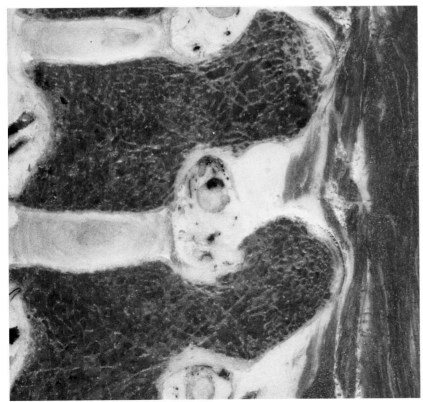

F

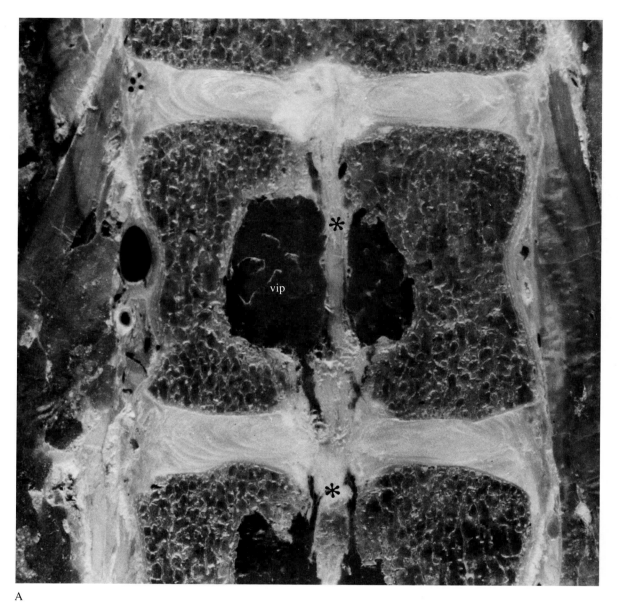

A

FIGURE 3.8 Coronal sections through the thoracolumbar junction (T12–L1–L2) and the conus medullaris. At the posterior border of the vertebral bodies, the ventral internal venous plexus (*vip*) and the posterior longitudinal ligament (*asterisk*) are exposed (**A**). The thecal sac is opened in **B**. The ventral root bundles of the cauda equina are seen in **C**. (*Figure continued* on pages 65–68.)

iliac crest by the strong iliolumbar ligaments. In many patients these processes articulate or are fused with the iliac bones, producing transitional vertebrae.

The lumbar spinal canal is ovoid or triangular, depending on the shape and size of the vertebral bodies, the pedicles, and the articular processes. Short lumbar pedicles, thick laminae, and prominent facets produce an increasingly triangular shape of the lumbar spinal canal toward the lower lumbar spine. The lateral recesses form rather acute angles at the base of the pedicles. The transverse diameter of the canal increases from L1 to L5, whereas the AP diameter decreases. The size of the thecal sac is inversely related to the amount of epidural tissue and varies within wide ranges. The location of the roots of the cauda equina depends on

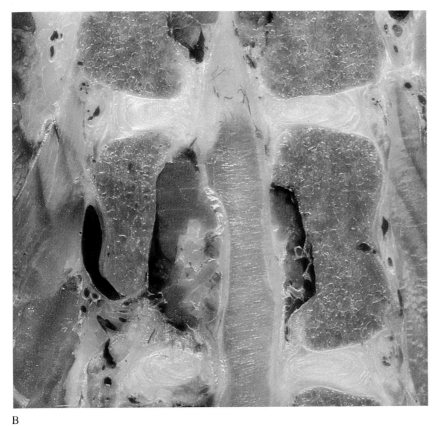

B

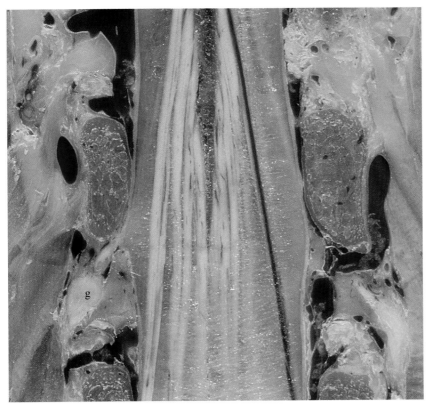

C

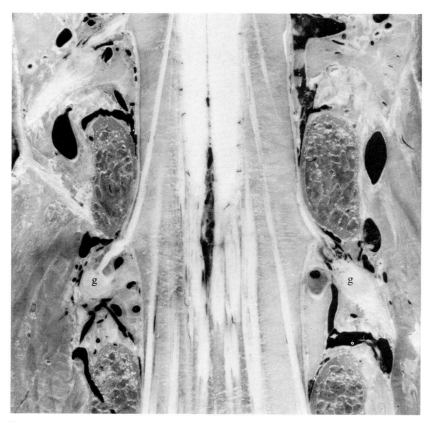

D

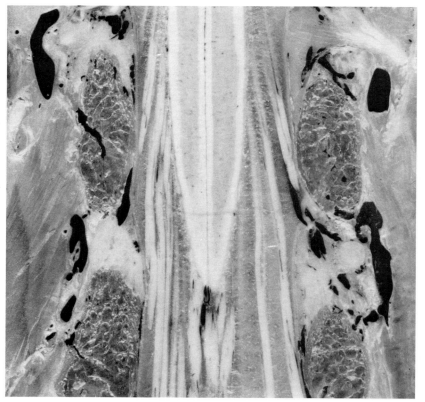

E

FIGURE 3.8 (*cont'd*) Coronal sections through the thoracolumbar junction (T12–L1–L2) and the conus medullaris. Note the steep course of the nerve roots (**D–G**) and their close contact with the pedicles. The thecal sac is wide in this specimen, and little fat and few veins are seen in the epidural space. In the foramina, segmental blood vessels and fat surround the nerve roots (**C–F**). The dorsal root ganglia (*g*) are small (**C** and **D**).

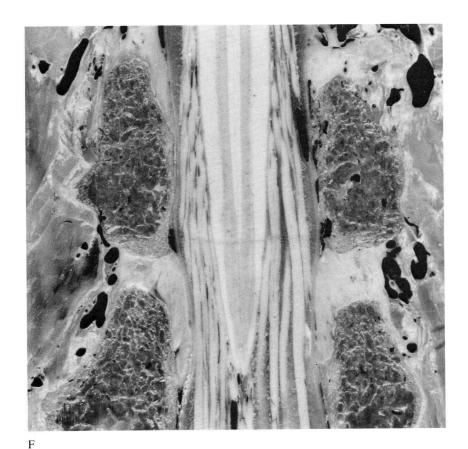

F

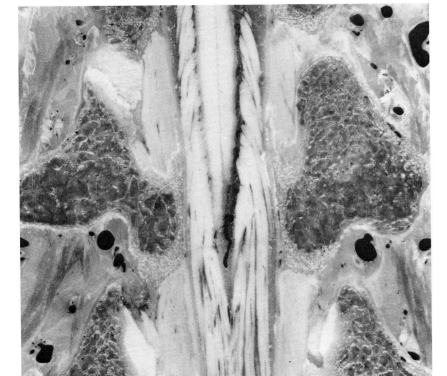

G

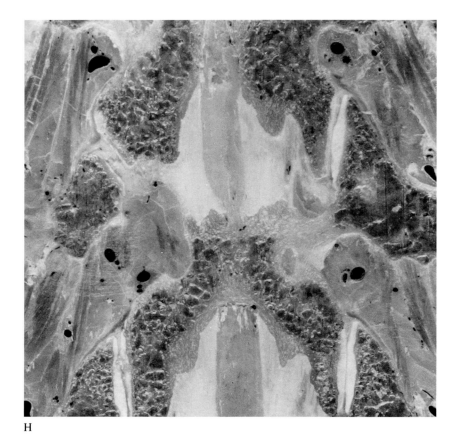

H

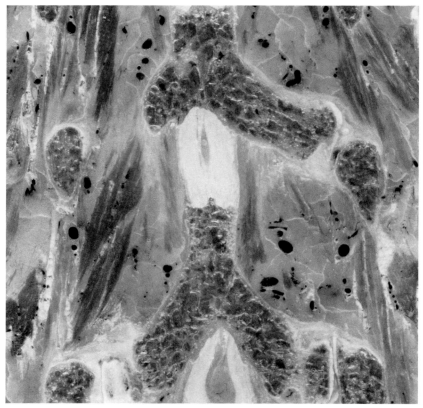

I

FIGURE 3.8 (*cont'd*)   Sections **H** and **I** demonstrate the closed neural arch and the posterior, sagittally oriented portions of the facet joints.

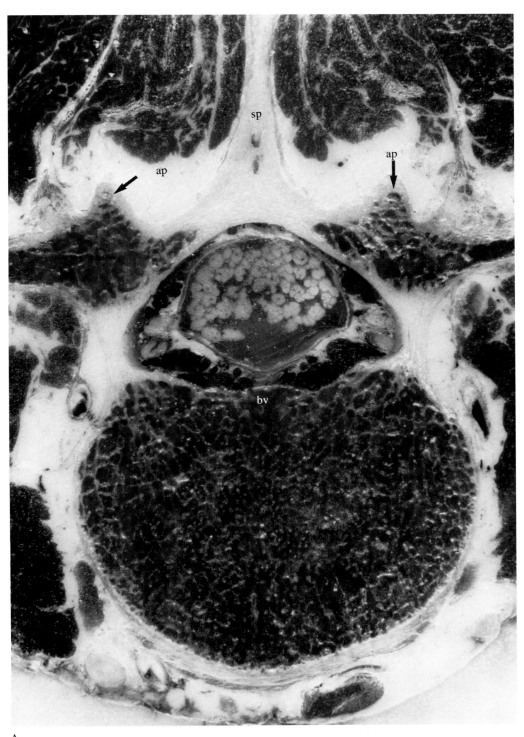

A

FIGURE 3.9 Axial sections through L4 and the L3–4 disc. The accessory process (*ap*) and the spinous process (*sp*) can be seen at the lower margin of the L4 pedicle (**A**). The midportion of the pedicle also displays the orifice of the basivertebral vein (*bv*) that anastomoses with the ventral internal venous plexus (*vip* in **B** and **C**). The epidural veins are less voluminous at the level of the intervertebral disc (**F**). The ligamenta flava merge posteriorly at an acute angle and form between them a triangular space that is constantly occupied by a poorly vascularized fat pad (*asterisks* in **B**, **D**, and **E**). The upper end-plate of L4, the midportion of the disc, and the lower end-plate of L3 are shown in **E**, **F**, and **G**, respectively. Note the cartilaginous end-plate and the dorsal root ganglion (*g* in **G**). (*Figure continued* on pages 70–74.)

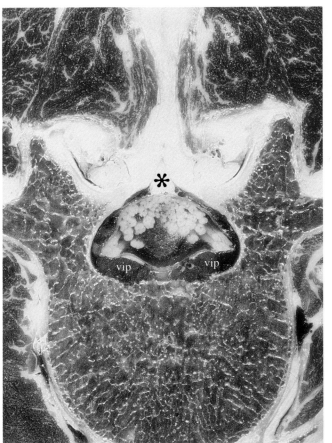

B

the position of the patient and does not seem to follow a strict pattern, except that exiting roots lie anterolaterally within the thecal sac. Posteriorly in the spinal canal, a triangular pad of fat containing the sparse veins of the dorsal internal plexus fills out the acute angle between the two portions of the ligamentum flavum. There is little fat in the notch of the lamina.

The posterior longitudinal ligament attaches to the midportion of the vertebral body. It therefore may bridge the posterior concavity of the vertebral body from one disc to another in a bowstring fashion. Because of this concavity and the large venous outlets at the midbody of the vertebrae, the spinal canal may assume a rather diamond-shaped configuration. In these cases the posterior longitudinal ligament projects within the spinal canal at a considerable distance from the posterior border of the vertebrae. Because the ligament is denser than the surrounding tissues, it is often visible on unenhanced CT scans.

The thick lumbar spinal ganglia occupy the upper portion of the intervertebral foramen. They are surrounded by connective and fat tissue and by fewer veins than in the cervical and thoracic spine. The spinal branch of the segmental artery and the sinuvertebral nerve traverse the upper portion of the foramen. The intervertebral veins are located mainly in the lower portion of the foramen, lying between the disc and the ligamentum flavum.

The dorsal muscle compartment in the lumbar region is delimited medially by the spinous processes. The anterior margin is a combination of the transverse processes, the

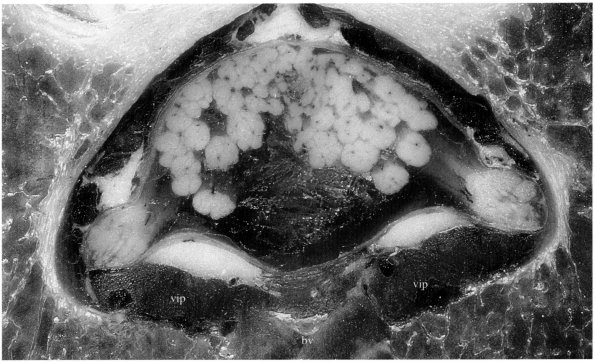

C

FIGURE 3.9 (*cont'd*)   See legend page 69.

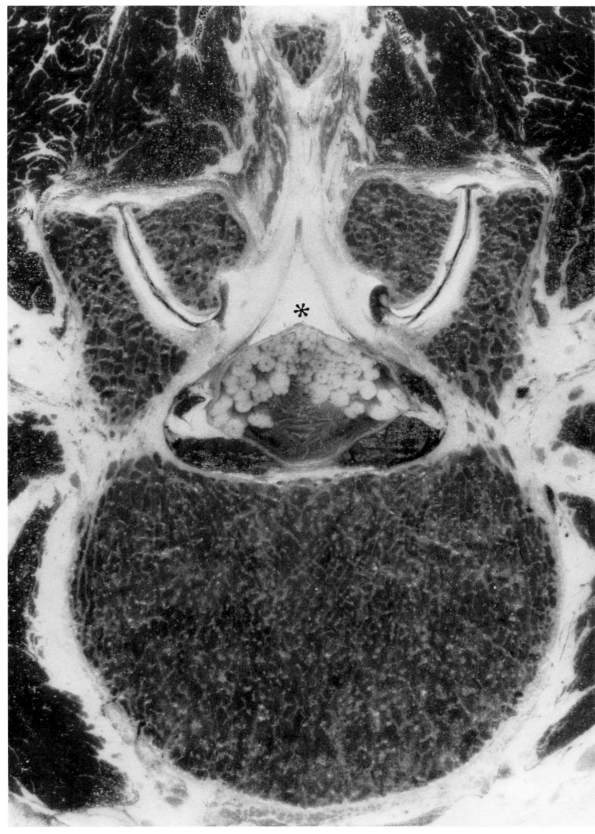

D

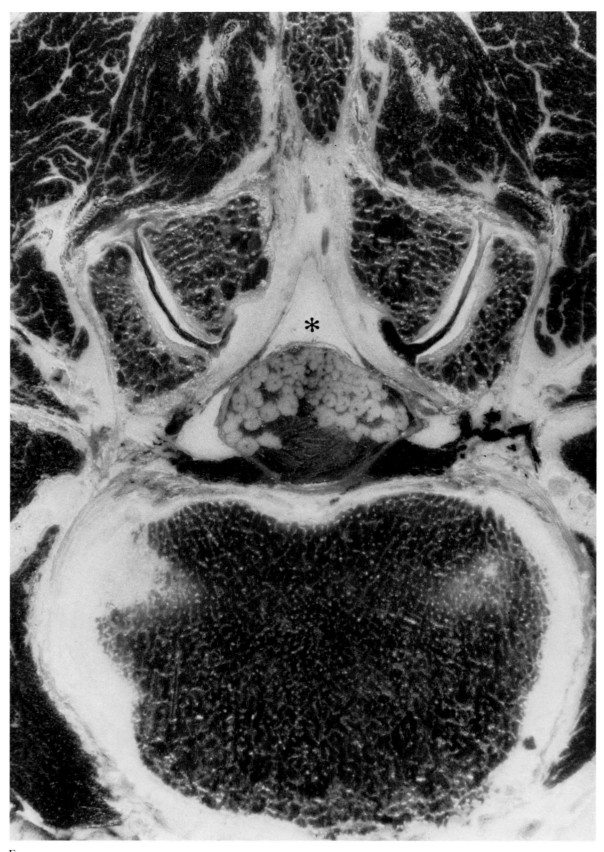

E

FIGURE 3.9 (*cont'd*) See legend page 69.

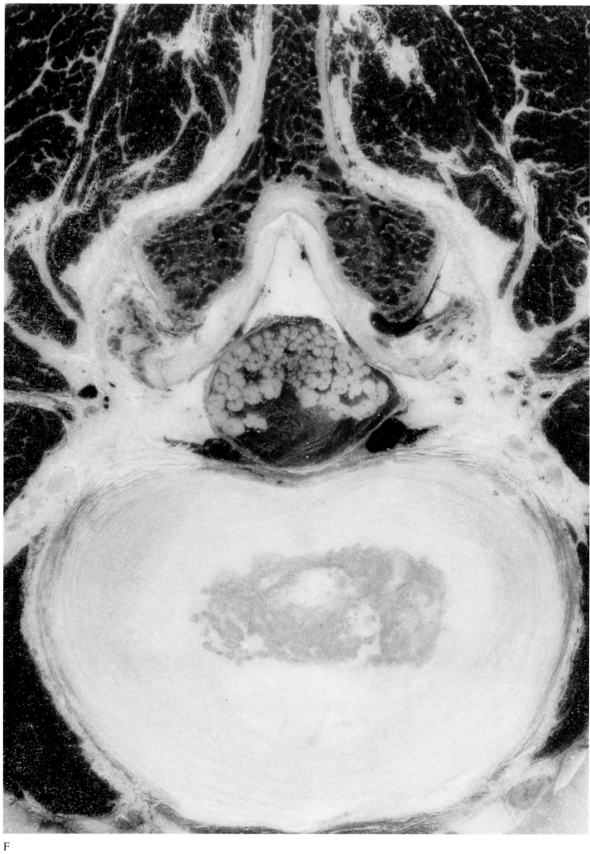

F

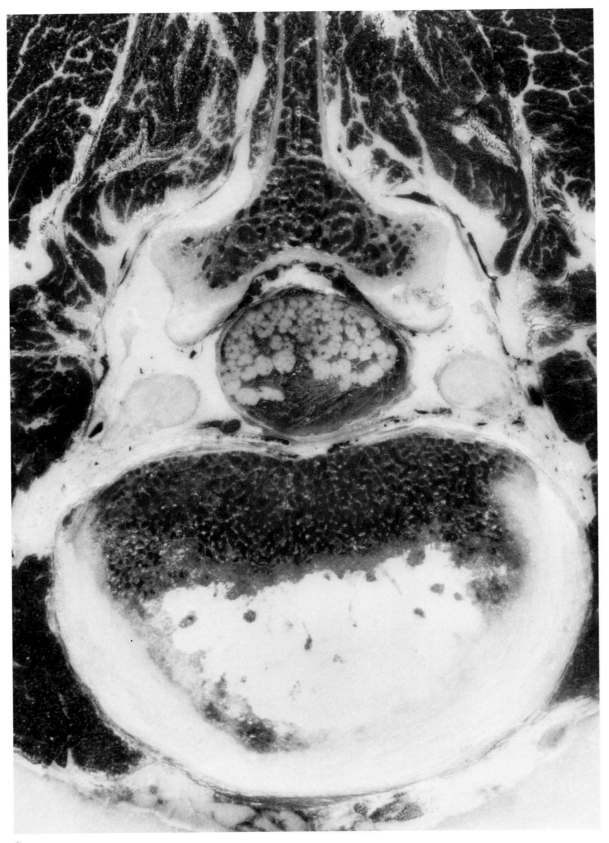

G
FIGURE 3.9 (*cont'd*)   See legend page 69.

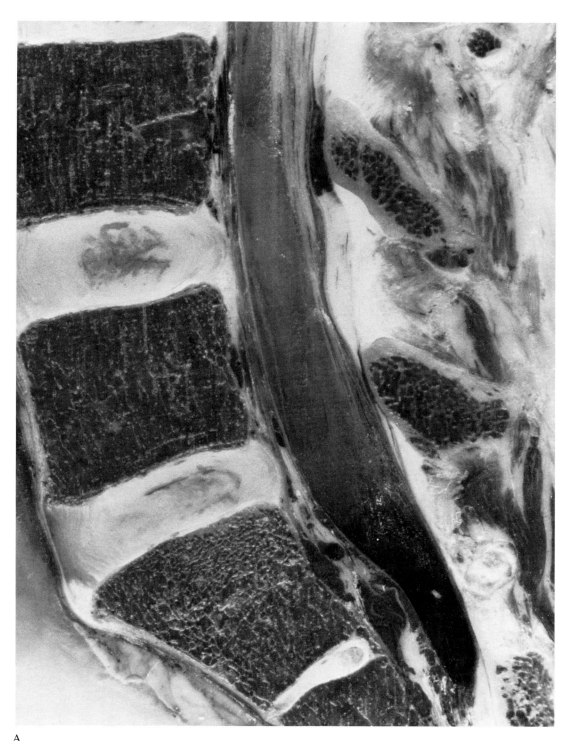

A

FIGURE 3.10 Sagittal sections through the lower lumbar spine (L4–L5–S1). Section A is slightly to the right of the midline, section B shows the nerve roots immediately before they take contact with the pedicle, beneath which they exit from the spinal canal. Note the slight physiological bulge of the discs. The anulus fibrosus extends some millimeters beyond the bony end-plates (*arrow* in **C**). (*Figure continued* on pages 76–79.)

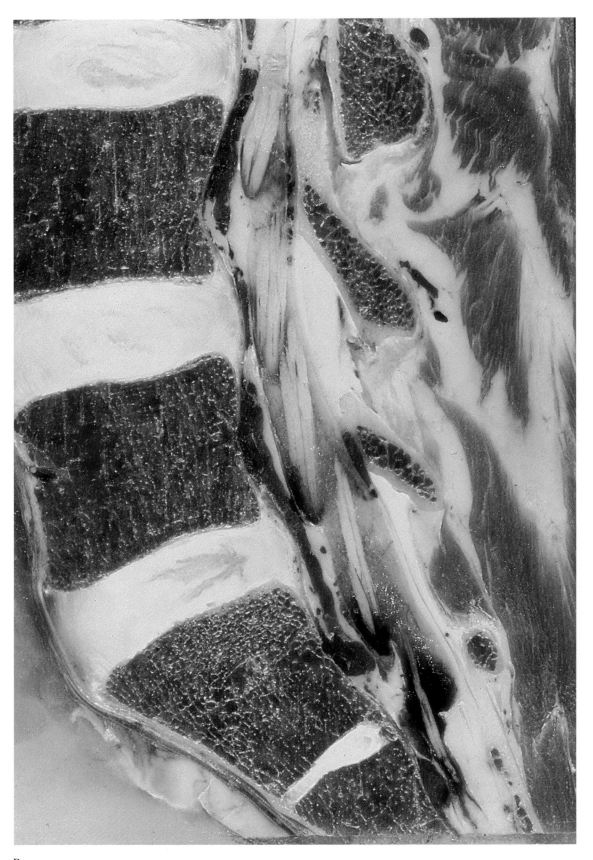

B
FIGURE 3.10 (*cont'd*)   See legend page 75.

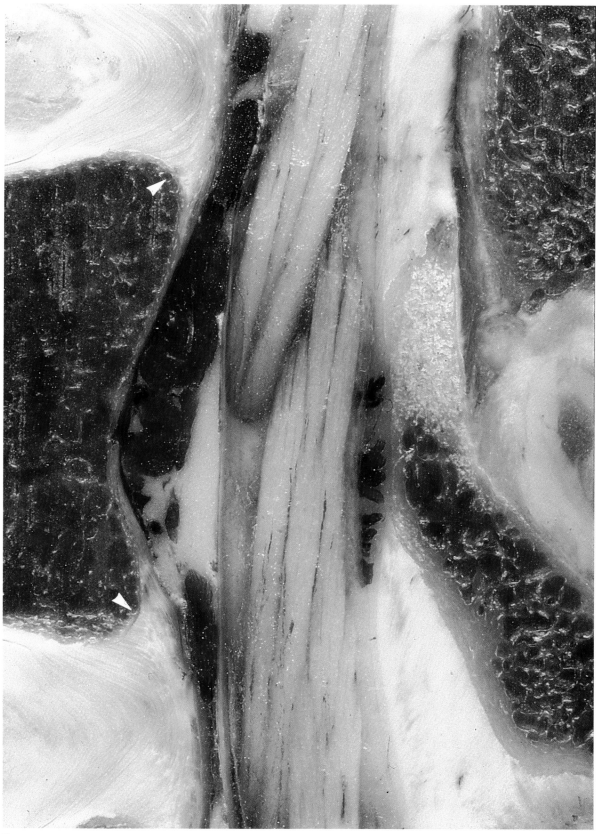

C

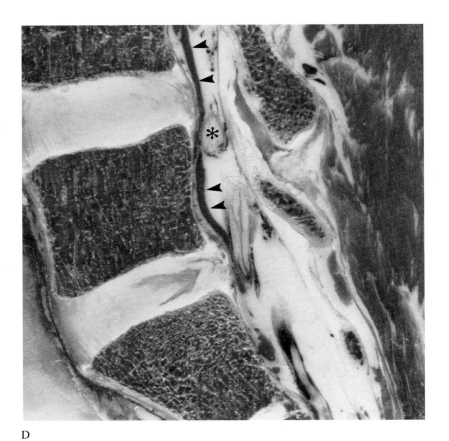

D

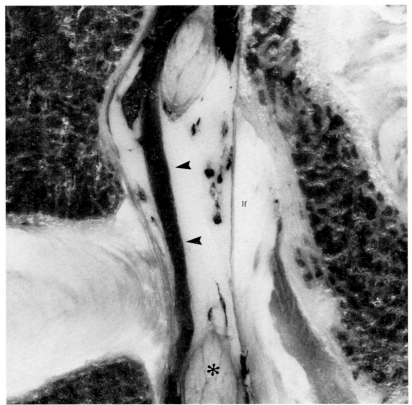

E

FIGURE 3.10 (*cont'd*) Sagittal sections through the lower lumbar spine (L4–L5–S1). The thick retrovertebral venous plexuses shown in **B** and **C** are connected by longitudinal ventral internal veins (*arrowheads* in **D** and **E**). Note also that the ligamentum flavum (*lf*) forms the capsule of the facet joint anteriorly (**E**). In the lateral recess, the exiting fifth lumbar nerve root (*asterisk*) encounters contact with the disc anteriorly and with the ligamentum flavum and the superior articular process of L5 posteriorly (**D** and **E**).

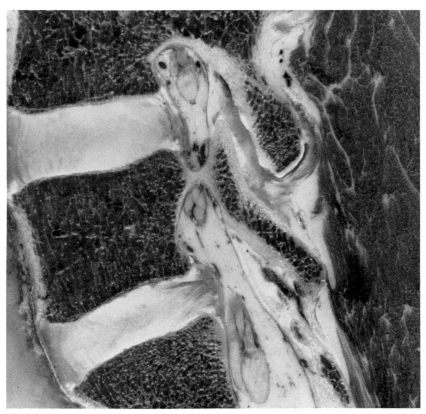

F

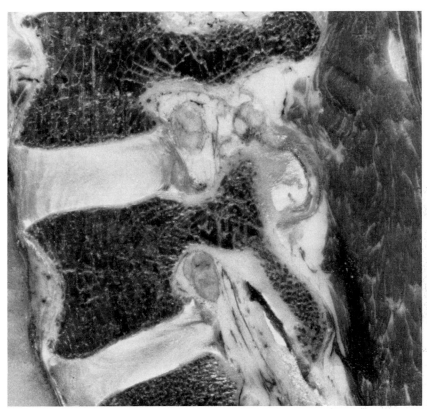

G

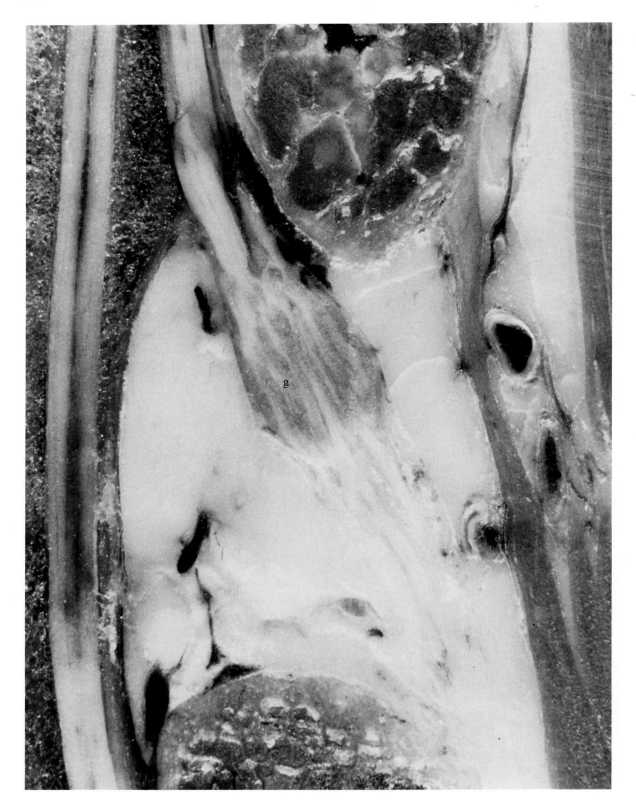

FIGURE 3.11.   High-power photograph of a coronal section through the left L2–3 neuroforamen. The dorsal and ventral roots of L2 closely follow the pedicle. The fusiform dorsal root ganglion (*g*) is embedded in foraminal fat. Segmental arteries and veins surround a thin muscle strand of the multifidus in the lateral portion of the neuroforamen.

middle layer of the lumbodorsal fascia, and the lumbar aponeurosis, which forms a strong membrane extending from the 12th rib to the iliac crest. The posterior border is the very coarse posterior layer of the lumbosacral fascia, which thickens distally and serves as an origin of the sacrospinalis and latissimus dorsi muscles. The transverse processes are interconnected by three short intertransverse muscles and the intertransverse ligament. The medial intertransverse muscles extend from the mamillary process of the inferior vertebra to the accessory process of the superior vertebra. The muscle strands of the multifidus overlying the posterior arch are separated by layers of fat tissue, which also contain the dorsal external venous plexuses. The more superficial layers of the sacrospinalis mainly consist of muscle tissue.

In the lumbosacral region, the erector spinae muscle masses are more homogeneous in cross section. In the upper lumbar spine, the more lateral portion (the iliocostalis), the intermediate portion (the longissimus), and a medial portion (the spinalis thoracis), may sometimes be distinguished on CT scans. The interspinalis muscle may present on either side of the spinous processes and interspinous ligaments. The quadratus lumborum is located anterior to the lumbar aponeurosis. The thick neural trunks of the lumbosacral plexus run obliquely downward and laterally between the quadratus lumborum and the lumbar aponeurosis and beneath the psoas major. The psoas major muscles lie on either side of the spinal column and are covered by the anterior layer of the lumbodorsal fascia—the internal abdominal fascia.

Sacrum

Refer to Figure 3.12.

The sacrum is a composite bone formed from five sacral vertebral segments. Its cranial surface bares the endplate for the lumbosacral disc and the superior articular processes. The thick pars lateralis (ala) has ear-shaped articular surfaces for the sacroiliac joint anteriorly.

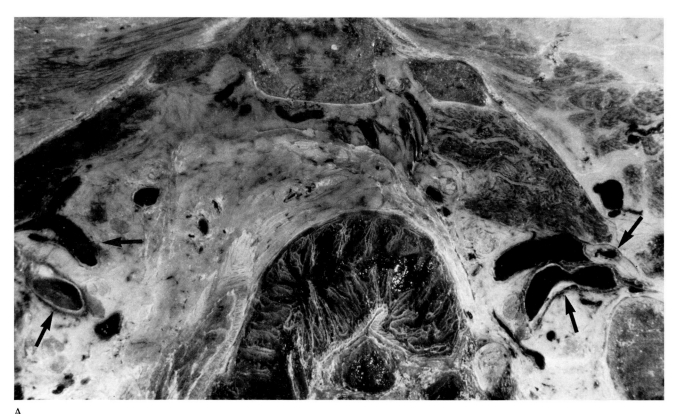

A

FIGURE 3.12 Axial sections from the tip of the sacrum (**A**) to the lumbosacral disc (**G**). The superior gluteal vessels exit through the superior gluteal notch (*arrows* in **A**). The sacroiliac joints are shown in **B–F**. The nerves of the lumbosacral plexus lie in close proximity to the lateral mass of the sacrum (*arrowheads* in **B–D**). The sacral canal and the large posterior and anterior (pelvic) neuroforamina are occupied by fat intermingled with small blood vessels. An accessory articulation between the sacrum and the posterior crest of the ilium is shown on the left side (*arrow* in **E**). Note the coarse lumbosacral fascia (*arrowheads* in **G**). (*Figure continued* on pages 82–84.)

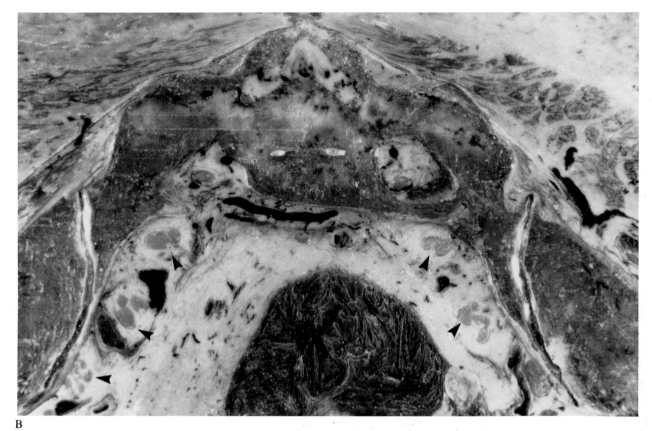

B

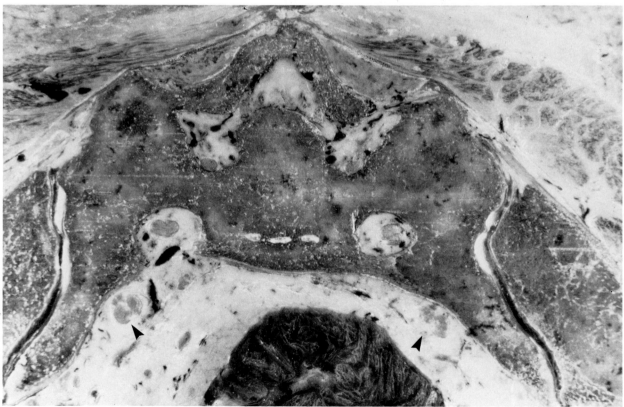

C

FIGURE 3.12 (*cont'd*)   See legend page 81.

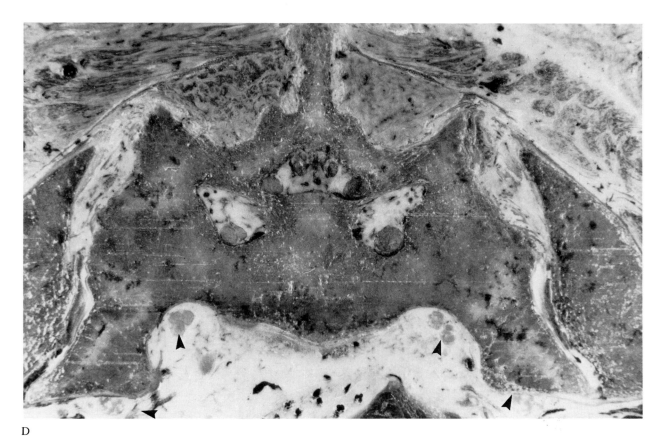

D

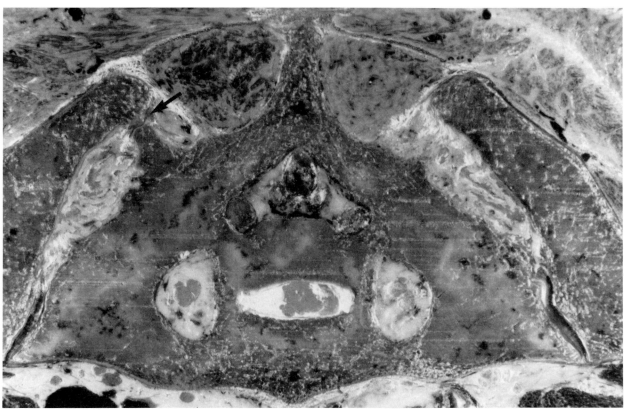

E

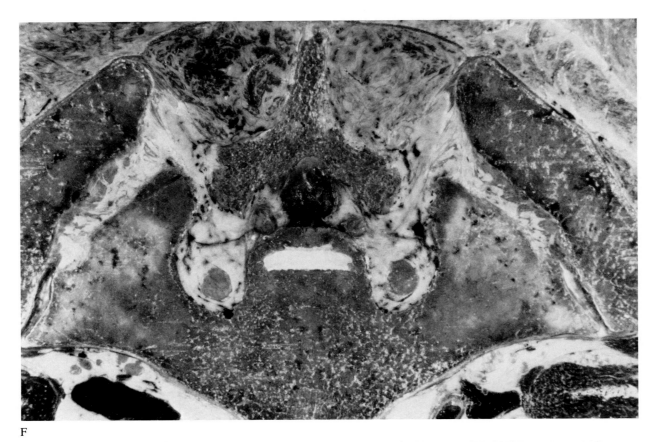

F

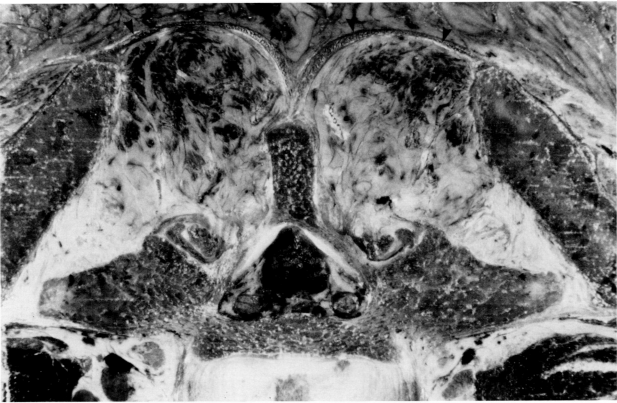

G
FIGURE 3.12 (*cont'd*)   See legend page 81.

The concave anterior surface of the sacrum contains ridges at the site of the remnants of the intervertebral discs. These ridges point at the wide, deeply grooved anterior (pelvic) foramina, which provide exits for the ventral rami of the sacral nerves. Corresponding posterior foramina are found on the convex posterior surface. A median crest of fused spinous tubercles forms a continuation of the spinous processes of the lumbar vertebrae. Less pronounced longitudinal crests on either side of the posterior foramina serve as attachments for the sacrospinalis muscle. The sacral canal is narrow in the AP view and curved or triangular in cross section.

The osseoligamentous space between the spinous crest, the iliac bone, and the thick thoracolumbar fascia contains the multifidus muscle and the origin of the sacrospinalis.

References

1. Rauschning W, Bergström K, Pech P: Correlative craniospinal anatomy studies by computed tomography and cryomicrotomy. J Comput Assist Tomogr 7:9-13, 1983
2. Rauschning W: Computed tomography and cryomicrotomy of lumbar spine specimens. A new technique for multiplanar anatomic correlation. Spine 8:170-180, 1983

Interpretation of Lumbar Spine CT: An Objective Grading System

4

The lumbar spine can be conveniently divided into five clinically important anatomic zones: foramina, facets, lateral recesses, intervertebral discs, and the bony canal. Specific deformity of any of these five zones may occur as isolated abnormalities, producing the signs and symptoms of radiculopathy or back pain.[1,2] Because the appropriate surgical approach for each of these potential sources of pain may be radically different, and it may be impossible to differentiate the precise cause of the symptoms, the responsibility to provide a precise preoperative analysis of each vertebral segment is placed on the radiologist. With this analysis, our clinical colleagues can tailor their surgery precisely to the anatomic causes defined by the CT scan.

Failed back surgery, unfortunately, is a common occurrence. In many cases it is due to inadequate or inappropriately conceived surgery, e.g., when patients undergo very small laminectomy and disc removal in the presence of prominent facets and recess stenosis. It is therefore important to prepare the surgeon for the type of spinal canal he will enter. He must be aware of the patency of the foramina, the status of the facet joints, and the shape and size of the laminae before he enters the operating room.

The 1–5 grading system was devised to code the amount of pathology in order to define surgically significant abnormalities. Specific measurements are not necessarily made in our schema. The assessment of anatomic abnormality may vary slightly with each observer, but definite guidelines, herein presented, allow objective definition and description of pathologic changes within each anatomic zone. When this system is used with a carefully conceived reporting form (Fig. 4.1), it provides an accurate, objective method to convey clinically useful anatomic information to the surgeon.

Evaluation of a Foramina

Anatomy

The lumbar intervertebral foramen has the shape of an inverted teardrop. The superior boundary is the pedicle of the upper vertebra. The anterior wall is formed by the posterior aspect of the vertebral body, the disc, and the body below. The inferior boundary is the pedicle of the lower body, which is situated caudal to the nerve root. The posterior wall, or roof, of the intervertebral foramen is formed by the pars interarticularis, the ligmentum flavum attached to it, and the apex of the superior articular process of the next lower vertebral body. Measurements made on lateral radiographs indicate that the average height of the first two lumbar foramina is 14–22 mm, whereas in the lower three lumbar foramina the measurement is 13–20 mm. The foraminal transverse diameter from ligamentum flavum to vertebral body is 7 mm.

The neural canal or tunnel begins in the spinal canal where the neural sheath emanates from the dural sac and ends where the nerve root emerges from the intervertebral foramen. The roof of the canal is formed by the ligamentum flavum and contiguous borders of the superior articular process and the superior margin of the lamina corresponding in number to the nerve root. Further laterally, the roof is formed by the pars interarticularis of this lamina and the ligamentum flavum related to it. The floor, or anterior aspect, of the canal is formed by the anulus fibrosus of the intervertebral disc, the posterior surface of the vertebral body, and occasionally also by the upper end-plate of the next lower vertebral body. The medial wall of the canal is formed by the dural sac and soft tissues of the epidural

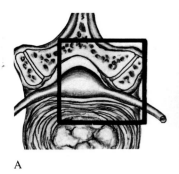

A

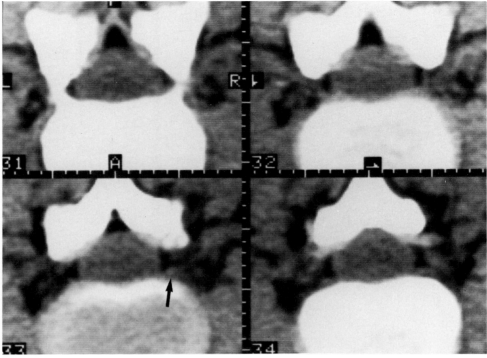

FIGURE 4.1 Normal neural foramen; axial view. **A.** Normal neural foramen, with its exiting nerve. **B.** Composite axial views demonstrate the ganglion and the nerve exiting in a normal-size neural foramen. Note the presence of small epidural veins (*arrow*) and the ganglion and root. There is a large amount of fat surrounding the exiting neural structures.

B

space (fat, blood, nerves). The lateral wall is formed first by the medial side and then by the inferior aspect of the pedicle. The nerve root exits in the superior portion of the intervertebral foramen. The neural covering of the nerve root ends at varying locations within the lateral recess or intervertebral foramen.

The intervertebral foramen is in actual fact a canal. When describing this canal, we must divide it into three clinically important zones: the medial third, which is continuous with the lateral recess; the central third, immediately below the center of the pedicle; and the outer third, beginning near the outer edge of the pedicle. In many patients the outer and middle portions of the foramen are normal whereas there may be very severe compression of the medial portion due specifically to hypertrophy or medial overgrowth of the superior articular process. In some patients broad lateral vertebral-body osteophytes may extend posteriorly and compress the exiting nerve root at the outermost end of the foramen.

CT Evaluation

Grade 1—normal foramina. The normal foramen may be assessed in axial, coronal, or sagittal views. The axial views demonstrate the anteroposterior dimension of the foramen (Fig. 4.1). It is this dimension that is reduced in the spinal stenosis syndrome due to congenitally short pedicles. One should see the normal foramen on at least three successive overlapping axial slices positioned in 3-mm intervals. The nerve root is usually coursing inferiorly through the foramen, and only a short segment is visualized on each axial image. The sagittal view best describes the cross section of the foramen (Fig. 4.2). Within every normal foramen one must identify the exiting nerve root, the surrounding perineural fat, the anulus fibrosus anteriorly, and the facet-joint capsule and ligamentum flavum posteriorly. Grade 1 normal foramina must be at least 1 cm high and 5 mm wide. There must be smooth bony walls. Perineural fat surrounding the nerve root should be clearly seen.

It must be pointed out that the grading system is used to judge only bony confines of the foramen. There may be functional foraminal stenosis causing nerve root entrapment due to abnormal soft tissue in the foramen. This soft tissue can be disc material, bulging anulus, swollen nerve root, scar, fibrocartilage (Fig. 4.3), or some combination of these possibilities. The presence or absence of abnormalities of a soft-tissue nature must be described specifically.

The coronal view is the only projection on which the entire extradural course of nerve can be seen (Fig. 4.4). One should be able to identify subtle swelling of the nerve at the ganglion at each level. The perineural and epidural fat should be symmetrical, and there should be no abnormal soft tissue indenting the exiting nerves. In situations of lateral disc herniation, the coronal images can be very helpful in accurately predicting just which nerve roots (exiting versus traversing) are likely to be affected.

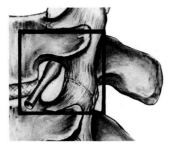

A

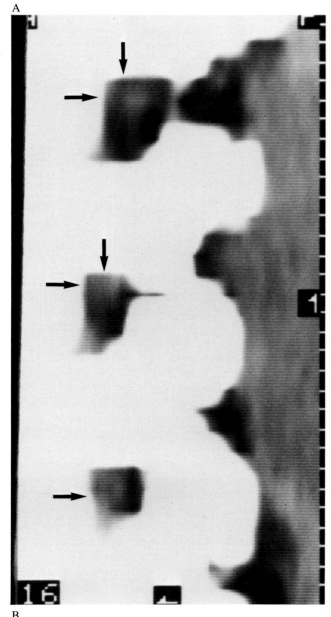

B

FIGURE 4.2 Normal neural foramen; sagittal view. **A.** Lateral view of the neural foramen. **B.** Sagittal reformation through the normal neural foramen. Note the normal exiting nerve in the superior anterior portion of the neural foramen (*arrow*). The inferior surface of the anterior wall of the foramen is formed by the margin of the disc.

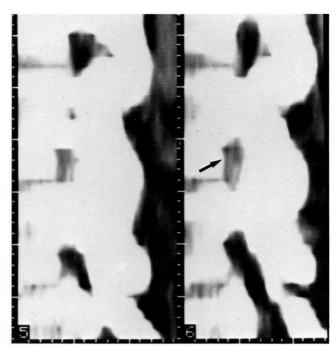

FIGURE 4.3 Normal-size neural foramen, filled with abnormal soft tissue. Note that the exiting nerve root cannot be seen because of the absence of surrounding fat (*arrow*).

Grade 2—slightly narrow but normal foramina. Anatomic studies of the lumbar neural foramen reveal that the nerve or ganglion occupies only one-sixth to one-fourth of the surface area of the foramen. Surrounding the nerve are blood vessels, lymphatics, nerves, and a variable amount of fat and connective tissue. Three-fourths of the foramen is a reserve space allowing for changes in size and shape of the foramen with normal motion. Grade 2 foramina are reduced in height to just under 10 mm but should be at least 5 mm in width. A canal this size is still capable of maintaining normal neural function throughout the complete range of motion (Fig. 4.5). When present, osteophytes are always minimal in size, and the facets are normally aligned in the sagittal views.

Grade 3—narrow foramin of questionable clinical significance. Grade 3 foramina are reduced in size more than are grade 2 foramina. In this borderline group we include those foramina in which some perineural fat can still be seen around the nerve on sagittal views (Fig. 4.6). Also included are those that are filled by abnormal soft tissue (disc or ligament) but that have bony confines larger than a normal nerve or ganglia (diameter approximately 5 mm).

The clinical significance of grade 3 foramina is difficult to assess. When they are filled with soft tissue or associated with upwardly directed spurs, they may produce symptoms. In these cases, coronal views are sometimes

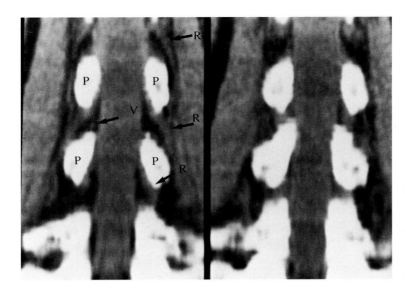

FIGURE 4.4 Sequential curved coronal reformations of a grade 1 normal neural foramen. The neural foramina are seen bilaterally on these views. The course of the exiting nerve roots (*R*) is clearly definable, surrounded by fat within both the canal and the exit foramina. Note also the epidural veins surrounded by fat (*V*). The root ganglia lies immediately beneath the pedicle (*P*).

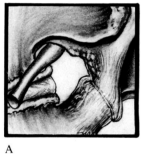

A

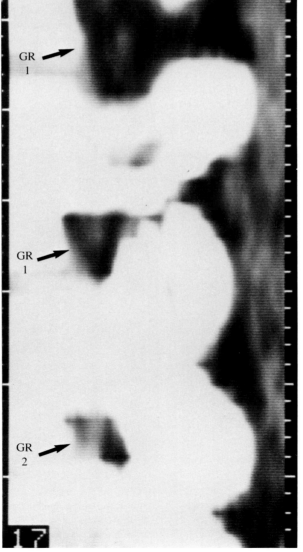

B

FIGURE 4.5 Grade 2 neural foramen; sagittal view. **A.** Diagram. **B.** Sagittal reformation demonstrates a neural foramen that is just less than 10-mm in height. The canal is slightly short but within normal limits.

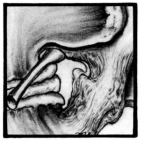

A

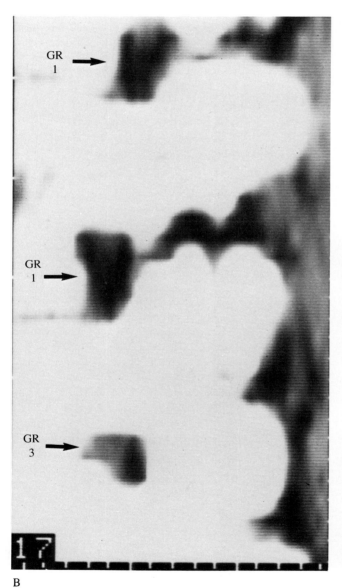

B

FIGURE 4.6 Grade 3 neural foramen. **A.** Diagram. **B.** Sagittal reformation demonstrating a somewhat short neural foramen narrowed by a degenerative ridge. A small amount of epidural fat is still seen around the exiting nerve. This is considered a borderline foramen.

extremely helpful. It is possible to define the relationship of the nerve to the pedicle and to the superior and inferior perineural fat. The coronal view is also helpful in cases where the canal is partially filled by herniated disc. In addition, on the coronal views it may be possible to see a fat plane between the nerve and a borderline bulging anulus, which indicates that the lesion is insignificant.

No reserve space is necessary in those spinal foramina where no motion can occur (notably, fused or transitional vertebral segments), and hence they are usually smaller than foramina at moving segments. These foramina measure in the grade 3 range, but because they do not become narrowed by osteophytes they are judged normal (Fig. 4.7).

Grade 4—moderately abnormal foramina. In this category we place those foramina that just fit a normal-size nerve; there is no reserve space (Fig. 4.8). Prominent osteophytes arising from the facet joints or the vertebral endplates may severely compress the nerve, particularly if motion further reduces the marginal dimensions seen on static CT images taken in a supine, unloaded (i.e., neutral) position. Facet hypertrophy and spurs tend to impinge on the nerve at the medial end of the foramen. End-plate spurs

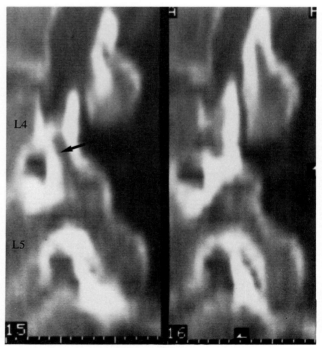

FIGURE 4.7 Congenital fusion, L4–5, with narrow foramen. Sagittal reformation demonstrates a small neural foramen at the level of a congenital fusion (*arrow*). The nerve root will not be entrapped in such a foramen because motion does not occur at the interspace.

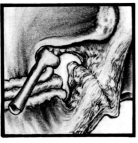

A

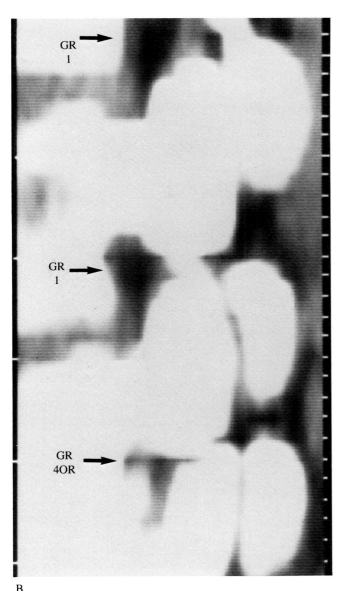

B

FIGURE 4.8 Grade 4 moderate foraminal narrowing. **A.** Diagram. **B.** Sagittal reformation on a patient with a grade 4 neural foramen. Note the degenerative ostophytic ridging arising from the vertebral end-plate. The coded diagnosis is 4 OR (osteophytic ridging).

may be found anywhere along the disc space, but they most frequently occur at the lateral and medial one-third of the foramen. It is quite likely that surgical intervention at a disc space with a grade 4 foramen should include a foraminotomy on the affected side. The sagittal view defines the precise area of impingement and the position and extent of contributing end-plate osteophytes or superiorly subluxed superior articular processes.

Grade 5—severe foraminal stenosis (Fig. 4.9). These patients have foramina with a physical diameter incapable of containing a normal nerve root even at rest. There is severe osteophyte formation, with bony indentation on the nerve. This is almost always associated with severe loss of height at the disc space and with arthritic degeneration at the facet joints.

Disc degeneration and subsequent disc-space narrowing can lead to facet subluxation. The tip of the superior facet of the inferior vertebral body moves upward toward the pedicle of the superior vertebral body. This results in a deformation of the intervertebral foramen and a shortening, thickening, or buckling of the ligamentum flavum into the foramen and nerve root canal (Fig. 4.10). The nerve root trapped in the foramen corresponds in number to the disc. The nerve compressed more medially in the lateral recess usually corresponds in number to the next lower segment, i.e., the number of the superior articular facet causing the problem. For example, narrowing of the L4 disc followed by subluxation of the L5 superior articular process usually traps the L5 nerve root between the inner margin of the L5 superior articular process and the remaining fibers of the L4 anulus.

There are repeated and frequent cases in which the correct decision regarding foraminal patency is best made from the sagittal view. Several obvious advantages can be cited. First, as has been mentioned, the sagittal view provides the most accurate estimate of foraminal size and shape. Second, in three-level studies the observer has available two other foramina on the same side for visual comparison. Third is speed of cognition. By simply glancing through the sagittal composite series from left to right, the observer quickly previews the presence of: (1) left foraminal stenosis (bone spur, soft tissue, etc.); (2) disc material protruding from the interspaces into the central canal; (3) right foraminal stenosis; and (4) the level and side at which these changes are located.

In addition to providing the best assessment of foraminal size and shape, the sagittal view also affords insight into the reason for a particular nerve root entrapment: congenitally small foramen; lateral ridging from sclerosis of the inferior end-plate; excess soft tissue within the foramen (lateral disc/anulus material versus swollen nerve root versus both); or subluxation of the superior articular process, thus trapping the exiting nerve root between the superior articular process and the pedicle. The latter situation is extremely difficult to diagnose from axial views alone.

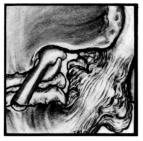

A

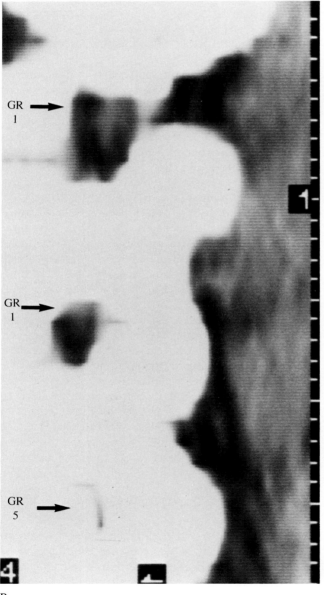

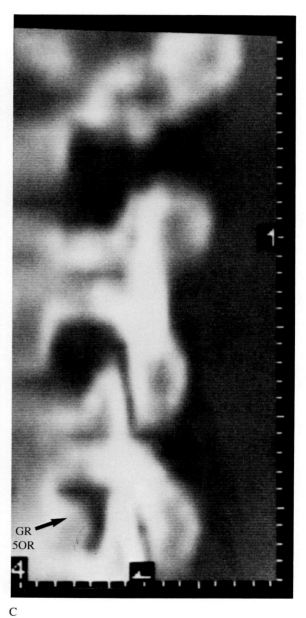

B

C

FIGURE 4.9 Severe foraminal stenosis. **A.** Diagram. **B.** Soft-tissue sagittal view demonstrates marked obliteration of the neural foramen at L5–S1. **C.** Bone-window sagittal view of the same patient.

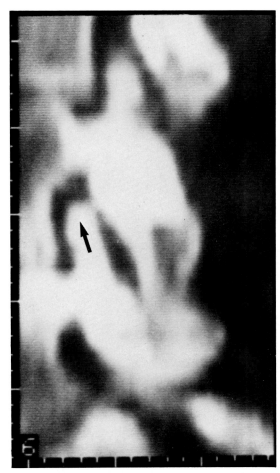

FIGURE 4.10 Foraminal encroachment due to upward subluxation of a facet. Sagittal reformation reveals a narrowed L4–5 intervertebral disc space. The superior facet of L5 is herniated upward into the neural foramen. The facet-joint space is abnormally widened as well.

Disc/Anulus Abnormalities

Anatomy and Pathophysiology

A detailed discussion of the anatomy and the pathophysiology of disc disease is found in Chapter 5, and so these subjects are not reviewed here.

CT Evaluation

Of all the anatomic zones of the lumbar spine, disc bulge or herniation is the easiest to quantitate objectively. The use of life-size images allows one to simply place a millimeter ruler on the film and measure the amount of protrusion. Measurements are made on the sagittal view, where even in normal patients the anulus can be seen as a structure of higher density than the dura or its contents. Surgeons

are most familiar with the lateral myelographic view. They have a clear mental picture of normal and pathologic anatomy based on the many years of practical experience and the large radiologic literature. It is obvious, therefore, that the view most easily correlated with the patient's pathology is the sagittal view.

Grade 1—the normal disc. Figure 4.11 demonstrates a normal disc in axial and sagittal planes. There is less than 1 mm posterior concavity as measured on the sagittal view. On the axial views the contour of the disc corresponds to the contour of the vertebral end-plate. Frequently we can identify normal epidural venous structures between the anulus and the dura.

Grade 2—normal disc with slight bulge. Posterior concavity of 2 mm is considered a grade 2 disc (Fig. 4.12), a variation of normal brought about by the aging process. This amount of extradural defect is rarely visible on myelography because of the presence of a normal anterior epidural fat plane. Symmetrical anulus bulge of this magnitude is very difficult to see on axial views, but it is quite obvious on the sagittal views.

Grade 3—mild disc bulge. An extradural defect of 3 mm is considered a grade 3 disc (Fig. 4.13). This is borderline between normal and pathologic. Myelography usually indicates the presence of a 3-mm extradural bulge, except at L5 where the epidural fat pad may be quite wide. Grade 3 discs are considered normal except under special circumstances, the most important of which is a narrow spinal canal. A 3-mm extradural defect is much more likely to cause root compression in an abnormally small canal than in a copious one. Discs with a 3-mm extradural defect are also considered abnormal where there is objective evidence of local nerve root compression, e.g., localized root displacement or swelling.

Grade 4—moderately abnormal disc. An extradural soft-tissue defect of 5 mm is called a grade 4 disc and is considered pathologic (Fig. 4.14). A grade 4 disc almost always produces an abnormal myelogram, even at the L5 interspace. In young patients there may be a 5-mm disc herniation without any associated osseous abnormality. In the older age group there frequently is spur formation at the end-plates associated with the soft-tissue extradural disc herniation. It is important to note the size of the spondylitic spurs and their precise localization, as their presence affects the surgical approach and outcome. A word of caution is necessary at this point: *The presence of 5 mm or more disc bulge or herniation is a pathologic condition; however, it may not be related to the patient's clinical complaints.* It has long been known that routine lumbar filming on patients undergoing cervical myelography has produced many examples of asymptomatic patients with objective myelographic abnormalities. CT is more sensitive than myelography for the definition of anatomic derangement. Consequently, it is even more important to be aware of the

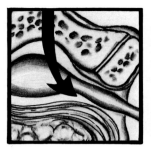
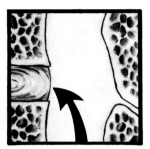

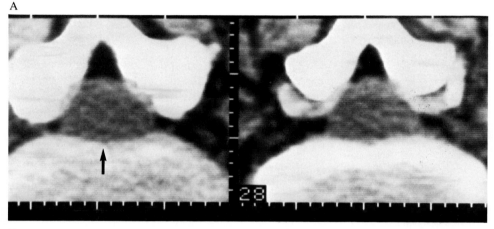

FIGURE 4.11 The normal disc. **A.** Axial and sagittal diagrams show a normal convex surface to the anulus in a young patient. **B.** Axial scan demonstrates a normal disc (*arrow*). **C.** Sagittal reformation demonstrates three normal discs (*arrows*). Note that on the sagittal view one can always see the high density of the anulus and the disc.

A

B

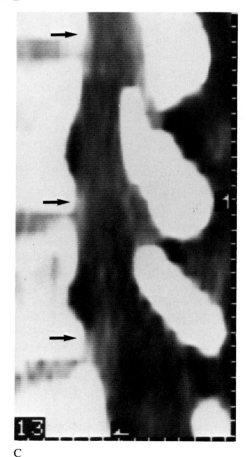

C

possibility that objective abnormalities may not cause symptoms. Careful clinical correlation is required in every case.

Grade 5—severe disc herniation. A disc bulge or herniation of more than 6 mm on the sagittal view is considered a grade 5 lesion and is surely pathologic (Fig. 4.15). As the amount of extradural defect increases, the certainty that the anatomic abnormality is causing the clinical symptoms also increases. Soft-tissue defects of grade 5 are more likely to cause symptoms than are 6-mm spurs, which are of a chronic nature.

Easy Measurements from Life-Size CT/MPR Images

Fast and accurate measurements represent a convenience rather than something that affects the identification of a disc abnormality per se. However, once a disc bulge or herniation has been found, an objective rating or measurement of soft-tissue protrusion may indeed affect patient management decisions regarding conservative treatment versus chymopapain injection or surgery. Moreover, comparison of accurate measurements over some time interval contributes to follow-up evaluations.

Measurements from life-size film images are very simple. Scan fields of different sizes (e.g., infant, medium adult, large adult) plus infinite magnification possibilities with either retrospective or prospective review are taken into account automatically by the

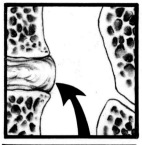

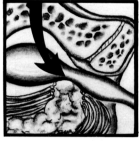

A

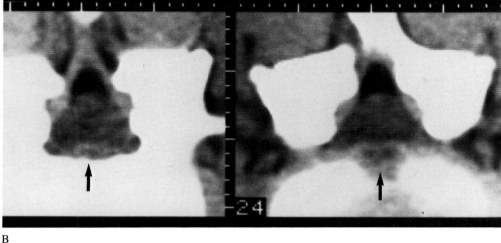

B

FIGURE 4.12 Grade 2 disc. **A.** Normal disc space with a 2–mm annular convexity. **B.** Axial scan showing a 2-mm diffuse annular convexity. **C.** Sagittal reformation demonstrates a 2-mm convexity of the anulus at L4–5. This is considered a normal finding.

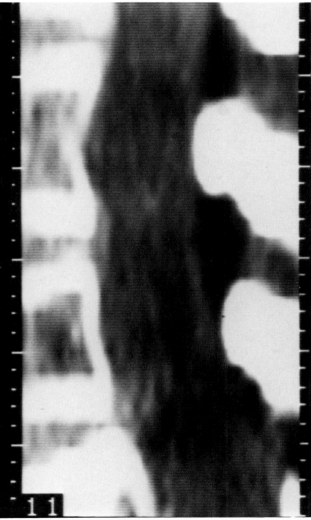

C

life-size CT/MPR processing technique. Similar measurements using nonlife-size images require a distance indicator on each filmed image or conversion factors for different scan fields—or such measurements must be made interactively on the CT display console. These alternatives are accurate but comparatively cumbersome.

Facet Joints

The lumbar facet joints have long been regarded as an overlooked cause of back and sciatic pain. It is now well established that disorders of the facet joints can cause all the physical signs and symptoms of disc herniation. However, it was Ghormley,[3] in 1933, who stressed the importance of facet disease in the diagnosis of back pain. Over the years, interest in the facet joints has waxed and waned. As myelography became more popular, disc herniation became the major focus of surgical attention.

Myelography, even in its most primitive form, produced easily understood high-contrast images of a definite anatomic derangement that could be easily repaired. The facet joints, on the other hand, because of the complexity of their structure, remained well obscured radiologically. The planes of the joints could be seen on frontal radiographs, and on oblique views (the best projection) the joint surfaces could be clearly identified. The bulk of the osseous mass of the facets and the area of abnormal hypertrophy remain extremely difficult to visualize by any conventional radiologic technique.

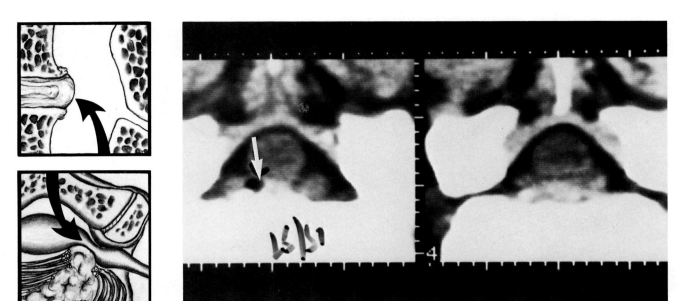

A

B

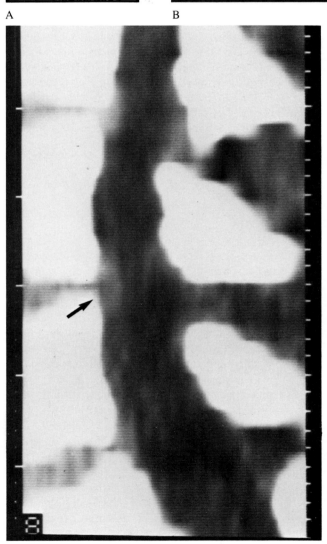

C

FIGURE 4.13 Grade 3 disc. **A.** Sagittal and axial diagrams of a 3-mm extradural defect. **B.** Axial scan demonstrates a 3-mm soft-tissue bulge of the disc associated with a bubble of gas in the epidural soft tissue; hence a code of 3 VC (vacuum change). **C.** Sagittal reformation also reveals a 3-mm extradural defect at the L4–5 disc space.

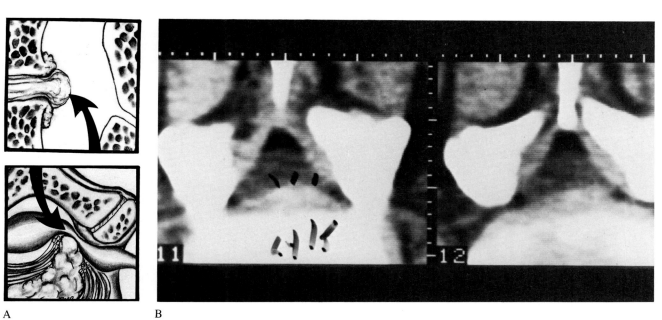

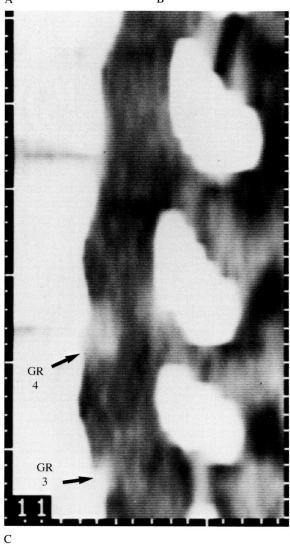

A

B

C

FIGURE 4.14 Grade 4 disc herniation. **A.** Sagittal and axial diagrams of a 5-mm disc herniation. **B.** Axial scan demonstrates a 5-mm central herniated disc. **C.** Sagittal reformation demonstrates a 5-mm L4–5 disc herniation and a 3-mm bulge of the anulus at L5–S1.

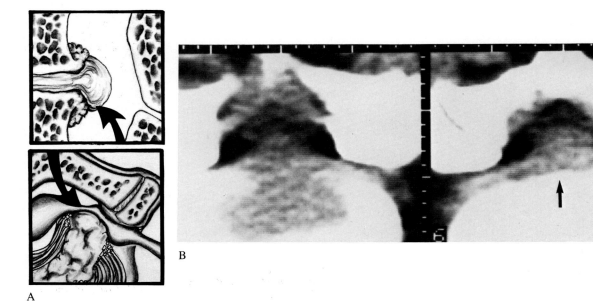

B

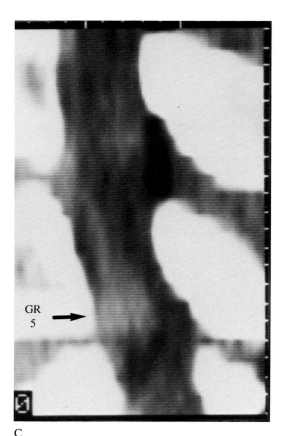

C

FIGURE 4.15 Grade 5 disc herniation. **A.** Sagittal and axial diagrams demonstrate more than a 6-mm disc herniation. **B.** Axial scan reveals a large central disc herniation (*arrow*). **C.** On sagittal view No. 10 one can measure a 10–mm soft-tissue extradural defect (*arrow*) at the L5–S1 intervertebral disc space.

It became obvious early on that CT scanning would be extremely useful in the diagnosis of anatomic derangement of the facet joints. Wide-window techniques using expanded attenuation scales made possible the first serious attempt at studying facet disease. High-resolution scanners provided the anatomic detail to make CT the primary radiologic examination in facet disorders.

CT/MPR provides the ideal way to study the facet joints. It produces high-contrast sagittal and coronal images that demonstrate the gross anatomy of the facet surfaces and the anatomic relationship between adjacent vertebral segments. Because the facet joints are both oblique to the sagittal plane and curvilinear, the axial plane is ideal for their delineation. This projection is also perfectly suited for the assessment of canal compression due to enlargement of the facets. The surgeon needs to know what space is available to the intradural contents and to exciting peripheral nerve roots, and this is best seen in the axial plane.

Anatomy

The superior articular facets project upward from the neural ring and have concave articular surfaces that face medially and slightly posteriorly at the first lumbar vertebra and more posteriorly and less medially in each lower vertebra. The inferior facets project downward and have a convex joint surfce that faces laterally and anteriorly in the upper lumbar spine and more anteriorly and less laterally in each successive vertebra. They are diarthrodial joints, with a capsule, synovium, and articular cartilage. The joint capsule is the ligamentum flavum.

CT Evaluation

As man proceeds into middle age, increasing degenerative changes result from cumulative stress placed on discs and facet joints due to a bipedal, upright habitus. In some patients the small joints are severely affected, out of proportion to the amount of disc collapse. As a general rule, degeneration of the facet joints is only one part of a generalized deformity of the vertebral segment. The CT analysis of the facet joints can be divided into two components: localized abnormalities of the joints themselves (e.g., spurs and erosions) and generalized abnormalities of the vertebral segments due to stenosis of the spinal canal from osteophytic hypertrophic spurs. It is this second deformity that has received the most attention in both the surgical and the radiologic literature. Expansion of the facet joints and laminae are key components in the spinal stenosis syndrome. This syndrome is becoming recognized universally as the major cause of back pain and of objective neurologic deficit in older people.

In an attempt to quantify and standardize the interpretation and reporting of facet abnormalities, a 1–5 scale has been chosen to define the spectrum from normal to severely pathologic. The schema is partially subjective in that it involves no routine measurements; however, it is useful because it provides a mental image orientation with which the surgeon is familiar. The numerical scale represents the size of the facets, together with the joint capsules and ligamentum flavum, and their relationship to the spinal canal and neural foramina. It does not quantify erosion, cyst formation, or capsule calcification—only size and canal or foraminal encroachment. Obviously those joints with severe cartilaginous destruction frequently contain large osteophytes that cause canal or foraminal encroachment.

Grade 1—normal facets. There is considerable variation in the normal facet joints, especially in the lumbosacral articulation. One must consider the lumbosacral level apart from the remainder of the lumbar spine because of the wide spectrum of transitional vertebrae that occur. This subject is covered in detail in Chapter 6. At one end of the spectrum is the truly sacralized fifth lumbar vertebra. In these patients the facets are small and may be completely fused. Because there is little or no motion at these joints, there is no significant spondylosis and the facets do not enlarge and compress the neural canal. Disc herniation does not occur at such an interspace. Asymmetry of the angle of inclination of the facets (facet tropism) (Fig. 4.16) may inhibit normal segmental motion and may be an important predisposing factor in disc herniation at this or the next higher interspace. The axial view provides the best visualization of this type of facet asymmetry. Above the L5 articulation the facets become more regular and symmetrical, with less variation between levels.

The normal facet-joint space measures approximately 1–3 mm, and it is smooth and well corticated (Fig. 4.17). There is a clear demarcation between the cortical and medullary bone of the articular process. The shape of the neural arch is semicircular or triangular, without any bony protuberances. There is a direct unbroken curve to the ventral surface of the lamina that terminates in the articular facet. In the sagittal plane the cartilaginous space is smooth and regular. The superior tip of the facet is sharp and separated from the undersurface of the pedicle. One should see a definite clear space between the superior tip of the superior

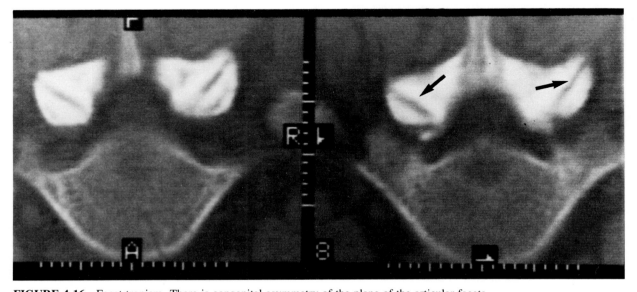

FIGURE 4.16 Facet tropism. There is congenital asymmetry of the plane of the articular facets. The left facet is more coronally oriented than the right facet.

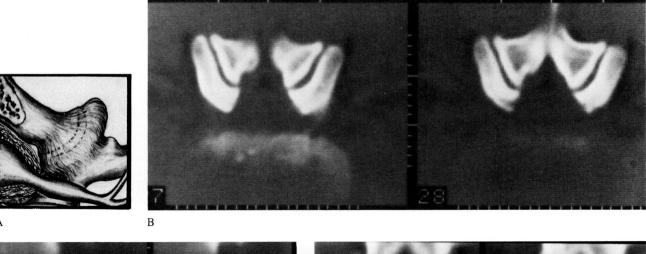

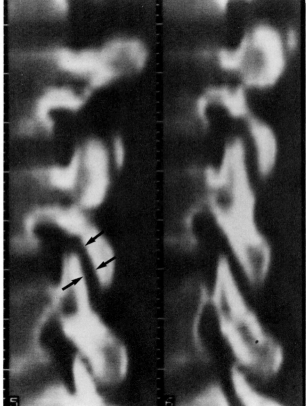

A

B

C

D

FIGURE 4.17 Normal grade 1 facet joints. **A.** Normal facet joint. **B.** Axial scans of normal facets. Note the dense cortical bone and the cartilaginous surface of the joint itself. **C.** Sagittal reformation reveals a normal joint space (*arrows*). **D.** Coronal reformation clearly defines the plane of the facets (*arrows*). Their surfaces can be accurately compared.

facet and the undersurface of the pedicle. Coronal scans are helpful in evaluating accessory ossification centers, fractures, or congenital fusion of the facets, and they are exceedingly important in assessing the continuity of lateral surgical fusions.

Grade 2—normal to slightly enlarged facets. With increasing wear and tear there is expansion and rounding of the superior articular facet. In the axial scans this is usually manifested by the medial overhanging of the medial

edge of the superior facet (Fig. 4.18). This breaks the smooth laminar curve as the facet projects into the canal. Frequently, osteoarthritic spurs project slightly into the canal. These spurs may arise from either superior or inferior facets, and they also cause slight indentation on the posterior aspect of the lateral recess. The amount of the degenerative change is usually mild. The joint surfaces may appear normal or slightly narrow. Because we are primarily quantitating facet size, there may be disproportionate degenerative change or severe erosive arthritis with minimal medial hypertrophic changes. We describe this disparity in the text of our report.

Grade 3—mildly pathologic facets (Fig. 4.19). In grade 3 lesions there is mild but definite indentation, by the ar-

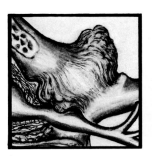

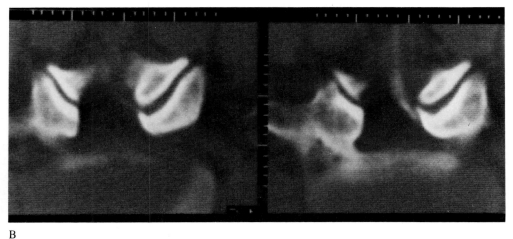

A
B

FIGURE 4.18 Grade 2 facet. **A.** Diagram. **B.** Axial scan. There is mild enlargement of the right facet, as compared with that on the left. This is a normal variant.

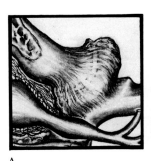

A

FIGURE 4.19 Grade 3 facets. **A.** Diagram. **B.** Axial scan of bilateral grade 3 facets. There is subtle indentation on the spinal canal. **C.** Grade 3 facet on the right, primarily due to an overhanging osteophytic spur. **D.** Grade 3 facet according to its size. However, there is disproportionate destruction of the articular bone and unusual widening of the joint space, perhaps due to facet effusion.

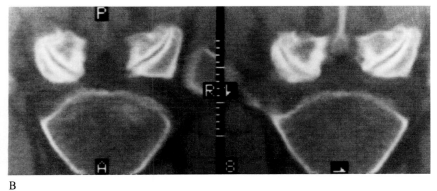

B

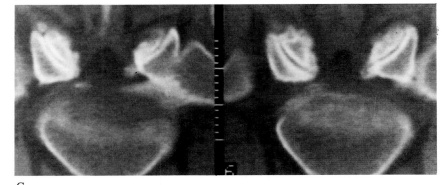

C

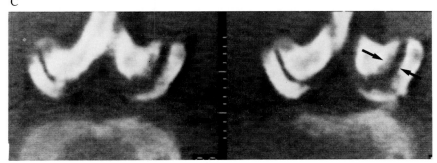

D

ticular process or by spurs arising from them, on the spinal canal and lateral recess. If the pedicles are congenitally short, the neural foramina may be narrowed, especially in the most medial portion. The degenerative change is usually mild. There are instances, however, where a severe destructive arthropathy may present with only minimal bony facet hypertrophy and canal compression (Fig. 4.19D). There may be additional canal encroachment caused by swelling or fibrous enlargement of the joint capsule and ligamentum flavum. Spurs that develop on the anterior aspect of the articular facets contribute to a trefoil shape of the spinal canal.

Grade 4—moderate facet hypertrophy. Joints that enlarge to produce moderate canal or foraminal encroachment are always abnormal. Joint surfaces may be partially smooth but are usually disorganized, pitted, sclerotic, and eroded (Fig. 4.20). Osteoarthritic spurs usually arise from both superior and inferior facets. Frequently they project in a spike-like manner into the canal, impinging on the dura laterally and encroaching on the posterior aspect of the lateral recesses. The joint capsules are often enlarged and occasionally calcified. The laminae may be hypertrophied, perhaps by abnormal tension on the periosteum by the ligamentum flavum or capsule.

Grade 5—severe facet hypertrophy. Patients with grade 5 facets always have disorganization of the articular surfaces (Fig. 4.21). There is gross erosion, pitting, and irregularity of the facet joint itself. Hypertrophic spur formation may be located at the anterior aspect of the facet joint, causing severe central canal and lateral recess stenosis, with concomitant foraminal narrowing. The spurs may also be seen posterolaterally and without effects of neural compression. The hypertrophic bone may become very thick and dense. Facets that have grown to grade 5 are likely to be associated with marked thickening and irregularity of the lamina. As the erosive process continues there is lateral rotation of the axes of the joint surfaces. The apices become flattened, and the ability of the facet to resist forward thrust is dramatically reduced. Anterior, posterior, or lateral subluxation of the facets can then occur, causing the syndrome of degenerative spondylolisthesis. Subluxation further compromises an already narrowed central spinal canal and lateral recess.

Specific CT Abnormalities

There are a number of specific abnormalities demonstrable on the scans that should be described specifically in the reporting of CT abnormalities.

The cartilaginous articular surfaces should be regular and smooth. They tend to be thickened in the center and at the periphery. Carrera et al.[4,5] found thinning of the articular cartilage in 25% of their cases, subchondral sclerosis in 22%, and subchondral cysts and erosions in 4%. These changes are often associated with osteophyte formation. A careful description is a surgical necessity because these spurs may cause root compression. In the absence of disc herniation or foraminal stenosis, articular irregularities, cysts, and degeneration may be a primary cause of back pain, and they often mimic sciatica.

Vacuum-joint phenomena are seen in approximately 20% of patients (Fig. 4.22). This is a much higher per-

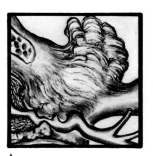

FIGURE 4.20 Grade 4 facets. **A.** Diagram. **B.** Enlargement of the right articular process is noted. There is marked pitting, irregularity, and destruction of the articular surface.

A

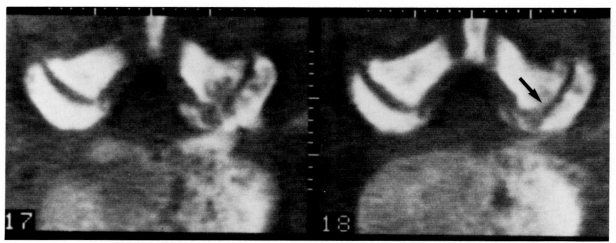

B

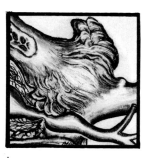

FIGURE 4.21 Grade 5 facets.
A. Diagram. **B.** Marked bony hypertrophy and overgrowth of the right facet joint are associated with spur formation.

A

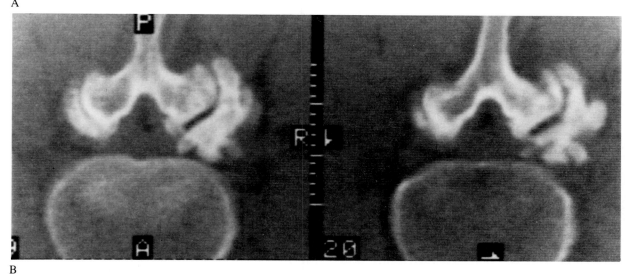

B

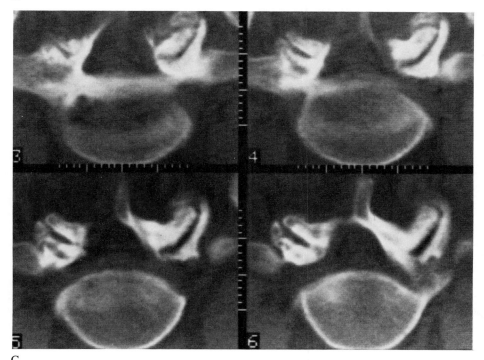

C

FIGURE 4.22 Vacuum joint phenomenon. Axial scans reveal severe degenerative change of both facets, with facet tropism. On the right there is gas within the joint space. Large posterior osteophytes are also noted. The right facet would be graded 4 Sp VC (Sp indicating posterior spurring and VC indicating vacuum change).

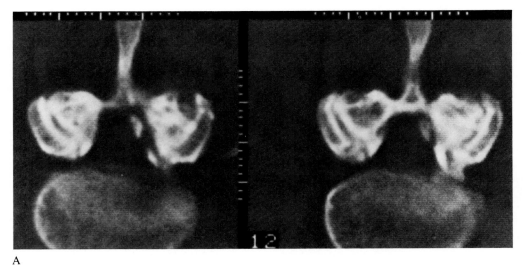

A

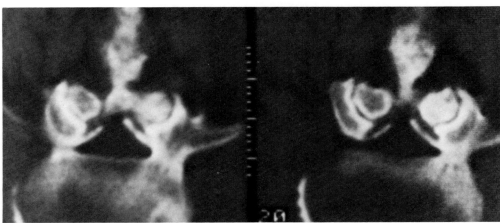

B

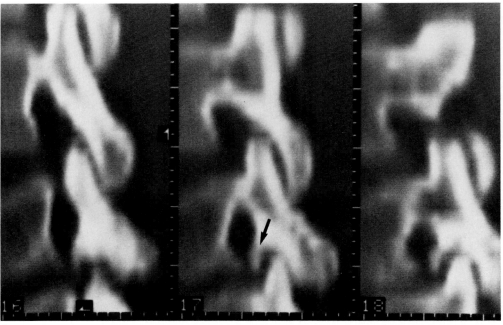

C

FIGURE 4.23 Periarticular calcifications. **A.** Axial scans at L4–5 demonstrate remarkable bony overgrowth of the facets, with ossification in the ligamentum flavum. **B.** Axial scans at L3–4 demonstrate dense calcification in the anterior fibers of the ligamentum flavum. **C.** Sagitally reformatted image reveals a characteristic deformity of calcification (*arrow*) in the apex of the joint capsule.

centage than that found on conventional radiographs. The significance of this finding is not clear. Carrera suggested that abnormally lax joints, uneven apposition of surfaces, or normal facets under distractive forces due to positioning may account for this finding.

Articular calcification—usually within the joint capsule but sometimes within the ligamentum flavum—can be found in as many as 16% of patients. Calcified plaques may indent nerve roots and compress lateral recesses. The sagittal view is most useful in diagnosing capsular calcification (Fig. 4.23).

Anatomic abnormalities are seen best in axial views, whereas the relationship of the facet is seen best in sagittal views. As the disc spaces narrow there is upward subluxation of the superior facets toward the pedicle, reducing the separation between the tip of the process and the undersurface of the pedicle. In severe cases there is grooving and indentation of the pedicle by the facet. Laxity of the joint capsule and the ligamentum flavum further adds to potential foraminal stenosis. This is due to the increased potential for the superior facet to sublux anteriorly and superiorly. Coronal reformation provides an excellent means of comparing pairs of the articular processes at two levels (Fig.4.24).

Lateral Recess

Anatomy

There is much controversy as to the precise definition of the term lateral recess stenosis. We prefer to separate lateral stenosis into foraminal stenosis and subarticular lateral recess stenosis. Our definition of the lateral recess is that cone-shaped portion of the bony spinal canal which extends laterally from the thecal origin of the nerve root to the medial end of the neural foramen.

CT Evaluation

Grade 1—normal lateral recess. In the axial view, the neural canal is triangular, without lateral compression in the area of the exiting nerve root. The pedicles are of normal length. On the sagittal view there should be at least a 5-mm space between the lamina and the vertebral body (Fig. 4.25A).

Grade 2—also a normal variant. The canal is trefoil in shape. The conical recess is well formed, but there is no compression of the exiting nerve. The distance between the buckled lamina and the posterior edge of the vertebral body is at least 5 mm (Fig. 4.25B).

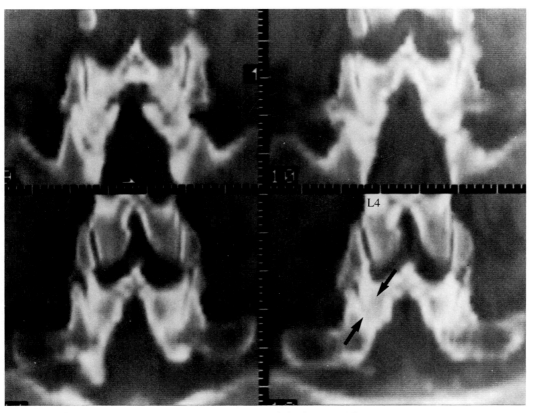

FIGURE 4.24 Coronal reformation on a patient with relatively normal facets at L4–5 and severely degenerated facets at L5–S1. Note that the entire articular processes are sclerotic, the cortical bone is eroded (*arrows*), and the left facet is slightly subluxed.

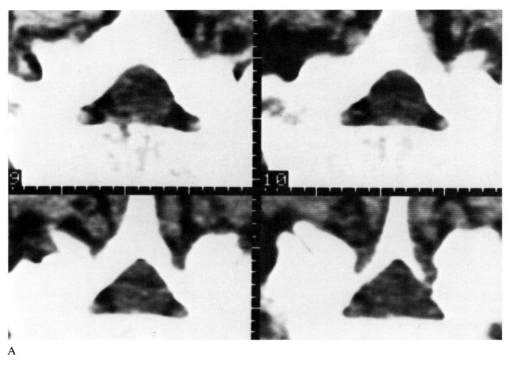

A

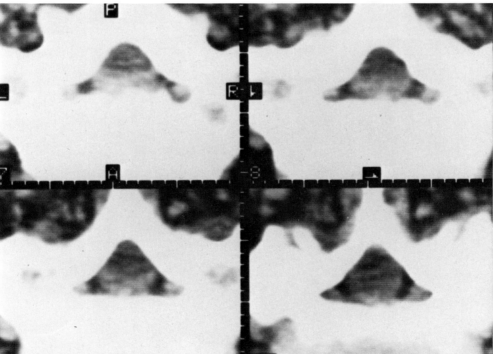

B

FIGURE 4.25 Lateral recesses; normal through abnormal. **A.** Grade 1. The bony canal is triangular, and the ascending nerve is surrounded by fat in a wide conical-shaped lateral recess. **B.** Grade 2. There is slight tapering of the lateral recess, which measures 5-mm. The nerve is normal in size. **C.** Grade 3. There is slight lateral buckling caused by the prominence of the facet. This is a borderline lateral recess. **D.** Grade 4. Axial scans demonstrate a large, protuberant bony spike arising from the medial end of a pars interarticularis defect narrowing the left lateral recess. (*Figure continued* on pages 107–108.)

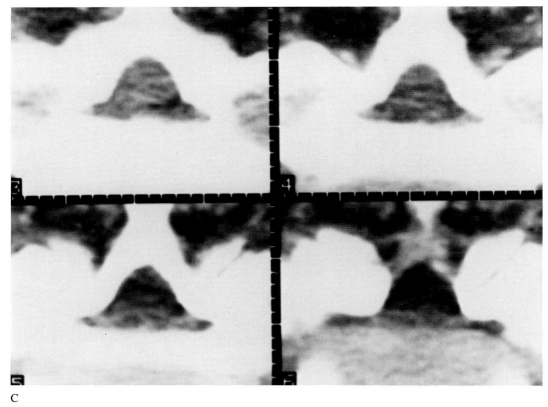

C

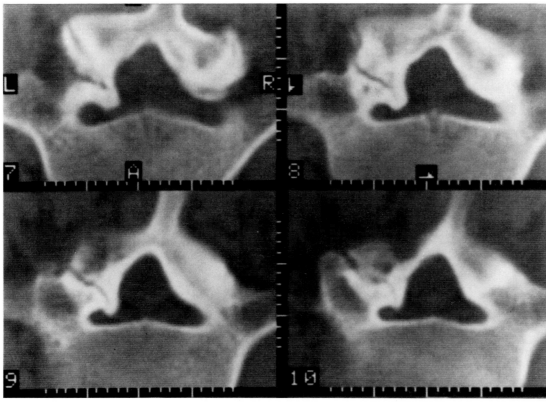

D

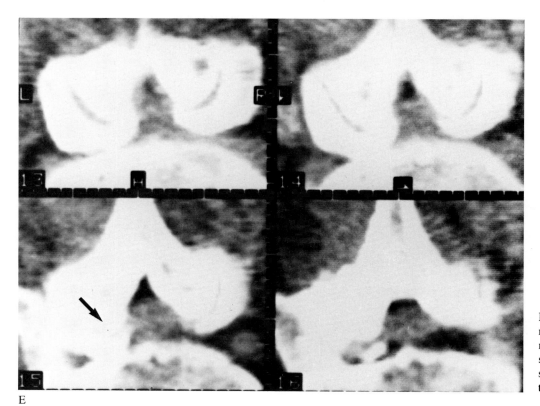

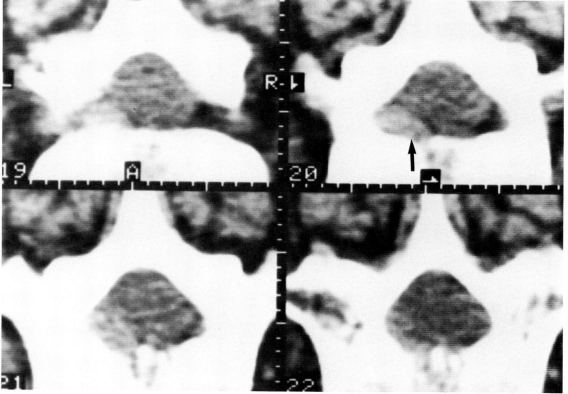

FIGURE 4.25 (*cont'd*) Lateral recesses; normal through abnormal. **E.** Grade 5. Severe recess stenosis caused by a congenitally short pedicle and prominence of the superior facet.

FIGURE 4.26 Disc in lateral recess. The bony spinal canal is normal in size, and the lateral recesses would be coded as grade 1. The descending nerve root is compressed in the lateral recess by a sequestered disc fragment. This would be graded 1*.

Grade 3—bony recess slightly narrower than 5 mm. This narrowing is usually due to expansion into the canal of the laminae and articular processes (Fig. 4.25C).

Grade 4—moderate recess stenosis. The recess is objectively narrow. This, in combination with enlargement of the facets, ligamentum flavum hypertrophy, and short pedicles, produces spinal stenosis.

Grade 5—severe recess stenosis. The exiting nerve is objectively compressed and may be impossible to identify within the recess (Fig. 4.25D). The foraminal component of the nerve may be swollen. It is quite common that recess stenosis is associated with central canal and foraminal stenosis as well.

The grading system describes only the bony confines of the canal. Entrapment of the descending nerve by soft-tissue masses (sequestered fragment or tumor) is indicated on the form by a star. The coding for the lateral recess in Figure 4.26 would be 1*, to indicate a recess of normal size but filled by a large disc fragment.

Central Canal

The subjective 1–5 grading of the central canal represents an expression of the cross-sectional area available for neural elements. Potential encroachments can be anterior, lateral, or posterior. Contributing structures are those that constitute the perimeter of the central canal at either the interspace or the interosseous portion of the vertebral segment. At the interspace, these structures include disc plus the vertebral end-plate and any associated spurs or ridges. Laterally, there are the articular facets plus their joint capsules and, again, any associated degenerative spurs. Posteriorly, the canal can be reduced by laminar thickening, ligamentum flavum hypertrophy, and bony overgrowth of posterior fusion masses.

Anatomy

At the interosseous level the anterior margin of the central canal is formed by the posterior cortical surface of the vertebral body plus ventrally located epidural venous structures. Laterally there are the pedicles and posteriorly the laminae. Because there are no joints or moving structures at the interosseous level, spurs or ridges are rare. Reduced central canal dimensions are most frequently on a congenital basis (i.e., short pedicles) or are due to the presence of abnormal soft tissue. The latter is most frequently caused by disc fragments located within, and possibly filling, the lateral recess. Less frequent encroachments include soft-tissue scarring or calcification of the posterior longitudinal ligament (more frequent in the cervical region).

CT Evaluation

In addition to the subjective graded assessment of central canal shape and size from various CT images, we attempt to indicate both the likelihood and the position of anticipated myelographic defects. This serves two purposes: correlation with existing or post-CT myelograms and reinforcement of the referring physician's confidence level regarding CT versus myelography. The more correct the correlations he receives, the easier is the transition from lumbar myelography to CT as the primary diagnostic imaging modality.

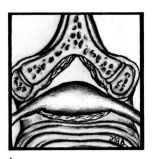

FIGURE 4.27 Normal central canal. **A.** Diagram. **B.** The normal spinal canal. Note that the theca is surrounded by fat, and there is adequate room for the exiting nerves.

A

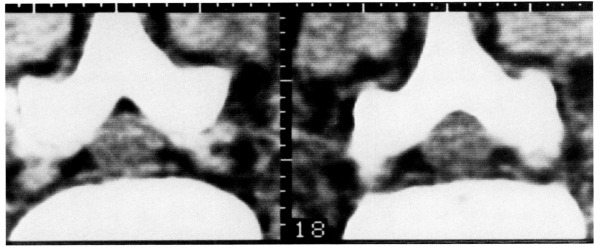

B

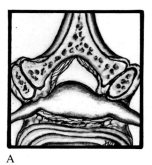

A

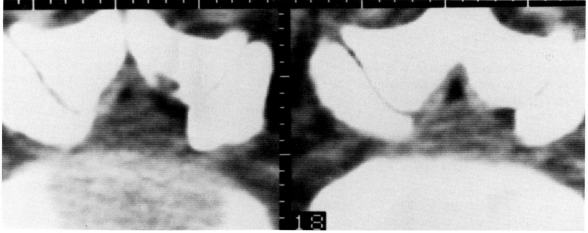

B

FIGURE 4.28   Grade 2 spinal canal. **A.** Diagram. **B.** This patient has a minimally narrowed bony canal after surgery. The left facet is slightly enlarged, and there is minimal bulging of the anulus. The overall space available for the theca is slightly reduced but still within normal limits, therefore this would be coded a grade 2.

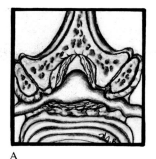

A

FIGURE 4.29   Mild central canal narrowing. **A.** Bony compression of the canal, of a mild nature. **B.** Axial scan demonstrates a spinal canal with normal bony confines; however, the surface area of the canal is reduced by a large central disc herniation. The overall space is mildly reduced. A myelographic defect would almost certainly be present. This is considered a grade 3 spinal canal.

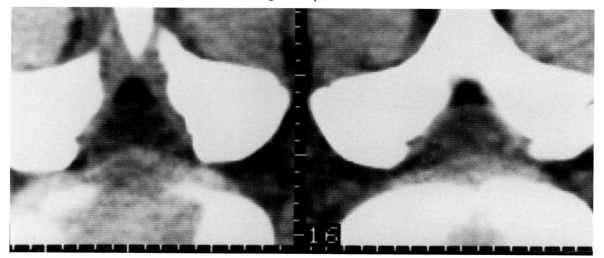

B

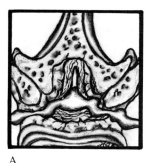

A

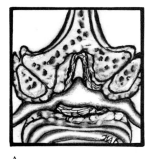

A

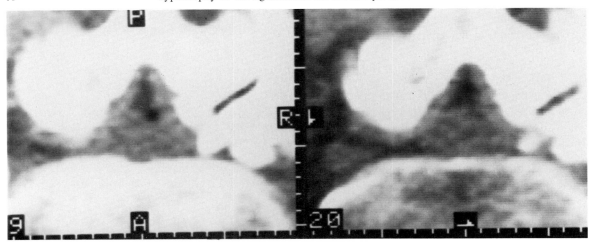

B

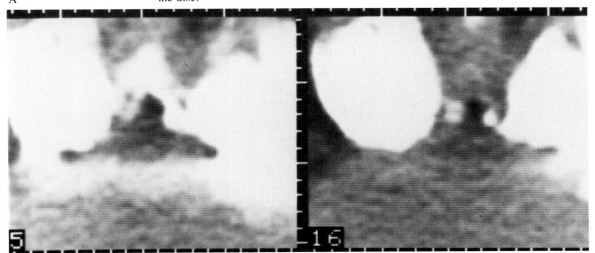

B

FIGURE 4.30 Grade 4 spinal canal. **A.** Diagram. . **B.** This spinal canal is narrowed. The pedicles are slightly short. The spinal canal is reduced in size primarily because of hypertrophy of the ligamentum flavum and periarticular soft tissues.

FIGURE 4.31 Severe central canal narrowing. **A.** Diagram. **B.** The central canal is remarkably reduced because of a combination of congenitally short pedicles, marked facet hypertrophy, periarticular soft-tissue swelling, and diffuse bulge or herniation of the disc.

Grade 1—normal central canal. Because there are variations in size and shape, ''normal'' is both subjective and relative. Measurements are not made routinely. Figure 4.27 shows a normal spinal canal in which there is ample room for the thecal sac—no obvious bony or soft-tissue encroachment is noted.

Grade 2—slight reduction of central canal. This is also normal but with smaller overall canal dimensions (Fig. 4.28).

Grade 3—mild reduction of central canal. At this point, overall dimensions are borderline, and minimal myelographic indentations are likely. The canal is considered ''snug.'' A congenitally small canal is often graded as mild stenosis over one or more levels. An otherwise normal canal with a large disc herniation within the canal is graded in the mild category (Fig. 4.29). Another example includes prominent ligamentum flavum, generous articular facets, and granulation or scar tissue from prior operative procedures.

Grade 4—moderate reduction of central canal. This category is used for definite abnormality with regard to both size and shape of the central canal. The structures that make up the perimeter of the spinal canal can all contribute, either alone or in combination. Moderate central canal stenosis implies definite myelographic defects and definite crowding of neural elements. The probability is high that a moderately stenotic central canal contributes symptomatically to the clinical problem (Fig. 4.30).

Grade 5—severe reduction of central canal. In this category the anticipated myelographic defect is high-grade stenosis or complete block. There is circumferential constriction at the interspaces. Severe disc herniations, degenerative changes of articular facets and facet joints, and spondylolisthesis are some of the leading causes for severe central canal stenosis (Fig. 4.31).

References

1. Glenn WV Jr, Rothman SLG, Rhodes ML: Computed tomography/multiplanar reformatted (CT/MPR) examinations of the lumbar spine. In Genant HK, Chafetz N, Helms CA (eds): Computed Tomography of the Lumbar Spine. University of California Printing Department, San Francisco, 1982, pp. 87-123

2. Rothman SLG, Glenn WV Jr: Spondylolysis and spondylolisthesis. In Post MJD (ed): Computed Tomography of the Spine. Williams & Wilkins, Baltimore, 1984, pp. 591-615

3. Ghormley RK: Low back pain with special reference to the articular facets with presentation of an operative procedure. JAMA 101:1773-1777, 1933

4. Carrera GF, Haughton VM, Syvertsen A, et al.: Computed tomography of the lumbar facet joints. Radiology 134:145, 1980

5. Carrera GF: Computed tomography of the lumbar facet joints. In Post MJD (ed): Computed Tomography of the Spine. Williams & Wilkins, Baltimore, 1984, pp. 485-491

Degeneration and Disc Disease of the Intervertebral Joint

5

The intervertebral joint can be described as two vertebral bodies with all of the associated ligamentous, muscular, and cartilaginous connections. Any discussion of back pain and its causes must deal with the intervertebral joint as a unit, because degeneration or disease of one segment is intimately connected with all other segments.

Degeneration of the Intervertebral Joint

The earliest degenerative changes of the intervertebral joint occur in the anulus. These take the form of small circumferential separations or clefts between the lamellae of the anulus. Such separations have been well documented in children as young as 8 years old. In the lowest spinal segments the clefts tend to occur in the posterior portion of the anulus and initially do not communicate with the nucleus pulposus. In the upper spine the clefts tend to be more anterior.

As the degenerative process progresses, increasing hyalinization and thickening of the lamellae occurs, and minor scarring and calcification are seen. By age 20, changes begin to occur within the nucleus itself. It is not clear how to differentiate the normal aging process from early degenerative change, which includes collagenation of the nucleus and deformity of the innermost annular fibers.

The nucleus contains approximately 88% water at birth, 80% at age 18, and approximately 70% at the end of the eighth decade. Adult discs become completely avascular, and they absorb water and nutrition by a direct fluid exchange between the nucleus and the extracellular space of the vertebral body. Charnley[1] demonstrated conclusively that the healthy nucleus absorbs large quantities of water against a pressure gradient. The fluid exchange of a normal disc occurs because the nucleus is a true chemical gel. The solid phase is a protein mucopolysaccharide. The dispersion medium is extracellular fluid. The physical interaction between the solid and liquid components of the gel causes the nucleus to imbibe water. An incompletely hydrated nucleus pulposus thus absorbs water from the vertebral extracellular space against a powerful pressure gradient—the force of gravity. The weight of the upper portion of the erect body squeezes water out of the disc. Relief of this pressure at night allows rehydration. This normal fluid flow takes place only in healthy discs. As degeneration occurs, there is chemical change in the protein-polysaccharide collagen matrix of the nucleus that prevents water absorption. The ultimate effect is a desiccated cartilaginous nucleus which is structurally incapable of acting as a fulcrum or cushion.

Clinically significant disc degeneration begins with the onset of radial cracks and fissures. These radial tears begin at the nucleus and extend outward toward the periphery of the disc. Farfan[2] pointed out that the shape of the disc and the structure of the facet joints affect the direction and location of these radial fissures. Discs with rounded posterior borders tend to develop midline tears, and discs with flat or concave posterior borders develop posterolateral radial lesions. Unilateral posterolateral tears tend to occur in patients with asymmetrical facet joints, whereas bilateral lateral fissures are more likely to occur in patients with symmetric facets. Anterior radial fissures can occur at all levels but seem to be more prevalent in the upper lumbar spine.

113

End-Plate Deformity

The cause of the radial fissuring is not clear. It may be related to compression of central annular fibers by a nucleus pulposus under stress. Radial fissures are occasionally associated with fracture through the cartilaginous end-plates. It is likely that these fissures are caused by a combination of torsion stress, compression, and flexion. It is Farfan's theory that the most important single force is that of torsion. As the degenerative process continues, osseous remodeling begins to occur—in two slightly different patterns. The first

is diffuse concavity of the bony end-plate, which may be due to bone modeling or end-plate fragmentation. Axial CT demonstrates a combination of disc density and bone density on the same section. This is difficult to interpret because of volume averaging, it is also difficult to diagnose compression that lies along the plane of the axial section, but coronal reformation clearly shows the concavity (Fig. 5.1). The second type of deformity has been termed ''Cupid's bow'' deformity[3,4] because of its biconcavity resembling a bow lying on its strings. This is also well seen on coronal reformation (Fig. 5.2).

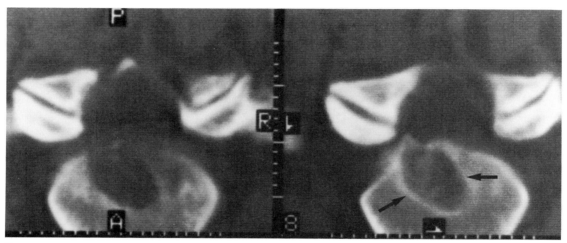

A

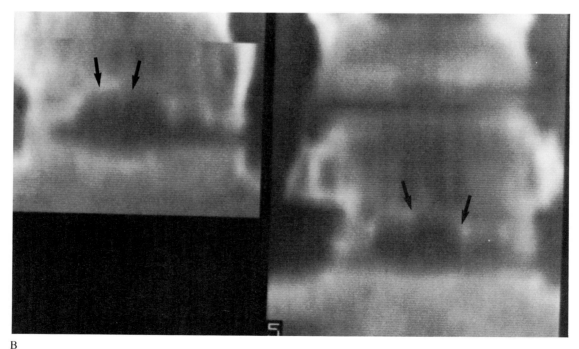

B

FIGURE 5.1   Concavity of the vertebral end-plate. **A.** Axial scan demonstrates lucency of the disc and density of the vertebral end-plate on the same scans. (*arrows*) **B.** Coronal view reveals upward convexity and sclerosis of the inferior end-plate of L5. (*arrows*).

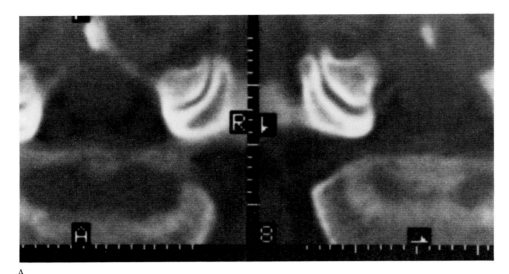

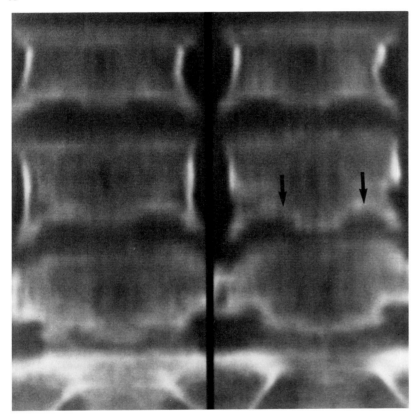

FIGURE 5.2 "Cupid's-bow" deformity. A. Axial views demonstrate symmetrical lucencies within the end-plate. B. Sagittal views reveal the typical "Cupid's-bow" deformity (*arrows*).

A

B

Schmorl's Nodes

Actual herniation of nuclear material through the vertebral end-plate into the body is called a Schmorl's node. In children the vertebral end-plates are fenestrated by blood vessels. With increasing age these vessels involute, leaving defects within the cartilaginous plate through which the nucleus can herniate. The number and size of these defects also tend to increase with age. Herniation may occur through these fissures or through fractures in the end-plate caused by trauma due to compression, alone or compression plus torsion.

The expansive pressure of the healthy nucleus and the stress of everyday life combine to produce tears in areas of developmental weakness within the cartilaginous end-plate. These tears allow herniation of anulus tissue and nucleus into the vertebral body. This incites resorption of the fine bony trabeculae beneath the end-plate, which in turn further accelerates the degenerative process. The small cavity that is produced allows continued herniation. Gradually, bony reaction occurs around the foreign material, producing first a cartilaginous then a bony lining. Enlargement of a Schmorl's node ceases when the elastic properties of the nucleus have been exhausted by nuclear degeneration due to a combination of desiccation and chemical change. The developmental stages of interbody herniation were shown very well in pathologic sagittal cross section by Schmorl and Junghanns[5] (Fig. 5.3).

CT scans show Schmorl's nodes as small lucencies with circumferential bone sclerosis. Within a sclerotic border, there may be several small Schmorl's nodes or one large cavity. Figure 5.4 represents a patient who demonstrates a well-defined lytic bone defect expanding through the vertebral end-plates which was not diagnosed radiographically before CT scanning. This well-marginated lytic defect is typical of a giant Schmorl's node.

Annular Bulging and Osteophyte Formation

Osteophytes form as a direct sequela to degeneration and are the most obvious anatomic anomalies, easily seen on analog radiographs. Schmorl found that spur formation was initiated by tears in the peripheral rim of the anulus through Sharpey's fibers. The separation leaves an abnormal attachment of disc to bone, which is then irritated by the continuous forces generated by a healthy nucleus pulposus. Repeated circumferential displacement of the healthy disc produces continuous overstrains, thereby inducing bony spur formation. This theory coincides with the clinical observation that patients with the largest bridging osteophytes have relatively normal disc heights.

The sequelae of separation of the peripheral rim of the anulus from the vertebra, as described by Schmorl, is striking on CT. When there is circumferential separation the entire low-density disc is seen to balloon over the edges

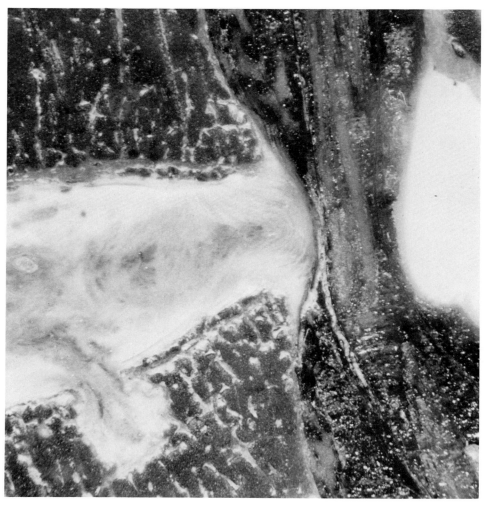

FIGURE 5.3 Schmorl's node, pathologic specimen. Sagittal section of an adult lumbar spine. Disc material is herniated through the end-plate into trabecular bone of the vertebral body.

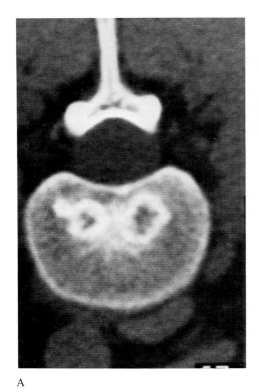

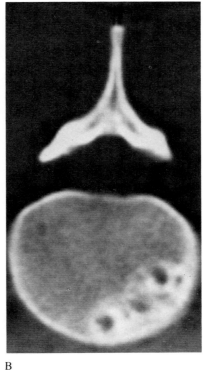

FIGURE 5.4 Schmorl's node. **A.** Axial scan of L3 with two lucent Schmorl's nodes in the posterior portion of the vertebral end-plate. **B.** Axial scan of L1. Interbody herniation has occurred in the anterior one third of the end-plate. **C.** Axial scan. Giant Schmorl's node. **D.** Coronal reformation. Giant Schmorl's node. There is a single lucency within the vertebral body, extending through the end-plate.

A

B

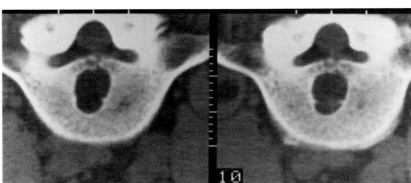

C

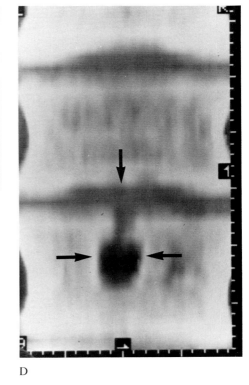

D

of the normal vertebral end-plate. Frequently, calcification is noted at the periphery of the circumferential bulge (Fig. 5.5).

Annular disruption need not be totally circumferential. In the upper vertebral segments, where the anterior fissures predominate, bulbous circumferential annular expansion may be seen only anteriorly. The anulus, conforming very closely to the normal (nonfissured) posterior portion of the disc, does not expand into the spinal canal. In the lower lumbar spine the central portion of the posterior disc margin in a young person has a concave or a flat appearance. As degenerative changes progress with age, desiccation of the nucleus results in further shrinkage and loss of height of the intervertebral space. The result is that the anulus fibrosis bulges outwardly.[5-7] This bulging is a re-

flection of both the degree and the rate of disc-space narrowing. The appearance on CT is a circumferential extension of the disc or anulus margin beyond the margins of the vertebral bodies, as shown in Figure 5.6. CT correctly

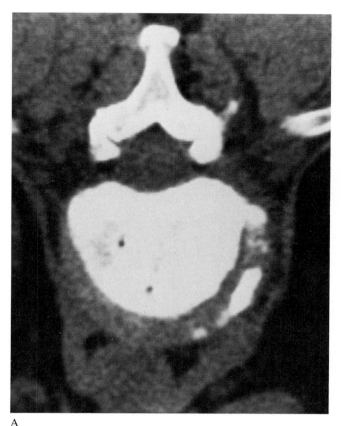

A

demonstrates the margins of the disc, but in an anatomic study CT was found to underestimate the severity of the degenerative changes within the nucleus and anulus.[6] On occasion the posterior border of the bulging anulus is concave. This is said to be due to buttressing by an unusually strong posterior longitudinal ligament[7] (Fig. 5.7).

The usual CT appearance of a desiccated bulging disc is that of posterior convexity instead of concavity in the midline. Symmetry of bulging is the rule and can be a helpful distinguishing point in differentiating bulging from disc herniation, which is typically posterolateral, focally localized to one side, and therefore asymmetrical. Patients require medical attention because of neural compression from the bulging anulus. Actually, these annular protrusions can occur anywhere along the vertebral ring. When they occur near the neural foramen, localized root compression can result.

Degeneration of the Facet Joints

Osteoarthritic deformity of the facet joint is a further manifestation of the degenerative process within the vertebral joint. In its earliest phases the articular cartilage becomes ulcerated, then with further wear and tear the cartilaginous surfaces become thin and the ulcerations deepen. The joint space becomes increasingly narrow (Fig. 5.8). Attempted

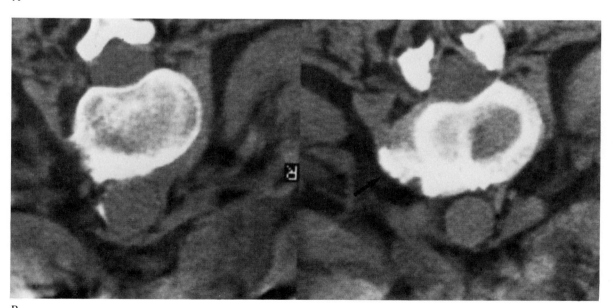

B

FIGURE 5.5 Diffuse bulging of the anulus. **A.** Calcification is present in the margin of this diffusely bulged anulus. **B.** Lateral bulging of the anulus, associated with a large lateral spur.

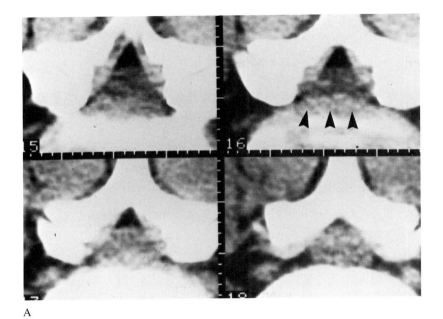

A

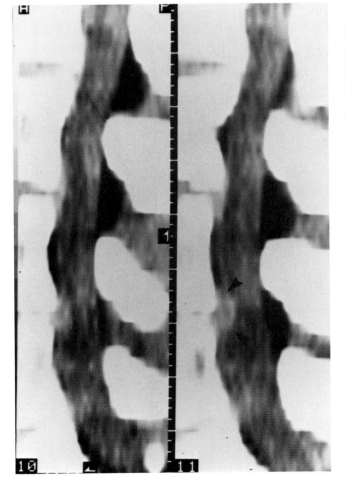

B

FIGURE 5.6 Concentric annular bulge. **A.** Axial views demonstrate symmetrical posterior bulging of the anulus (*arrowheads*). **B.** Sagittal view reveals a 5-mm anterior extradural defect (*arrowheads*) compressing the spinal canal by almost 50%.

FIGURE 5.7 Annular bulge with posterior concavity (*arrowheads*).

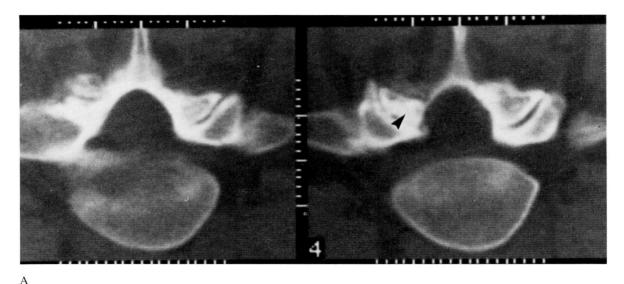

A

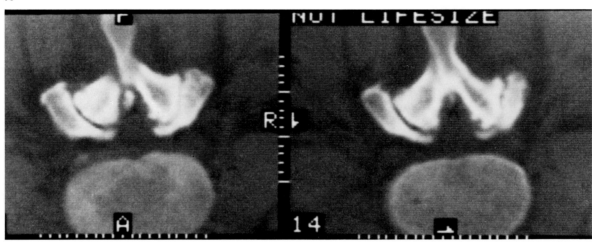

B

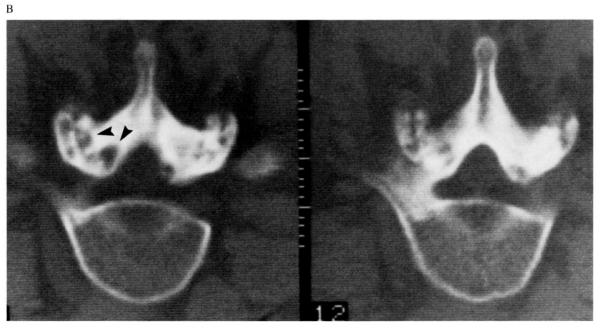

C

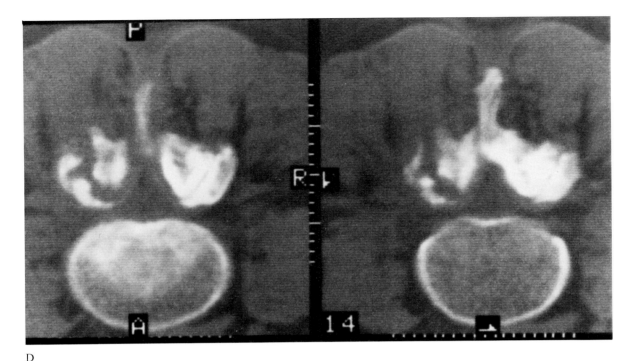

D

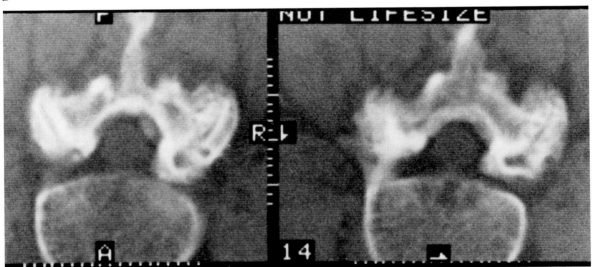

E

FIGURE 5.8 Facet disease; five patients. **A.** The right facet is almost totally normal. The left cartilaginous space is narrow. **B.** Both joint spaces are narrow. The cortical subarticular bone is thinned. **C.** Bilateral erosion of the subarticular bone is noted. There are large cystic cavities in the facets. **D.** Marked distraction of the left joint, with soft-tissue swelling and probable joint effusion. **E.** Bilateral hypertrophic spur formation.

healing of the cartilage produces a fibrous reaction. The normal relationship of the opposing cartilaginous surfaces is disturbed, causing injury to the encapsulating soft tissues. Healing of the joint capsule produces osteophytes at a joint margin; simultaneously, when the cartilaginous cap of the facets become eroded, there may be loss and thinning of the underlying trabecular bone, with significant subchondral bone resorption and cyst formation. Ligamentous laxity can cause a paradoxical enlargement of the joint space.

Notable changes occur within the neural arch with increasing degeneration of the intervertebral joint. The arches may become osteoporotic and lose the ability to resist torque. A peculiar type of compression stress fracture has been shown to occur, which is seen as a buckle on the lateral surface of the lamina at the base of the articular process. These fractures can alter the position and orientation of the facet surface and therefore predispose to degenerative spondylolisthesis with intact pars.

Abnormalities of the facet joints are discussed more extensively in Chapter 4.

Disc Herniation

Lumbar disc herniation is a common cause of nerve-root compression. Disc protrusion is preceded by well-defined structural changes in the anulus and nucleus. Radiating cracks in the anulus fibrosis develop centrally and extend peripherally, thus weakening resistance to nuclear herniation.

Herniation occurs more frequently in the young because they usually have a turgid nucleus—the type that is more likely to herniate. With age the nucleus loses its turgor and becomes desiccated and fibrotic. Herniation can be severe, with rupture of the anulus and the posterior longitudinal ligament, resulting in disc fragments in the central canal; but more commonly there is prolapse of disc material beneath the posterior longitudinal ligament (Fig. 5.9).

Simple bulging of the anulus can give rise to the same problems encountered with herniation. Prolapse of the intervertebral disc can occur in any direction. Those that occur in the posterolateral direction generally give rise to nerve-root compression syndromes (Fig. 5.10). A far-lateral prolapse of the disc into the foramen at a level where the articular processes are normal usually results in

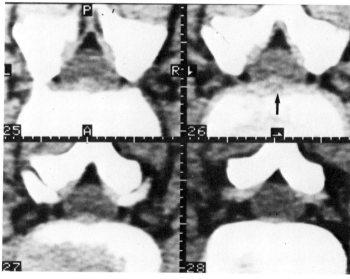

A

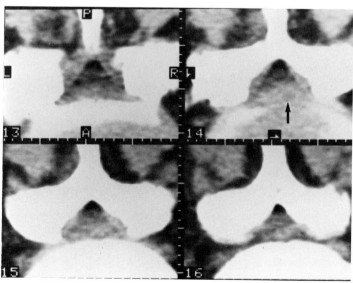

B

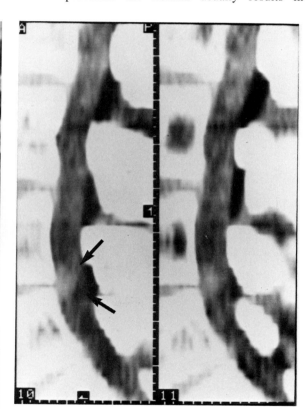

C

FIGURE 5.9 Central disc prolapse. **A.** Patient 1. Small central disc prolapse (*arrow*). **B.** Patient 2. Large central disc herniation (*arrow*). **C.** Sagittal view of patient 2. Note that the extradural mass nearly fills the spinal canal (*arrows*).

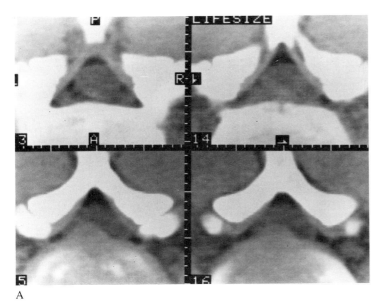

A

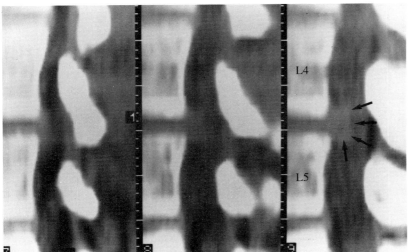

B

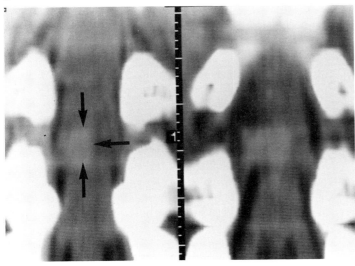

C

FIGURE 5.10 Posterolateral disc herniation. **A.** Axial scan shows large posterolateral disc herniation. **B.** Sagittal reformation shows a 7-mm disc protrusion from the L4–5 disc space. **C.** Coronal view shows the disc fragment, with smooth borders and contours, compressing the L5 and S1 roots (*arrows*).

compression of the nerve root exiting at that level; that is, the nerve root corresponds in number to the disc (i.e., a far lateral L5-S1 interspace herniation irritates the L5 root). A posteromedial herniation of the disc into a normal canal usually results in compression of the most lateral nerve root within the dural sac, i.e., the nerve root exiting at the next lower foramen (an L5-S1 posteromedial herniation usually affects the S1 root). A posterolateral prolapse of the disc into a canal with coexisting hypertrophy of the articular processes will probably result in compression of multiple nerve roots.

There is considerable confusion regarding the terminology used to describe disorders of the disc. It is therefore useful to define several commonly used descriptive terms.

Disc protrusion or *disc bulging* refer to instances where there is either localized or diffuse bulging of the anulus fibrosis. The annular fibers are intact, and at surgery there is no extrusion of nuclear material.[8]

Disc prolapse refers to those instances where there is displacement of nuclear material which is confined by the outer fibers of the anulus.

Extruded disc refers to those cases where a portion of the disc material extends outward through an annular tear. This fragment is still in contact with the disc space and is usually partially retained within the annular defect.

Disc sequestration refers to those instances where the herniated nuclear fragment is *separate* from the disc space. This *free nuclear fragment* may migrate anywhere in the spinal canal and may even perforate the dura.

The relationship of the posterior disc margin to the posterior bony surface of the end-plates immediately above and below needs to be characterized, whether the abnormality is a diffuse bulge or a focal herniation. When the disc margin is further posterior than the bone margin, the possibility exists for encroachment and therefore nerve-element entrapment. Even though a central bulge—from either a focal central herniation or as part of a generalized, posteriorly convex, bulging annular margin—is usually of less consequence than a similar more lateral bulge or herniation, it is important that even these central abnormalities be properly characterized, as they can cause ventral myelographic defects if they indent the dural sac. Large central disc herniation is dangerous in the sense that it can produce cauda equina compression with bowel and bladder problems. The lack of sciatic pain in midline herniation may dangerously mislead the physician away from a serious problem. It is helpful to measure objectively, when possible, the amount of central protrusion beyond the bony margin. This can be done by paying careful attention to the posterior margins of both adjacent end-plates. The sagittal plane facilitates this best and does not confuse the viewer by partial-volume averaging effects or oblique angulation of the axial slices.

Noting the positions of both end-plates avoids confusion, and therefore overreading, when one vertebral segment is displaced either anteriorly or posteriorly onto an-

other. Accurate quantification of real disc bulge in cases of spondylolisthesis best illustrates this point. What seems to be a significant anulus bulge in the axial view may actually be of little conseqence when evaluated more accurately on the sagittal view. The same is true at many normal L5-S1 interspaces, where because of the lower lumbar lordosis the posterior border of the disc slopes posteriorly. The angled axial section may be confusing with regard to the respective positions of the posterior margins of the inferior L5 end-plate, the L5 disc, and the superior S1 end-plate. Tilted-axial images may help, but in more than 15% of cases the gantry simply does not tilt to accommodate the L5-S1 interspace angle. The sagittal view provides a simple and effective solution to this problem.

The farther from the midline that the disc herniation occurs, the greater the possibility for irritation and/or displacement of nerve roots traversing the interspace in the lateral recess of the central canal. The typical situation is encroachment of the anterior aspect of the lateral recess at one level, with irritation or entrapment of the nerve roots exiting not at that level but at the next inferior one or two levels. The most common site is the L4-5 interspace, with the L5 and S1 roots being affected. Coronal images are often the most helpful in predicting affected nerve roots (Fig. 5.10C).

Proceeding away from midline to the lateral recess, the disc margin forms the anterior inferior portion of the nerve-root canal or foramen. In this position a disc bulge or herniation is often insignificant because the encroachment affects neither the traversing nerve root (more medial) nor the exiting nerve root, which is located more superiorly in the anterior superior quadrant of the nerve-root canal or foramen (Fig. 5.11). To avoid either undercalling or overcalling the presence of disc or anulus material within the foramen, it is important to have a series of axial images through the entire foramen. We advise using 3-mm intervals and 5-mm thicknesses.

Occasionally, far lateral disc herniations present as soft-tissue abnormalities either within or lateral to the foramen itself[9-11] (Figs. 5.12, 5.13). These are relatively infrequent, but they represent the situation for which myelography is useless or misleading. In these cases CT can accurately provide the diagnosis, but *only if the CT spine pictures are not coned down too tightly.*

The extruded, sequestered, or free disc fragment poses a special diagnostic and therapeutic problem, especially to those who routinely scan only vertebral interspaces using the tilted-gantry approach.[12] It is not rare for the disc fragment to migrate away from the interspace, in which case the axial slices through the interspaces will appear totally normal, and the fragments are missed (Figs. 5.14, 5.15). Teplick and Haskins stated, "A small fragment may be overlooked or misinterpreted if no disc herniation is seen at the disc space. In view of the not insignificant incidence of sequestered fragments, when indicated it might be pru-

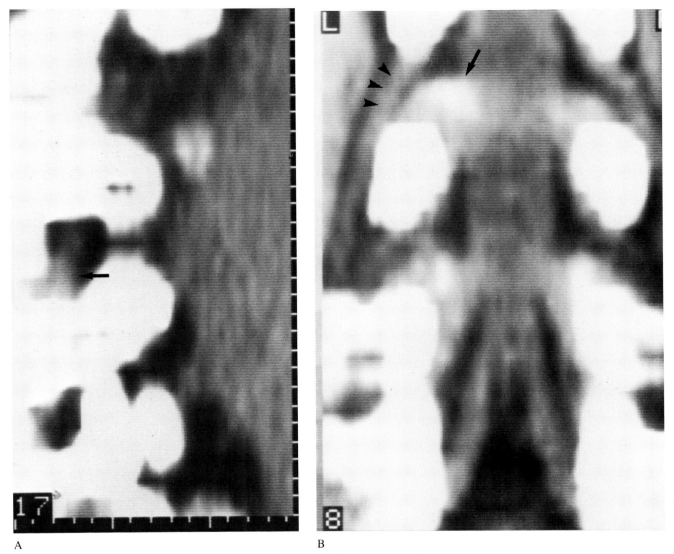

A   B

FIGURE 5.11 Diffuse disc bulge below exiting root. Sagittal (**A**) and coronal (**B**) views. Note the shadow of a diffusely bulging anulus (*arrows*) below the exiting nerve root (*arrowheads*).

dent to take sufficient CT sections to cover the entire canal between the interspaces."[13] How, in prospect, do you determine which patients need complete CT examinations and which need only incomplete tilted-gantry examinations? We believe that all need the complete study.

According to Dillon et al.,[14] 34 of 40 extruded disc fragments migrated 6 mm or more from the involved disc space. In their series, 50% of migrating discs descended in the spinal canal, 40% ascended, and 10% of the extrusions occurred in both directions. Fries et al.[15] found a higher percentage of fragments migrating cephalad. Both groups acknowledged that superiorly migrating fragments tend to travel the greatest distances—an important observation, as it is these small superior fragments that hide in the axillary pouch and are missed at surgery.

Specific CT Findings

Certain specific abnormalities strongly suggest a symptom-producing disc herniation. Localized posterior displacement of a nerve root by lateral herniation is one of the more clear-cut abnormalities—it almost always correlates well with the side and level of the clinical symptoms. Nerve-root swelling associated with displacement or as an isolated finding also strongly suggests a significant lesion and correlates well with clinical complaints (Fig.5.16). The least specific abnormality is asymmetry of the epidural fat. Although this may suggest a relationship between the CT abnormality and the clinical findings, prior surgery may cause fibrotic scar that can obliterate the normal fat planes. Careful correlation of the clinical findings with all three projections usually provides the correct diagnosis.

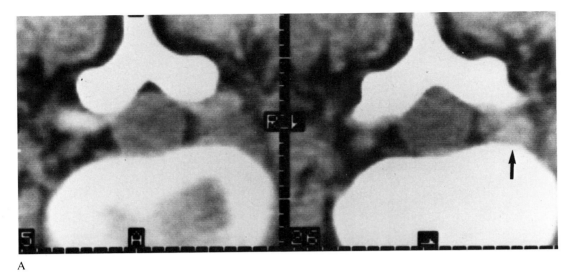

A

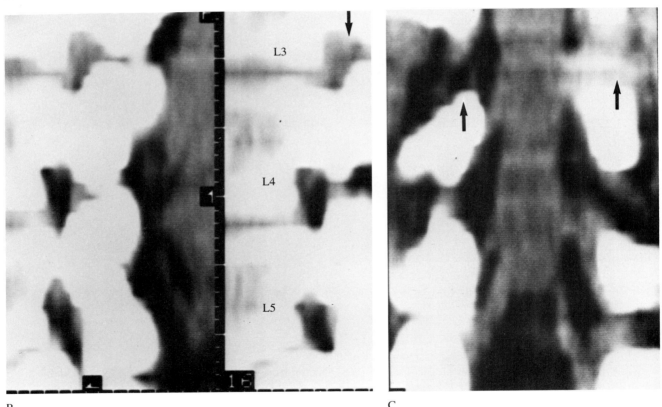

B   C

FIGURE 5.12 Foraminal disc herniation. **A.** Axial scan shows a large soft-tissue mass filling the L3–4 foramen. **B.** Sagittal view shows the L4 and L5 roots surrounded by fat. At L3–4 the foramen is filled with disc (*arrow*). **C.** Coronal view. Note the asymmetry of the two foramina (*arrows*) and the loss of the exiting right L3 root.

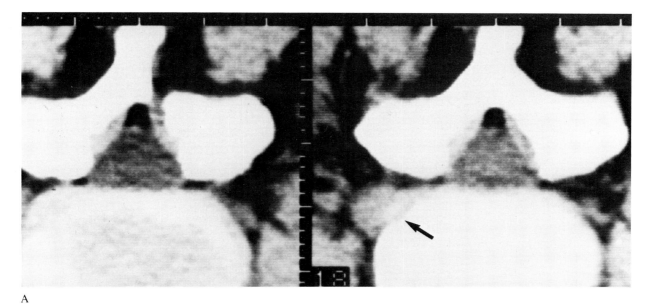

A

B

FIGURE 5.13 Extraforaminal disc herniation. Axial (**A**) and coronal (**B**) views demonstrate a localized mass (*arrows*), which is extruded disc lateral to the neural foramen.

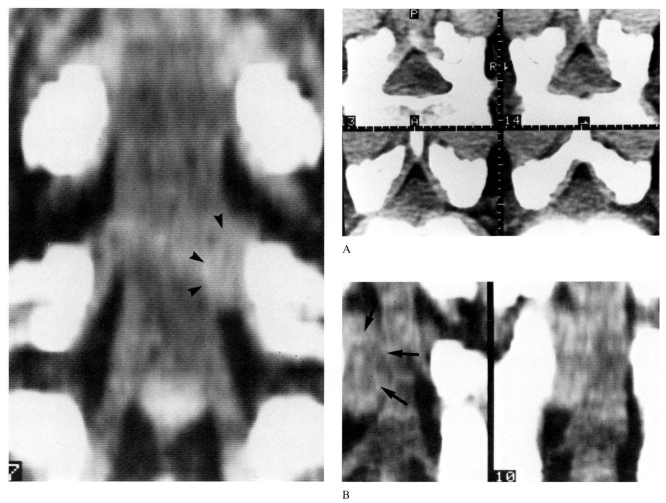

A

B

FIGURE 5.14   Small, sequestered disc fragment. Coronal views reveal a small localized disc herniation (*arrowheads*). Note the subtle widening of the extradural space on the side of the disc. There is slight shift of the nerve root medially (*arrow*).

FIGURE 5.15   Massive sequestered disc. Axial (**A**) and coronal (**B**) views demonstrate a huge extradural mass of disc. The fragment displaces the roots and the theca and widens the epidural spaces on the side of the lesion.

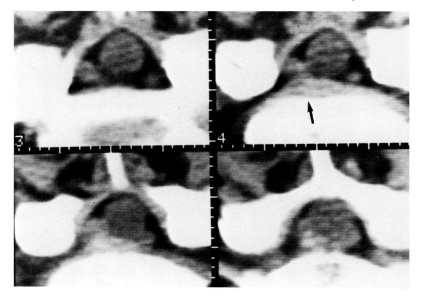

FIGURE 5.16   Lateral disc herniation with displaced swollen root. Left lateral disc herniation has displaced the left S1 root. The root is twice as large as its contralateral mate.

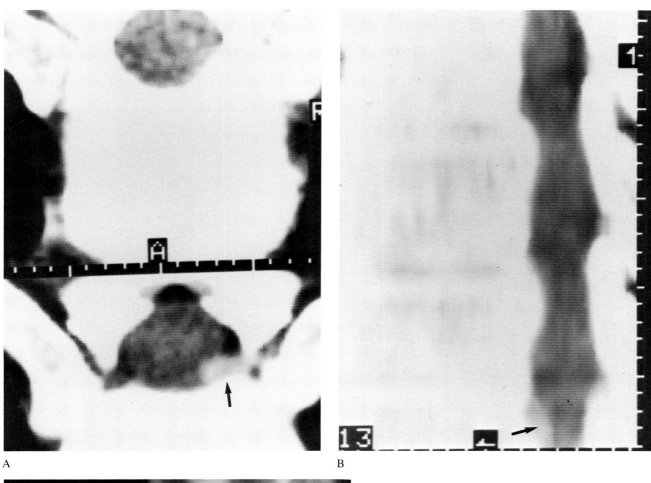

A

B

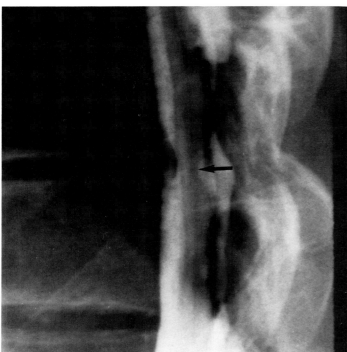

C

FIGURE 5.17 Thoracic disc herniation. **A, B.** Axial and sagittal views on a patient with many years of pain radiating to the scapula. There is a soft-tissue disc herniation (*arrows*). **C.** Myelogram on the same patient. The herniation is indicated (*arrow*). (*Figure continued on page 130.*)

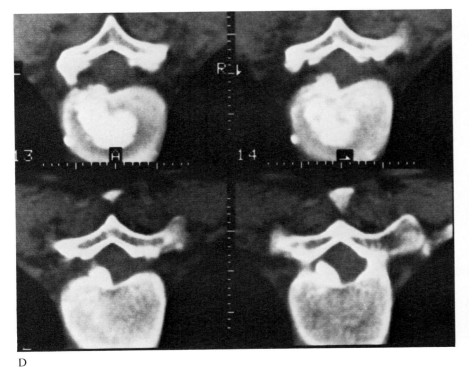

D

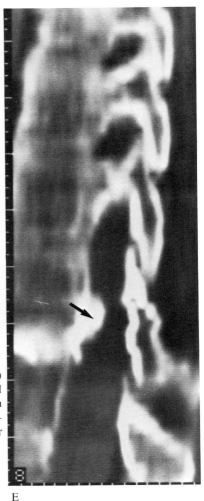

FIGURE 5.17 (*cont'd*) **D, E.** Axial and sagittal views on a patient with herniation of a large totally calcified nuclear fragment (*arrow*).

E

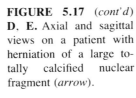

FIGURE 5.18 Vacuum disc. Axial scan shows a small amount of gas in the center of the disc.

Thoracic disc herniation, because it is so unusual, poses specific diagnostic problems. These lesions may present because of myelopathy and cord compression or long-standing thoracic root radiculopathy. Plain films are usually of no value. CT demonstrates the same types of abnormality in the thoracic spine as it does in the lumbar and cervical areas. Discs are higher in attenuation than the cord or epidural fat. They may, on occasion, calcify (Fig. 5.17).

Degeneration of the Intervertebral Disc

With increasing desiccation of the nucleus, retraction and fibrosis of the disc occur. Clefts can develop within the disc, which fills with gas.[16] This is termed the vacuum effect. This gas has been found to contain 90-92% nitrogen.[17] Vacuum changes have been found in up to 20% of patients.[18] The vacuum phenomenon of severely degenerated discs is typically noted in the central portion of the interspace (Fig. 5.18). Because the gas can migrate any-

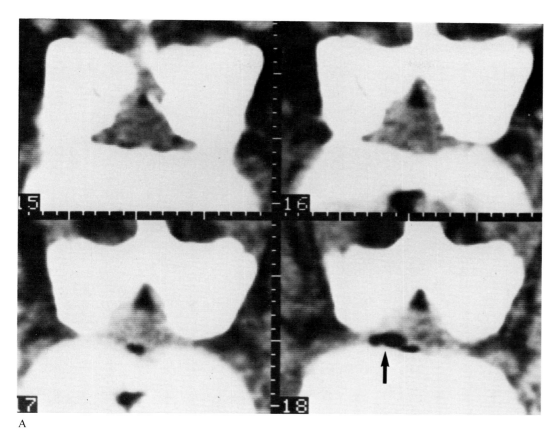

A

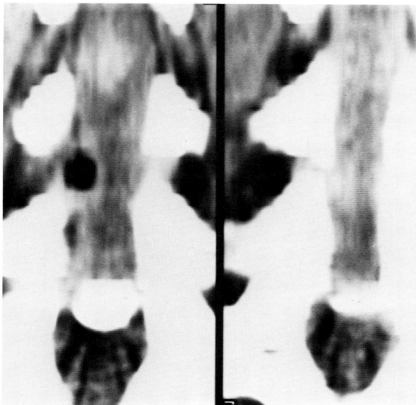

B

FIGURE 5.19 Vacuum disc effect. **A, B.** Patient 1. Axial and coronal scans demonstrate gas within the L4–5 disc space extending into the extradural space (*arrow*). The bubble of gas extends into the medial end of the neural foramen. The associated herniated disc compresses the descending L5 root. Note also a large L5–S1 bony ridge with associated disc herniation. (*Figure continued* on page 132.)

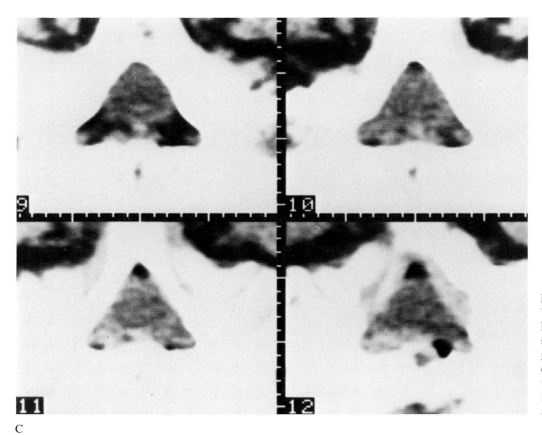

C

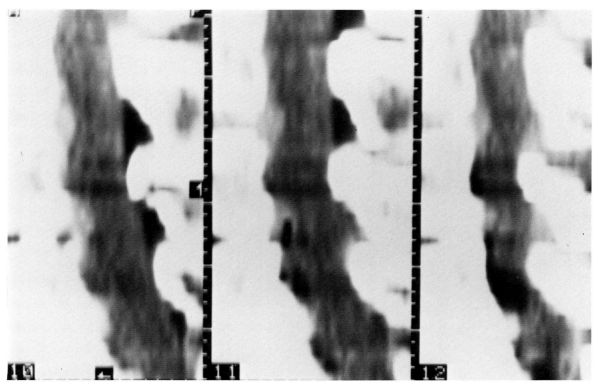

D

FIGURE 5.19 (*cont'd*) Vacuum disc effect. **C, D.** Patient 2. Axial and sagittal views demonstrate gas with a diffusely bulged disc. Note on the sagittal view that there are prominent extradural defects at all three levels.

where within the fissured interspace, it can present along the anterior margin of the central canal in the midline, in the lateral recess, or even in the foramen. The gas itself is of no consequence. It is an important sign because it indicates that there is either displacement of the posterior ligamentous structures posterior to the gas or actual disc herniation (Fig. 5.19). Gas from a vacuum phenomenon must be distinguished from air introduced by a recent lumbar puncture, myelographic procedure, or epidural injection (Fig. 5.20). Iatrogenically introduced air is resorbed, but the gas in a degenerated disc may be bounded posteriorly by stretched annular fibers, and this bulging anulus may cause neural compression.

Degenerative Ridging and Spur Formation

A common manifestation of the advancing degenerative process of the intervertebral disc is osteophytic spur formation. Vertebral-body spurs form at the bony attachment of Sharpey's fibers. Occasionally they are large enough to buttress the disc space and prevent collapse. Often they occur posteriorly and posterolaterally, and frequently they extend into the neural foramina. Huge buttressing lateral and anterior osteophytes rarely cause symptoms. In fact, because they frequently mimic spine fusion, they may ac-

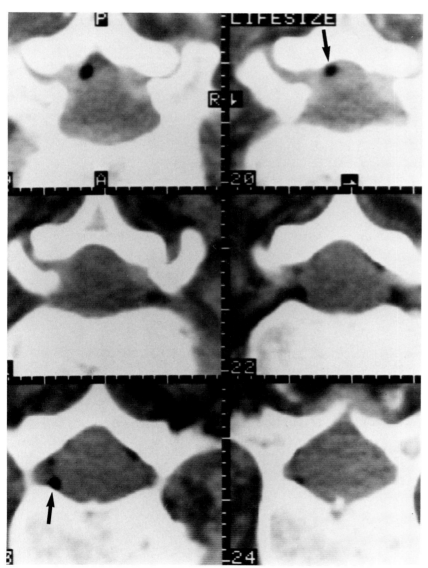

FIGURE 5.20 Iatrogenically placed air. CT scan performed several days after lumbar puncture reveals gas (*arrows*) in the epidural space.

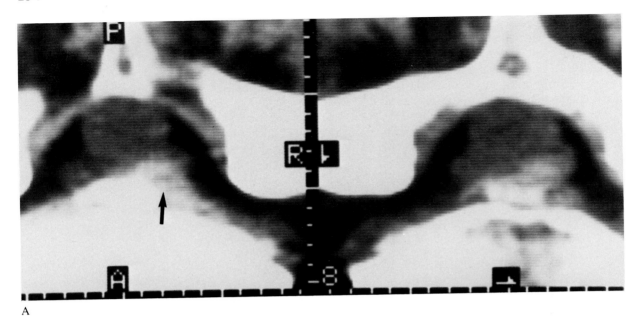

A

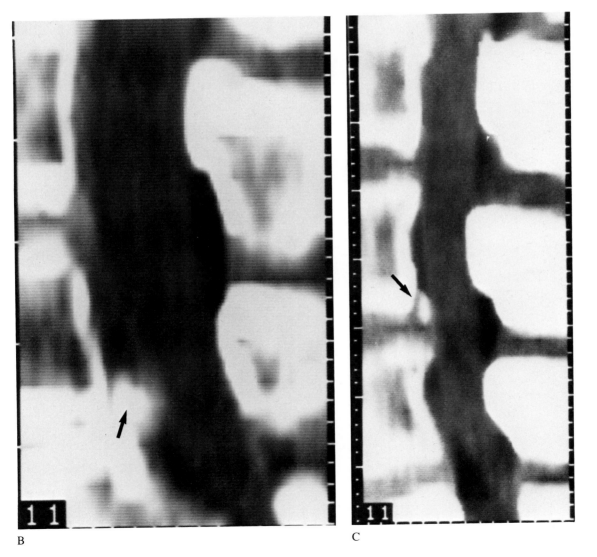

B

C

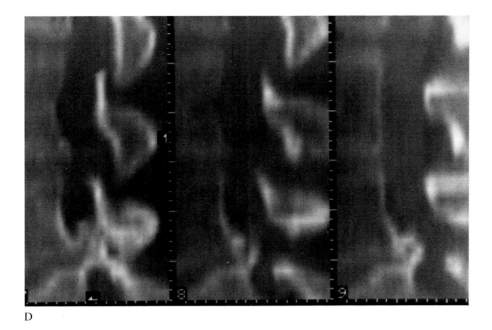

D

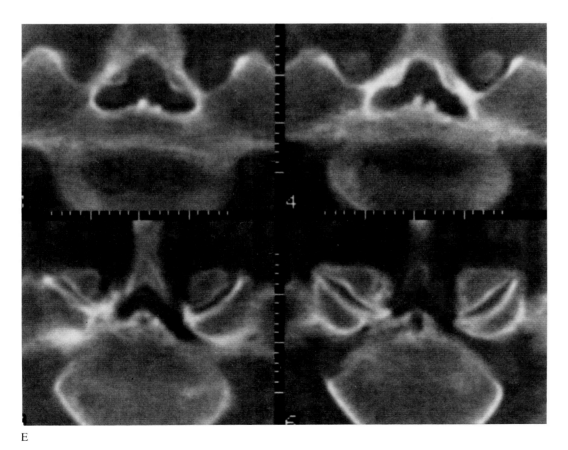

E

FIGURE 5.21 Calcified anterior extradural lesions. **A, B.** Axial and sagittal views on a patient with a large calcified herniated disc (*arrows*). The anterior extradural calcification is separate from the vertebral end-plate. **C.** Patient with calcification (*arrow*) in the posterior anulus. **D** Sagittal views on a patient with a pair of large end-plate osteophytes. See axial view (**E**).

tually prevent symptoms. Small posterior vertebral end-plate spurs arising from severely degenerated disc spaces are much more likely to produce symptoms caused by canal, recess, or foraminal compression. On occasion, calcification of the posteriorly bulging anulus may mimic osseous spur formation. The distinction is actually of little consequence. In fact, if there is a substantial calcified extradural mass causing neural compression, it makes little surgical difference whether one calls it a spur or a calcified anulus. Its physiological consequences are the same.

Axial and sagittal views of three patients with calcified anterior extradural masses impinging on the spinal canal are shown in Figure 5.21. The first lesion (Figs. 5.21A, B) a calcified herniated disc, is fairly localized. Calcified disc fragments may occur anywhere, but the calcification tends to be focal. On the sagittal view one should be able to see that the calcification, although in close association with the disc space, is not continuous with the vertebral end-plates. The second patient (Fig. 5.21C) has calcification in the posterior edge of a diffusely bulging anulus, which is best seen in the sagittal view. The crescentic calcification conforms to the posterior annular fibers. The third patient (Figs. 5.21D, E) has a typical degenerative ridge osteophyte. Note that the ridge osteophyte is continuous with the vertebral end-plate. In each case, although the pathology is slightly different, there is substantial extradural mass, which is compatible with the clinical history. The surgical implications are the same.

Ridges and spurs frequently coexist with soft-tissue disc herniation. They may be immediately adjacent to the disc fragment or may be at some distance (Fig. 5.22). Microsurgical removal of a disc fragment in the presence of a large bony ridge may not relieve the patient's symptoms. We have seen instances where soft-tissue herniated fragments have been removed but the surgery failed to relieve all of the symptoms because the extent of spurs was not appreciated intraoperatively. It is therefore our obligation when analyzing CT spine scans to make careful note of the presence, location, and size of all associated osteophytes.

We may conceptualize the ridges as occurring in three separate locations: central, lateral, and foraminal. Although it is common for these ridges to traverse two or even all three areas, we define them on the basis of the area of the spinal canal that is likely to be compressed. Medial ridges indent the theca and may cause symptoms of spinal stenosis. Lateral ridges may compress descending nerve roots, producing symptoms in the root that exits one level below the affected disc space. Foraminal spurs compress the root exiting within the foramen and are frequently misdiagnosed clinically as a disc herniation one disc space higher up. It is important, therefore, when describing of these ridges in the CT report to indicate where neural compression is most likely occurring. This frequently alter the surgical approach to the disc space.

At the L5-S1 interspace one commonly encounters a clearly definable pair of end-plate ridges. The appearance on CT is so typical it needs to be described. These end-plate ridges tend to be long, commonly extending out from beyond the neural foramina toward the midline. Sometimes they traverse the entire disc space, but occasionally they are discontinuous centrally. The axial scans reveal two curvilinear ''railroad-track'' ridges. The more anterior ridge arises from the posterior inferior end-plate of L5 and the posterior ridge arises from the posterior superior end-plate of the sacrum. These railroad tracks are always pointed upward in an arc not dissimilar from that of the bulging anulus. The ridges are best viewed in the sagittal plane. The spikelike superior tips often extend into the anterior medial quadrant of the neural foramen and impinge on the exiting root (Fig. 5.23).

One interesting abnormality must be differentiated from degenerative ridging because of its potential medicolegal implications. This is the uncommon entity called posterior limbus vertebra.

According to Schmorl and Junghanns,[5] anterior intrabody herniation that occurs in close proximity to the ring apophysis may in actuality fracture off from this apophysis.[19] They showed several anatomic specimens with disc material extruded forward through the anterior end-plate defect. Similar changes may rarely occur posteriorly.[20] We have studied three such patients and have seen two others, (R. Cloward, personal communication), all of whom had sustained significant trauma. The individual in Figure 5.24 fell from a ladder and was complaining of pain and radiculopathy. On the axial scan a dense bony ''ridge'' extends across the spinal canal. A herniated disc fragment is also obvious. Coronal reformations through the vertebral end-plate reveal typical changes of intravertebral disc herniation. The key finding is on the sagittal view, where a cleavage line is noted between the ring apophysis and the vertebral body. It thus seems that posterior limbus vertebra is likely to be a true traumatic lesion. Differentiating posterior limbus vertebra from degenerative disc disease therefore has major medicolegal significance. It is one of the very few instances of disc herniation that is almost definitely related to a traumatic event. The diagnosis can be made with certainty on the sagittal view.

Chemonucleolysis

Early studies suggested that herniated disc material might be chemically digested in order to relieve the symptoms of disc herniation. Initial clinical trials during the 1960s and 1970s indicated that chymopapain was useful in treating disc herniation, but the treatment was withdrawn from use in 1975. Various other enzyme derivatives have also undergone clinical trials over the past several years. Early in 1983 chymopapain was released for general usage in the continental United States and seems to be well received, despite

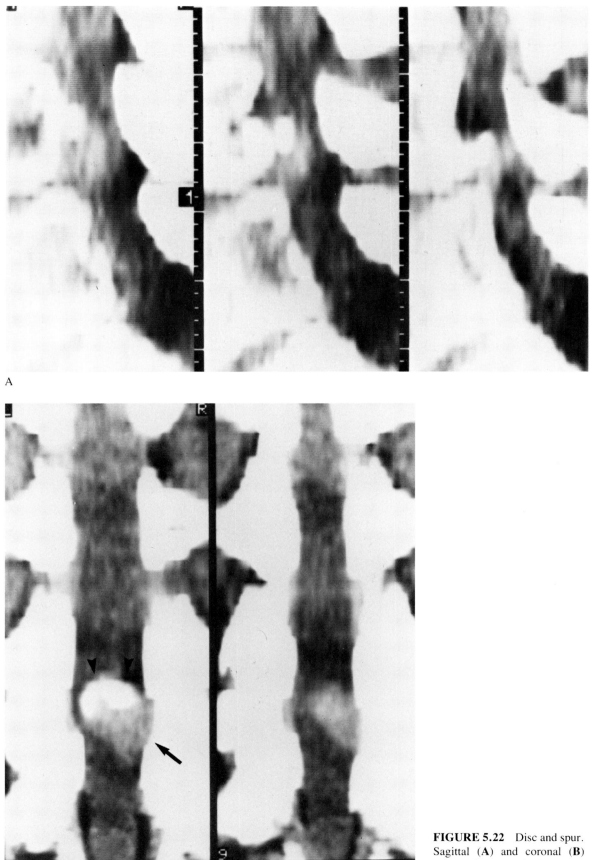

A

B

FIGURE 5.22 Disc and spur. Sagittal (**A**) and coronal (**B**) reformations reveal a large prolapsed disc associated with prominent osteophytic ridging.

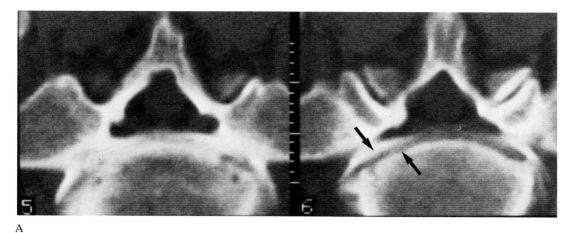

A

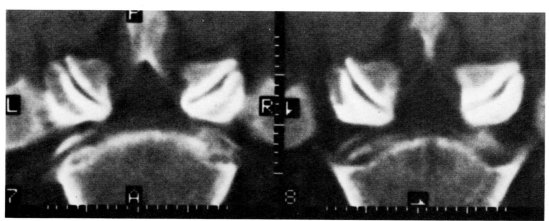

B

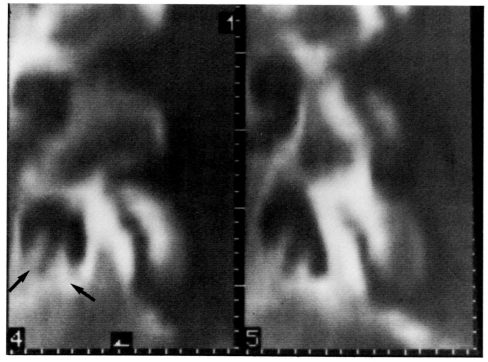

C

FIGURE 5.23 ''Railroad-track'' osteophytes. **A–C** End-plate osteophytes extend superiorly and produce a characteristic railroad-track appearance. The posterior ''rail'' is the spur rising from the superior end-plate of the sacrum; the anterior ''rail'' is the spur from the inferior end-plate of L5.

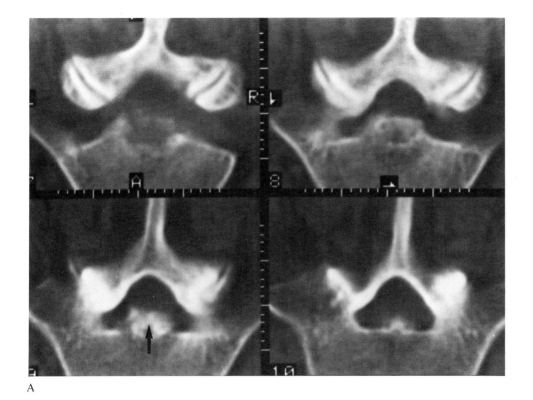

A

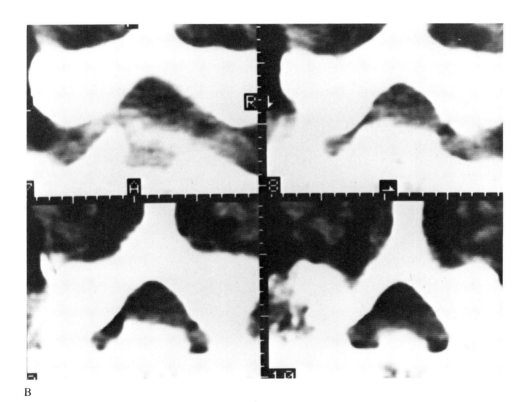

B

FIGURE 5.24 Posterior limbus vertebra. **A.** Axial bone-window view reveals a prominent bony ridge (*arrow*) across the disc space. **B.** Axial soft-tissue view shows a disc fragment associated with the ridge. (*Figure continued* on page 140.)

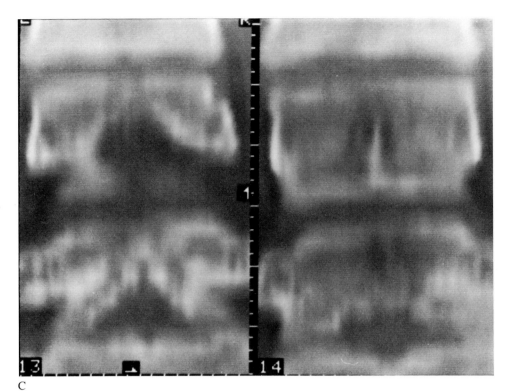

C

FIGURE 5.24 (*cont'd*) Posterior limbus vertebra. **C.** Coronal reformation demonstrates compression of the posterior margins of the vertebral end-plate; these are typical changes of interbody disc herniation. **D.** Sagittal reformation defines a linear cleavage plane between the fractured apophyseal ring and the vertebral body (*arrow*).

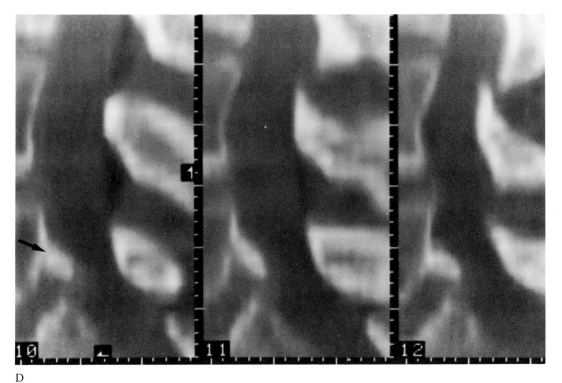

D

some problems. Early CT studies demonstrated an objective decrease in the size of herniated discs after chymopapain injection.[21] Now, as expected, the number of patients scanned after chymopapain failure has begun to increase. It is important therefore to be aware of the CT changes one might see.

During the first several weeks after chymopapain injection the disc margin loses definition and soft-tissue infiltrate appears around the nerve roots. The latter finding may be due to edema from the chemical irritation of the enzyme, but it generaly resolves within a matter of weeks.[21] In our experience, some blurring of the disc margin may remain for months (Fig. 5.25). The first objective change in the injected disc is a decrease in the CT attenuation values, probably because of liquefication or chemical change within the disc. It may take up to 6 months for actual resorption of extruded disc material (Fig. 5.26). There is a good correlation between relief of symptoms and objective decrease in size.[21] No change in the radiographic appearance of the disc is almost always associated with failure of therapy.

Chymopapain injection is not the preferred treatment for migrated disc fragments, but even large free fragments occasionally disappear. The elderly gentleman shown in Figure 5.27 had symptoms of spinal stenosis. His original CT scan showed remarkable bony canal stenosis and a large disc herniation. Although spinal stenosis is usually a contraindication to chemonucleolysis, this patient was a poor surgical candidate; therefore it was decided that enzyme injection might be beneficial in that it would reduce the soft-tissue component. Indeed, the postchymopapain scar demonstrated remarkable shrinkage of this huge disc fragment (Fig. 5.28).

After chemonucleolysis, the disc space frequently collapses. This happens most commonly when discs of normal height are injected. Because decreasing the disc-space height always decreases the vertical diameter of the neural foramen, it is important to evaluate the foramen on preinjection CT to exclude significant osteophytes.

The place of chymopapain in the treatment of lumbar disc disease is still unclear. There are those who advocate strict criteria for patient selection,[21,22] but some inject one or more disc spaces without a formal set of objective selection criteria. It is important for those who read lumbar CT scans to be aware of the great responsibility that rests with them. First, one must have objective evidence of disc disease and be wary of overreading abnormalities of the L5-S1 intervertebral disc. Second, one must warn the surgeon of potential pitfalls, e.g. free fragments at great distances from the disc, or, most important, preexisting recess or foraminal stenosis.

Intradiscal injection is not always a totally benign procedure. Leakage of the enzyme may cause severe neural irritation. Contamination of the disc space may also lead to bone necrosis and infection. The patient in Figure 5.29 developed marked pain in the right leg within weeks of chemonucleolysis. Right-sided radiculopathy became intense. Follow-up CT revealed soft-tissue epidural abscess and vertebral end-plate erosion caused by osteomyelitis.

Marked destruction of the vertebral end-plates is also noted in Figure 5.30. This patient had chemonucleolysis at two levels. There is no associated soft-tissue epidural abscess here, which somewhat reduces the likelihood that infection is present. We have now seen or heard of three similar cases of what seems to be noninfectious chemical destruction of the vertebral end-plates.

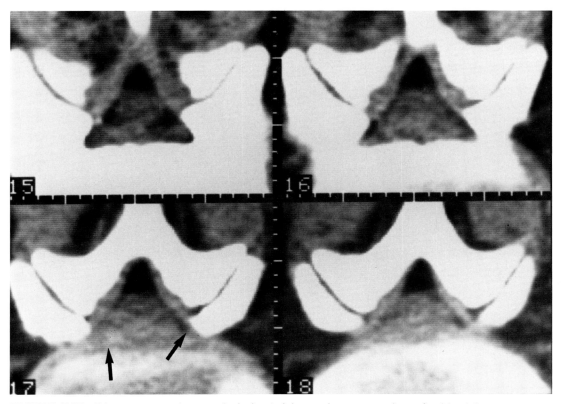

FIGURE 5.25 Disc space postchemonucleolysis. Axial scan demonstrates loss of epidural fat planes around the theca (*arrows*).

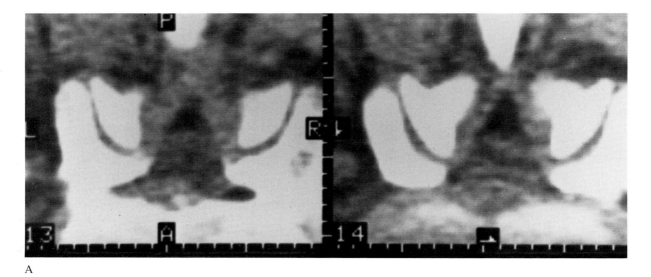

A

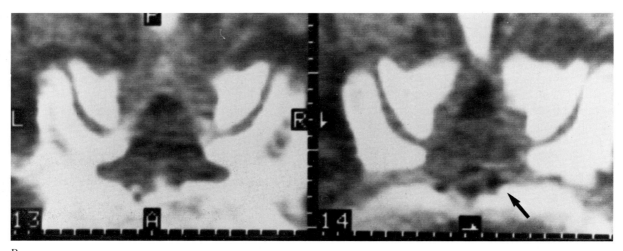

B

FIGURE 5.26   Postchemonucleolysis changes. **A.** Axial scan before chemonucleolysis demonstrates 5-mm central bulging of the L4–5 disc. **B.** Axial scan after chemonucleolysis demonstrates marked lucency (*arrow*) within the injected disc.

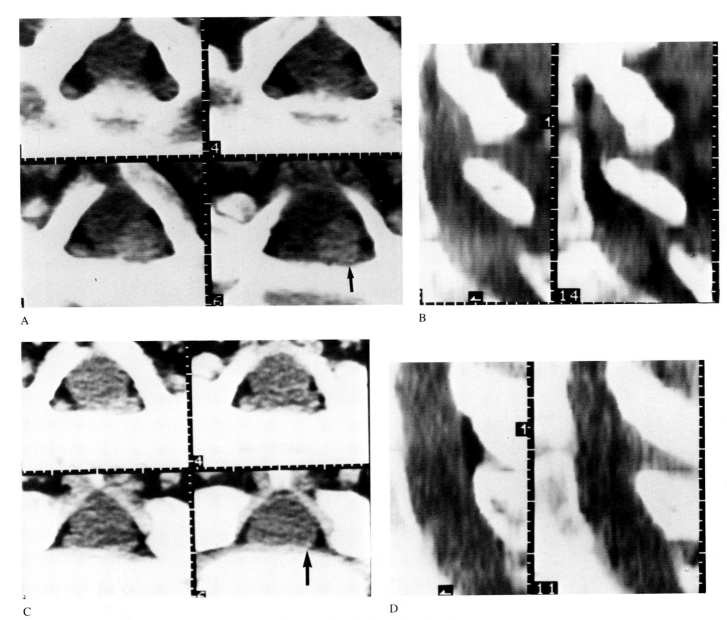

FIGURE 5.27 Dissolution of disc material with chymopapain. **A, B.** Axial and sagittal views before chymopapain reveal a large (10-mm) herniated disc (*arrow*). **C, D.** Axial and sagittal views after chemonucleolysis reveal that the disc fragment is gone (*arrow*).

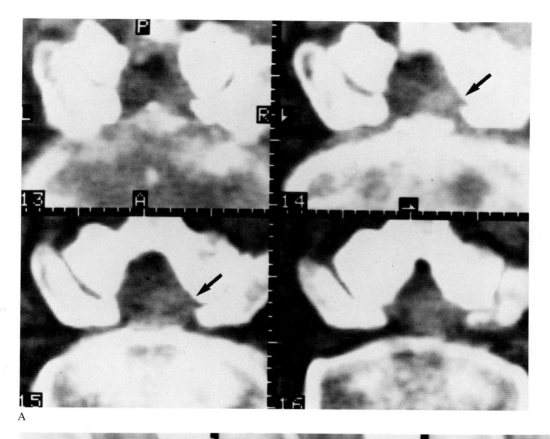

A

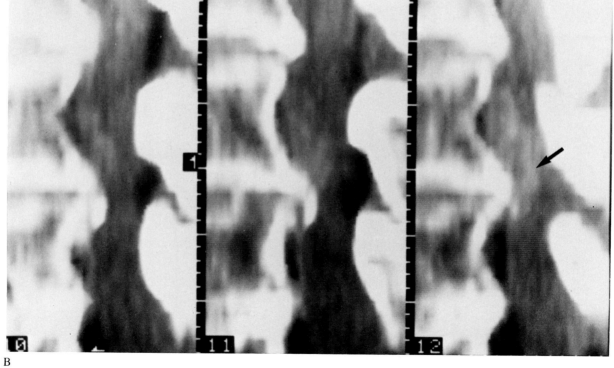

B

FIGURE 5.28   Dissolution of a soft-tissue disc in patient with spinal stenosis. **A–C.** Axial, sagittal, and coronal views before chemonucleolysis demonstrate large osteophytes and a huge soft disc herniation (*arrows*). **D–F.** Same patient after chemonucleolysis. The disc fragment is no longer present. (*Figure continued* on pages 145–146.)

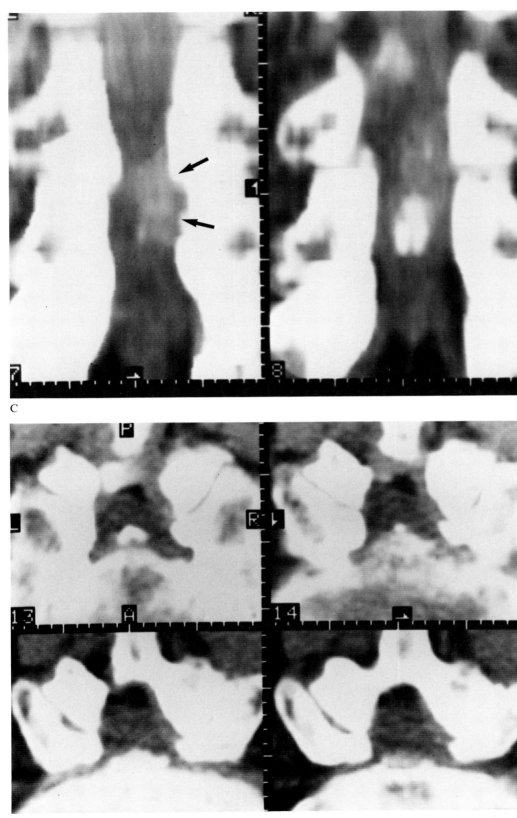

C

D

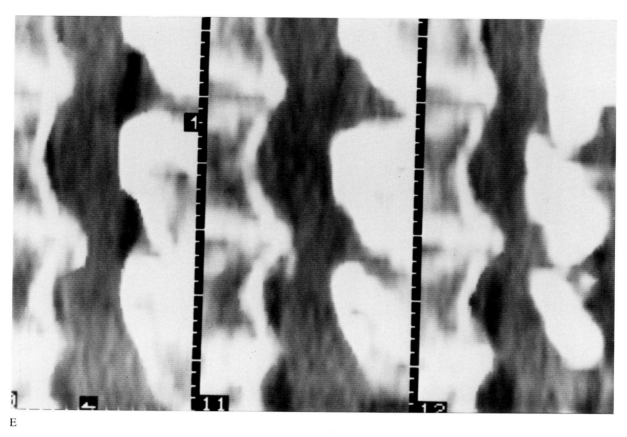

E

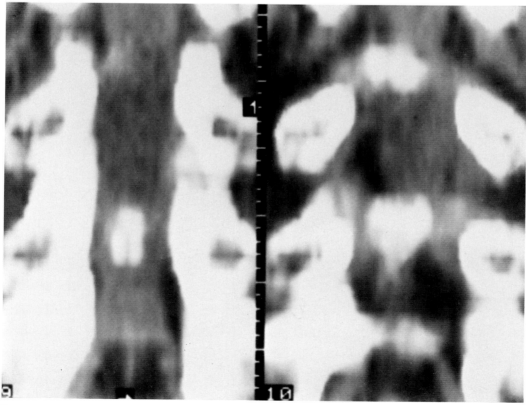

F

FIGURE 5.28 (*cont'd*)   See legend page 144.

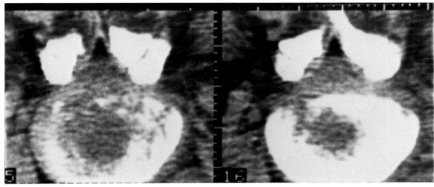

A

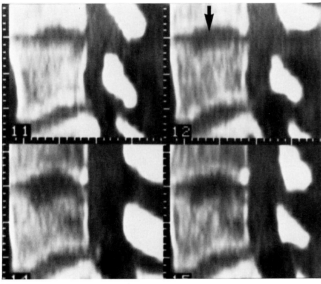

B

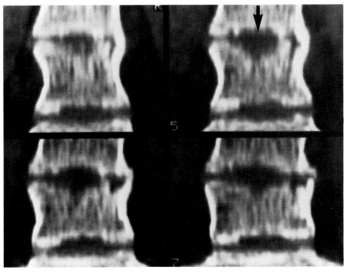

C

FIGURE 5.29 Disc-space infection after chemonucleolysis. **A.** Axial soft-tissue views showing an epidural soft-tissue mass extending into the neural foramen. **B**, **C.** Sagittal and coronal reformations reveal erosion of the end-plates (*arrows*).

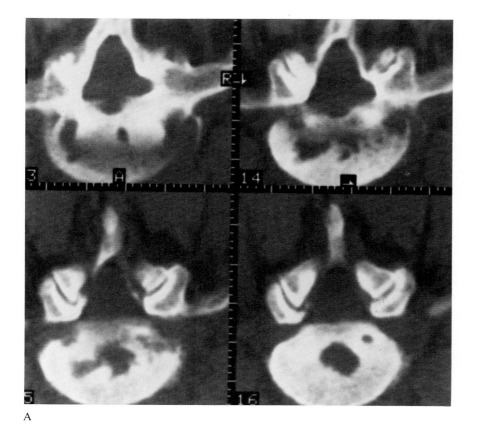

A

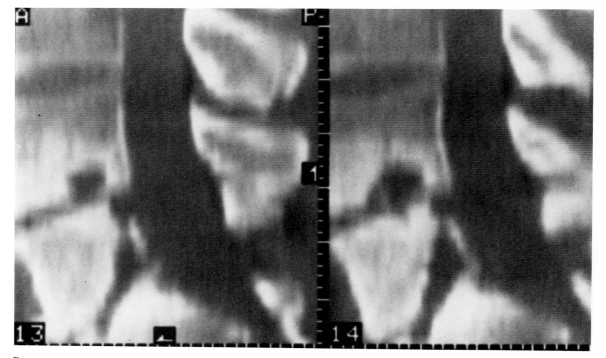

B

FIGURE 5.30   Disc-space destruction after chemonucleolysis. Axial (**A**) sagittal (**B**) and coronal
(**C**) reformations demonstrate marked destruction of the vertebral end-plates of both injected disc
spaces.

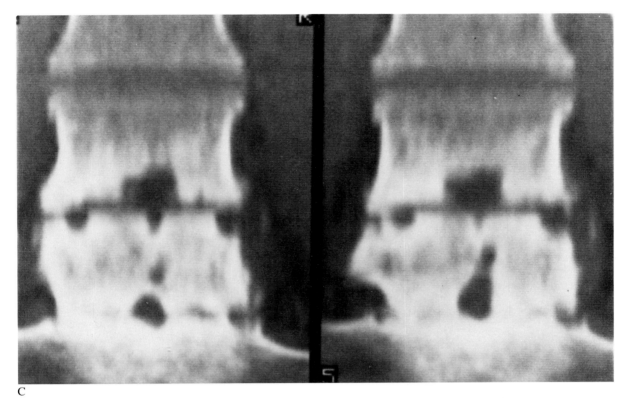

C

FIGURE 5.30 (*cont'd*)

Differential Diagnosis of Disc Herniation

A number of entities may be mistaken for disc disease on axial CT. Many are significant diagnostic problems, but some are diagnostic problems only in the absence of the appropriate views.

Anomalies and irregularities of the theca or nerve-root sheaths are frequently cited as potential pitfalls in the diagnosis of herniated disc.[12–14,23–25] The most common of these is the conjoined nerve root, or composite root sleeve. In this anomaly two adjacent roots share a common origin from the dural sac. Composite root sleeves tend to be unilateral and usually involve L5 and S1. They almost always arise at some level between the two normal contralateral roots. The normal symmetrical pattern of paired exiting roots is broken. The conjoined pair arise lower than the normal L5 roots and slightly higher than the contralateral S1 roots. Therefore on axial CT one sees a prominent soft-tissue bulge on one side with little or no surrounding epidural fat. On the normal side the root has already exited and there is a large amount of fat (Fig. 5.31). This axial soft-tissue asymmetry is not always obviously root rather than disc. Measuring the attenuation usually indicatesit to be of the same density as cerebral spinal fluid (CSF). Some

have advocated using ''blink mode'' when available,[24] but we have not found this of value.

Because the important anatomic information is the symmetry of the exiting roots, the coronal view is critical in making the diagnosis. Figure 5.32 shows a patient with asymmetry of the termination of the theca. Note the asymmetry of the origin of the roots in each case. Nowhere is there a hint of an extradural mass (disc fragment). Similarly, other dural anomalies have given problems on axial-only CT. Unilaterally dilated root sheath and dural diverticula may produce similar axial CT findings: asymmetry of the theca and epidural fat simulating lateral disc herniation. The diagnosis is obvious, however, on coronal views (Fig. 5.33). The epidural veins are prominent in some patients and therefore may pose a diagnostic problem. With experience, the specific anatomic arrangement of the epidural venous plexus allows correct diagnosis of epidural fat.

Herniated discs are, of course, only one type of anterior extradural mass. Because they are so common, it is relatively easy to forget the less common ones: tumor and infection. Most epidural tumor is associated with intraosseous metastasis, i.e., bone destruction; therefore the diagnosis should be obvious. However, localized metastatic deposits within the spinal canal may not be obvious. Also,

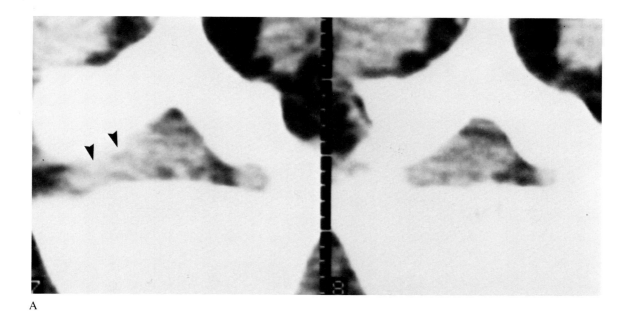

A

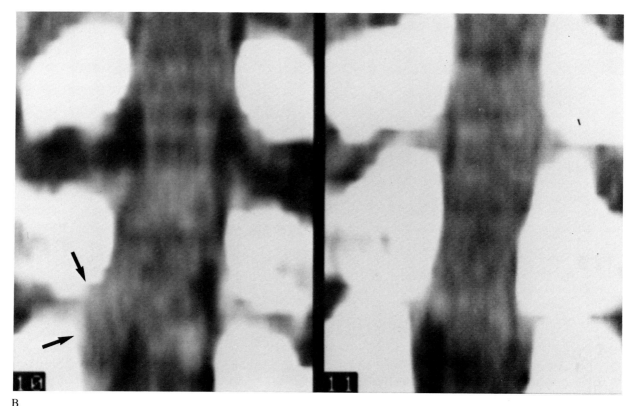

B

FIGURE 5.31   Conjoined nerve root. **A.** Axial scan demonstrates asymmetry of the epidural fat. The pair of conjoined roots exit together on the left. **B.** Curved coronal reformation demonstrates definite asymmetry of the extradural portions of the root (*arrows*). **C.** Coronal view on a second patient with conjoined roots (*arrows*). (From Rothman SLG, Dobben GD, Rhodes ML, et al: Computed tomography of the spine: curved coronal reformations from serial images. Radiology 150:185–190, 1984. With permission.)

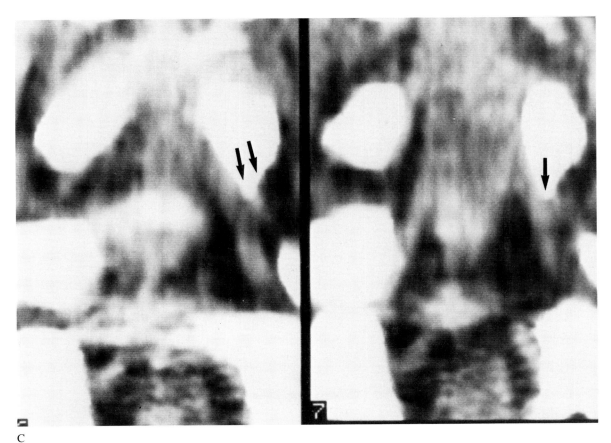

C

FIGURE 5.31 (*cont'd*)

lymphoma may infiltrate the epidural space and spare the bone. Epidural infection may masquerade as disc herniation, especially in the early stages of disc-space infection. These disorders therefore pose a significant diagnostic problem, which is compounded by many patients being treated with chemonucleolysis without operative confirmation of the diagnosis before therapy. Axial views show epidural tumor or infection to look much like disc herniation. However, the sagittal view differentiates most epidural tumors and infections because they tend to extend a longer distance along the spine and they are rarely confined to the disc space (Fig. 5.34). One may have more difficulty differentiating them from migrating fragments, but the latter tend to be more localized masses. It should be possible, using high-quality sagittal images, to distinguish nearly all tumors and infections, or at least to raise the consciousness of the referring physician so that on these high-risk patients chemonucleolysis is not the primary treatment.

Two very rare nonneoplastic conditions that can easily be mistaken for disc sequestration are ganglion cyst and localized nodular swelling of the roots. Figure 5.35 demonstrates a small high-attenuation density in the right lateral recess. The coronal view reveals that the mass extends down into the S1 neural foramen. This patient was explored, and because of a right S1 radiculopathy, localized expansion of the ganglion was noted. Biopsy failed to reveal neoplasia. A local decompression was performed which relieved the patient's radiculopathy.

Actually, the most common pseudodisc is the anulus fibrosis itself. As previously mentioned, vertebral displacement caused by subluxation or spondylolysis appears on axial CT as a disc bulge or herniation. Similarly, patients with steep lordotic curves seem to have prominent bulging discs. The sagittal view provides the diagnosis in these patients.

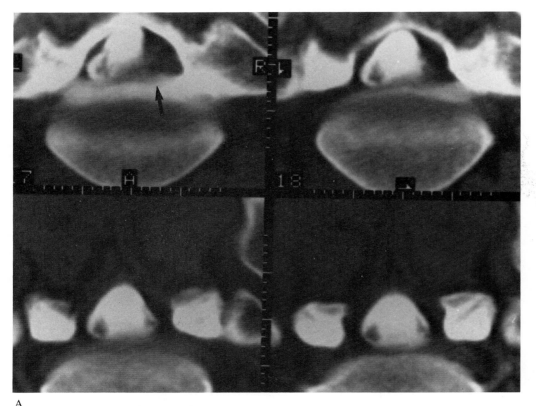

A

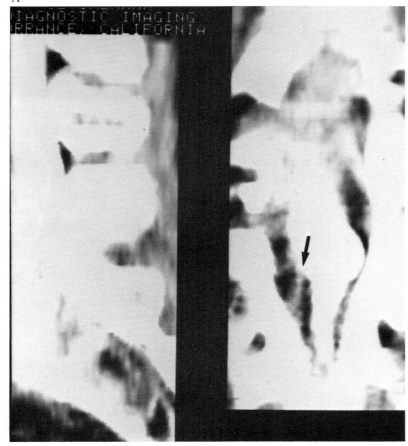

B

FIGURE 5.32 Asymmetrical nerve roots. **A.** Axial metrizamide CT scan showing failure of filling of the right root sleeves (*arrow*). **B.** Coronal reformation demonstrates that the roots on the right lie extradurally, whereas those on the left are intradural. (Reprinted with permission from Rothman SLG, Dobben GD, Rhodes ML, et al: Radiology 150:185–190, 1984.)

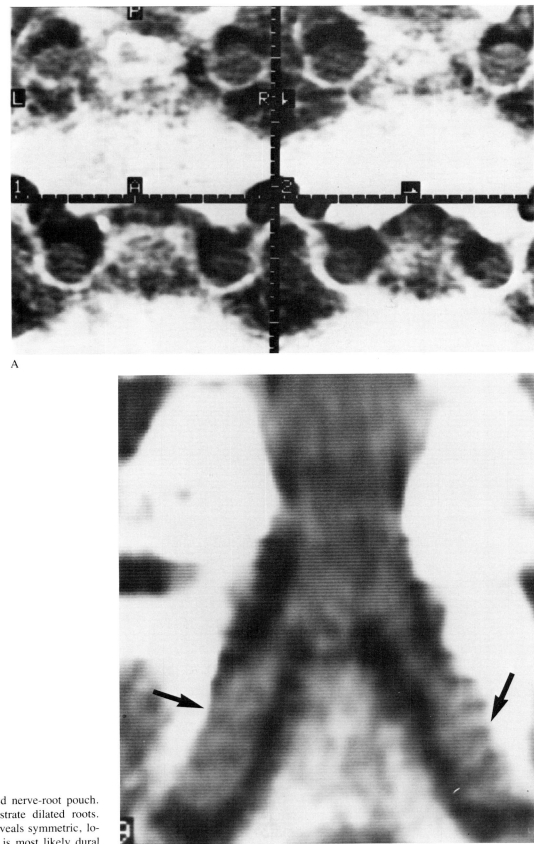

FIGURE 5.33 Dilated nerve-root pouch. **A.** Axial scans demonstrate dilated roots. **B.** The coronal view reveals symmetric, localized dilation, which is most likely dural dilation (*arrow*).

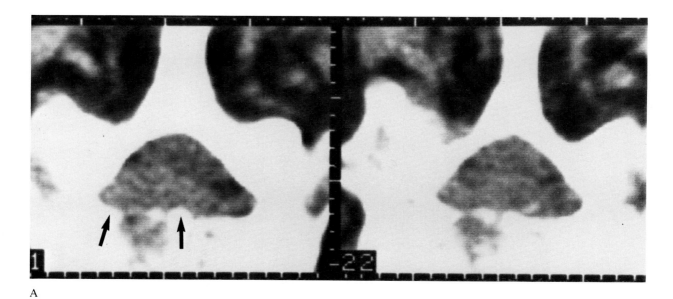

A

B

FIGURE 5.34   Epidural tumor. **A.** Axial view demonstrates a small soft-tissue epidural mass (*arrows*), which looks like a herniated disc. **B.** Sagittal reformations define a long epidural mass behind the vertebral body. This type of picture should strongly suggests tumor.

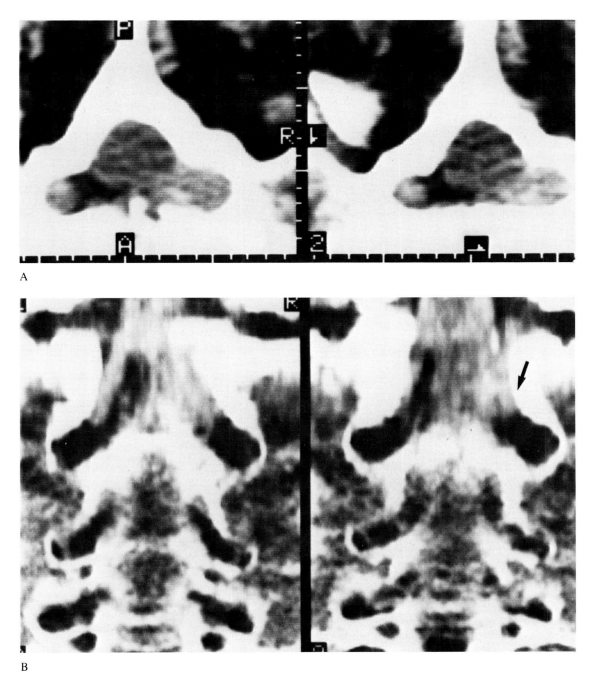

A

B

FIGURE 5.35 Benign expansion of the S1 ganglion. **A.** Axial views demonstrate loss of fat in the right lateral recess by a mass of high density. **B.** Coronal reformation shows this to be localized expansion of the exiting root.

Summary

One of the primary elements of CT spine examination is the careful evaluation of the disc and anulus and their relation to central canal, lateral recesses, and foramina. The fact that CT offers at least as effective an evaluation of disc/anulus abnormalities as does myelography has been documented in the literature.[26–29] The extent to which noninvasive CT becomes the primary diagnostic procedure— and lumbar myelography the secondary diagnostic procedure—depends heavily on the accuracy with which various changes of the disc/anulus can be characterized with CT. We can find no evidence in the literature that the detractors of nonmetrizamide lumbar CT have ever compared complete multiplanar reformation techniques with CT myelography.[30] We hope that this will soon be accomplished, and that most patients can be spared an unnecessary lumbar puncture and instillation of contrast agent.

References

1. Charnley J: The imbibition of fluid as a cause of herniation of the nucleus pulposus. Lancet 1:124-127, 1952
2. Farfan HF: Mechanical Disorders of the Low Back. Lea & Febiger, Philadelphia, 1973
3. Volger JB III, Helms CA, Dorward RH, Wall SD: Variations in the CT appearance of the vertebral end-plates: Schmorl's nodes and other processes. Presented at the 69th Radiological Society of North America meeting, 1983
4. Ramirez H Jr, Navarro JE, Bennett WF: "Cupid's bow" contour of the lumbar vertebral endplates detected by computed tomography. J Comput Assist Tomogr 8:121-124, 1984
5. Schmorl G, Junghanns H: The Human Spine in Health and Disease. Grune & Stratton, New York, 1971
6. Williams AL, Haughton VM, Meyer GA, Ho K-C: Computed tomographic appearance of the bulging annulus. Radiology 142:403-408, 1982
7. Williams AL, Haughton VM: Disc herniation and degenerative disc disease. In Newton TH, Potts DG (eds): Computed Tomography of the Spine and Spinal Cord. Clavadel Press, San Anselmo, 1983, pp. 231-249
8. Chafetz N: Computed tomography of lumbar disk disease. In Genant HK, Chafetz N, Helms CA (eds): Computed Tomography of the Lumbar Spine. University of California, San Francisco, 1982, pp. 125-138
9. Abdullah AF, Ditto EW III, Byrd EB, Williams R: Extreme-lateral lumbar disc herniations: clinical syndrome and special problems of diagnosis. J Neurosurg 41:229-234, 1974
10. Williams AL, Haughton VM, Daniels DL, Thornton RS: CT recognition of lateral lumbar disk herniation. AJNR 3:211-213, 1982
11. Novetsky GJ, Berlin L, Epstein AJ, et al: The extraforaminal herniated disk: detection by computed tomography. AJNR 3:653-655, 1982
12. Williams AL, Haughton VM, Daniels DL, Grogan JP: Differential diagnosis of extruded nucleus pulposus. Radiology 148:141-148, 1983
13. Teplick JG, Haskins ME: CT and lumbar disc herniation. Radiol Clin North Am 21:259-288, 1983
14. Dillon WP, Kaseff LG, Knackstedt VE, Osborn AG: Computed tomography and differential diagnosis of the extruded lumbar disc. J Comput Assist Tomogr 7:969-975, 1983
15. Fries JW, Abodeely DA, Vijungco JG, et al: Computed tomography of herniated and extruded nucleus pulposis. J Comput Assist Tomogr 6:874-887, 1982
16. Larde D, Mathieu D, Frija J, et al: Spinal vacuum phenomenon: CT diagnosis and significance. J Comput Assist Tomogr 6:671-676, 1982
17. Ford LT, Gilvia LA, Murphy WA, Gadom A: Analysis of gas in vacuum lumbar disc. AJR 128:1056-1057, 1977
18. Resnick D, Niwayama G, Guerra J, et al: Spinal vacuum phenomena: anatomical study and review. Radiology 139:341-348, 1981
19. Lindblom K: Discography of dissecting transosseous ruptures of intervertebral discs in the lumbar region. Acta Radiol (Stockh) 36:12-16, 1951
20. Radberg CT: Plain film examination of the spine. In Post MJD (ed): Radiographic Evaluation of the Spine: Current Advances with Emphasis on Computed Tomography. Masson, New York, Publishing USA, Inc., 1980, pp. 424-468
21. Heithoff KB, Burton CV, Salib RM: Computed tomographic evaluation in chemonucleolysis. In Genant HK (ed): Spine Update 1984: Perspectives in Radiology, Orthopaedic Surgery, and Neurosurgery. Radiology Research and Education Foundation, San Francisco, 1983
22. McColloch JA: Chemonucleolysis: state of the art. In Genant HK (ed): Spine Update 1984: Perspectives in Radiology, Orthopaedic Surgery, and Neurosurgery. Radiology Research and Education Foundation, San Francisco, 1983, pp. 127-130
23. Mani JR: Pitfalls in the computed tomographic diagnosis of herniated disc. In Genant HK (ed): Spine Update 1984: Perspectives in Radiology, Orthopaedic Surgery, and Neurosurgery. Radiology Research and Education Foundation, San Francisco, 1983
24. Helms CA, Dorwart RH, Gray M: The CT appearance of conjoined nerve roots and differentiation from a herniated nucleus pulposus. Radiology 144:803-807, 1982
25. Teplick JG, Teplick SK, Goodman L, Haskins ME: Pitfalls and unusual findings in computed tomography of the lumbar spine. J Comput Assist Tomogr 6:888-893, 1982
26. Haughton VM, Eldevik OP, Magnaes B, Amundsen P: A prospective comparison of computed tomography and myelography in the diagnosis of herniated lumbar disks. Radiology 142:103-110, 1982
27. Eldevik OP, Dugstad G, Orrison WW, Haughton VM: Effect of clinical bias on the interpretation of myelography and spinal computed tomography. Radiology 145:85-89, 1982
28. Rashkin SP, Keating JW: Recognition of lumbar disk disease: comparison of myelography and computed tomography. AJNR 3:215-221, 1982
29. Anand AK, Lee BCP: Plain and metrizamide CT of lumbar disk disease: comparison with myelography. AJNR 3:567-541, 1982
30. Dublin A, McGahan JP, Reid MH: The value of computed tomographic metrizamide myelography in the neuroradiological evaluation of the spine. Radiology 146:79-86, 1983

CT of the Sacrum

6

Lesions of the sacrum are among the most difficult to diagnose by routine radiography. It is not uncommon for large destructive lesions to be rendered invisible because of the undulating sacral contours and masking by overlying bowel gas shadows. Sacral CT, however, provides ideal visualization of both bony and parasacral soft-tissue lesions. This brief chapter reviews the normal anatomy of the sacrum and several of the more common abnormalities that involve it and the lumbosacral junction.

Anatomy

The sacrum is a large triangular bone consisting of five fused vertebral segments.[1,2] It sits like a wedge between the iliac bones, which are attached on its two lateral surfaces by two long, irregular, synovial sacroiliac joints. These joints are encapsulated by strong interosseous sacroiliac ligaments. Inferiorly, the pointed apex articulates with the coccyx; superiorly, the broad base articulates with the fifth lumbar vertebra. Its biconcave pelvic surface faces downward and forward. Between the sacral vertebral segments are parallel ridges of cortical bone that mark the planes of fusion between the individual sacral segments. There are four pairs of large, trumpet-shaped ventral sacral foramina through which pass the ventral rami of the first four sacral nerve roots. Lateral to the foramina are the costal elements that unite with each other and fuse to the central vertebral segments. The dorsal surface is biconvex backward and upward. In the midline is relatively smooth median crest

from which emanate three or four spinous tubercles. Below the spinous processes is a small posterior gap (the sacral hiatus), the result of failure of central fusion of the laminae of the fifth sacral segment. Just lateral to the medial sacral crest lie four pairs of small dorsal foramina through which pass the smaller dorsal rami of the sacral roots. Medial to the foramina, immediately below the superior sacral facets, are parallel rows of four small tubercles that represent the fused intrasacral articular process. These tubercles form a ridge called the intermediate sacral crest. Lateral to the foramina are a second row of tubercles that arise from the fused transverse processes. These tubercles make up the lateral sacral crest.

The lateral surface of the sacrum is formed medially by fused transverse processes and laterally by the costal elements, and it is much broader superiorly than inferiorly. The flat, smooth, ear-shaped auricular surface anteriorly articulates with the ilium. The posterior rough portion serves as the attachment for the ligaments. Within the sacrum lies the sacral canal, through which descend the sacral and coccygeal nerve roots, the meninges, and the filum terminale, which descends through the sacral hiatus to the coccyx. The upper four sacral roots exit through the four pairs of foramina. The fifth sacral roots exit between the sacrum and the coccyx.

The tapering sacral canal is triangular in the upper segments and flat or crescentic in the lower levels (Fig. 6.1). The dural sac usually terminates within the sacrum, but this is variable. When the thecal sac ends at or above the L5–S1 disc space there is a large amount of epidural

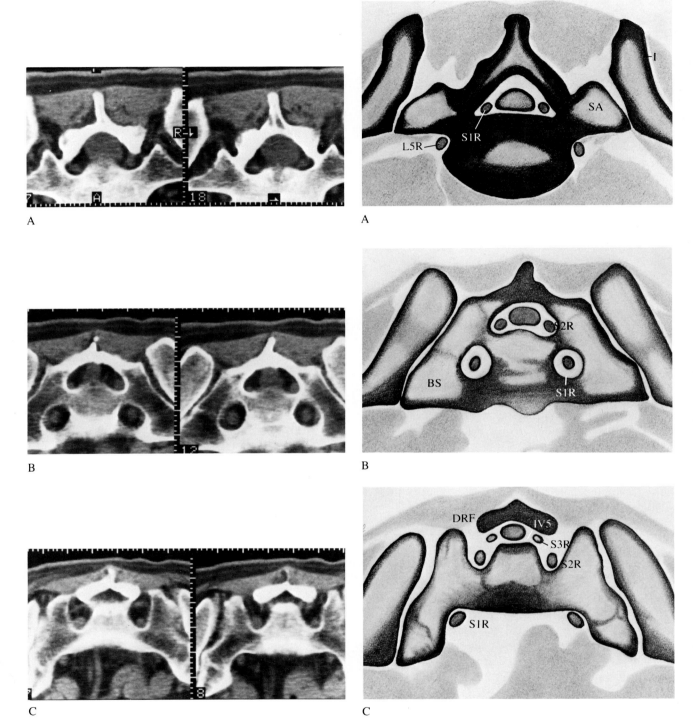

FIGURE 6.1   Normal axial views. **A.** Upper sacrum. **B.** Lower S1 segment. **C.** Upper S2 segment. **D.** S2–3 segment. **E.** S3 segment.

Anatomic key for Figures 6.1–6.3:   (I) iliac bone. (SA) sacral ala. (BS) body of sacrum. (L5R) L5 root. (S1R) S1 root. (S2R) S2 root. (S3R) S3 root.

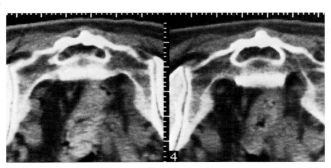

D

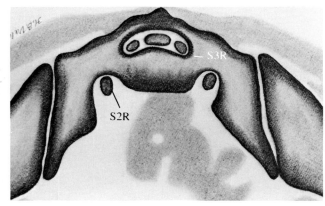

D

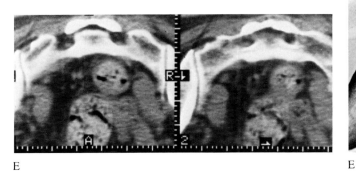

E

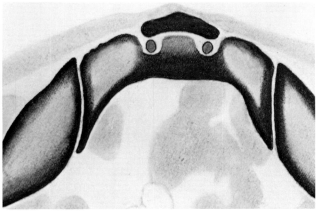

E

fat anterior to the exiting nerve roots. It is in these cases that myelography is normal in the face of rather marked disc herniation (Fig. 6.2).

The base of the sacrum is formed by the osseous endplate of the superior sacral segment. In cross section the first sacral body is almost indistinguishable from that of L5. The anterior surface (the promontory) is convex. The posterior surface is flat or convex. The sacral canal is triangular at this level because of the short pedicles. There is great variability in the size, shape, and direction of sacral facets (Fig. 6.3). In most patients the facets are oriented 45–60 degrees to the midsagittal plane. The costal elements and transverse processes fuse to form the sacral ala.

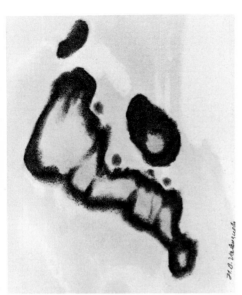

A

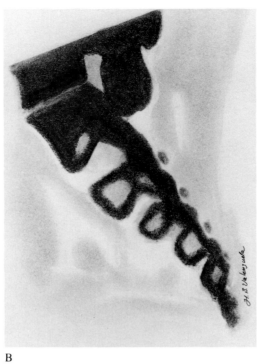

B

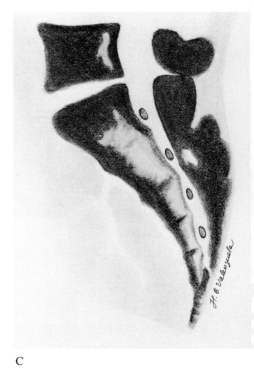

C

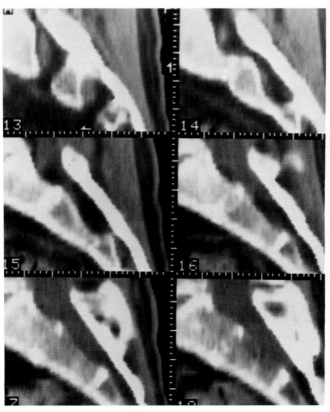

D

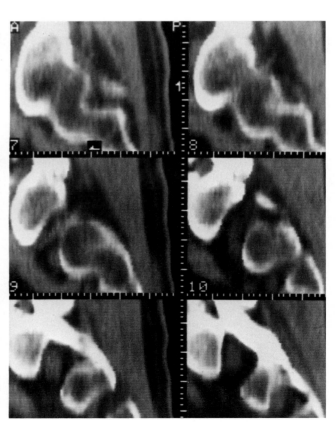

E

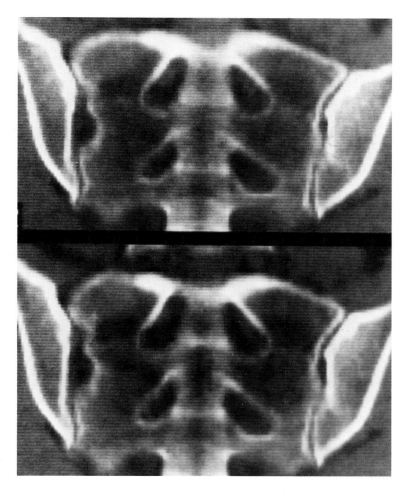

FIGURE 6.2 Normal sagittal views. **A.** Far lateral view. **B.** Lateral sagittal view through exit foramina. **C.** Sagittal view just off the midline. **D, E.** Twelve comparable sequential sagittal images.

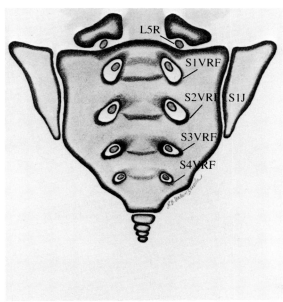

A

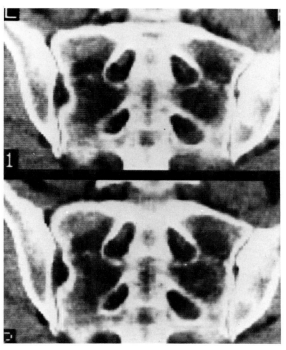

FIGURE 6.3 Normal coronal views. **A.** Coronal view through ventral root foramina. **B.** Central coronal view. **C.** Coronal view through dorsal root foramina. (*Figure continued* on page 162.)

A

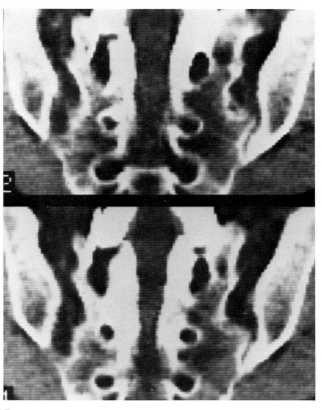

B

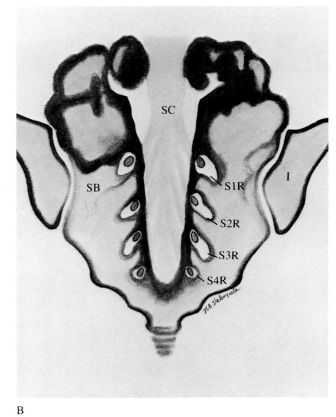

B

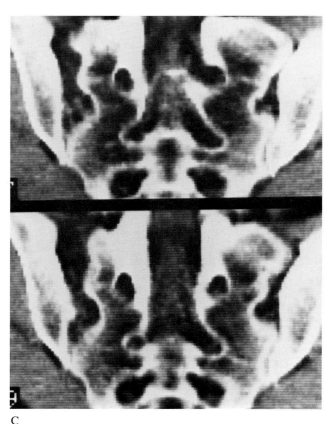

C

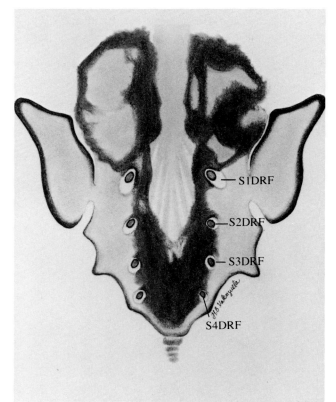

C

FIGURE 6.3 (*cont'd*)   See legend page 161.

CT of the Lumbosacral Articulation

Transitional Vertebral Segments

The lumbosacral articulation is one of the most variable areas in the body. In fact, Vesalius described six rather than five sacral segments as the normal pattern.[3] In most people the sacrum begins with the 25th vertebra, but patients exist with many anatomic combinations: four lumbar vertebra with six fused sacral segments; six lumbar segments with four fused sacral segments; four lumbar segments with a transitional fifth vertebral segment; and five lumbar segments with a sixth transitional lumbosacral vertebra. The terms "lumbarization" of a sacral segment or "sacralization" of a lumbar segment are commonly used, but we prefer the more generic term "lumbosacral transitional vertebra." These anatomic variations can be of considerable clinical significance, mainly because fused transitional segments alter the biomechanical stability of the base of the spine. This is most obvious in the clinical setting of degenerative spondylolisthesis. Degenerative subluxation occurs most often in patients with transitional lumbosacral vertebrae. Disc herniation is also more common at the level above a fused transitional lumbosacral vertebra. Lumbari-

zation or sacralization may be unilateral or bilateral, asymmetrical or symmetrical.

For the radiologist evaluating CT scans, a simple practical problem commonly arises: At which level is the disc herniation? How should we accurately communicate to our surgical colleagues the appropriate level to operate for patients in whom there may be legitimate ambiguity because of an anatomic variation? This problem is compounded on CT, because we are looking at very similar-appearing cross-sectional slices rather than an overview, as in a frontal radiograph of the spine. Even the digital ScoutView may not help when the lowest ribs are difficult or impossible to identify. A simple rule is to be very precise with anatomic discription. First, one must clearly indicate that there is a transitional vertebra and that, for the purpose of the scan, the counting begins from the lowest visible disc space. Accurate description of the lowest disc space includes a comment as to its relationship to the iliac crest, and it describes the relative size of the transverse processes. Counting up from this carefully described disc space allows the surgeon to correlate the CT report with the patient's routine radiographs and eliminates the possibility of operating at the wrong level.

A typical example of a symmetrically articulated transitional lumbosacral vertebra is shown in Figure 6.4. Note

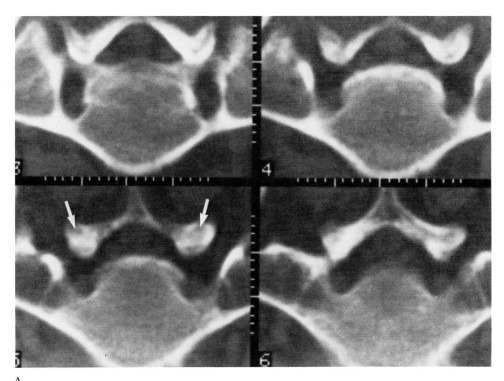

A

FIGURE 6.4 Symmetrical transitional vertebra. Axial view (**A**) and sagittal reformation (**B**) demonstrate a narrow, fused, transitional L5–S1 vertebral segment. The facets are hypoplastic and fused (*arrows*). The transverse process resembles the top of a normal S1 segment. (*Figure continued* on page 164.)

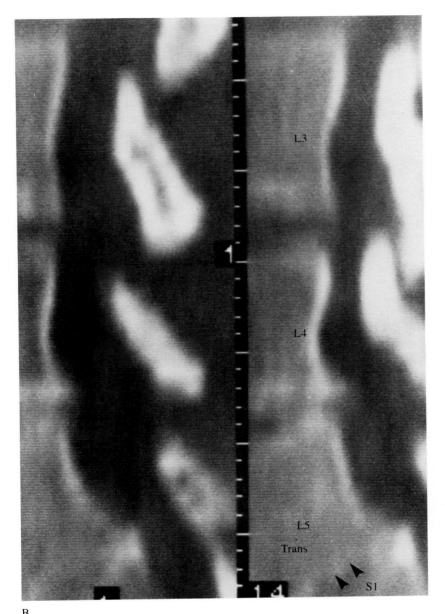

B

FIGURE 6.4 (*cont'd*)   **B.** Sagittal reformation.

the large transverse processes and hypoplastic facets. The disc space is diminutive but not diseased. Figure 6.5 shows an asymmetric transitional vertebra. Note that one transverse process is similar to a lumbar vertebra and one is similar to the sacrum. Coronal reformation demonstrates a neural foramen on one side. A true pseudarthrosis develops in some individuals, and degenerative spurs that can compress the exiting nerve root may form (Fig. 6.6).

Transitional vertebral segments are occasionally associated with congenital deformities in adjacent vertebra. The patient in Figure 6.7 has a transitional lumbosacral articulation. The lowest two lumbar segments are congenitally fused. Above the fusion there is degenerative narrowing that has caused the formation of a lateral osseous bridge.

Facet Anatomy

There is great variability in the size, shape, and direction of the lumbosacral facets. In the majority of patients the facets are obliquely oriented, measuring 45–60 degrees (Fig. 6.8A). Examples exist where the surfaces of the facets lie

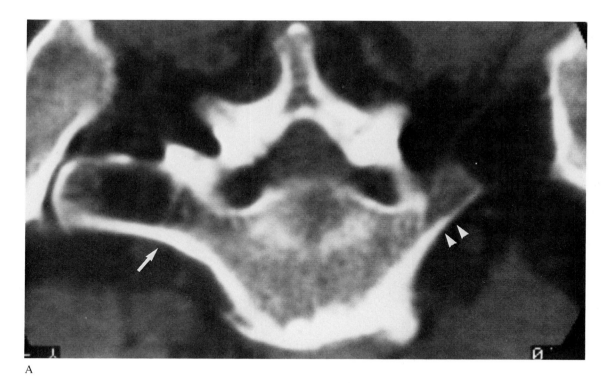

A

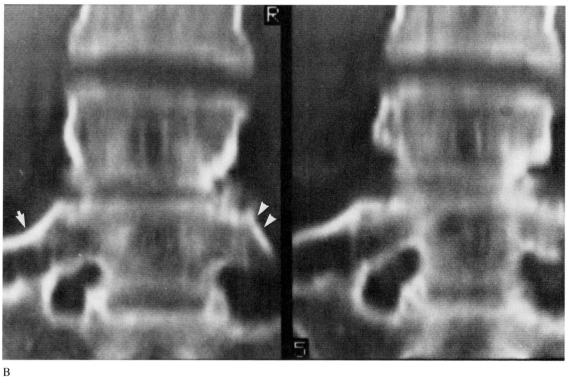

B

FIGURE 6.5 Asymmetrical transitional vertebra. Axial view (**A**) and coronal reformation (**B**). The left transverse process resembles a sacral vertebral segment (*arrow*). The right transverse process resembles a lumbar segment (*arrowheads*). There is a well-formed bony foramen surrounding the distal portion of the exiting nerve root on the side of the broad transverse process. (*Figure continued* on page 166.)

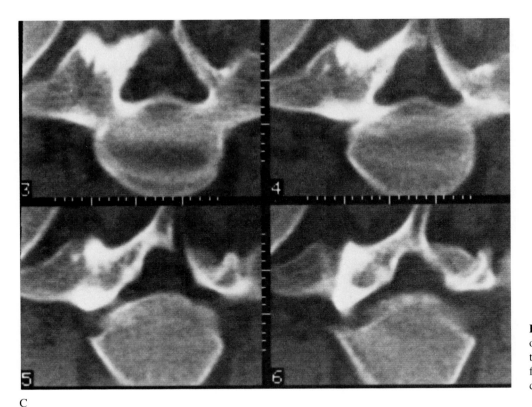

C

FIGURE 6.5 (*cont'd*) **C.** Another patient with asymmetrical transitional vertebra. Note a well-formed right-sided articular pair and dense left-sided bony fusion.

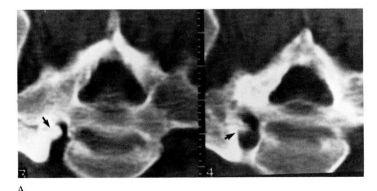

A

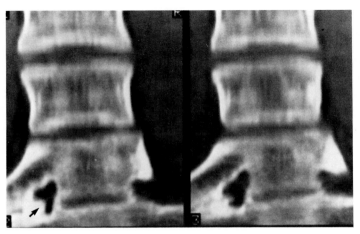

B

FIGURE 6.6 Pseudarthrosis. Axial view (**A**) and coronal reformation (**B**). Degenerative spurs have developed at the site of lateral pseudarthrosis of the transverse process. These spike-like projections may compress the exiting nerve root.

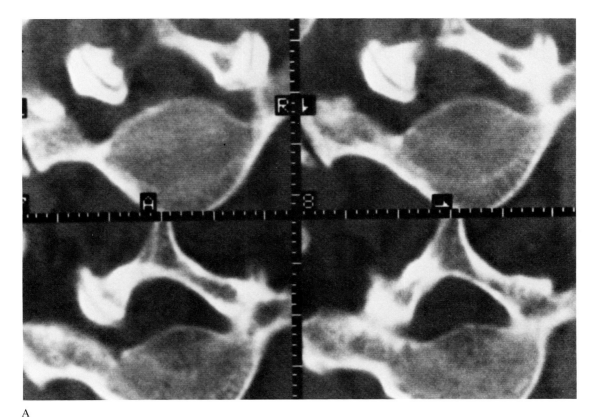

A

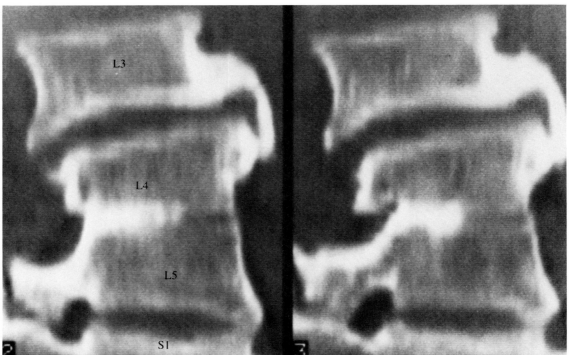

B

FIGURE 6.7 Asymmetrical transitional vertebra with congenital fusion above. **A.** Axial scan demonstrates asymmetrical transverse processes and facets. **B.** Coronal reformation reveals the transitional segment, as well as congenital fusion of the lower two lumbar segments. There is degenerative narrowing of the interspace above the congenital fusion, with a large buttressing lateral osteophyte.

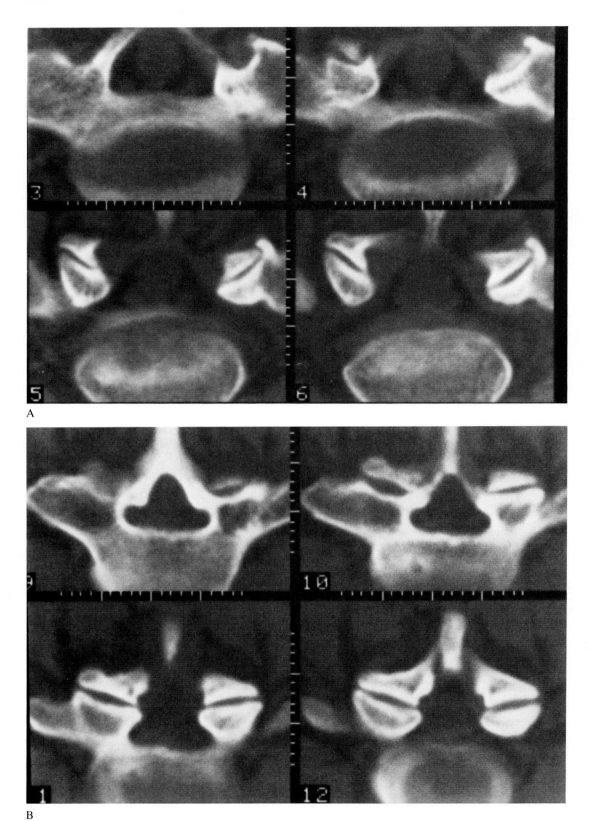

FIGURE 6.8 Variations in facet orientation at the lumbosacral junction. **A.** The usual situation, where the facets are obliquely oriented. **B.** Coronally oriented facets. **C.** Sagittally oriented facets. **D.** Asymmetrical facets (facet tropism).

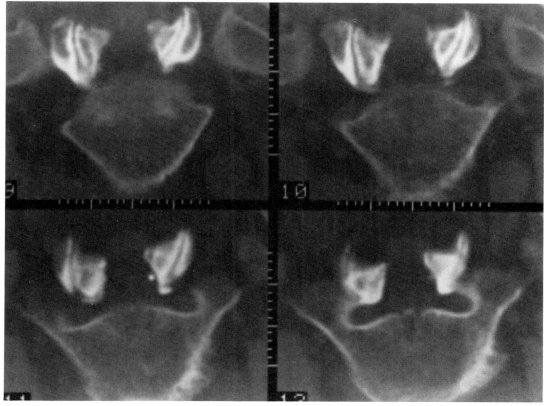

C

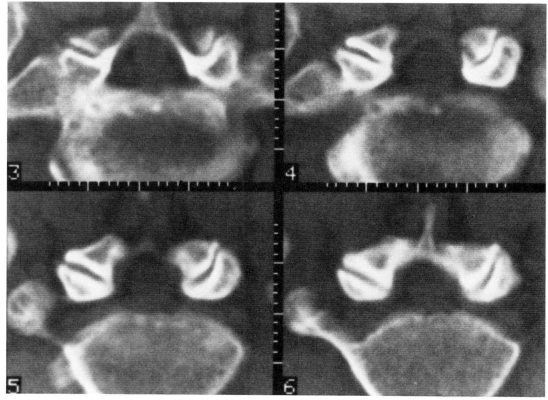

D

almost totally in coronal orientation (Fig. 6.8B) and, more rarely, in nearly sagittal orientation (Fig. 6.8C). Facet tropism (asymmetry of angulation) is relatively common at this level (Fig. 6.8D). The anatomic orientation of the facets correlates with various clinical disorders. Sagittal orientation and facet tropism are associated with disc herniation and degenerative spondylolisthesis. Coronal facet orientation is associated with lateral-recess stenosis caused by compression of the descending S1 root between the flat coronally oriented superior facet and the vertebral body of L5. The entire shape of the neural canal is related to the roundness of the vertebral body and the orientation of the facets. Note that in patients with coronally oriented facets the laminae produce a more markedly trefoil spinal canal. It is in these patients that lateral stenosis occurs. In patients with sagittally oriented facets the neural canal is much more round, the lateral recesses do not have a trefoil appearance, and the roots do not become entrapped.

It is important to realize that lateral stenosis is exceedingly rare in some anatomic forms of the spinal canal. One should not be tempted to describe spinal stenosis when no anatomic deformity exists. *Not all small spinal canals*

are "stenotic." The diagnosis of "spinal stenosis" on a CT report tempts the surgeon to perform facetectomy as part of his decompressive operation. We must not suggest by our report that this will be useful when the facets are not actually causing root compression. Removing all or part of the facets unnecessarily may lead to spinal instability or stress fracture, two clinically significant iatrogenic complications.

It was observed in our series of 450 patients with spondylolysis that the superior articular facets of the sacrum were often unusually short when compared with patients without spondylolysis (Fig. 6.9). The facets above the pars defect tended to be prominent and broad. It is interesting to speculate that the fulcrum of rotation of the neural arch, which is usually drawn through the center of the pars interarticularis, may be unusually low in patients prone to pars fracture. Consequently, the stress on the pars might be greater than normal during flexion.

Neural arch abnormalities of L5 are also associated with facet asymmetry and transitional lumbosacral articulation. This type of deformity is commonly noted in patients with unilateral spondylolisthesis (Fig. 6.10).

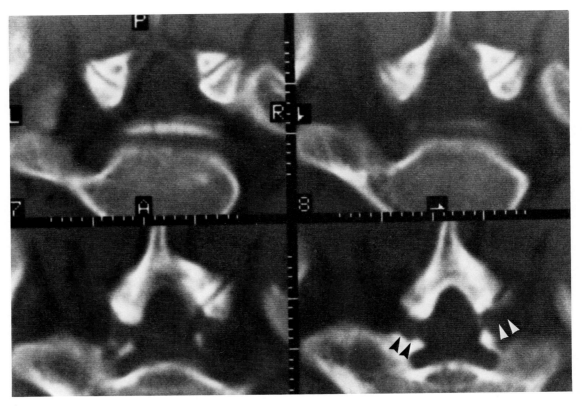

A

FIGURE 6.9   Facets in spondylolysis. **A.** Axial scan revealing a small but otherwise normal articular process (*arrows*) and typical pars interarticularis defects (*arrowheads*). **B.** Sagittal view through the left pars interarticularis defect (*arrowheads*). There is an unusually short superior sacral facet (*arrows*). **C.** Sagittal view of a normal S1 facet, for comparison.

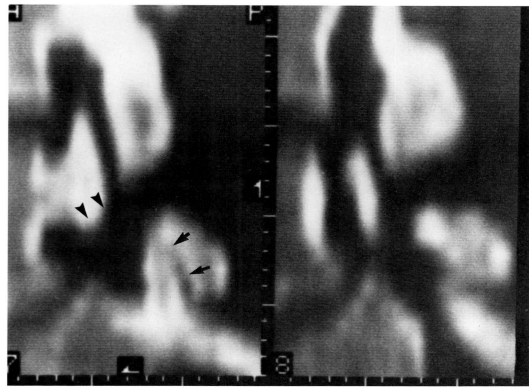

B

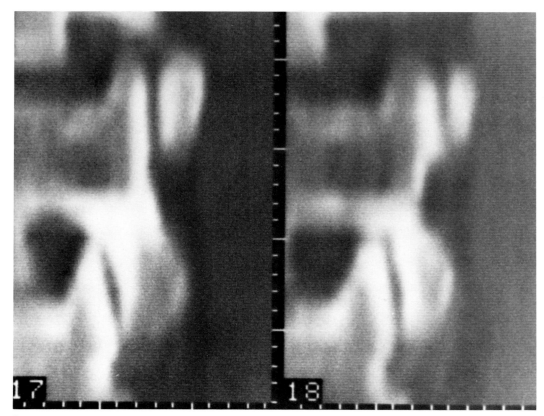

C

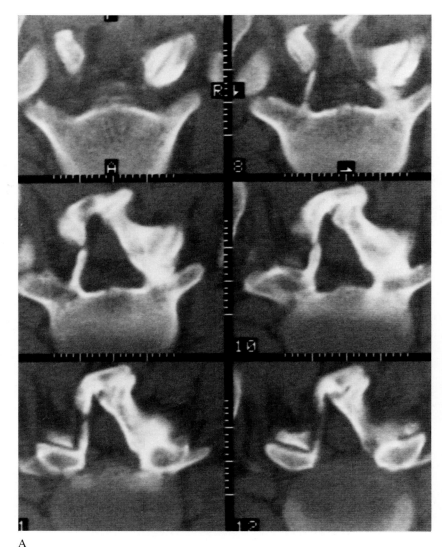

A

FIGURE 6.10 Anomalous lumbosacral facets. **A.** Unilateral spondylolysis, with associated deformity of the neural arch and spina bifida occulta. The left facet is markedly hypoplastic, as compared with the right. **B.** Asymmetry of the posterior elements associated with deformity of the right facet (*arrow*). **C.** Facet tropism, with multiple ossification centers for the S1 superior articular process. (*Figure continued on pages 173, 174.*)

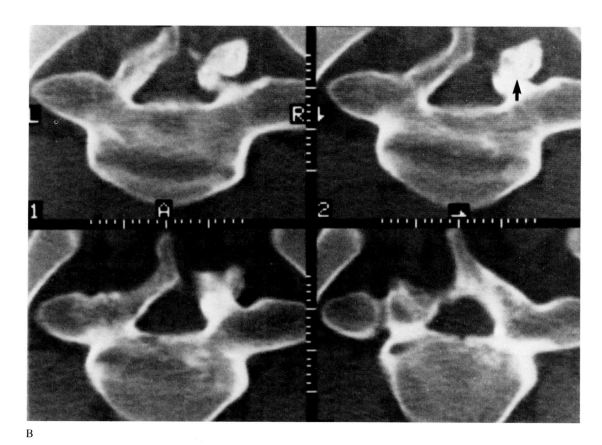

B

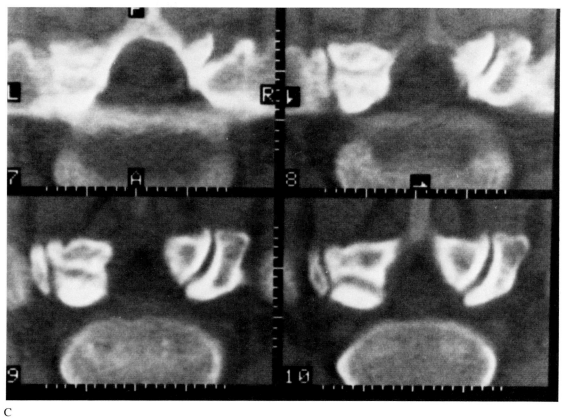

C

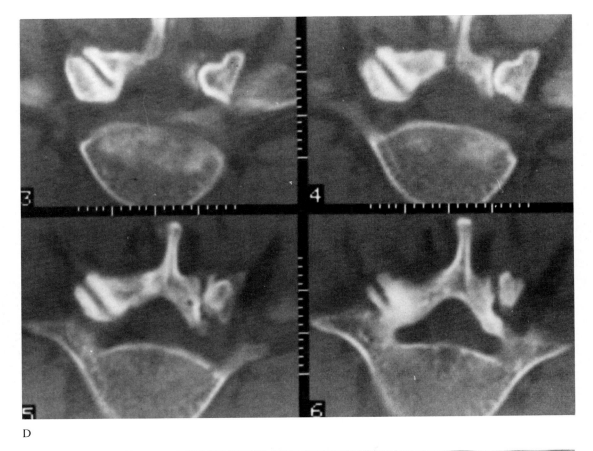

D

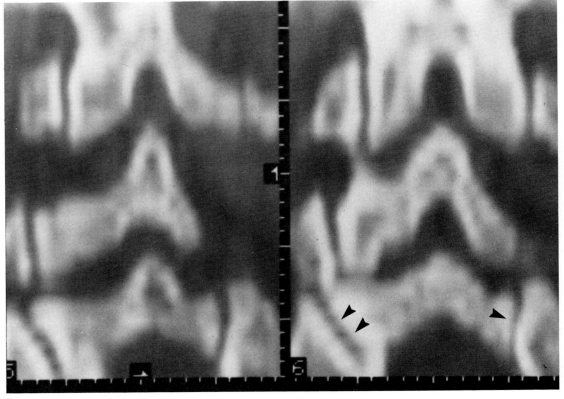

E

FIGURE 6.10 (*cont*
Axial view (**D**) and
ronal reformation
demonstrating facet tr
ism, with deformity a
malrotation of the right
ticular processes.

Bifid Spine and Neural Arch Anomalies of the Lumbosacral Level

The vertebral arch of the first sacral segment is often rudimentary, and it is occasionally developed unilaterally. The two halves may nearly meet in the midline at the same level, but occasionally they are at different levels (Fig 6.11A). A separate spinous process ossification center is sometimes seen within the posterior cleft (Fig. 6.11B). Although there is no established causal relationship between spina bifida occulta and disc herniation syndromes, Gillespie[4] found the incidence of spina bifida three times more common in his series of patients with operated discs than in the general population. There is also a well-established relationship between spondylolysis and neural arch defects of the lumbosacral junction.

More severe forms of spinal dysraphism are frequently associated with meningocele, myelocele, and intradural lipomatous lesions. The most severe cases present early in life, but small sacral lipomas with tethered spinal cord and roots frequently present during adult life because of increasing neurologic deficit (Fig 6.12). This topic is discussed in greater detail later in the chapter.

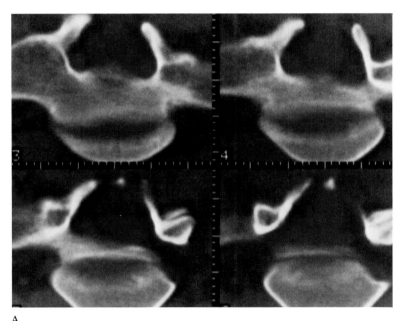

A

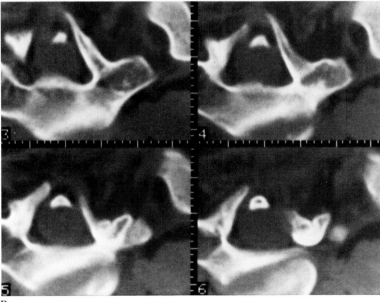

B

FIGURE 6.11 Spina bifida occulta. **A.** Wide central bifid spine. **B.** Wide bifid spine with central spinous process ossification center. (*Figure continued on page 176.*)

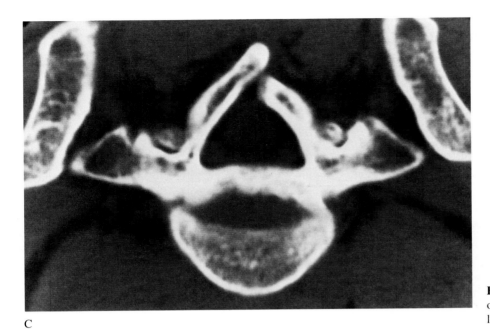

C

FIGURE 6.11 (*cont'd*) **C.** Spina bifida occulta. The two halves meet at different levels off the midline.

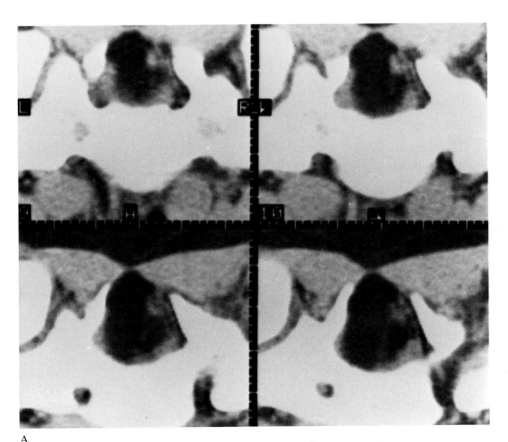

A

FIGURE 6.12 Intradural lipoma. **A.** Axial scan demonstrating a large intradural lipoma associated with tethered nerve roots. **B, C.** Sagittal and coronal views on the same patient

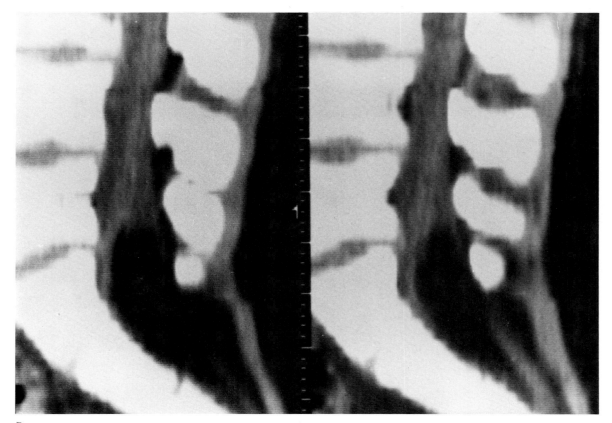

B

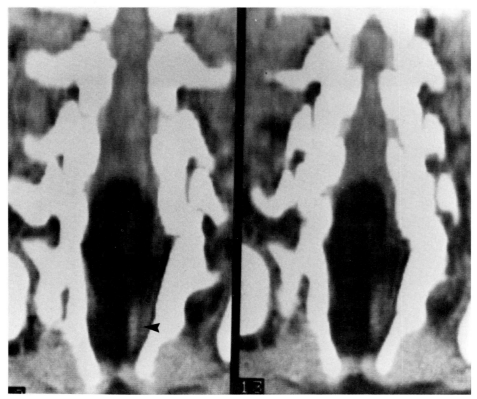

C

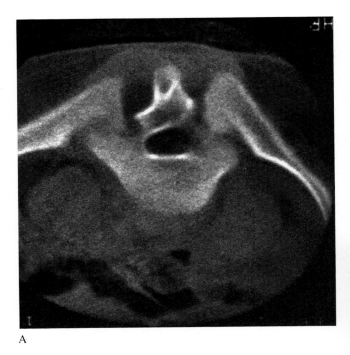

A

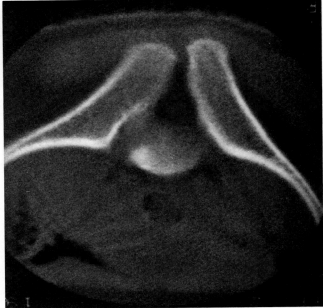

B

FIGURE 6.13 Sacral agenesis. **A, B.** CT at the L5 level reveals marked narrowing of the spinal canal. L5 articulates with the iliac wings in an abnormal manner. Lower down, the two iliac wings articulate with each other. (Reprinted with permission from Naidich et al.[6]).

Major congenital abnormalities of the sacrum are uncommon and generally manifest early in life. Total sacral agenesis presents most commonly at or soon after birth, associated with a variety of orthopedic deformities, neurologic deficits, and urologic dysfunctions. Types defined by Renshaw[5] are: type I—total or partial unilateral sacral agenesis; type II—partial sacral agenesis with symmetrical defect and a stable articulation between the iliac bones and a normal or hypoplastic S1; type III—variable lumbar and total sacral agenesis, with the ilia articulating with the lowest existing vertebra; and type IV—variable lumbar and total sacral agenesis, with the lowest vertebra resting on fused ilia (Fig. 6.13).[6]

Minor developmental anomalies of the sacrum may cause diagnostic problems. The patient in Figure 6.14 was involved in an automobile accident. An axial-only lumbar CT scan was misinterpreted as demonstrating a fracture of the sacrum and a disc herniation. Careful analysis of the images, especially in the coronal view, define a partial failure of fusion of the S1 vertebral segment. The cleft is asymmetrical, extending toward the left S1 anterior neural foramen. Note the asymmetry of the two halves of S1 and the neural foramina. The most important finding on the axial scan is that the neural arch is intact. This certainly excludes the possibility that this is a traumatic lesion. The peculiar appearance of the disc space is due to soft tissue that fills the bony defect between the two nonfused sacral ossification centers. The same end-plate deformity is found in patients with "butterfly" vertebrae at other levels (see Figure 12.11).

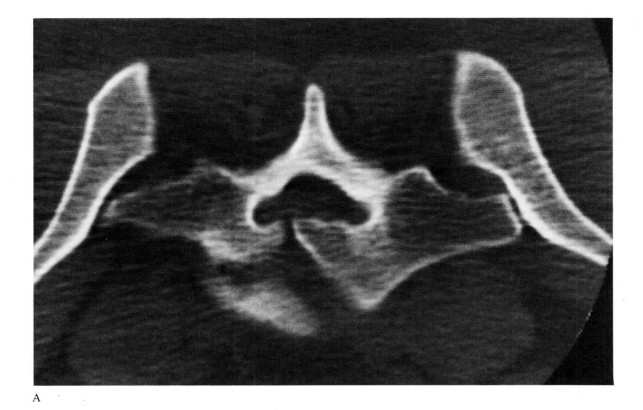

A

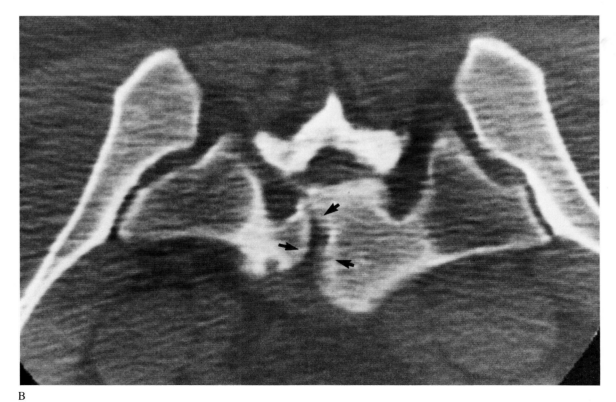

B

FIGURE 6.14 Congenital failure of fusion of the first sacral segment. **A, B.** Axial views demonstrate a well-corticated bony cleft in the S1 segment (*arrows*). The posterior elements are intact. (*Figure continued* on page 180.)

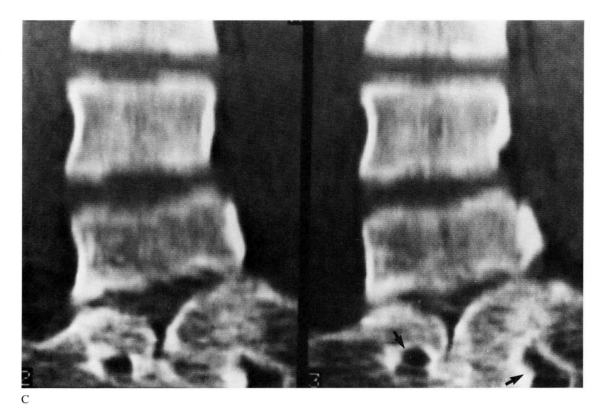

C

FIGURE 6.14 (*cont'd*)   **C.** Coronal reformation shows hypoplasia of the left half of S1. The left neural foramen is smaller than the right half. In the coronal plane, there is no mistaking this for a traumatic lesion.

Compare the appearance of the congenital fusion defect with that of an actual healed sacral fracture (Fig. 6.15). Note the irregularity of the bone defect and the bone sclerosis at the site of healing. Acute fracture of the sacrum must involve the entire body. It must traverse the sacral canal and encompass the posterior elements. Figures 6.15B, C show a recent fracture of the sacrum, with the inferior segments displaced anteriorly.

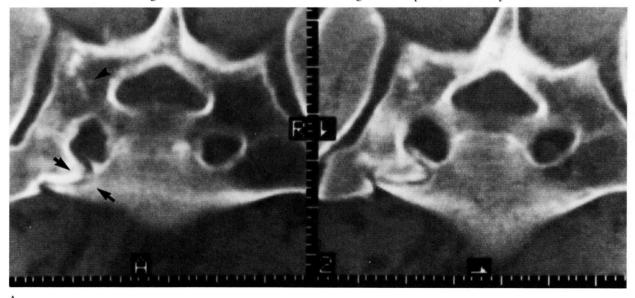

A

FIGURE 6.15   Healed fracture of the sacrum. **A.** There is an old fracture of the left sacrum. The lower portion of the fracture is healed and sclerotic (*arrowhead*). The upper portion is still visible as an irregular lucent line (*arrow*). **B, C.** Axial and sagittal views on a patient with a recent fracture. The inferior segments are displaced forward (*arrows*).

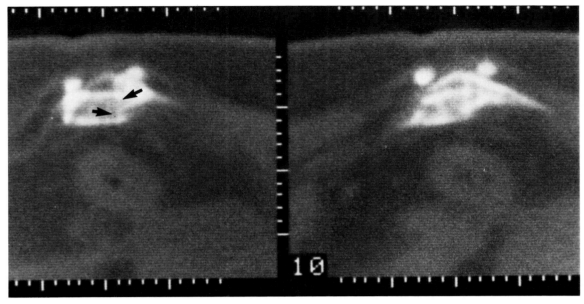

B

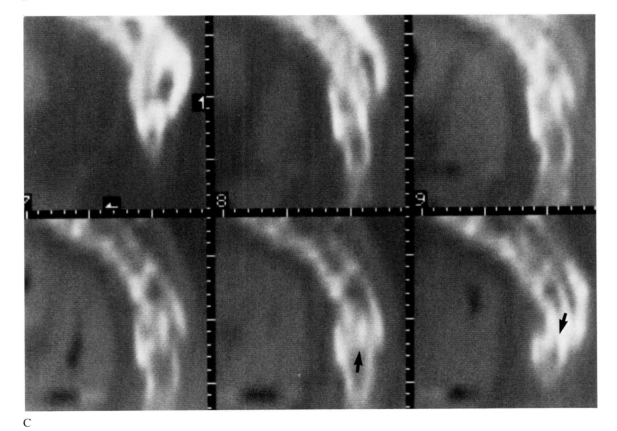

C

Tumors of the Sacrum and Their Differential Diagnosis

Tumors involving the sacral nerve roots or the sacrum may arise within the pelvis, the bone, or the spinal canal. Rectal carcinoma and posterior peritoneal metastasis may produce sizable presacral lesion, which may cause considerable pain. The scan in Figure 6.16 demonstrates a prominent mass behind the contrast-filled colon but in front of the sacrum. This is seen to advantage on the sagittal reformation.

Osseous sacral lesions are most often metastatic. They

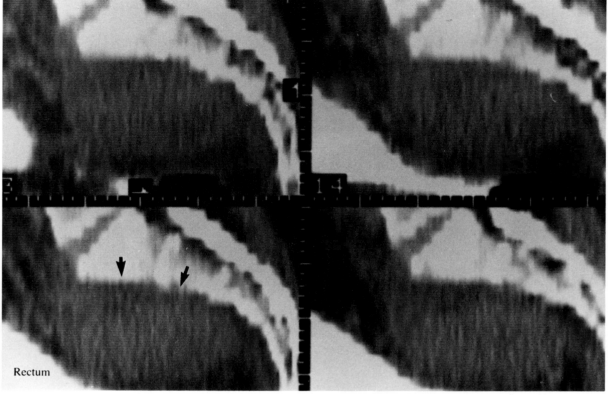

A

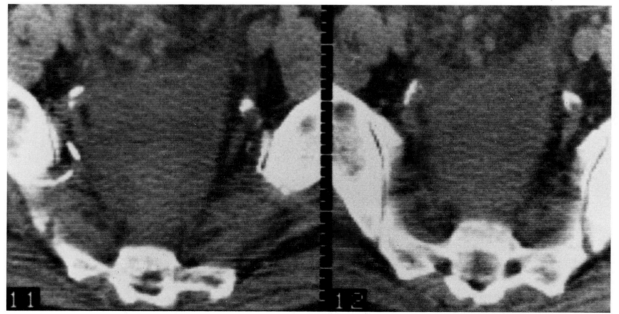

B

FIGURE 6.16   Presacral tumor. Axial view (**A**) and sagittal reformation (**B**) reveal a large soft-tissue tumor mass (*arrows*), which does not invade the sacrum. The colon is filled with water-soluble contrast medium.

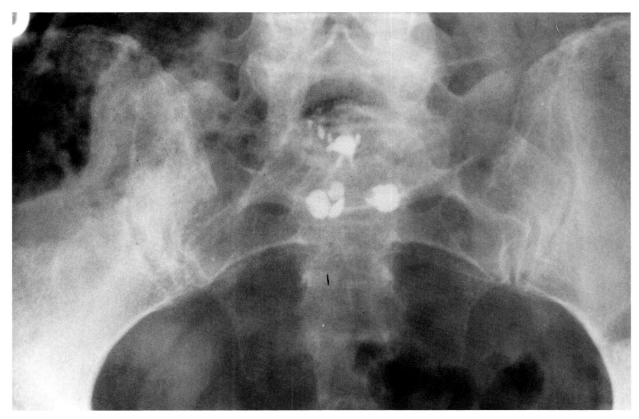

A

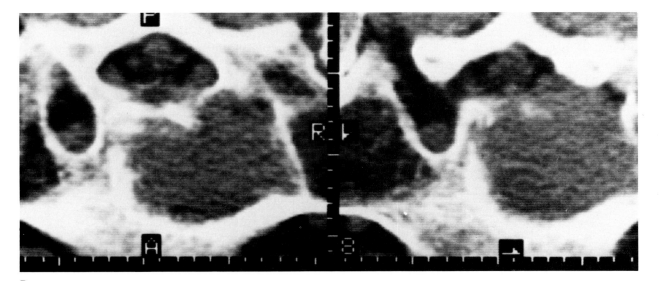

B

FIGURE 6.17   Metastatic sacral lesion. **A.** Radiograph that appears normal; there is no obvious bone destruction. **B.** Axial CT demonstrates a large lytic defect in the sacrum, extending into the right neural foramen. (*Figure continued* on page 184.)

are usually lytic lesions with substantial intrapelvic mass (Fig. 6.17), and they typically cause bone pain. When the tumor mass extends into the neural foramen or to the sacral spinal canal, radiculopathy may ensue. The coronal view is most helpful in defining the relationship of the tumor mass to the descending nerve roots. Osteosarcomas and chondrosarcomas are diagnosed easily because they typically contain abnormal tumorous bone. Estimation of the

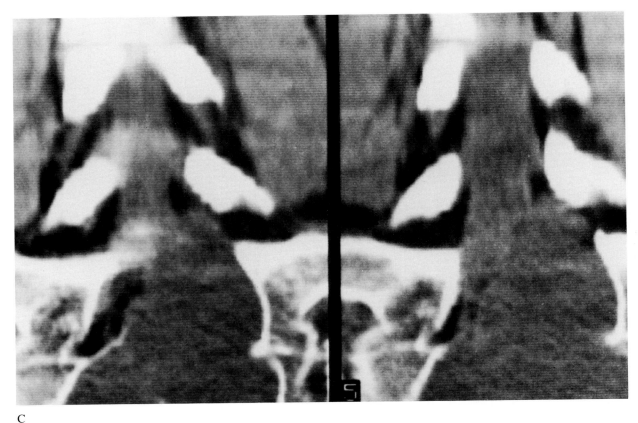

C

FIGURE 6.17 (*cont'd*) **C.** Coronal reformation shows the full extent of the tumor mass. Note the relationship of the mass to the exiting roots.

size and scope of the lesion is crucial when radical resection of a portion of the pelvis is contemplated.

Chordomas involve the bony sacrum as well as the sacral canal and the neural foramina (Fig. 6.18). In some cases the mass may extend ventrally and dorsally through the foramina.[7,8] Neurofibromas and schwannomas that arise from the sacral roots may be unilateral or bilateral. They may extend from the sacral canal through the neural foramina into the pelvis, producing smooth, regular enlargement of the involved foramina. The attenuation values are

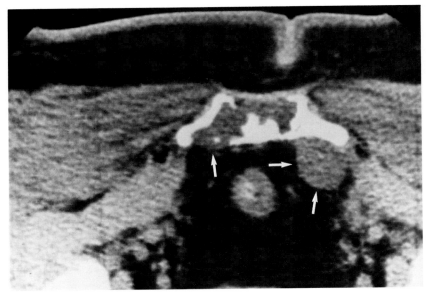

A

FIGURE 6.18 Chordoma. **A, B.** Axial scans demonstrate a soft-tissue intrasacral tumor that is growing through the ventral sacral wall. A small soft-tissue tumor is noted within the pelvis. The aggressive nature of the tumor suggests the diagnosis of chordoma.

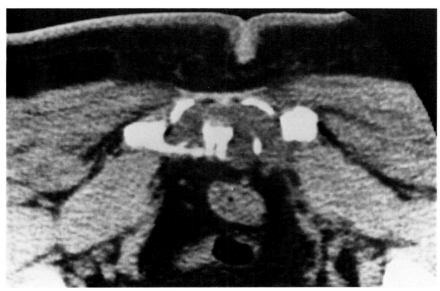

B

usually the same as for the paraspinal musculature. A specific diagnosis of a nerve root or root sheath lesion can be made if only the foramina are expanded by mass without the spinal canal being involved.[7]

Intradural tumors may be so small they cause no bony expansion of the spinal canal. Some patients presenting with radiculopathy due to small masses may be mistakenly operated for disc herniation. Myelography, especially when performed with Pantopaque, may fail to clearly define subtle lesions.

The patient in Figure 6.19 had had two previous spinal operations: disc removal and fusion. He was reevaluated because of continued pain. Metrizamide myelography was misinterpreted as showing a recurrent disc bulge and scar from the previous surgery. A CT scan revealed two discrete tumor nodules in the sacral canal, which proved to be ependymoma. Large, slow-growing intrasacral tumors are usually gliomas; most often they are ependymomas. They typically expand the sacral canal and the exiting neural foramina (Fig. 6.20). The anterior wall of the sacral canal may be scalloped by the enlarging tumor. The attenuation values of these lesions are also similar to those for the paraspinal musculature. This must be contrasted with the one pseudotumor of the sacrum, the intrasacral meningocele.

Intrasacral meningocele is caused by expansion of the dura and arachnoid within the sacral spinal canal. The ectatic dural pouch or pouches frequently behave as mass lesions. The cerebrospinal fluid (CSF) filled sac may displace nerve roots and distort the lower lumbar or lumbosacral roots on a myelogram. The sacral canal is expanded, as are affected neural foramina. The dural pouches may produce large intrapelvic masses that are frequently mistaken for solid tumors. Because the CT attenuation of these pouches is that of CSF rather than of soft tissue, it is often possible to suggest a specific diagnosis from the scans. The patient in Figure 6.21 has a large intrasacral and intrapelvic meningocele. The spinal canal is enlarged, and there is extension of the sac into the pelvis. Myelography performed after the CT scan demonstrates deformity of the theca. As in many examples of this disorder, the neck of the meningocele is very narrow and only a small volume of contrast medium enters the cavity. It is important to realize that films performed immediately after contrast-medium instillation often do not demonstrate any myelographic contrast. Typically, filming must be delayed and follow a period of ambulation in order to completely fill the cavity with contrast medium. Because of this, it is very important that there be a high index of suspicion that a meningocele exists; otherwise, it may be misdiagnosed as a solid tumor.

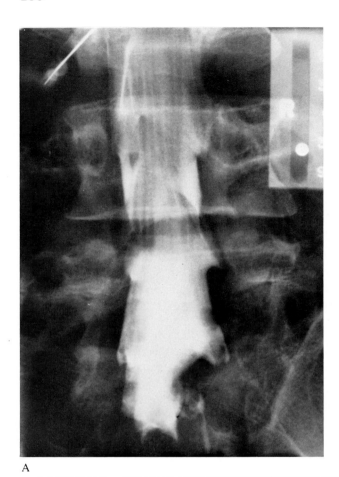

A

FIGURE 6.19 Intradural ependymoma. **A.** Metrizamide myelogram misinterpreted as showing postoperative scarring. **B.** Axial
scans show a well-demarcated soft-tissue mass surrounded by
metrizamide (*arrows*). **C.** Coronal reformation demonstrating at
least two intradural masses (*arrows*). **D.** Sagittal view.

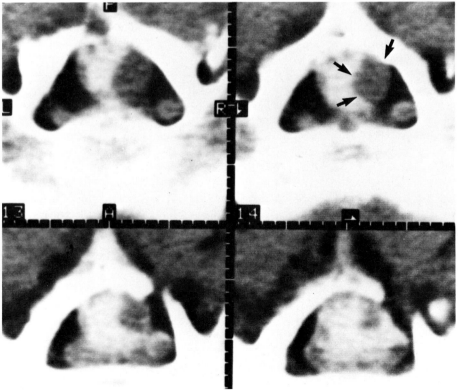

B

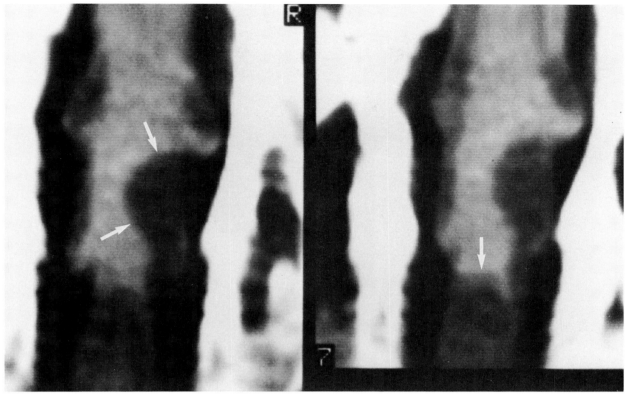

C

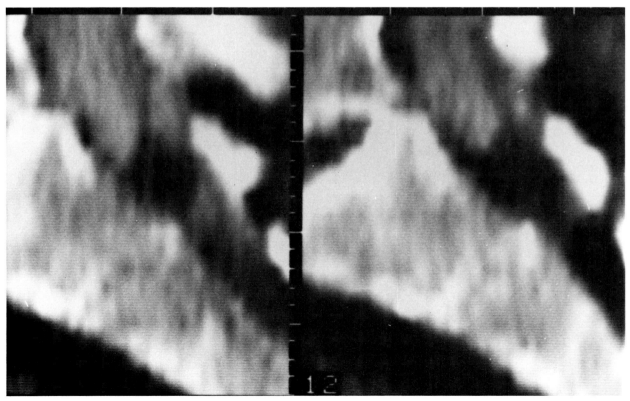

D

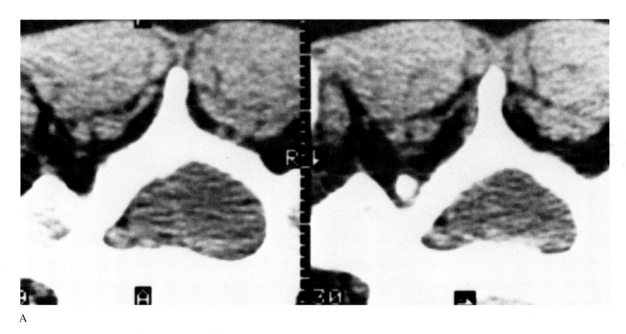

A

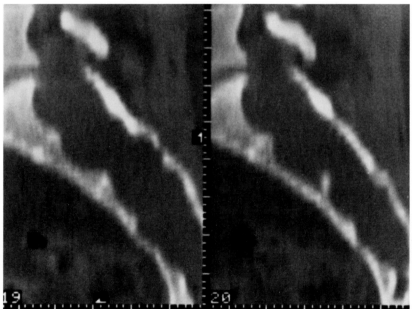

B

FIGURE 6.20 Intrasacral tumor. **A.** Axial views demonstrate asymmetrical widening of the spinal canal by a mass on the right side. **B.** Midsagittal reformations reveal typical scalloping of the sacrum. **C, D.** Coronal reformations show the tumor that expands the sacral canal and neural foramen. Note the normal left S1 root.

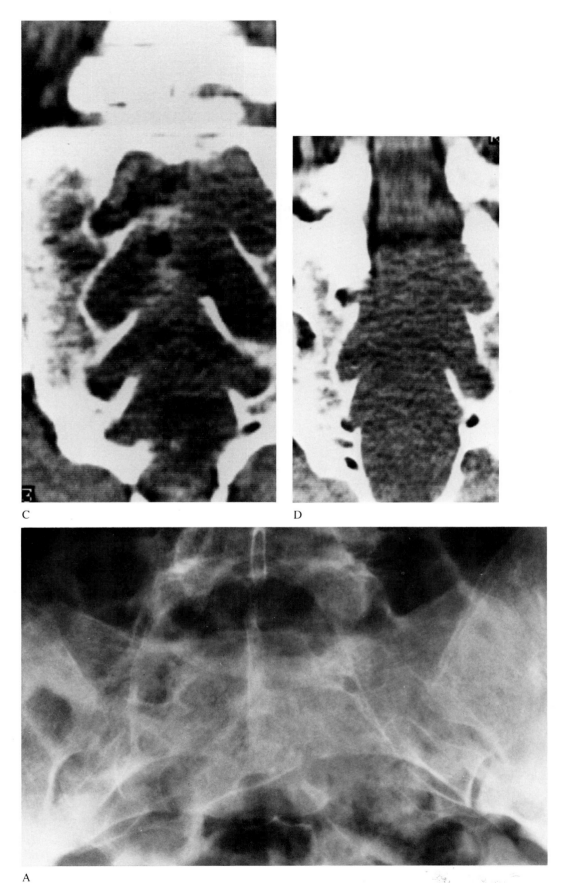

C

D

A

FIGURE 6.21 Intrasacral meningocele. **A.** Radiograph of the sacrum showing subtle asymmetry of the sacral nerve roots. (*Figure continued* on page 190.)

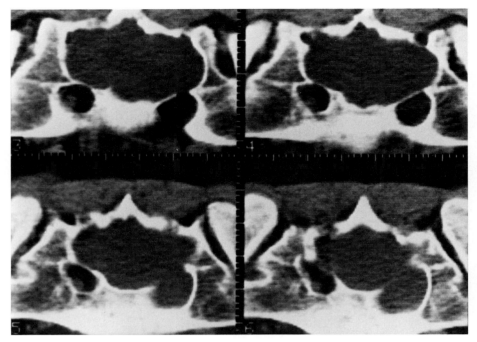

B

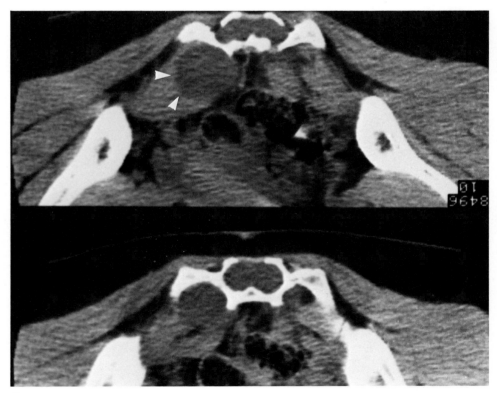

C

FIGURE 6.21 (*cont'd*) **B.** Axial CT. The sacral canal and the right neural foramen are dilated by a mass of low attenuation. **C.** Axial scans through the lower sacrum demonstrate a low-attenuation mass (*arrowheads*) in the parasacral soft tissues. This is an intrapelvic meningocele. **D.** Sagittal view demonstrates an expanded sacral canal with scalloping of the ventral wall. **E, F.** Frontal and lateral metrizamide myelogram performed after the CT diagnosis. Delayed films reveal deviation of the sacral canal to the right and two small contrast collections in the meningocele.

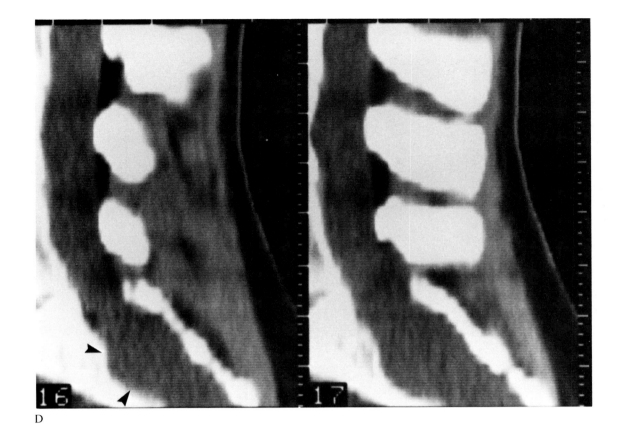

D

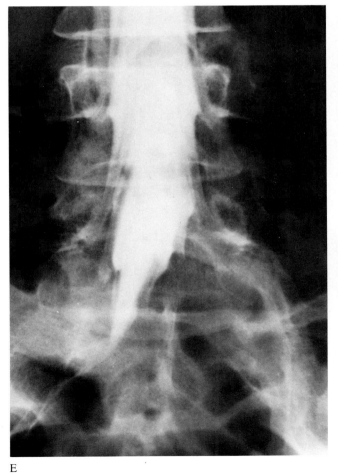

E

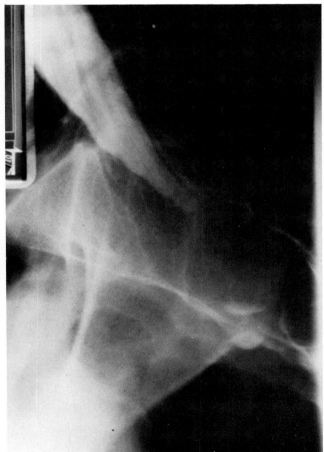

F

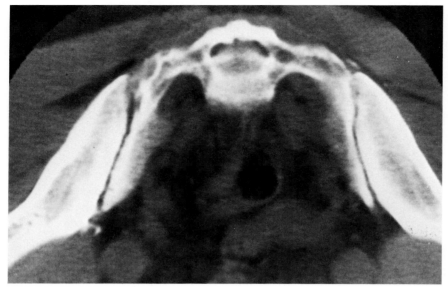

A

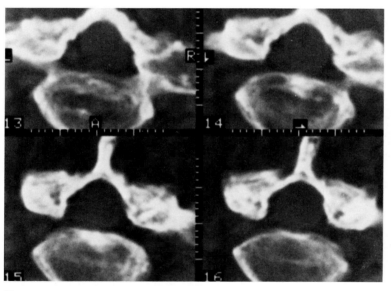

B

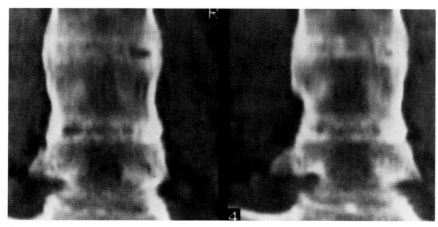

C

FIGURE 6.22 Ankylosing spondylitis.
A. Early changes with subtle erosion of the
periarticular bone. **B.** Axial view shows end-
stage ankylosing spondylitis. Note total fusion of the L5–S1 facets. **C.** Coronal reformation showing total bony ankylosis of
the spine. **D.** Sagittal reformation showing
bony changes of diffuse dural ectasia.

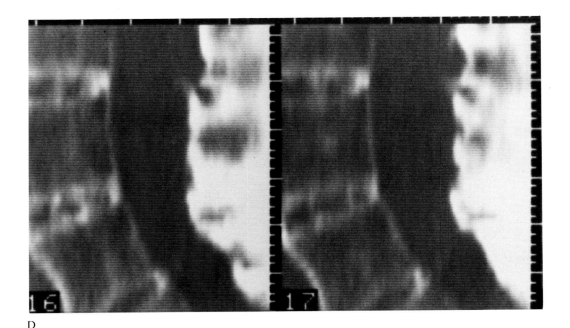

D

Sacroiliac Joint Abnormalities

The sacroiliac joint has two components: a synovial portion and a ligamentous portion. Either may become involved in a variety of arthropathies, the most important of which are the seronegative spondyloarthropathies, ankylosing spondylitis, Reiter's syndrome, psoriatic arthritis, and enteropathic spondyloarthritis.

Sacroiliitis is the hallmark of ankylosing spondylitis. Although it may seem unilateral very early in its clinical course, it most commonly is bilaterally symmetrical in distribution.[9,10] Radiographically and on CT scans the arthropic changes occur most severely on the iliac side of the joint. Earliest changes are those of periarticular demineralization. This is followed by erosion of cortical bone (Fig. 6.22), which is most severe on the iliac side of the joint. Later, the subchondral bone becomes sclerotic. Bony bridges ultimately form across the joint, leading to total bilaterally symmetrical fusion (Fig. 6.22).

Ankylosing spondylitis may be distinguishable from Reiter's syndrome and psoriatic arthritis because of its symmetry. The other seronegative spondyloarthropathies are more likely to be asymmetrical. CT changes within this group of disorders are otherwise nearly indistinguishable (Fig. 6.23).

Degenerative arthritis of the sacroiliac joints is quite different. Changes may be unilateral or bilateral (Fig. 6.24). The joint space narrows because of erosion and degeneration of the cartilage. Although these abnormalities may diffusely involve a joint, localized lesions commonly occur in the inferior portion.[9] Bony erosion is relatively uncommon and, when present, is usually localized. Osteophyte for-

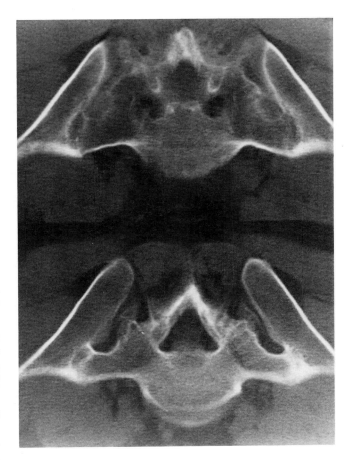

FIGURE 6.23 Reiter's syndrome. Axial views on a patient with symmetrical end-stage Reiter's syndrome. This is indistinguishable from end-stage ankylosing spondylitis.

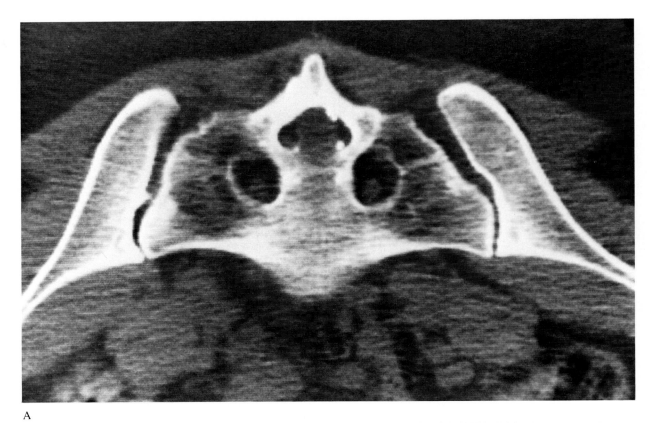

A

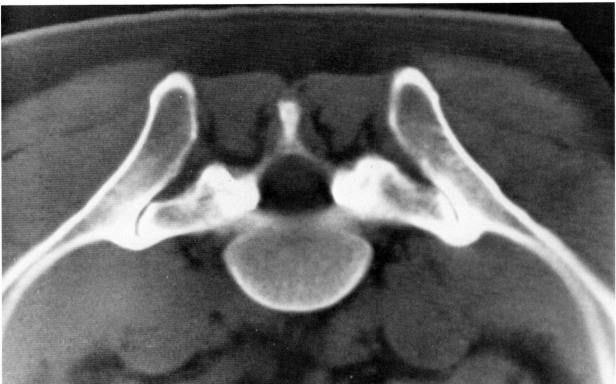

B

FIGURE 6.24   Degenerative arthritis of the sacroiliac joints. **A.** Early changes. **B.** Late periarticular bony ridging across the ligamentous portion of the joint.

mation is common, predominantly at the anterior superior and inferior portions of the joint, when very prominent periarticular bony ankylosis may occur. There may also be ligamentous calcification and ossification.

References

1. Warwick R, Williams PL: Gray's Anatomy, 35th British edition. Saunders, Philadelphia, 1973
2. Whelan MA, Gold RP: Computed tomography of the sacrum: 1. Normal anatomy. AJNR 3:547-554, 1982
3. Vesalius. Quoted in Schmorl G, Junghanns H: The Human Spine in Health and Disease. Grune & Stratton, New York, 1971, p. 60
4. Gillespie H: The significance of congenital lumbosacaral abnormalities. Br J Radiol 22:257, 1949
5. Renshaw TS: Sacral agenesis: classification and review of twenty-three cases. J Bone Joint Surg 60A:373-383, 1978
6. Naidich TB, McLone DG, Harwood-Nash DC: Spinal dysraphism. In Newton TH, Potts, DG (eds): Modern Neuroradiology, Vol. 1: Computed Tomography of the Spine and Spinal Cord. Clavadel Press, San Anselmo, California, 1983, pp. 299-353
7. Whelan MA, Hilal SK, Gold RP, et al: Computed tomography of the sacrum: 2. Pathology. AJNR 3:555-559, 1982
8. Whelan MA: Computed tomography of the sacrum. In Post MJD (ed): Computed Tomography of the Spine. Williams & Wilkins, Baltimore, 1984, pp. 94-118
9. Resnick D, Niwayama G: Diagnosis of Bone and Joint Disorders, Vol. 2. Saunders, Philadelphia, 1981
10. Carrera GF: Sacroiliitis. In Newton TH, Potts DG (eds): Modern Neuroradiology, vol. 1, Computed Tomography of the Spine and Spinal Cord. Clavadel Press, San Anselmo, California, 1983, pp. 281-284

Lumbar Spinal Stenosis
7

Spinal stenosis, which has attracted increasing attention in recent years, represents an important group of clinical and radiologic entities. Recognition and ultimate surgical management of the many abnormalities found in this group require precise preoperative delineation of the morbid anatomy. Conventional radiography and tomography have been very disappointing in providing the necessary deliniation of canal compression. Measurement of the interpeduncular distance, although quite precise on conventional radiographs, is the least important measurement. Midsagittal measurement is very imprecise because of the difficulty in estimating the location of the anterior surface of the laminae. Conventional axial tomography provided the first accurate picture of the sagittal dimension, but it was limited by poor contrast resolution. Computerized tomography[1-3] and ultrasound[4] have finally provided the means for accurate measurement of midsagittal diameter and surface area. It is now possible to provide a preoperative assessment of bony and soft-tissue canal compression and to guide surgical decompression by objective anatomic measurements.

Although there is some disagreement about precise nomenclature of the various syndromes, it is useful to divide spinal stenosis into two broad classes: central and lateral stenosing syndromes. Verbiest in 1949[5] and again in 1954[6] described central canal compression based on the impeded passage of myelographic contrast medium during myelography. Compression of spinal nerve roots within the lateral recess was described in 1955 by Schlesinger[7].

According to Verbiest,[8] true spinal stenosis of the lumbar vertebral canal is a form of compression produced by the walls of the vertebral canal. It involves the whole of the vertebral canal by exerting compression at two of its opposite surfaces. He described two types of stenosis: (1) transport stenosis, wherein the clinical manifestations are due to impeded flow of fluid, which is dependent on the available cross-sectional area of the canal surface of the stenotic structure, and (2) compressive stenosis, which includes abnormal compression of opposing surfaces only. According to these definitions, indentation on the spinal canal by disc protrusion or localized tumor is not considered true spinal stenoses. In this chapter we discuss only those conditions that produce true canal stenosis. Soft-tissue lesions that compress neural structures but are unrelated to canal narrowing are excluded.

Congenital Stenosis

The term "congenital stenosis" is limited to those cases where narrowing of the spinal canal is related to or is part of congenital malformation of the lumbar spine. It may be associated with spina bifida, diastematomyelia, or other localized malformations. The classic example of congenital stenosis is achondroplasia, which is characterized by a defect in enchondral bone formation and includes the entire spine (Fig. 7.1). The spine presents with a long kyphotic curve and an accentuated lordosis. The pedicles are short because of the defect in enchondral growth. The anteroposterior diameter of the spinal canal is reduced dramatically to about one-half its normal size. Typically, the interpeduncular distance diminishes at each successively lower spinal site. In this disorder both the midsagittal and interpeduncular distances are reduced severely. Epidural fat is reduced and the neural structures, which develop normally,

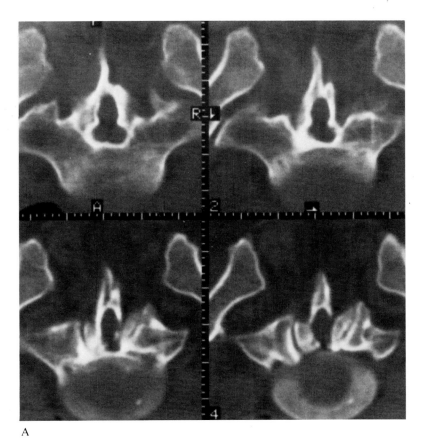

A

FIGURE 7.1 Achondroplasia. **A.** Axial scans reveal the typical deformity of achondroplasia. The lateral diameter of the canal is greatly reduced. This can be most easily proved by measuring the interpedicular distance. **B.** Coronal view. Note that the spinal canal seems to taper at the lowest lumbar levels. (*Figure continued* on page 198.)

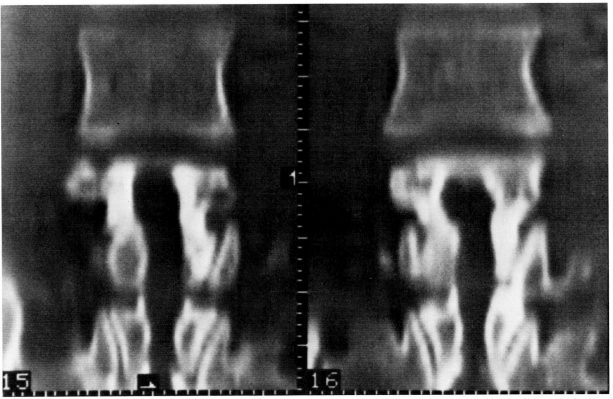

B

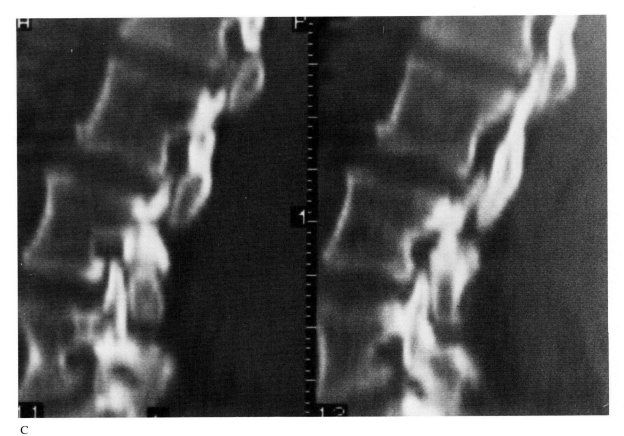

C

FIGURE 7.1 (*cont'd*)   **C.** Sagittal reformation reveals a slightly narrow anteroposterior dimension of the spinal canal.

are disproportionately large compared to the canal size. Very minor degenerative arthritis produces profound neurologic signs and symptoms.

Idiopathic Developmental Spinal Stenosis

Verbiest[9] defined idiopathic developmental spinal stenosis as a disorder of unknown etiology showing a growth disturbance of the bony walls of the vertebral canal during the pre- and postnatal periods. This category specifically excludes congenital lesions. It is characterized by reduction in the sagittal diameter of the spinal canal. The interpeduncular distance is usually normal.

''Absolute stenosis'' is said to occur when the midsagittal diameter is 10 mm or less. In these patients, the cauda equina syndrome or compression may occur. ''Relative stenosis'' is a condition wherein the midsagittal diameter is 10–12 mm (the lowest limits of normal) and the reserve capacity in the spinal canal is so reduced that slight degenerative change may cause symptomatic compression.

When evaluating the sagittal diameter one must consider two distinct CT planes. In the sublaminar plane the posterior wall of the spinal canal is completely bony. In the interlaminar segment the posterior wall is formed primarily by the ligamentum flavum and the medial expansion of the articular processes. Because in normal patients the inner surface of the lamina slopes posteriorly in relation to the anterior wall of the spinal canal, the ratio of the midsagittal diameter of the upper border of the lamina to the lower border of the lamina is less than one. In idiopathic spinal stenosis this ratio may be equal to or greater than one (Fig. 7.2). When measuring these diameters on axial scans, it is important that the plane of section be perpendicular to the vertebral end-plates and that measurements be made at the caudal and cephalad ends of the lamina. When measurements are made on sagittally reformatted images, the specific canal deformity and the midsagittal diameter ratios can be measured. More important, in the sagittal plane one can actually measure the narrowest point of the spinal canal, wherever it may be.

Scans through the articular processes demonstrate hypertrophy and degeneration of the facet surfaces and disc or anulus bulging. The severity of symptomatic stenosis is usually related to the secondary degenerative changes obvious at these levels.

Idiopathic developmental stenosis appears in young people but does not become symptomatic until superimposed degenerative changes occur. The vertebral bodies are normal in height. The pedicles are short and the laminae relatively flat. The intervertebral foramina are moderately

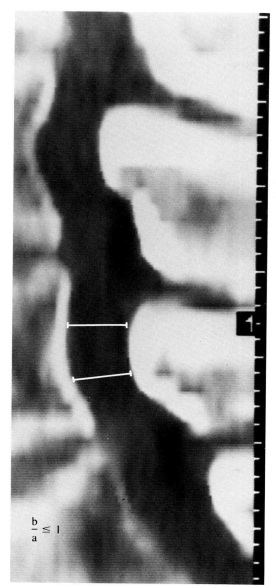

$$\frac{b}{a} \leq 1$$

FIGURE 7.2 Laminar deformity in spinal stenosis. Sagittal bone-window reformation on a patient with a flat lamina.

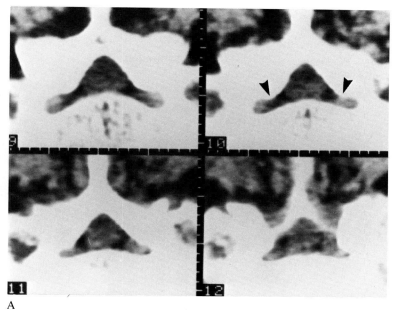

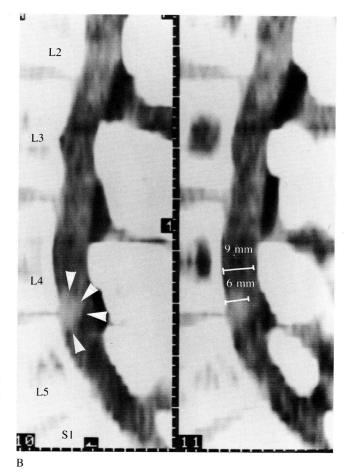

narrowed in the anteroposterior diameter and are normal in height (Fig. 7.3). The anatomic deformity may exist for many years before discs degenerate and spurs form along with concomitant hypertrophic enlargement of the facets and contraction of the foramen circumferentially.

Patients with lumbar stenosis are usually asymptomatic until the end of the third decade, although symptoms may occur at a younger age because of minor disc herniation. There is an increasing incidence of symptoms with age, even into the seventh decade. When planning appropriate decompressive surgery, it is extremely important to study adequately the entire lumbar spine.

FIGURE 7.3 Developmental central stenosis. **A.** A sequence of axial scans demonstrate congenitally short pedicles and lateral canal indentation (*arrows*) by prominent superior articular processes and lamina. **B.** Midsagittal reformation demonstrates a narrow spinal canal and an L4–5 disc (*arrowheads*).

Central Canal Stenosis

In patients with either congenitally or developmentally small spinal canals, the clinical syndrome of central canal stenosis with cauda equina compression is produced by enlargement of the inferior articular facet, which bulges posteromedially into the spinal canal and thereby causes formation of a small medial recess. In central stenosis the canal is further reduced in size by prominent osteophytic ridges arising from the vertebral end-plates[10] (Fig. 7.4). Stenosis is further complicated by swelling and fibrosis of the periarticular soft tissues, hypertrophy, and occasionally calcification of the ligamentum flavum (Fig. 7.5). The laminae frequently are hypertrophied and demonstrate an irregular whiskering of

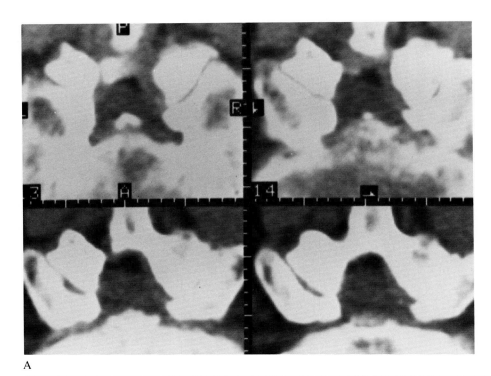

A

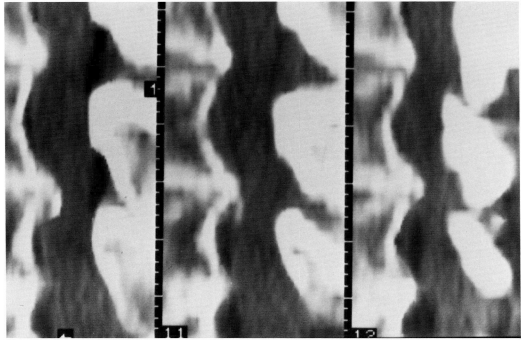

B

FIGURE 7.4 Central stenosis—central ridging. (**A**) Axial and sagittal (**B**) views on a patient with claudication. Note the marked central canal stenosis caused by central osteoarthritic ridging and a prominent articular process.

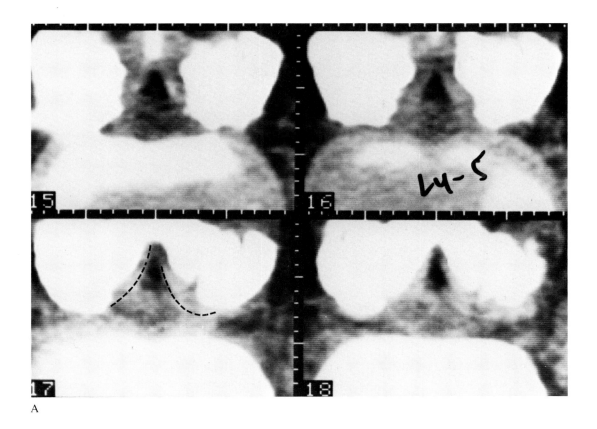

A

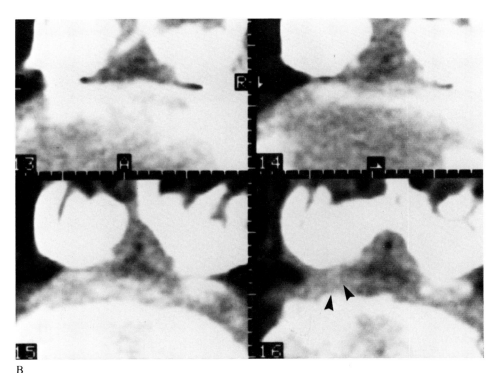

B

FIGURE 7.5 Central canal stenosis—soft-tissue component. **A.** Sequence of axial scans demonstrate marked stenosis. Pedicles are short and facets are enlarged, but there is a major component of ligamentum flavum hypertrophy. **B.** Central stenosis caused by prominent periarticular soft-tissue swelling (*arrowheads*). (*Figure continued* on page 202.)

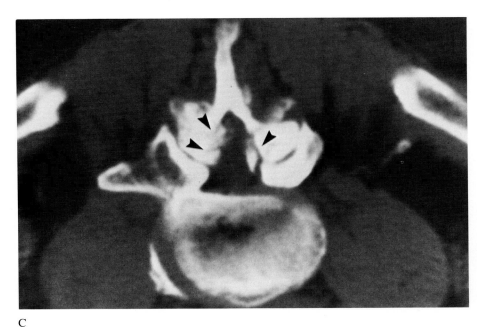

C

FIGURE 7.5 (*cont'd*) **C.** Central stenosis caused by lateral ossification and calcification of ligamentum flavum and calcified callus at the level of a pars interarticularis defect.

new bone. Degenerative spondylolisthesis (Fig. 7.6) produces the most severe central canal stenosis, a detailed discussion of which can be found in Chapter 8.

An unusual cause of central canal stenosis is seen in Figure 7.7. On the axial scans the lamina seems to be too close to the disc space, accounting for this patient's claudication, although the lamina does not reach the level of the disc space. We must therefore explain what abnormal bone is compressing the roots. Note the severe erosive arthropathy of the left facet. There seems to be a joint effusion present. The key to explaining this complex case is found on the coronal images. Note the inferior articular processes and the very remarkable expansion of the joint spaces (Figs. 7.7C, D). On these views it is obvious that the midline bridge of bone is actually distrophic bone arising from the articular processes. This is medial "whiskering," which is most likely a sequel to the aggressive arthritis of the facets. It seems appropriate for the radiologist to suggest treating the facet joint pathology in an attempt to reduce the nerve root compression.

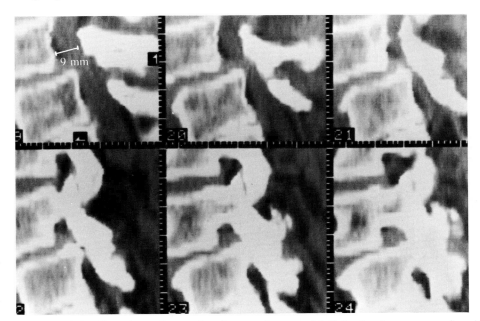

FIGURE 7.6 Central canal stenosis—degenerative spondylolisthesis. A sequence of sagittal reformations demonstrates 9-mm forward degenerative spondylolisthesis. Severe central canal stenosis is caused by compression of the spinal canal between the posterior surface of the upper endplate of L5 and the anterior surface of the L4 lamina.

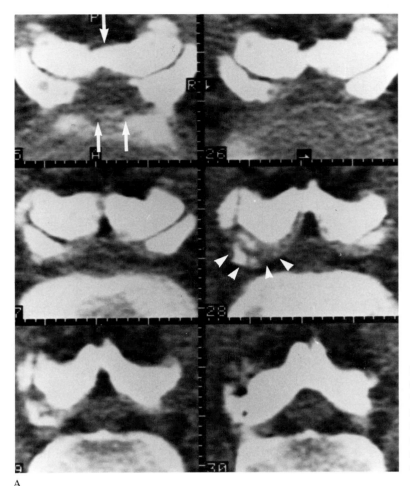

A

FIGURE 7.7 Central canal stenosis caused by facet disease. Axial soft-tissue (**A**) and bone-window (**B**) views reveal a narrow canal at the level of the disc space (*arrows*). The facet joints are markedly abnormal, and there is a suggestion of a joint effusion (*arrowheads*). The bone-window views reveal cystic disorganization of the subarticular bone (*arrow*). (*Figure continued* on page 204.)

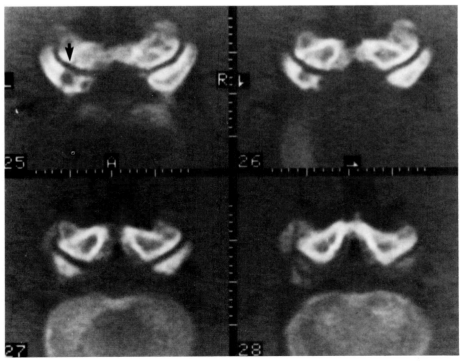

B

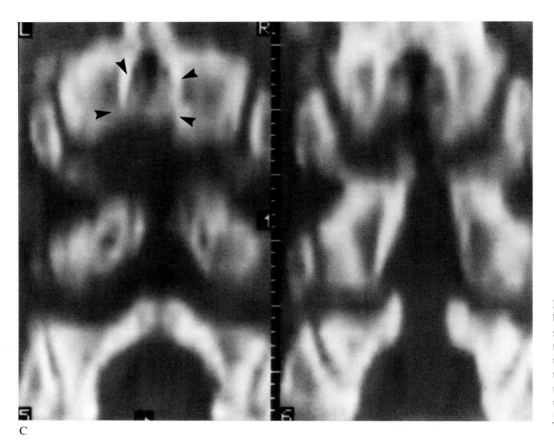

FIGURE 7.7 (*cont'd*) Coronal bone windows (**C**) and soft-tissue (**D**) coronal views prove that the posterior ridge of bone is not the lamina but reactive bone extending medially from the articular processes (*arrowheads*). Note the abnormal widening of the joints (*arrows*).

C

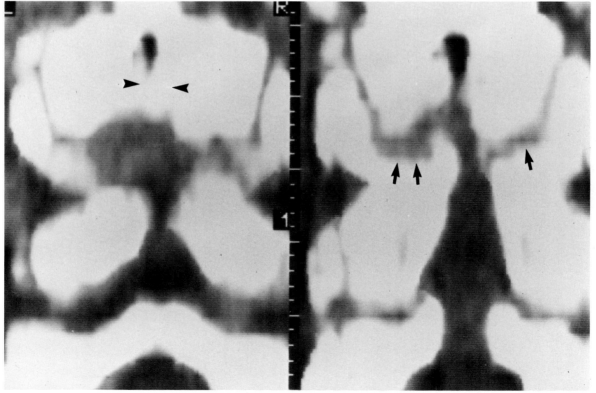

D

Lateral Spinal Stenosis

Lateral spinal stenosis was described in detail by Schlesinger in 1955.[7] He presented two patients in whom the superior facets of the sacrum, oriented in the coronal plane, formed the posterior wall of a recess, the anterior wall of which was the fifth lumbar vertebral body and disc. The first sacral nerve was lying laterally within this lateral recess and was compressed by bone. Epstein et al.[11] presented 15 patients with lateral recess syndrome and used the term "superior facet syndrome" in contradistinction to central spinal stenosis, which is "inferior facet syndrome." They described the typical trefoil appearance of the canal with a normal midsagittal diameter and specific narrowing of the lateral recesses by hypertrophy of the superior facet (Fig. 7.8). Heithoff[12] defined two distinct entities: (1) Lateral stenosis, which by his definition represents compression of an exiting root in its neural foramen (nerve root canal). The compressing structure is the superior articular process that herniates upward into the foramen. (2) Subarticular recess stenosis, which is the entity described by Schlesinger and Epstein. The superior facet entraps the exiting root just below the disc space in patients with short pedicles and indentation on the lateral spinal canal by the subarticular portion of the lamina.

Although we have drawn a clear distinction here between the central and the lateral compressive syndromes, they frequently occur concurrently. We prefer to further divide the groups into central stenosis, lateral recess stenosis (subarticulr stenosis), and foraminal stenosis. Because the treatment for foraminal narrowing is very different from the treatment for lateral recess or central stenosis, we believe it is useful to clearly distinguish between these entities when possible. When there is coexisting central, lateral, and foraminal stenosis, we prefer to describe the deformity in precise anatomic terms so the surgeon knows exactly what he is dealing with and what approaches he should take.

Epstein's group of patients with pure lateral stenosis syndrome (subarticular recess stenosis) were, for the most part, younger than were those with central stenosis, and the presenting complaint was almost always intense sciatica. There was nothing in the clinical presentation to distinguish this group of patients from those with central disc herniation. Straight leg raising caused severe pain in every case

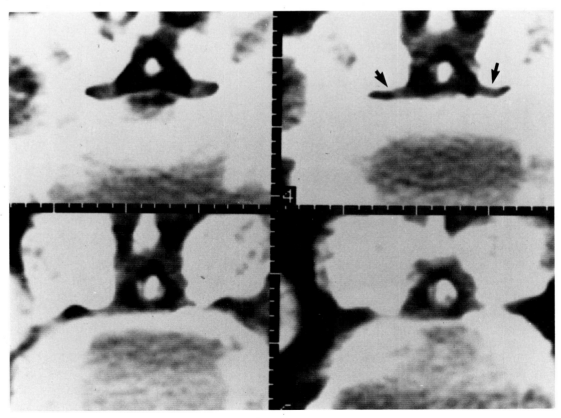

A

FIGURE 7.8 Lateral canal stenosis (subarticular recess stenosis). (**A**) Axial soft-tissue views demonstrate prominent lateral subarticular stenosis. The descending roots are compressed between the superior articular process and the disc space. (*Figure continued* on page 206.)

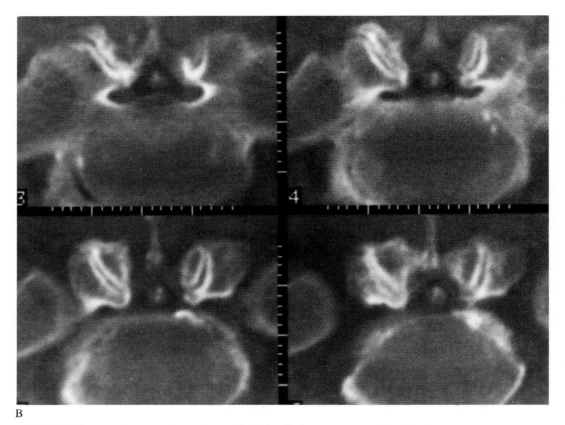

B

FIGURE 7.8 (*cont'd*)   Lateral canal stenosis (subarticular recess stenosis). (**B**) Bone window views demonstrate prominent lateral subarticular stenosis. The descending roots are compressed between the superior articular process and the disc space.

(this is relatively uncommon in pure central stenosis). Neurologic deficit was minimal and did not allow interspace localization. Myelography was strikingly normal in this series because the affected roots were compressed extradurally.

The axial CT view is diagnostic. The spinal canal commonly demonstrates a typical trefoil appearance caused by encroachment by the superior articular process. Spinal canal or nerve root compression is compounded by osteoarthritic facet spurs or dense calcification of the facet joint capsule (Figs. 7.9, 7.10). In most of these cases the nerve roots are difficult to see within the stenotic lateral recesses. Sagittally reformatted images demonstrate narrowing of the medial portion of the foramen, caused primarily by prominence of the medial expansion of the superior facet. In some cases the medial expansion of the facet may be quite striking.

Kirkaldy-Willis et al.[13,14] further divided this entity into two varying forms: (1) that caused by fixed deformity at one or two levels; and (2) that caused by dynamic recurrent rotation or extension deformities.

The dynamic form of stenosis is described first, because it is a precursor of the static form. At degenerating intervertebral segments, abnormal rotatory and flexion/extension motions may occur either independently or together. The superior facet shifts, narrowing the lateral recess. The compression is therefore intermittent. Rotation-produced entrapment can be seen on axial CT scans performed in the supine position with hips elevated. When abnormal rotation is present, the foramen on the elevated side becomes narrowed.

Entrapment resulting from abnormal flexion/extension motion is seen most frequently at L4–5. At the degenerated intervertebral segment hyperflexion causes anterior subluxation of the superior facet up into the neural foramen, with compression of the nerve within the foramen (Fig. 7.11). Sagittally reformatted views may demonstrate widening of the joint space and a "vacuum effect" within the joint. Rotation deformity and mixed rotation and extension deformity involve narrowing of the disc space, anulus bulging, and vertebral osteophyte formation. As the spinous process rotates toward one side, the superior facet on that side subluxes forward and the opposite facet (the posterior one) widens. The lateral recess on the side of the spinous process becomes narrowed, with concomitant root compression. Combinations of rotational and hyperextensional motion tend to cause the most severe symptoms of entrapment.

In "fixed" lateral entrapment the abnormally increased motion no longer takes place. The joint capsules become fibrotic and calcified, and the disc space collapses.

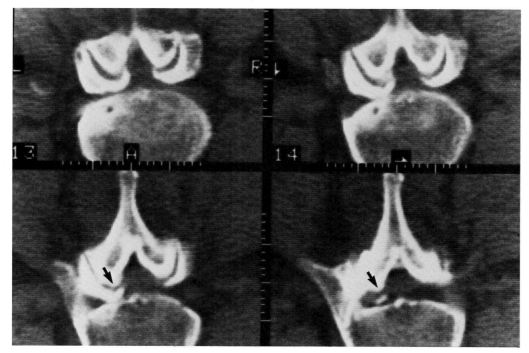

A

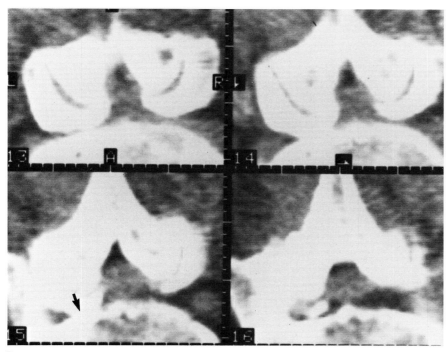

B

FIGURE 7.9 Lateral canal stenosis. Axial bone (**A**) and soft-tissue (**B**) views. The superior articular processes are large. The medial lips extend well into the spinal canal. The left side is more severely affected than the right. There is marked lateral recess compression. (*Figure continued* on page 208.)

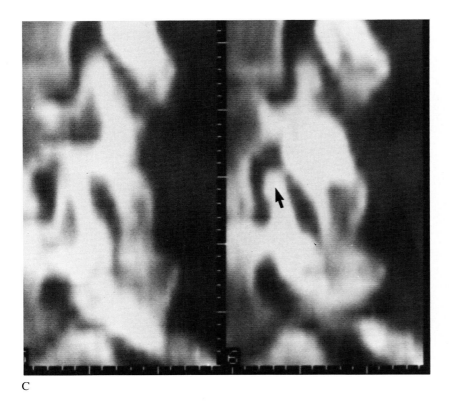

C

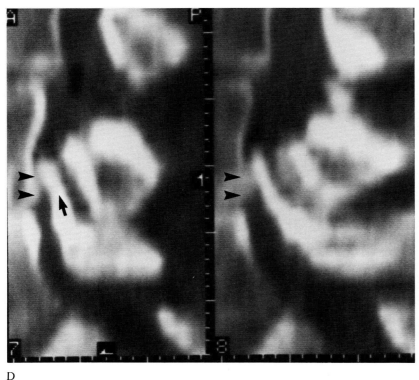

D

FIGURE 7.9 (*cont'd*)   **C, D.** Sagittal reformations through the left neural foramen and lateral recess demonstrate both lateral and subarticular recess stenosis. The apex of the superior facet of L5 is herniated upward into the neural foramen (*arrows*), and the subarticular recess is compressed by the anterior face of the broad horizontal extension of the superior facet more medially (*arrowheads*).

Typically, the vertebral end-plates are eroded and sclerotic. The superior facets become fixed in an abnormally high position, causing fixed foraminal and recess compression. Although the superior articular process is sometimes displaced upward into the pedicle, grooving its inferior surface, this does not often cause entrapment of the exiting nerve. Lateral recess compression of the next lowest nerve root predominates.

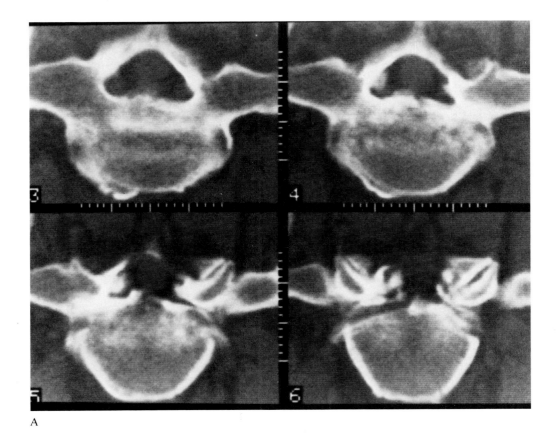

A

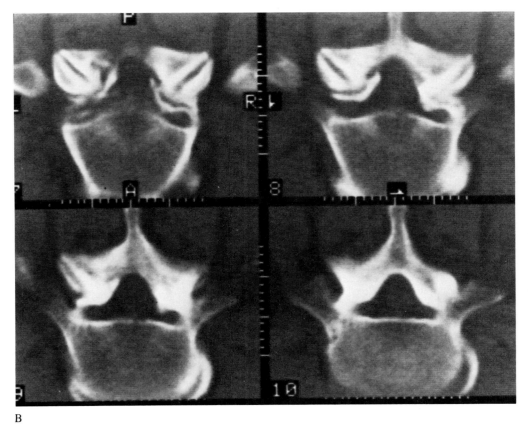

B

FIGURE 7.10 Lateral canal stenosis. **A, B.** Sequential axial scans demonstrate severe lateral recess stenosis. The apical capsules of the joints are densely calcified (*arrow*). The lateral recesses are narrowed. There is a large degenerative ridge extending across the canal that further compromises the left neural foramen. **C, D.** Sagittal reformations reveal dense capsular calcification and degenerative ridging that compresses the exiting nerves in the neural foramina. (*Figure continued on page 210.*)

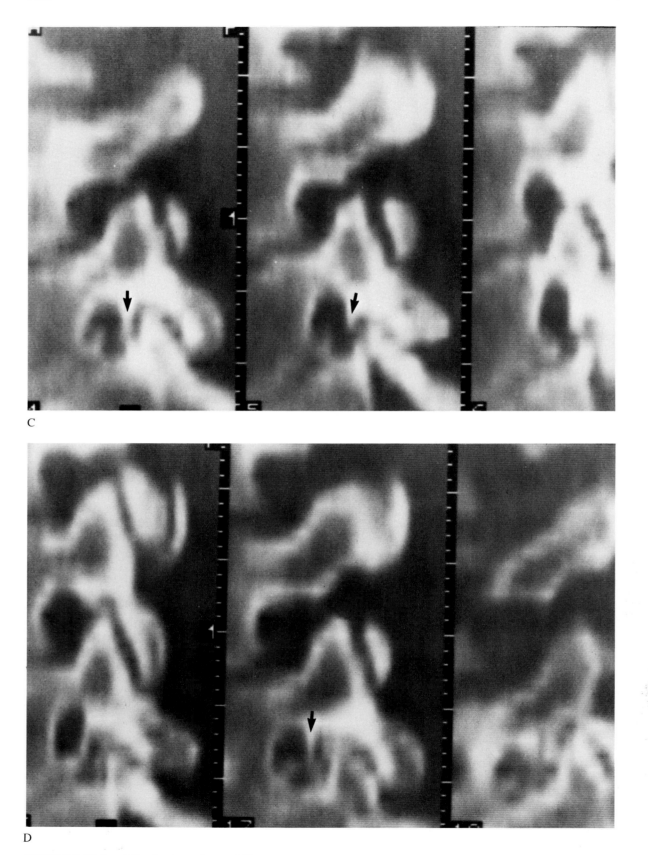

C

D

FIGURE 7.10 (*cont'd*)   See legend page 209.

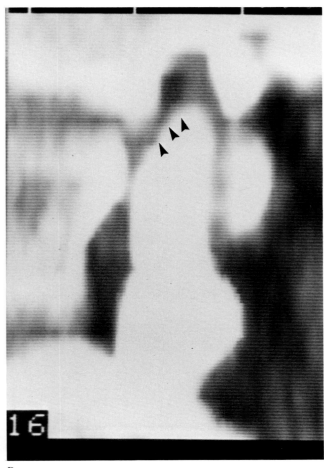

B

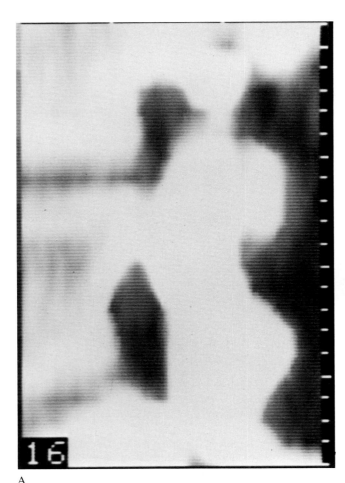

A

FIGURE 7.11 Dynamic stenosis. **A.** Sagittal reformation in neutral position. **B.** Sagittal reformation in hyperextension. Note the difference in the size of the L4–5 neural foramen (*arrowheads*).

Overreading Spinal Stenosis

The main problem when evaluating spine CT for spinal stenosis is the tendency for people with limited experience to overcall the diagnosis. Not all narrow spinal canals are stenotic. It is important to remember the obvious: Small people have small spinal canals. It is unreasonable to assume that the surface area of the spinal canal is the same in a 7-foot basketball player and a 5-foot woman. One should reserve the diagnosis of stenosis for those patients who have asymmetrical developmental deformity—mainly pedicles that are *disproportionately* short or facets that are *disproportionately* large. The patients in Figure 7.12 have narrow canals of varying shapes but do not have symptomatic spinal stenosis. Simply stating that a patient has ''spinal stenosis'' on a CT report produces a specific reaction in the mind of a surgeon: He will think about radical laminectomy, facetectomy, and possibly foraminotomy. It is inappropriate to perform that much surgery when it is not absolutely necessary. The incidence of surgical scar and adhesions is related in part to the amount of surgery performed. In any case, one should never do anything to mislead a surgeon into operating.

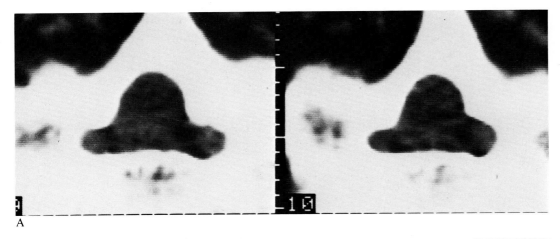

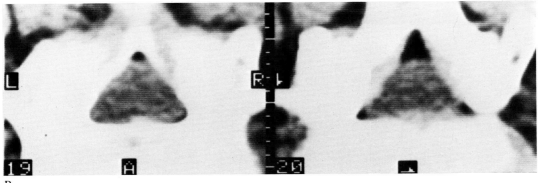

FIGURE 7.12 Commonly misinterpreted spinal canals. **A.** Axial scan through the pedicles. Symptomatic stenosis rarely involves this level. Note that although the canal is narrow the round theca is not distorted. **B.** Trefoil canal shape, but the roots are not compressed.

References

1. Lee BCP, Kazam E: Computed tomography of the spine and spinal cord. Radiology 128:95-102, 1978

2. Ullrich CG, Binel EF, Sanecki MG, Kieffer SA: Quantitative assessment of the lumbar spinal canal by computed tomoraphy. Radiology 134:137-143, 1980

3. Ullrich CG, Kieffer SA: Computed tomographic evaluation of the lumbar spine: quantitative aspects and sagittal-coronal reconstruction. In Post MJD (ed): Radiographic Evaluation of the Spine: Current Advances with Emphasis on Computed Tomography, Masson, New York, 1980

4. Porter RW, Hibbert C, Wellman P: Backache and the lumbar spinal canal. Spine 5:99-105, 1980

5. Verbiest H: Sur Certaines Formes Rares de Compression de la Guere de Cheval. I. Les Stenoses Osseuses du Canal Vertebral in Hommage a Clovis Vincent, Maloine, Paris, 1949, pp. 161-174

6. Verbiest H: Radicular syndrome from developmental narrowing of the lumbar vertebral canal. J Bone Joint Surg 36B:230-237, 1954

7. Schlesinger PT: Incarceration of the first sacral nerve in a lateral bony recess of the spinal canal as a cause of sciatica. J Bone Joint Surg 37A:115-124, 1955

8. Verbiest H: Fallacies of the present definition, nomenclature, and classification of the stenoses of the lumbar vertebral canal. Spine 1:217-224, 1976

9. Verbiest H: The significance and principles of computerized axial tomography in idiopathic developmental stenosis of the bony lumbar vertebral canal. Spine 4:369-371, 1979

10. Sheldon JJ, Leborgne JM: Computed tomography of central lumbar stenosis. In Post MJD (ed): Computed Tomography of the Spine. Williams & Wilkins, Baltimore, 1984, pp. 570-590

11. Epstein JA, Epstein BS, Rosenthal AD, et al: Sciatica caused by nerve root entrapment in the lateral recess: the superior facet syndrome. J Neurosurg 36:583, 1972

12. Heithoff KB: High resolution computed tomography and stenosis: an evaluation of the causes and cures of the failed back surgery syndrome. In Post MJD (ed): Computed Tomography of the Spine. Williams & Wilkins, Baltimore, 1984, pp. 506-535

13. Kirkaldy-Willis WH, Heithoff K, Bowen CT, Shannon R: Pathological anatomy of lumbar spondylosis and stenosis, correlated with the CT scan. In Post MJD (ed): Radiographic Evaluation of the Spine: Current Advances with Emphasis on Computed Tomography. Masson, New York, 1980

14. Kirkaldy-Willis WH, Heithoff K, Tchang S, et al: Lumbar spondylosis and stenosis: correlation of pathological anatomy with high resolution computed tomographic scanning. In Post MJD (ed): Computed Tomography of the Spine. Williams & Wilkins, Baltimore, 1984, pp. 546-569

Spondylolysis, Spondylolisthesis, and Pseudospondylolisthesis

8

These three disorders, although generally discussed as a unit, are really separate entities. They occur in patients within different age groups; they are caused by different stresses; they are treated differently. They all share one common feature: vertebral subluxation or the propensity for subluxation.

Cleavage Abnormalities of the Pars Interarticularis

Primary among the defects of the lumbar spine is spondylolysis, which is found in approximately 5–7% of the general population.[1] The vertebral arch is divided into two segments by a fibrous cleft within its isthmus (the pars interarticularis). The anterosuperior segment consists of the pedicles, the transverse processes, and the superior facets. The posterior inferior segment consists of the inferior facets, the laminae, and the spinous process.

Most pars interarticularis defects occur at L5 (approximately 60%) and L4 (approximately 30%); only a very small percentage occur at other lumbar levels. Clefts occur bilaterally far more often than unilaterally.

There is wide disagreement in the literature as to the nature of the pars interarticularis defect. Some authors favor a congenital or developmental theory; others consider it an acquired cleft. Wide racial differences in incidence have been noted. In one series[2] the incidence was found to be: in white males 6.4%; in American blacks 2.8%; and in Alaskan Eskimos 27.4%.

Histologic examination of several infantile spondy-

lolyses revealed that the fibers filling the cleft extend from one bone surface to another and deeply penetrate the adjacent osseous structures, similar to Sharpey's fibers. The osseous surfaces abutting the cleft also showed the typical surface features of juvenile apophyseal centers with groove elevations and indentations.[1] Spondylolysis is frequently associated with other ring anomalies and congenital maldevelopment of the accompanying facets.

The most popular theory is that spondylolysis is due to minor trauma. Radionuclide bone scans are usually positive in the acute phase of back pain. The high incidence of pars defects in young athletes, gymnasts, and divers strongly suggests that pars defects are actually fractures, probably fatigue fractures.

In support of the fracture theory, Wiltse et al.[3] described 17 patients with lumbar spine radiographs that were originally read as normal. Later radiographs, however, revealed pars interarticularis defects. All but one of these patients had been involved in some type of vigorous physical exercise. Long-term follow-up showed that in five of these patients the defect progressed to significant spondylolisthesis. Some of the patients in this series who were treated with body casts or corsets were followed to complete healing.

In isthmic spondylolisthesis there is true anterior slippage of one vertebra on its next lowest mate because of a defect in the pars interarticularis. Isthmic spondylolisthesis occurs most commonly at L5. Its clinical significance, aside from the obvious malalignment and malformation, rests mainly on the extent of functional disability and impairment of activity.

Classification

The following classification of spondylolysis was suggested by Wiltse [4,5]:

1. *Dysplastic*. In this disorder a congenital abnormality of the upper sacrum and/or the neural arch of L5 allows the lower lumbar vertebra to slide forward on the sacrum. The pars interarticularis usually becomes elongated and the facets dislocate because of insufficient strength to withstand the forward force of the weight of the upper half of the body. This entity is very rare.
2. *Isthmic*. This is divided into three types.
   a. *Type A*. The primary lesion is due to stress fracture of the pars interarticularis and is the most common type. The lesion starts to appear between the ages of 5.5 and 6.5 years and is more common in females. The exact traumatic mechanism is not clear. Although forward slippage occurs, it seems likely that the major force would be in the direction of extension.
   b. *Type B*. Here the pars interarticularis is elongated and thinned but not fractured. This type is thought to be caused by healed stress fracture. The abnormality is occasionally found in family members of patients with signs of classic pars defects.
   c. *Type C*. This is acute, traumatic vertebral injury. It is the least common type of the group.
3. *Degenerative*. This is a disorder of late middle age. It is primarily due to severe degeneration of the facet joints, which produces intervertebral joint instability. The affected segment may be subluxed forward or backward, producing cauda equina compression.
4. *Traumatic*. This is due to an acute fracture and is an unstable injury.
5. *Pathologic*. In this type, subluxation is caused by some generalized disorder of bone.

To Wiltse's list, we suggest an additional classification:

6. *Iatrogenic*. Dislocation of vertebrae may occur as a sequel to laminectomy with facetectomy. It may also be caused by postoperative stress fracture of the facets.

Patient Population

Over the last 30 months, more than 700 patients with various types of spondylolisthesis were evaluated in our clinic by routine reformatted CT.[6] Of these, 450 had pars defects; 225 with degenerative spondylolisthesis and 25 with iatrogenic subluxation. There were no examples of acute trauma or the rare dysplastic types. These cases were all reviewed and the abnormalities were quantitated on a scale of 1–5. In each case the amount of dislocation was measured on the view that looked the worst. Midsagittal views were used for patients with asymmetrical subluxation, and more lateral sagittal views were used for those with asymmetrical or rotatory subluxation.

The amount of foraminal stenosis was also measured on the appropriate sagittal films. A value of one was assigned to a normal foramen, and 5 was allotted to a foramen reduced in both height and transverse diameter.

Spinal canal compression caused by soft-tissue or bony callus at the site of the pars defect was estimated from the axial images. This abnormality is not well known to the radiologist but is often an important cause of symptoms.

Pars Interarticularis Defects —Spondylolysis

Isthmic defects were noted in 450 patients: 92% were at L5 and 7% were at L4. Unilateral clefts were demonstrated in 68 patients (Table 8.1). Disc protrusion or herniations defined as an anterior extradural defect of 5 mm or more, as seen on sagittally reformatted images, were noted in 86 patients. Significant herniation was noted more frequently at L4–5 than at L5–S1. Characteristic deformity of the neural foramina—best described as a flattening of the foramen with anteroposterior deformity—was encountered in 142 patients.

Congenital anomalies of the upper sacrum or the affected vertebral arch were noted in 160 cases. The actual incidence may be slightly higher because the posterior elements of the sacrum were not visualized in many of the examinations. Lateral indentation or compression due to soft tissue or bony callus was demonstrated in 68 patients, in half of whom it was believed to be potentially significant. Bony stenosis of the lateral recesses was defined in 10 cases.

Discussion

In the past, assessment of patients with low back pain has included both radiographs and myelography, and occasionally conventional tomography as well. All or much of the information produced by the above group of examinations is available on multiplanar spine CT.

The CT appearance in the axial and sagittal planes of bilateral pars interarticularis without spondylolisthesis is demonstrated in Figure 8.1. Nondisplaced pars fractures appear just anterior to the facets. They are seen as horizontal irregular lucencies extending medially into the spinal canal. In the sagittal plane, the pars defect is seen as a

TABLE 8.1 Summary of Radiologic Review of 700 Patients

Disorder	L5	L4	L3	L2	L1
Pars defect, bilateral[a]	355	27	11	1	
Pars defect, unilateral	64	4			
Forward degenerative spondylolysis[b]	20	128	21		
Degenerative retrolisthesis		37	38	16	2

[a]Multiple levels in eight cases.

[b]Multiple levels in 33 cases.

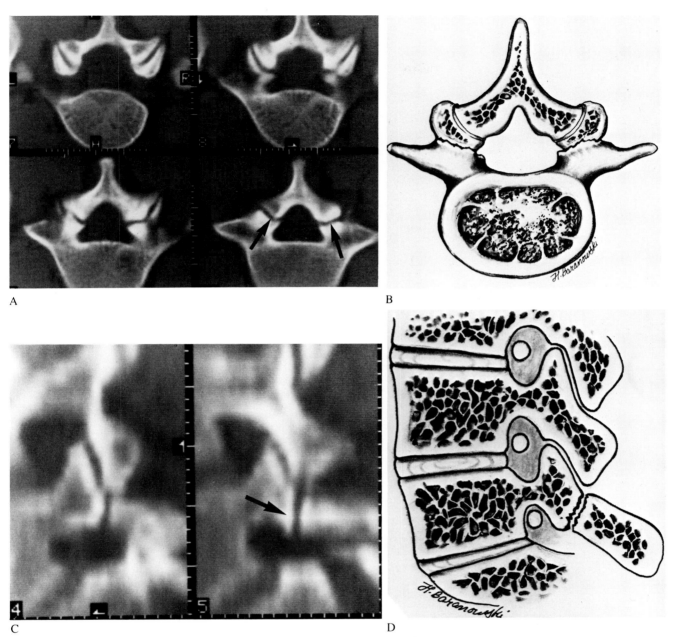

FIGURE 8.1 Bilateral pars interarticularis defects. **A.** Axial scans show symmetrical irregular pars defect (*arrows*). **B.** Diagram of **A**. **C.** Series of sagittal reformations showing the pars defect (*arrow*). **D.** Diagram of **C**. (Reprinted with permission from Rothman and Glenn.[13])

jagged defect separating the vertebral body pedicle and superior facet from the inferior facet.

CT is rarely performed in the young patient with acute back pain. Localized positive bone scan in a 6 to 14-year-old is most often due to spondylolysis. The patient in Figure 8.2 is an exception. This child, with 2 weeks of back pain, had a normal radionuclide bone scan. Both axial and sagittal

views revealed a definite thin pars defect, which was undoubtedly an acute pars fracture.

Nathan[7] suggested that many defects in the pars interarticularis of L5 are produced by upward pressure of the inferior facet of the sacrum and downward force from the inferior facet of L4 (Fig. 8.3). We have observed that the inferior facets of L4 tend to be very large, and the superior

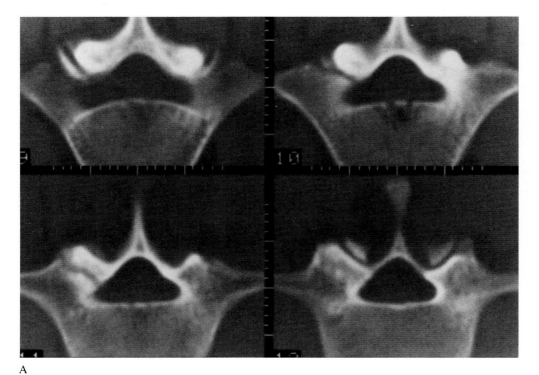

A

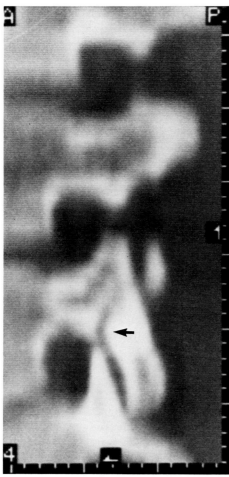

B

FIGURE 8.2   Acute pars fracture. Axial (**A**) and sagittal (**B**) views show an acute pars fracture. Note the thin crack traversing the pars interarticularis on the sagittal view (*arrow*).

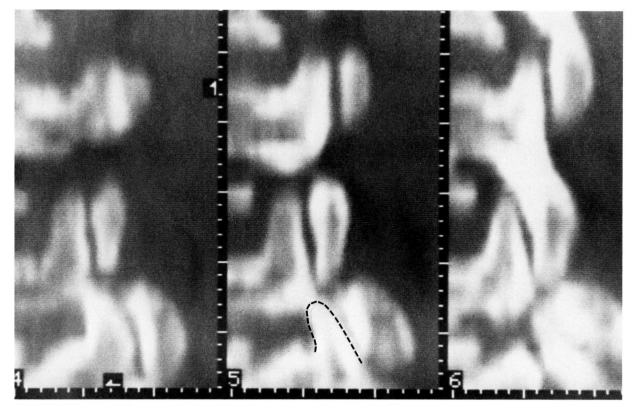

FIGURE 8.3 Pars defect, sagittal view. There is an apparent "pinching" of the pars. Downward pressure from the inferior facet of L4 and upward pressure from the hypoplastic superior facet of L5 are noted.

facets of S1 tend to be short. This may exaggerate the abnormal stress on the pars. As L5 slips forward on the sacrum, the pars defects widen. The axial views take on a "double-canal" appearance. Geometric distortion of the spinal canal is due to a combination of forward slippage and increase in lordosis that accompanies spondylolisthesis. The L5 disc space is so anteriorly tilted that even maximal gantry angulation is unable to produce scans parallel to the disc space. Sagittal images give an undistorted view of the pars defect and allow accurate measurement of the diameter of the spinal canal (Fig. 8.4).

It may be difficult to diagnose L4 and L3 pars defects; on axial-only CT as they may be confused with sagittally oriented facets. The pars defects are lower in the neural arch, and they tend to be irregular, whereas normal facets are usually smooth and curved.[8] Of course, the sagittal view provides the diagnosis (Fig. 8.5).

Sixty-eight unilateral pars defects were studied in our series. These are frequently associated with anomalies of the neural arch or sacrum (Fig. 8.6). It is not clear whether unilateral defects are fractures, with the associated anomalies predisposed to undue stress on the pars, or true cleft anomalies. Assuming that unilateral pars defects are also fractures, one must explain why these fractures occur in only one pars. It is probable that, in fact, there may have originally been bilateral fractures and one has healed. Some support for this hypothesis is found in patients similar to the one in Figure 8.7. This shows a typical right-sided pars defect, but the left pars and lamina are hypertrophied and sclerotic. The sagittal reformations demonstrate loss of definition of the corticomedullary junction of the pars on the enlarged side. This is thought to represent healing of microfractures and hypertrophy of bone along lines of stress. Bone sclerosis opposite a unilateral pars defect is the rule rather than the exception.[9] It is not uncommon for the diagnosis of osteoblastoma to be made incorrectly on plain radiographs.

Spondylolisthesis with intact pars (type 2,B) is rare. The pars is never really normal. It is almost always deformed and sclerotic (Fig. 8.8). Subluxation is usually only slight. In several young patients in the series, scans were performed within 6 months of the onset of back or radicular pain. Within this time frame, it is possible to see radiographic evidence of healing of the pars fracture (Fig. 8.9).

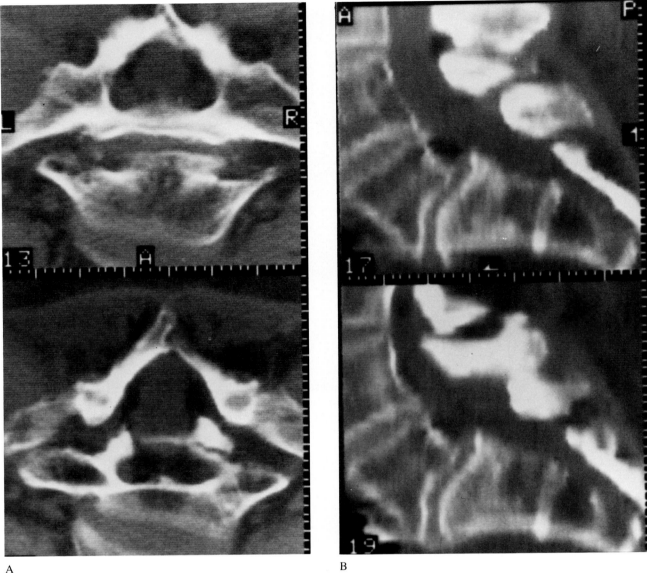

A   B

FIGURE 8.4   Bilateral pars interarticularis defect, with spondylolisthesis. **A.** Axial views reveal a wide pars interarticularis defect. There is a ''double-canal'' appearance due to simultaneous sectioning of two vertebrae. **B.** Sagittal view demonstrates 7-mm spondylolisthesis.

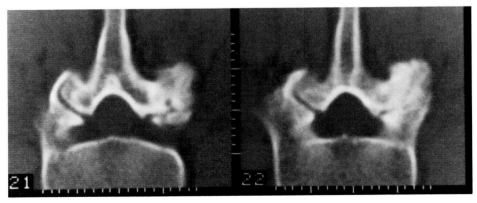

A

FIGURE 8.5   Spondylolisthesis of L4 and L3. **A.** Axial scan on a patient with L4 pars interarticularis defect. At the levels above L5, the defects look quite like articular facets. They can be distinguished because the border of the pars defect appears irregular and some callus is occasionally noted.

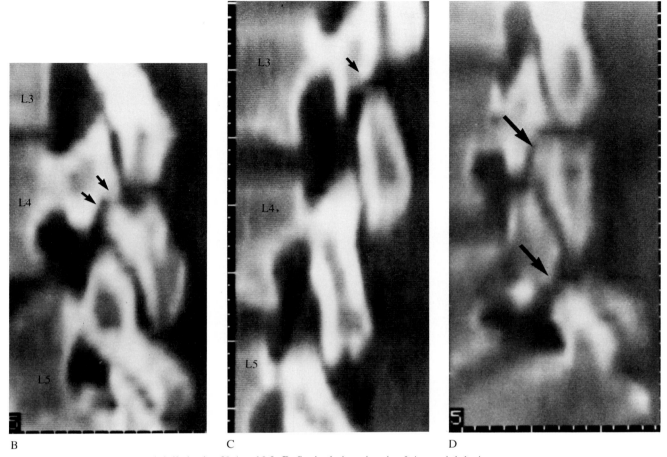

B   C   D

FIGURE 8.5 (*cont'd*)   Spondylolisthesis of L4 and L3. **B.** Sagittal view showing L4 spondylolysis (*arrows*). **C.** Sagittal view showing L3 spondylolysis (*arrow*). **D.** Sagittal view showing both L4 and L5 spondylolysis (*arrows*) in a different patient.

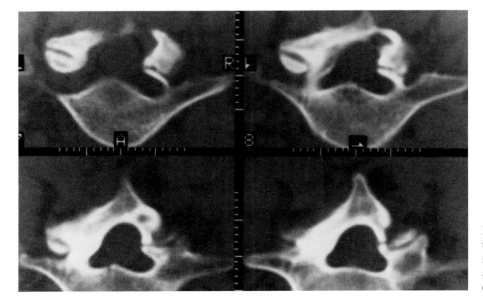

FIGURE 8.6   Unilateral pars interarticularis defect, with anomaly. Axial scans demonstrate unilateral pars interarticularis defect on the right. The facets and laminae are asymmetrical.

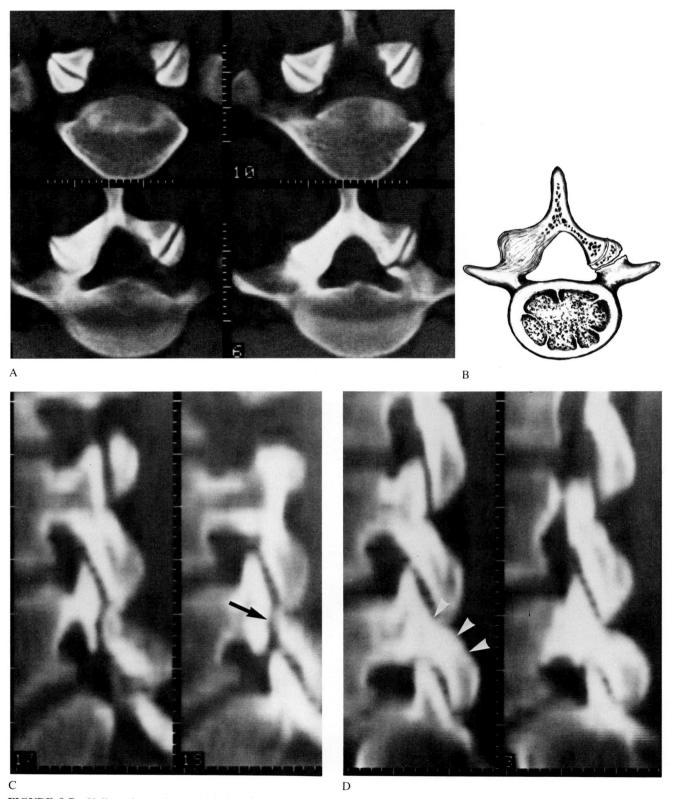

FIGURE 8.7 Unilateral pars interarticularis defect. **A.** Axial scan on a patient with unilateral right pars interarticularis defect. **B.** Diagram of A. **C.** Sagittal reformation through the right pars defect (*arrow*). **D.** Sagittal reformation through the thickened pars (*arrowheads*). (Reprinted with permission from Rothman and Glenn.[13])

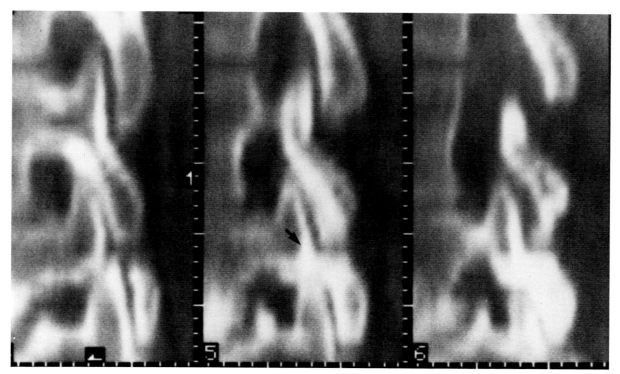

FIGURE 8.8 Spondylolisthesis with intact pars interarticularis. Sagittal views demonstrate a typical elongated deformed pars (*arrow*).

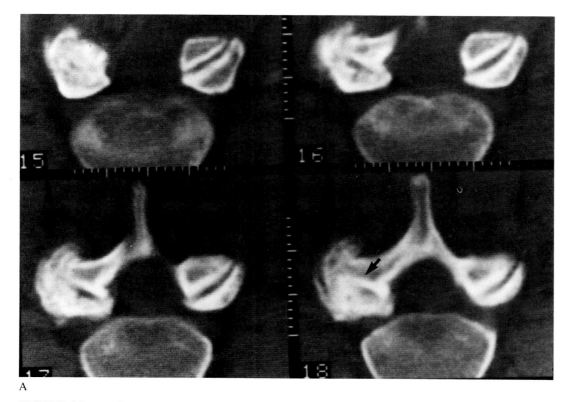

A

FIGURE 8.9 Healing pars interarticularis fracture. **A.** Axial scans on a patient several months after the onset of low back pain seems to show degeneration of the left facet (*arrow*). There is no obvious pars defect. (*Figure continued* on page 222.)

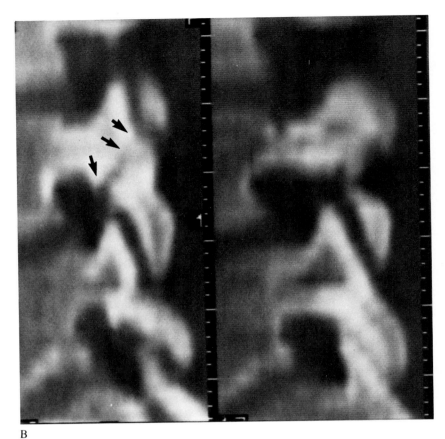

B

FIGURE 8.9 (*cont'd*) **B.** Sagittal reformations demonstrate healing of a pars interarticularis fracture with exuberant callus formation (*arrows*). The facet is actually normal.

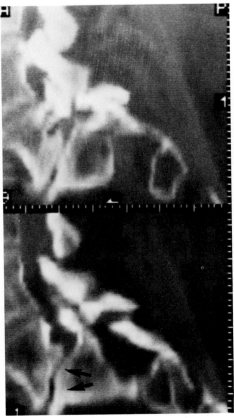

FIGURE 8.10 Degeneration of the L5–S1 disc space. Sagittal reformation demonstrates spondylolisthesis and considerable degeneration of the disc. The inferior end-plate of L5 is compressed, and there is a small collection of gas within the disc space (*arrows*).

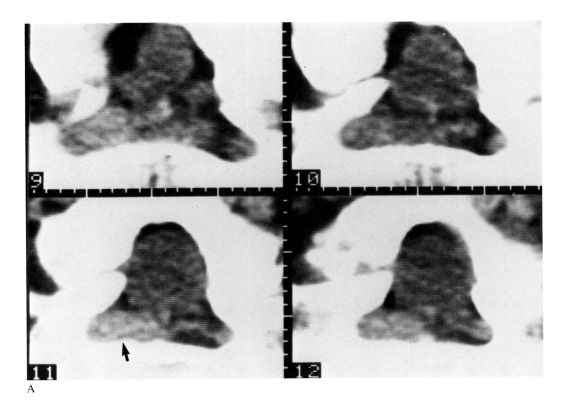

A

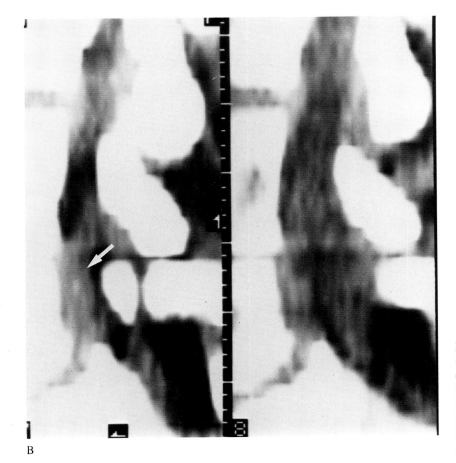

B

FIGURE 8.11 Disc herniation above spondylolisthesis. **A.** Axial scans demonstrate a free disc fragment lying in the left lateral gutter, (*arrow*). **B.** The sagittal views define high-density disc material extending almost all the way down behind the vertebral body of L5, (*arrows*).

Disc Herniation

Many patients with spondylolysis and spondylolisthesis demonstrate radiographic abnormalities without ever having significant back pain. It is clear, therefore, that the mere demonstration of the defect on CT scanning does not necessarily indicate that the anatomic deformity is the cause of the patient's pain. In fact, it is as important to define the associated abnormalities that produce symptoms as to diagnose the pars defect.

According to Wiltse,[5,10] pain in children is caused by either an acute pars fracture or a painful degenerated disc at the level of the spondylolisthesis. He suggested that many, but not all, degenerating discs are painful.

There are many causes for back pain in adults with spondylolisthesis. It behooves us to seek out diligently the anatomic causes for each of these potential sources of back pain. Degeneration of the disc space almost always occurs at the level of spondylolisthesis. Vacuum disc effect is a common finding in older patients. It is possible for these degenerated disc spaces to be the cause of significant pain (Fig. 8.10).

It is noteworthy that disc herniation is quite uncommon at the level of the pars defect; most series suggest an incidence of approximately 4%.[11] Removal of the offending disc in these patients, with or without concomitant spine fusion, may be curative.

Disc herniation is much more common at the interspace above the pars defect. In MacNab's series,[12] herniated L4 discs were diagnosed in 31% of patients with L5 spondylolisthesis. Significant disc herniation on the CT scan probably signifies that the pars defect is less important and that simple L4 discectomy could be curative. This is one of the two most common causes of L5 radiculopathy.

The most sensitive radiographic procedure for the estimation of disc protrusion or herniation is CT. Sagittal reformations allow one to measure the extradural defects caused by bulging of the anulus, even if it is invisible in myelography. This is especially true in patients with wide epidural space. When assessing the disc spaces in the patients in this series, we used fairly strict criteria for diagnosing significant disc herniation. We included only those patients with an anterior epidural bulge of 5 mm or more. We do not mean to imply that severe symptoms of disc herniation may not occur with lesser degrees of herniation, or that all 5-mm bulges cause symptoms. Clinically, however, our experience has shown that patients operated for 5-mm discs have significant pathology. In our series, 86 patients had 5 mm or more of disc herniation. A pair of scans on a patient with left-sided disc herniation is shown in Figure 8.11. The extent of the epidural defect may be measured on the sagittal views. A large free fragment compressing the descending L5 nerve root is seen on the axial scans.

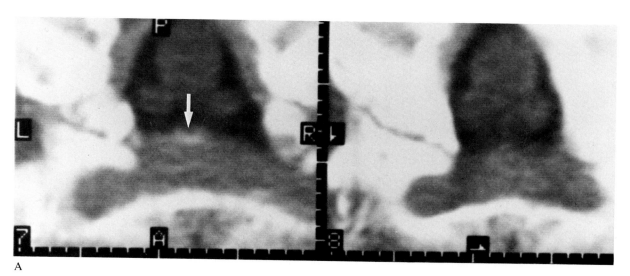

A

FIGURE 8.12   Overestimation of disc herniation. **A.** Axial views apparently show prominent bulge of the L5 disc (*arrow*). **B.** Sagittal views indicate that no disc material protrudes beyond the posterior edges of the sacrum, (*arrows*). This is due to the marked angulation of the L5–S1 disc space in patients with spondylolisthesis.

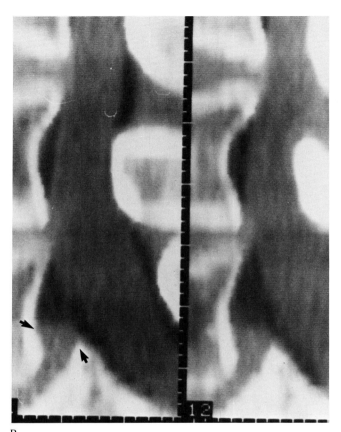

B

Extreme caution must be used if the amount of disc herniation is being estimated from only the axial scans. In many patients with steep lumbar lordosis and ''double-canal'' artifact, the axial views grossly overestimate the amount of canal compression by disc herniation. On the axial view of Figure 8.12 there seems to be a very prominent extradural defect due to disc herniation. The sagittal images clearly demonstrate that the anulus is distorted, but no disc material bulge is posterior to the plane of the back of the sacrum.

Neural Foramina

There is a characteristic deformity of the neural foramina in patients with L5 spondylolisthesis.[13,14] The height of the L5 foramen is reduced, and the pedicle forming the roof of the foramen is abnormally close to the sacrum, causing the orientation of the foramen to be horizontal rather than vertical. This deformity may be seen in patients with little or no forward listhesis, but the degree of flatness of the foramen seems to parallel the amount of listhesis in most instances. In our series, 31% of patients with L5 spondylolisthesis had foraminal stenosis graded moderate to severe.

The flattened foramen is further compromised because of a combination of anterior and posterior bony indentation. Typically, there is indentation on the superior aspect of the foramen by the inferior tip of the base of the fractured pars (Fig. 8.13). The foramen takes on a horizontally bilobed appearance. The descending inferior tip of

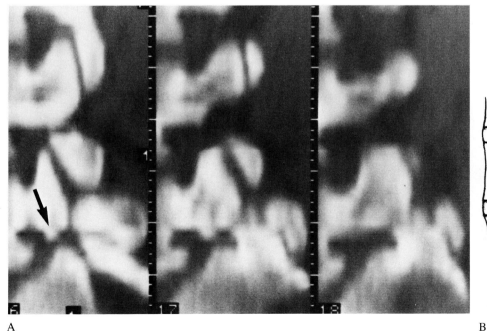

A

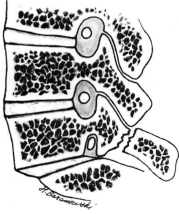

B

FIGURE 8.13 Characteristic foraminal deformity. **A.** Sagittal reformation reveals a horizontally oriented foramen with a central ridge due to downward projection of the inferior tip of the pars fracture (*arrow*). **B.** Diagram of **A**.

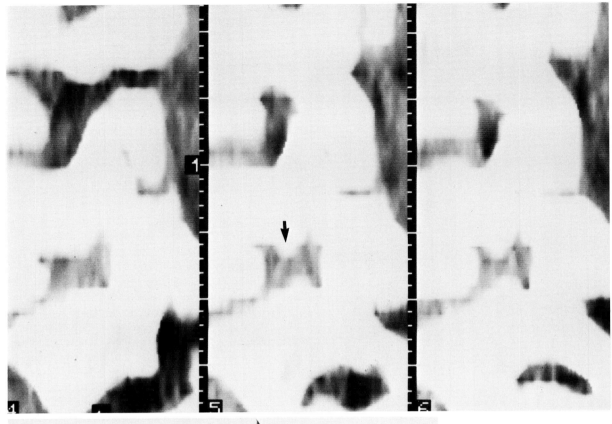

A

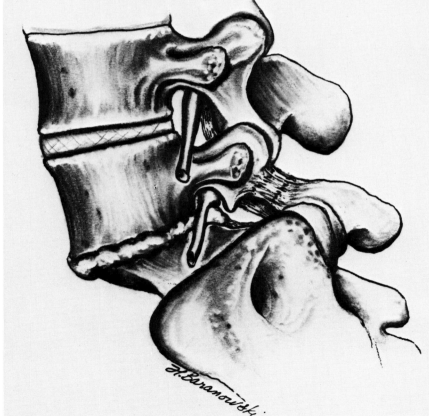

B

FIGURE 8.14 Foraminal deformity with abnormal interforaminal soft tissue. **A.** Sagittal reformation demonstrates normal L3 and L4 foramina. The L5 foramen is narrow and filled with abnormal soft tissue (*arrow*). **B.** Diagram of **A.** (Reprinted with permission from Rothman and Glenn.[13])

the fractured pars forms a central bony ridge within the horizontal canal. As the amount of listhesis increases, or the height of the affected disc space decreases, the central indentation on the foramen becomes more severe. In many of our cases it seems that the foraminal narrowing is due to downward herniation of the inferior pole of the fractured pars rather than to the floating neural arch.

MacNab[12] stated that downward and forward spondylolisthesis places the exiting L5 nerve roots on stretch. The pedicles descend and slide forward, flattening the nerve roots and increasing the angle of egress from the canal. He also noted that significant slippage does not occur without degeneration of the disc. He depicted a patient in whom the disc has bulged around the periphery of the vertebral body, compressing the exiting nerve. There is a striking correlation between the pathologic changes in MacNab's diagram and the soft-tissue abnormalities demonstrated by our soft-tissue-window sagittal views. He further described a "corpora-transverse ligament" that runs from the transverse process to the side of the vertebral body. The fifth lumbar root runs between the ligament and the ala of the sacrum. He suggested that as L5 descends the ligament acts as a guillotine and may entrap the root against the sacrum.

Woolsey[15] suggested that the the free-floating lamina of L5 is a frequent cause of root compression, usually at S1. The S1 root, and to a lesser extent the L5 root, is entrapped by forward rotation of the lamina. This has prompted some surgeons to perform total removal of the free laminar fragment and all associated fibrocartilaginous mass.[16] The sagittal CT views are ideal for evaluating this type of deformity.

Foraminal stenosis is aggravated by the presence of lateral osteophytes. Degenerative osteophytic ridging is a common sequel to the narrowing and deformity of the disc space, which almost always occurs with significant spondylolisthesis. On sagittal images optimized for soft tissue (Fig. 8.14) one can almost always see that the deformed foramen is filled with abnormal soft tissue replacing the normal perineural fat. This abnormal soft tissue most likely represents lateral bulging of the anulus fibrosis, "callus" surrounding the pars defect, or a combination of the two.

Associated Congenital Anomalies

Spondylolysis is associated with many minor congenital anomalies of the facets and neural arches. The most common include spina bifida occulta, hypoplasia of the facets, and anomalous laminae, alone or in various combinations. A series of axial images demonstrating a dysplastic right L5–S1 facet joint is seen in Figure 8.15. A unilateral pars defect is seen on the right with associated hypoplasia of the left pars. The spinous process is deviated to the left, and the laminae are asymmetrical.

A more complex anomaly is shown in Figure 8.16. Actually, this patient was sent for evaluation to "rule out L5 osteoblastoma." The neural arch is markedly abnormal.

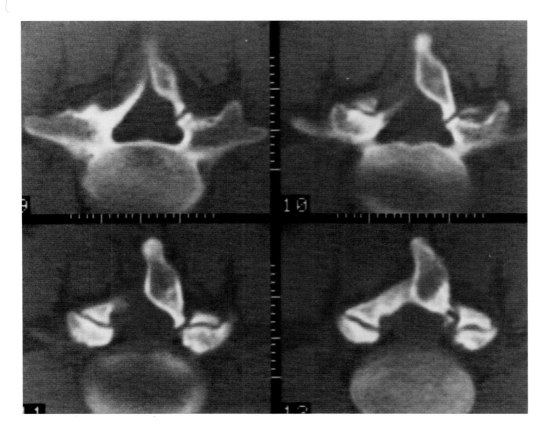

FIGURE 8.15 Spondylolysis with congenital anomaly. There is congenital asymmetry of the laminae and facets. The spinous process is deviated to the left.

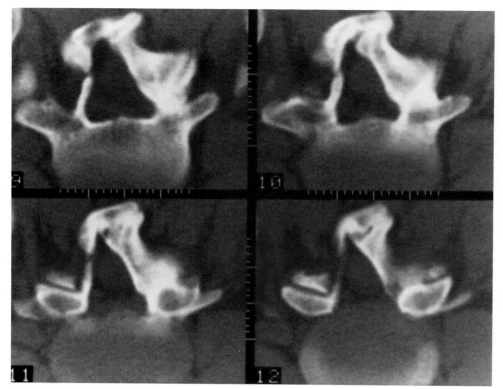

FIGURE 8.16   Major anomaly of the posterior arch. **A.** Axial scan on a patient who was thought to have osteoblastoma of the spine in the right pedicle. The scan reveals a tilted, deformed, cleft spinous process. The laminae are asymmetrical.

There is hypoplasia of the right lamina and spina bifida occulta, which is projecting laterally toward the right. The left lamina is grossly hypoplastic, with a wide pars defect, seen best on the sagittal views. The right facet joint is present, but the left is completely missing.

A still more complex anomaly in a patient with bilateral pars defects is shown in Figure 8.17. A prominent lateral bulge indenting the theca is noted on the soft-tissue views. A prominent cleft is noted through the left half of the neural arch, there is asymmetry of the posterior elements, and a free-floating bone fragment is seen posteriorly on the coronal scans.

There are two types of congenital cleft that are associated with spondylolysis. The first type occurs within the neural arch, behind the pars interarticularis, and medial to the spinous process (Fig. 8.18); this has been termed a "retroisthmic defect." The second type occurs anterior to the pedicle, in the fusion plane of the pedicle with the vertebral body; this is called a "retrosomatic cleft" (Fig. 8.19). The retroisthmic defect is probably of no consequence, but the retrosomatic cleft has been associated with degeneration of the disc and spondylolisthesis.[17]

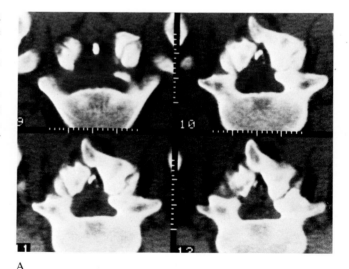

A

FIGURE 8.17   Bilateral pars defect and anomaly. **A.** Axial views demonstrate a neural arch cleft and bilateral pars interarticularis defects. **B.** Soft-tissue axial scans reveal prominent fibrocartilaginous mass compressing the theca. **C.** Coronal view on the same patient. (Reprinted with permission from Rothman and Glenn.[13])

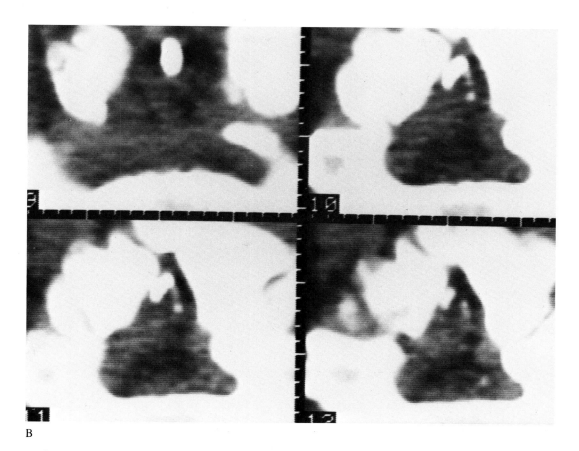

B

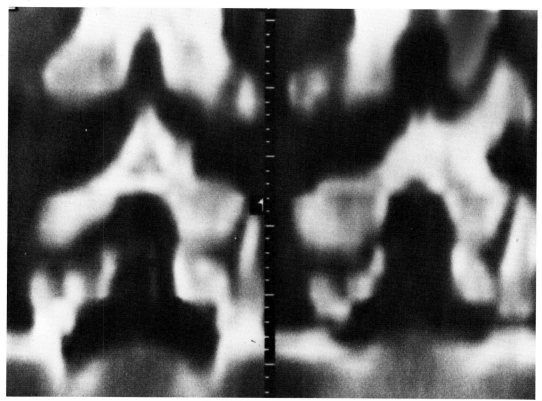

C

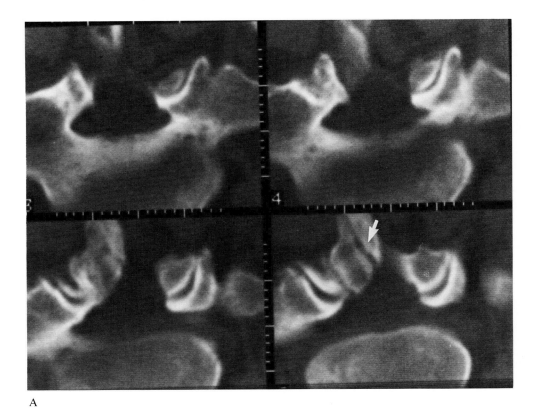

A

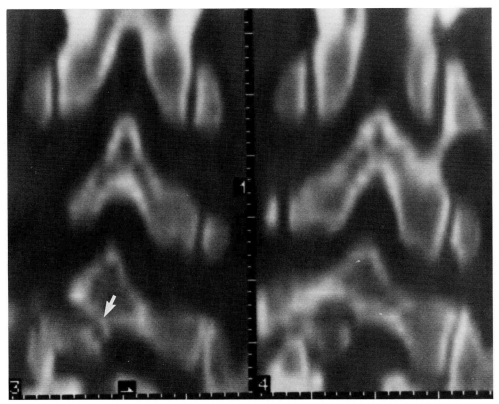

B

FIGURE 8.18   Retroisthmic cleft. Axial (**A**) and coronal (**B**) views reveal clefts within the left lamina (*arrows*).

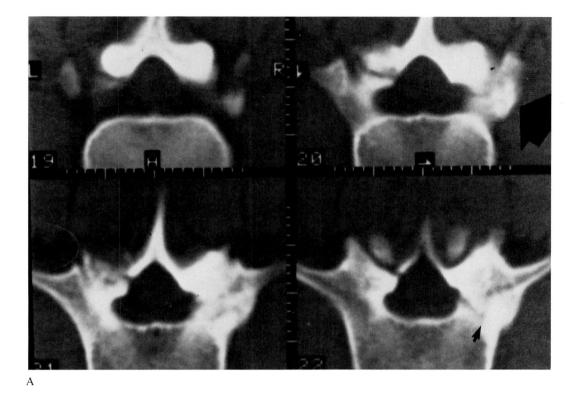

A

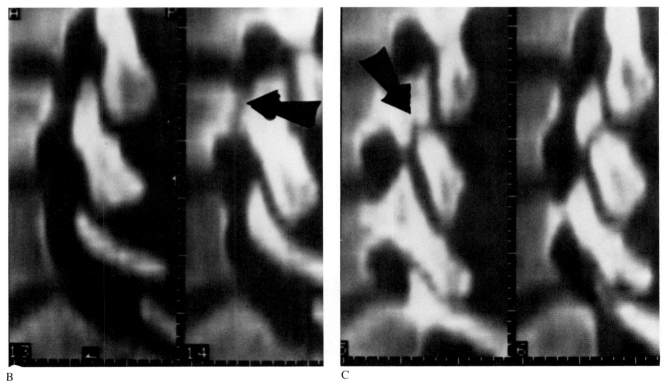

B

C

FIGURE 8.19 Retrosomatic clefts. **A.** Patient 1. Axial scan with pars defect on the left (*arrow*) and a retrosomatic cleft on the right. **B.** Sagittal view through the retrosomatic cleft, which lies anterior to the pedicle. **C.** Sagittal view of the opposite side through a typical pars defect (*arrow*). (*Figure continued* on page 232.)

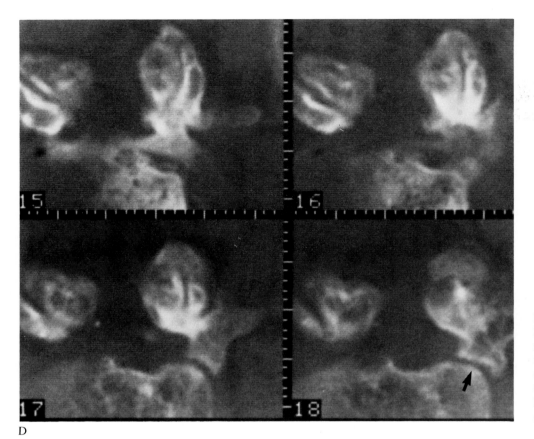

D

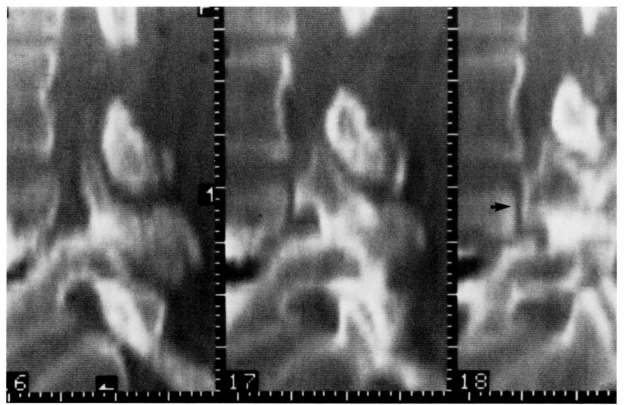

E

FIGURE   8.19   *(cont'd)*
D. Patient 2. Axial scan shows retrosomatic cleft on the right *(arrow)*. **E.** Sagittal reformation demonstrates marked degeneration of the disc space, spondylolisthesis, and foraminal stenosis *(arrow)*.

Lateral Canal Compression

Soft-tissue or bony indentation or compression of the lateral surface of the spinal canal was noted in 68 patients. This defect has not been emphasized previously in the radiologic literature. Typically, a prominent soft-tissue bulge projects medially from the anterior margin of the pars defect (Fig. 8.20). In some patients there is calcification or true ossification within or abutting the pars defect. These lateral soft-tissue or bony masses may indent the dura and occasionally severely compromise the spinal canal (Fig. 8.21). These changes are thought of as callus formed at the fracture site—the soft-tissue or bony sequelae to pseudarthrosis formation. The axial plane is best for evaluating this process.

Lateral Recess

Bony indentation of the lateral recesses was seen in 10 cases (Fig. 8.22). Recess compression was usually at the site of the pars defect, and it was frequently, but not always, associated with callus formation.

Degenerative Spondylolisthesis

In our clinical series there were 225 cases of degenerative spondylolisthesis with intact neural arch. This entity has been well known for many years, but Junghanns[18] studied

it carefully in 11 spines and described the pathologic changes in detail. He coined the term "pseudospondylolisthesis." The terms "degenerative spondylolisthesis" or "degenerative spondylolisthesis with intact neural arch" are more correct linguistically and descriptively[19] because "spondylolisthesis" really means downward vertebral sliding.

The L4–5 intervertebral joint is the most commonly affected, followed by L3–4 and L5–S1 (Table 8.1). The amount of anterior slippage is generally less than 1 cm, but the effect on the neural elements may be severe. Because the pars is intact, the subluxated vertebral body draws its lamina with it. The cauda equina becomes compressed between the anteriorly subluxated lamina and the vertebral body below (Fig. 8.23). Sacralization of L5 is four times more common in patients with degenerative spondylolisthesis than in the general population. The incidence of degenerative spondylolisthesis is more common in blacks and almost exactly parallels the increased incidence of sacralization of L5.

The disorder is one of middle age. It is seen infrequently in patients under the age of 40. Females are affected four times as frequently as males. A straight, stable lumbosacral joint seems to be a predisposing factor because of the abnormal stress placed on the L5 intervertebral joint. Hypermobility leads to disc degeneration and ligamentous laxity. This produces degenerative remodeling of the articular facets, with flattening of the superior facet of L5 and forward subluxation of the inferior facet of L4.

The weight of the upper body is borne by the L5

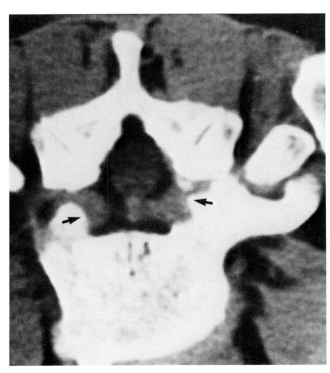

FIGURE 8.20 Soft-tissue callus from pars fracture. Axial view demonstrates two large soft-tissue masses (*arrows*) extending centrally from the anterior into the pars defect.

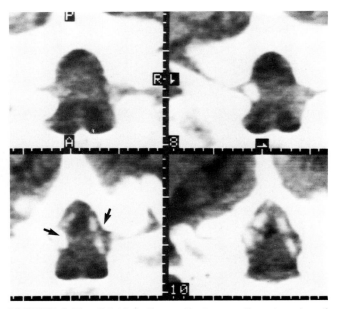

FIGURE 8.21 Calcified fibrocartilaginous callus. A series of axial scans demonstrate prominent calcified callus and calcification of the ligamentum flavum compressing the theca (*arrows*).

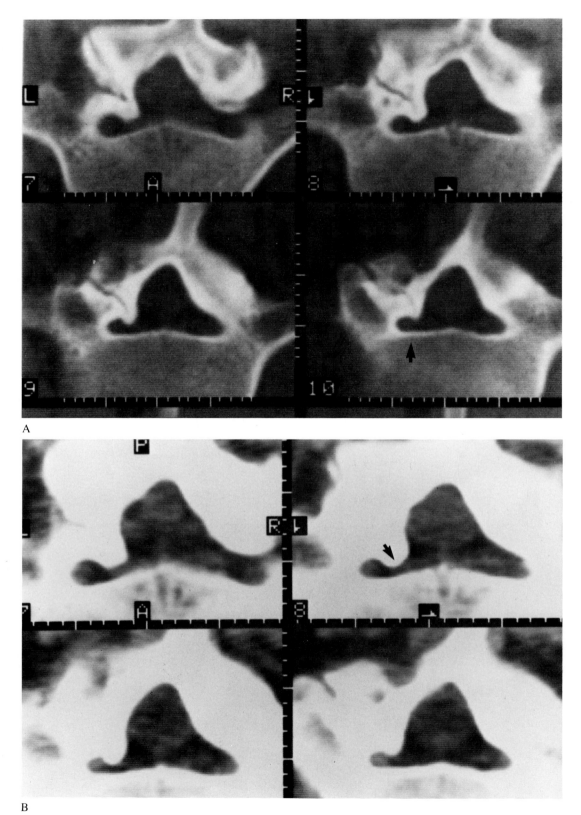

FIGURE 8.22 Lateral recess stenosis. **A.** Bone window axial scans demonstrate lateral recess stenosis at the level of a pars interarticularis defect (*arrow*). **B.** Soft-tissue axial views on the same patient.

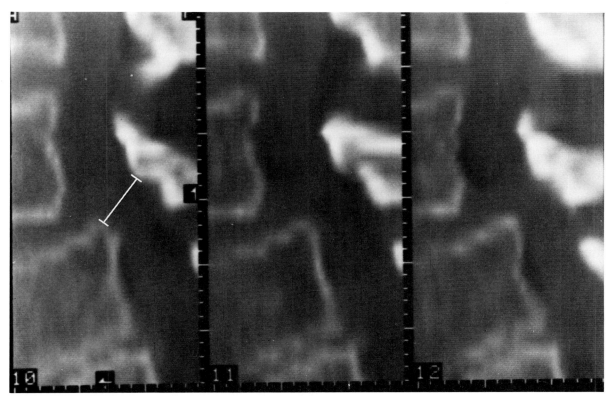

FIGURE 8.23 Degenerative spondylolisthesis, L4–5. Sagittal reformations reveal 8-mm forward subluxation of L4 on L5. The diameter of the spinal canal is reduced to 8-mm. This is measured from the posterior lip of the superior end-plate of L5 to the undersurface of the L4 lamina.

level. This produces a forward and downward force, which is resisted by the muscles, ligaments, and posterior articulations of the spine. When the plane of the facets is oriented sagittally, there is relatively less bony resistance to this force than when the orientation is oblique or coronal

(Fig. 8.24). The joint surfaces tend to be curved so that they are sagittal posteriorly but curved like a ''J'' anteriorly. It is this curved articular surface that resists forward displacement, similar to more oblique or coronal joints. Articular tropism is extremely common in these patients

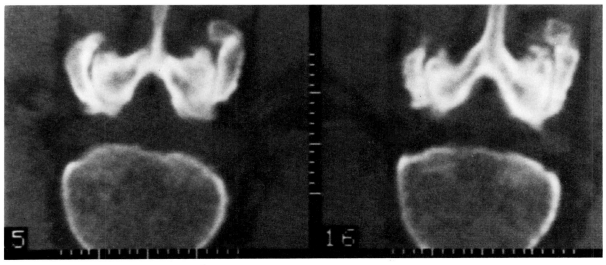

FIGURE 8.24 Degenerative spondylolisthesis, L4–5. Axial views demonstrate sagittally oriented facets that have dislocated. Cartilaginous surfaces are irregular and eroded.

and is likely a very important predisposing factor leading to dislocation.[20] In these cases the angle between the pedicle and the facet tends to be closer to 180 degrees than to the more usual 90 degrees.

We believe that a relatively simple mechanism leads to degenerative spondylolisthesis. Degeneration of the disc increases with advancing age. This, coupled with congenital malalignmnent, leads to increasing abnormal mobility. Anterior displacement is increased by flexion. The usual rocking motion of the joint is accompanied by forward and backward sliding. This abnormal motion adds to the eroding stress on the facets, further aggravating the slippage. It has been suggested that the anterior slippage is due only to disc degeneration. This seems very unlikely because narrowing of the disc with normal facet orientation should lead to downward and posterior subluxation.

Severe symptoms requiring surgery are relatively uncommon.[21] Patients most often present with prolonged, chronic central low back pain; intermittent at first but more persistent and severe with passing time. Symptoms tend to be present for long periods of time before definitive therapy is contemplated. Unilateral or bilateral sciatica may be present and associated with motor neuropathy as well as weakness and atrophy of the lower extremities. Lasegue's sign (pain on straight leg raise) is not commonly present.

In patients with severe subluxation, intermittent neural claudication is a relatively common sign. Pain and paresthesia tend to increase upon walking or even standing with the back straight or extended. This pain is relieved by rest and by lying supine. Surgical intervention is prompted by evidence of cauda equina compression, which is similar to that produced by any other type of severe spinal stenosis.

CT Analysis

Routine radiographs and digital ScoutViews demonstrate the presence and amount of forward subluxation. The amount of abnormal motion at the intervertebral segment can be assessed by fluoroscopy or by flexion/extension films. Myelography has always been required for complete assessment of cauda equina and nerve root compression. However, CT/MPR can replace myelography in the majority of these cases: It allows excellent visualization of the bony and soft-tissue deformity. CT analysis must include: (1) evaluation of the size and shape of the stenotic spinal canal; (2) assessment of the amount of disc or anulus anterior soft-tissue extradural mass; (3) delineation of the anatomy of the facet surfaces and osteophytes; (4) notation of the lateral or rotatory laminar subluxation; (5) evaluation of the amount of ligamentum flavum and periarticular soft-tissue hypertrophy; and (6) evaluation of foramina for bony or soft-tissue encroachment.

One word of caution is necessary. There is one normal anatomic variant that on sagittally reformatted CT seems to show subluxation when none is actually present. For this

to occur, the S1 body must be round or ovoid posteriorly and the L5 body must be concave or flat inwardly. This peculiar combination of anatomic variants cause L5 to seem to be displaced forward on S1 on the midline CT reformations. In fact, however, the L5 body is shorter than S1, and no subluxation exists (Fig. 8.25). This can be proved by looking at lateral sagittal views. On these images the lateral surfaces of the bodies always line up correctly on both sides, even though the central views demonstrate offset.

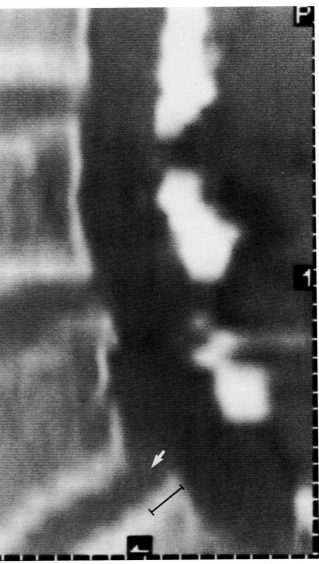

A

FIGURE 8.25 True pseudospondylolisthesis. **A.** Sagittal views along the midline appear to show forward subluxation of L5 on the sacrum (*arrow*). **B.** Axial views demonstrate a round sacral body and a flat L5 body (*arrows*). L5 is unusually short along its midsection, giving the appearance of spondylolisthesis. **C.** Lateral sagittal view shows that the vertebral end-plates align properly (*arrows*).

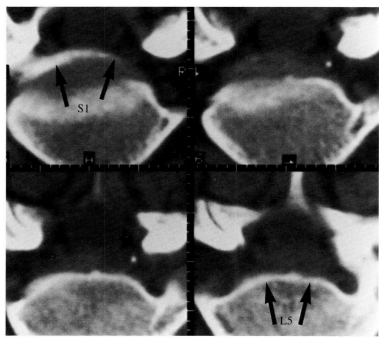

B

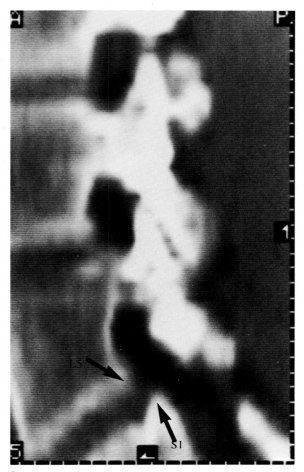

C

Assessment of Spinal Canal Compression

The patient whose sagittal scans are depicted in Figure 8.26 has a normal-size spinal canal. There is 8 mm forward subluxation of L4 on L5. The narrowest area of this patient's spinal canal is an oblique line drawn from the inferior tip of the lamina of L4 to the posterior rim of the superior end-plate of L5. Forward dislocation of the lamina of the upper vertebral body compresses the cauda equina against the superior lip of the lower vertebral body. In this typical case there is no significant soft-tissue extradural mass and no evidence of disc herniation.

Narrowing of the intervertebral disc space with bulging of the anulus fibrosis is noted frequently in patients with degenerative spondylolisthesis. Disc herniation, however, is less commonly associated with degenerative spondylolisthesis than with isthmic spondylolisthesis. These facts correlate well with the overall incidence of disc herniation, which tends to be a disorder of early middle-aged people. Its incidence increases through the fourth decade of life and then tends to decrease. The extrusion of disc material is more likely to occur in the young, where the nucleus retains more of its gel like character. Collapse of the desiccated disc space usually occurs without free-fragment herniation in the middle-aged and elderly.

The patient in Figure 8.27 demonstrates an 8-mm anterior subluxation of L4 and L5. Unlike the previous case, there is a large amount of soft-tissue bulge of the disc and the anulus into the spinal canal. The sagittal diameter of the spinal canal is reduced markedly by the anulus bulge, ligamentum hypertrophy, and expansion of the facet joints. There is severe soft-tissue spinal stenosis, further compro-

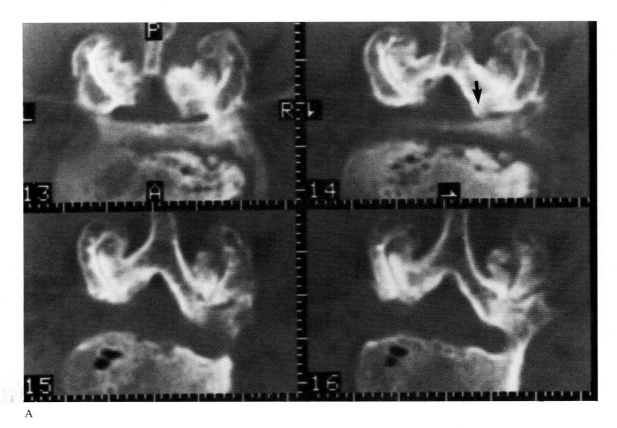

A

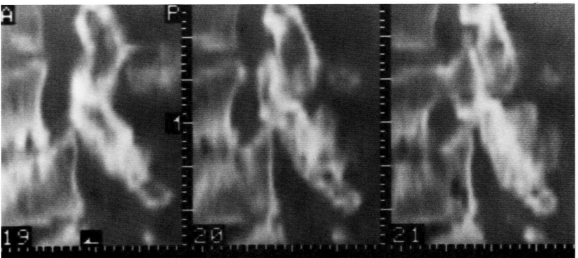

B

FIGURE 8.26 Articular tropism and degenerative spondylolisthesis. **A.** Axial views demonstrate considerable tropism of the facet joints. The plane of the right facet is nearly sagittal, and that of the left facet is more curved and coronal. The subluxation is more on the side of the sagittally oriented facet. The inferior articular process of L4 has subluxated forward and medially (*arrow*). **B.** Sagittal reformation shows 10-mm forward subluxation of L4 on L5, with severe degeneration of the disc space, with a vacuum disc effect. The joint surfaces are irregular and eroded. Note that the neural foramen is relatively well maintained.

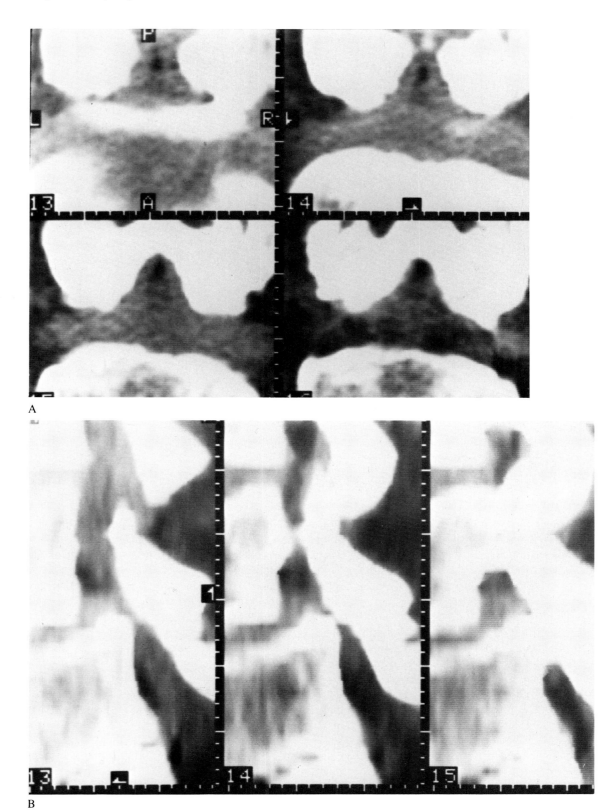

A

B

FIGURE 8.27 Spondylolisthesis associated with soft-tissue bulging of the disc and anulus. Axial views (**A**) and sagittal reformations (**B**) demonstrate prominent bulge of the disc and anulus into the spinal canal. The canal is profoundly narrowed because of a combination of the subluxation and the soft-tissue bulge.

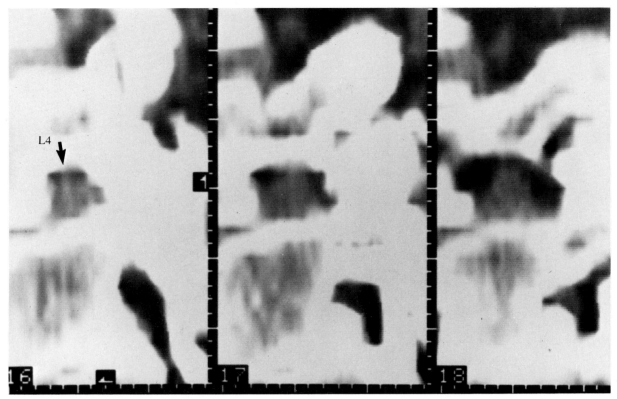

FIGURE 8.28   Foraminal occlusion caused by herniation of disc material. Three sagittal views on a patient with 8-mm spondylolisthesis reveals that the neural foramen is normal in size. The foramen is, however, filled with disc material. Note the exiting L3 nerve in the foramen above.

mised by the anterior bony dislocation. On the sagittal view in Figure 8.28 the neural foramina are of normal size, but they are almost completely filled with herniated disc and bulging of the anulus.

Assessment of Facet Pathology

The hallmark of spondylolisthesis with intact neural arch is severe erosion and degeneration of facet joints. These changes may manifest in many ways. The patient whose scans are portrayed in Figure 8.29 has an asymmetrical severe destructive arthropathy that has destroyed the cartilaginous surface of the left joint. The joint space seems unusually widened because of the severe erosions that have occurred on both articular surfaces. Sagittal and coronal views similarly demonstrate this abnormal articular complex. There is a relative paucity of hypertrophic spondylitic spurs. The patient in Figure 8.30 is one of the few in our clinical series with degenerative spondylolisthesis at L5–S1. In this situation the facet joints are oriented sagittally. The joint surfaces are severely degenerated; they are irregular, pitted, and grooved. These films demonstrate a relatively large amount of hypertrophic spurring on both axial and sagittal

views. Note especially the severe destruction of the apex of the superior facet of the sacrum and the grooving and destruction of the undersurface of the pars interarticularis.

A vacuum joint effect is often noted in degenerative spondylolisthesis. The patient in Figure 8.31 demonstrates very severe hypertrophic degenerative changes of the L4–5 facets. Both joint spaces are expanded and filled with gas. There is very little asymmetry of the facets in this patient. The articular surfaces are coronally oriented. This accounts for the fact that although there is severe osteoarthritic erosion of the joints there is only 3 mm forward subluxation.

The most severe clinical symptoms may occur when there is unrestricted anterior dislocation of the inferior facet of the upper vertebral body, beyond the confines of the anterior limb of the superior facet. This may occur bilaterally, causing forward dislocation, or unilaterally, causing rotatory subluxation (Fig. 8.32). Rotatory subluxation can produce severe compression of the lateral recess and marked narrowing of the neural foramen on the affected side. In the patient in Figure 8.33 there is marked degeneration, destruction, and erosion of both pairs of articular process. The sagittal view clearly defines degenerative disc disease and vacuum changes at L4 and L5. The spinal canal is

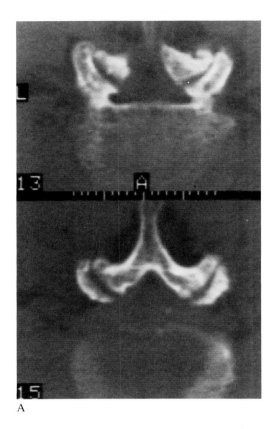

A

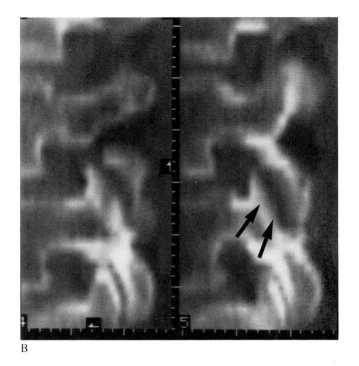

B

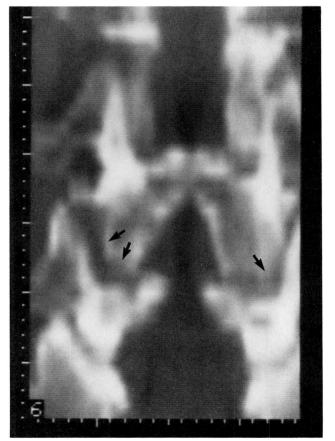

C

FIGURE 8.29 Arthropathy in degenerative spondylolisthesis. **A.** Axial scan demonstrates severe erosive arthritis of the facet joints, especially on the left. There is erosion of the cartilage and the joint space is widened. **B, C.** Sagittal and coronal views similarly show a widening of the joint, with destruction of the articular surfaces (*arrows*).

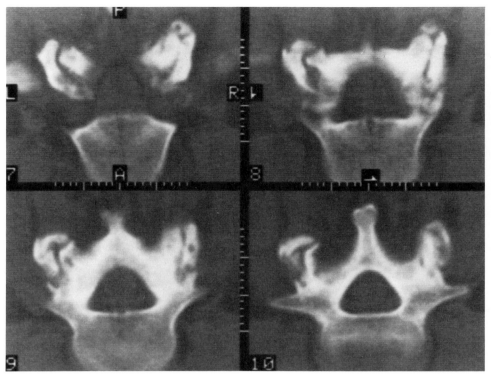

A

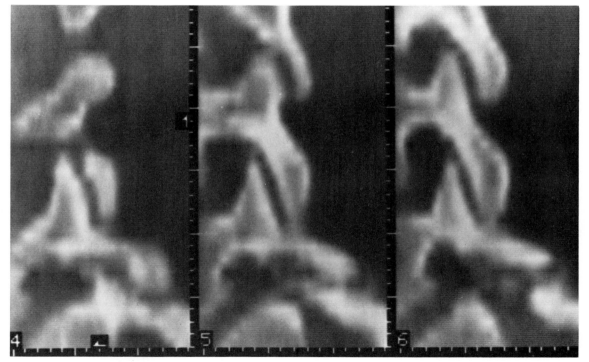

B

FIGURE 8.30   Degenerative spondylolisthesis, L5–S1. Axial (**A**) and sagittal (**B**) views demonstrate sagittally oriented facets bilaterally. There is a minor degree of facet tropism. The cartilaginous surfaces of the joints are remarkably eroded, irregular, pitted, and destroyed. There is a considerable amount of hypertrophic bony change. The neural foramen is only moderately reduced in size.

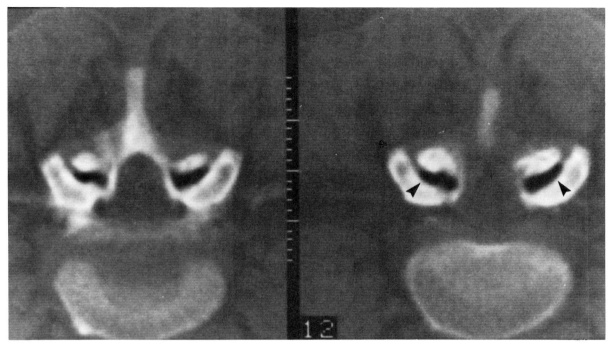

A

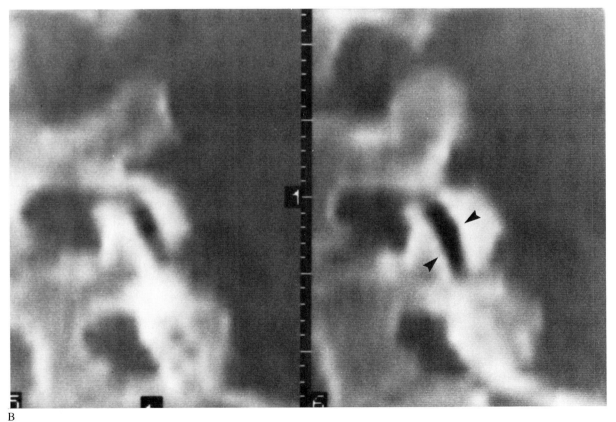

B

FIGURE 8.31 Gas effect in facet joints. Axial (**A**) and sagittal (**B**) views reveal arthropathy of the joints, which are expanded by gas. (*Figure continued* on page 244.)

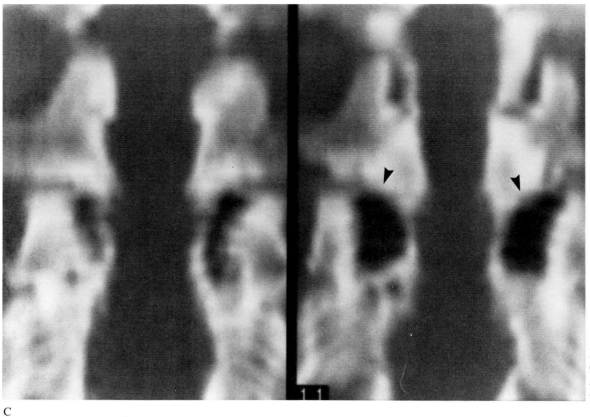

FIGURE 8.31 (*cont'*
C. Coronal views reve
arthropathy of the join
which are expanded by g

C

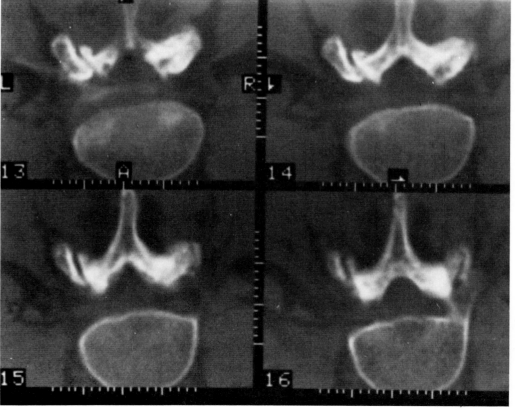

A

FIGURE 8.32 Rotatory
subluxation. Soft-tissue (**A**)
and bone-window (**B**) axial views demonstrate subluxation of the left facet
and severe left-sided canal
and recess stenosis.

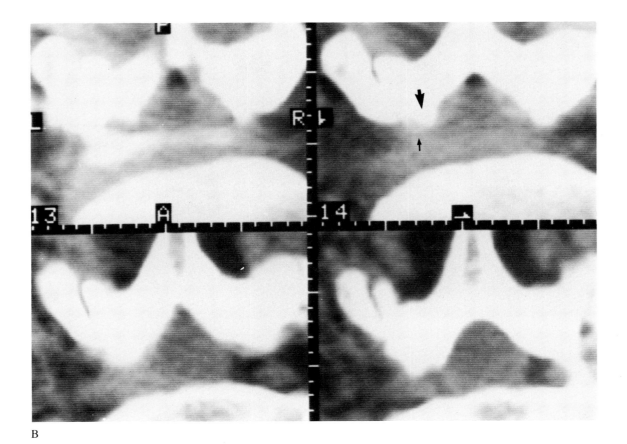

B

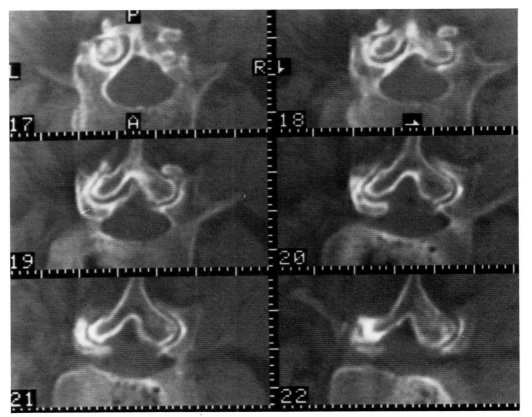

A

FIGURE 8.33 Rotatory subluxation. **A.** Axial scan demonstrates rotatory subluxation. There is marked deformity of the facet joints bilaterally. **B.** Sagittal view demonstrates vacuum disc effect at the lower two levels. Also clearly visible is 11 mm forward subluxation of L4 on L5. The spinal canal is considerably narrowed because of the subluxation. **C.** Coronal view demonstrates vacuum effects at three levels, with lateral rotatory dislocation at several levels. (*Figure continued on page 246.*)

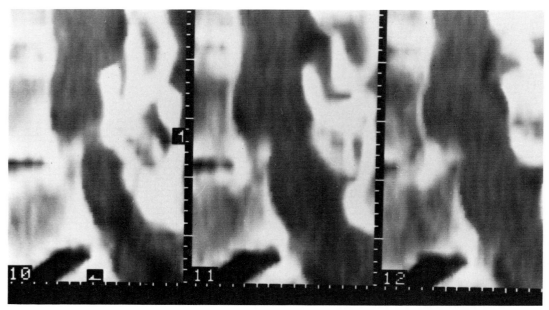

B

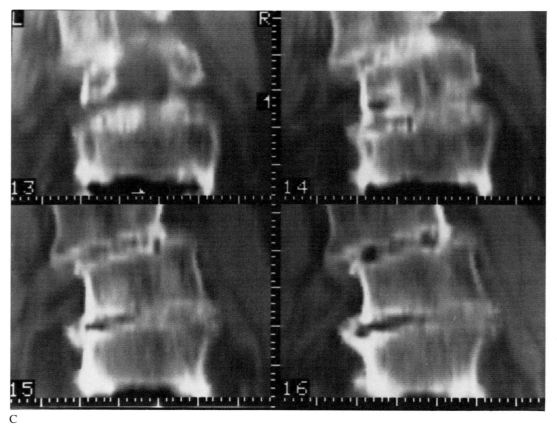

C

FIGURE 8.33 (*cont'd*)
See legend page 245.

narrowed because of 11 mm forward subluxation. On the coronal view, however, we best appreciate the lateral and rotatory component of this deforming arthropathy.

Lateral subluxation tends to occur when the joint surfaces are oriented in the coronal plane. This is the least common type of degenerative spondylolisthesis. The anter-oposterior diameter of the spinal canal may be normal, but there is compression of the lateral surface of the theca by the subluxating facet (Fig. 8.34).

Ligamentum flavum hypertrophy and periarticular soft tissue are frequently found in patients with severe arthritis of the facet joints. These abnormally hypertrophied soft-

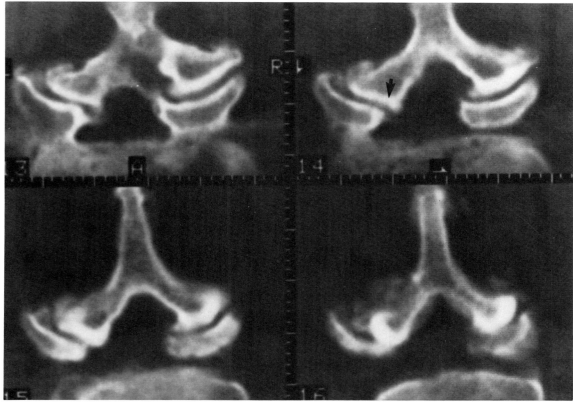

A

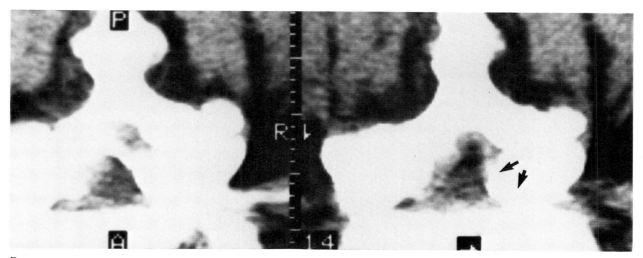

B

FIGURE 8.34 Lateral subluxation. Axial scans windowed for bone (**A**) and soft tissue (**B**) reveal coronally oriented facets. There is considerable lateral subluxation of the facets, causing prominent compression of the left lateral recess. The space available for the theca and cauda equina is remarkably reduced.

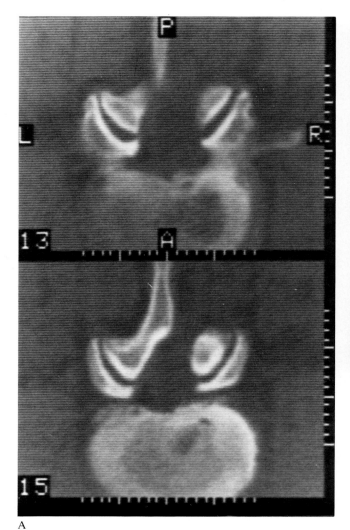

A

FIGURE 8.35   Retrolisthesis. **A.** Axial views demonstrate degeneration of the intervertebral disc, with some degenerative spurs in the neural foramina on this postoperative patient. Note that the articular surfaces are normal. **B.** Sagittal view demonstrates erosion of the end-plate, with 3-mm retrolisthesis of L4 on L5.

tissue structures tend to compress the cauda equina profoundly in what is an already severely compromised canal. On occasion, the ligamentum flavum calcifies. When this calcification is unduly thick, it may also cause posterolateral spinal canal compression.

Neural foraminal encroachment is less a factor in forward degenerative spondylolisthesis than is lateral-recess and canal stenosis. Foraminal narrowing is caused by downward displacement of the pedicle due to the subluxation. Stenosis becomes severe when there are large spurs or bulging of the anulus fibrosis laterally into the neural foramen. These changes may account for some patients' severe radiculopathy.

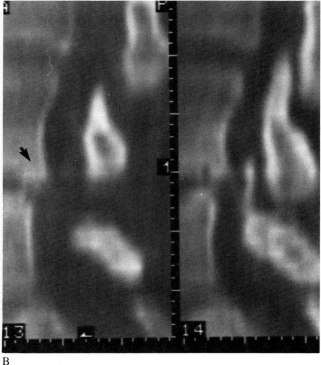

B

Retrolisthesis (Reverse Spondylolisthesis)

Retrolisthesis, or reverse spondylolisthesis, is another condition that is manifested by abnormal vertebral alignment. In this disorder, one vertebra subluxates posteriorly on its next lowest mate. The primary predisposing factor is disc degeneration. The facet joints are usually normal (Fig. 8.35).

With increasing degeneration of the nucleus, the disc space narrows. The weight of the body acts to displace the inferior facet of the upper vertebra down the inclined surface of the superior facet of the lower vertebra, producing true retrospondylolisthesis. Traction of the erector spinatus muscles and the ligamentum flavum may play some role in this displacement. Retrolisthesis is most likely to occur at L3–4 and L4–5, which are the most mobile portions of the lumbar spine. The cartilaginous surfaces of the facet usually appear relatively normal, allowing downward slippage. Cartilage erosion, which is the hallmark of forward degenerative spondylolisthesis, is less evident when posterior subluxation occurs.

CT usually reveals all of the signs of disc degeneration: disc narrowing, spur formation, sclerosis and erosion of the end-plates, and facet-joint laxity (Fig. 8.36). In some patients posterior dislocation is seen only during hyperextension. This is called ''primary instability'' and may be one of the first radiologic manifestations of disc degener-

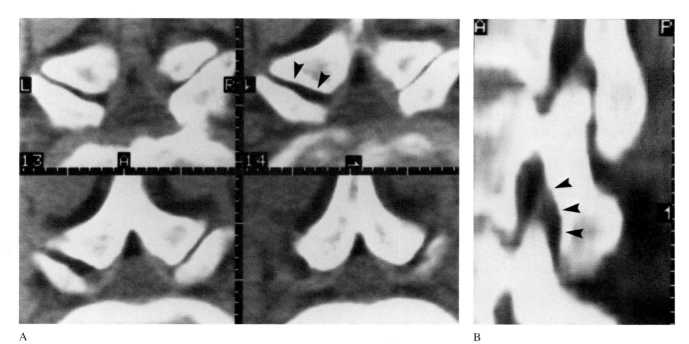

A   B

FIGURE 8.36   Retrolisthesis, with laxity of the facet joint. Axial (**A**) and sagittal (**B**) views demonstrate widening of the facet joint on the left side, without evidence of erosion of the joint surfaces or loss of cartilage (*arrowheads*).

ation. There is rarely more than 5–6 mm posterior subluxation, and spinal stenosis symptoms are less common than in patients with forward subluxation. One of the important features of retrolisthesis is foraminal stenosis, which is caused by upward displacement of the superior facet of the lower vertebra into the neural foramen (Fig. 8.37). On sagittal

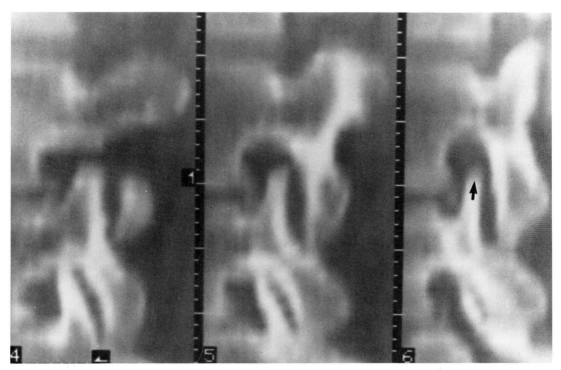

FIGURE 8.37   Retrolisthesis, with foraminal stenosis. A series of sagittal views demonstrate upward herniation of the superior facet at L5 into the neural foramen (*arrow*).

reformations one often sees that the exiting root is impressed by the articular process. One must realize that supine CT images tend to underestimate the amount of foraminal stenosis in this entity because encroachment is accentuated in the upright and hyperextended positions. Frequently, prominent lateral anulus bulge further compromises the already diminished foramen.

The diagnosis of retrolisthesis is obvious on spine films. One can easily measure the amount of retrolisthesis on well-positioned lateral radiographs. There are two pitfalls that should be noted: (1) Rotation and tilting of the central ray of the x-ray beam may produce the appearance of mild retrolisthesis when none is actually present; and (2) there is an anatomic variant of the lumbosacral junction that mimics retrolisthesis. In instances where the top of the sacrum is ovoid and the anteroposterior diameter of the L5 vertebral body is increased or kidney shaped, the lateral posterior rim of the L5 end-plate tends to extend over the plane of the top of the sacrum. On conventional radiographs this condition appears to be retrolisthesis. Measuring the anteroposterior diameter in these patients proves that L5 is actually deeper than the sacrum and is not displaced. Sagittal CT views will demonstrate that only the lateral surface overrides the sacrum whereas the center of the bones align properly.

CT Examination

CT examination of these patients includes the following:

1. Assessment of the amount of sagittal canal reduction
2. Evaluation of the amount of soft-tissue compression
3. Evaluation of foraminal patency

Spinal stenosis is relatively uncommon in patients with retrolisthesis. When present, compression occurs between the inferior end-plate of the superior vertebra and the lamina of the inferior vertebra.

The patient in Figure 8.38 is rather typical of our clinical series. There is severe degeneration of the disc at the L3–4 level, with minor amounts of disc bulging at L4–5 and L5–S1. The sagittal diameter of the canal is reduced at the level of the dislocation. The major abnormality is within the neural foramen and the lateral recess, where the exiting nerve is compressed between the posterior portion of the vertebral end-plate and the superior facet.

As with degenerative spondylolisthesis with forward subluxation, disc herniation is relatively rare. When it does occur, the neural canal may be compromised severely because of the relatively narrow spinal canal.

The patient in Figure 8.39 is unusual in that he demonstrates both forward spondylolisthesis at L4–5 and retrolisthesis at L3–4. This is not as uncommon as is generally

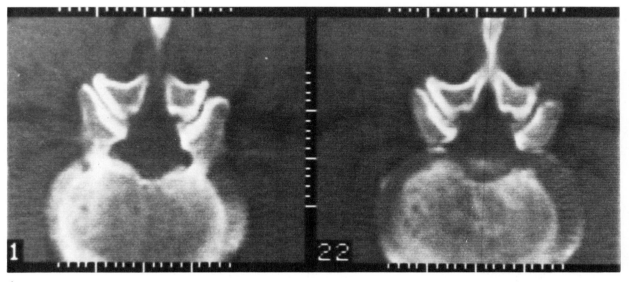

A

FIGURE 8.38   Retrolisthesis, with recess stenosis. **A.** Axial scan demonstrates degenerative change of the L3–4 level, with diffuse bulge of the anulus across the disc space. Calcification in the posterior anulus wall appears to abut the anterior portion of the superior facet. **B.** Sagittal reformation demonstrates 7-mm retrolisthesis of L3 on L4. Note the apposition of the posterior edge of the inferior end-plate of L3 to the superior facet of L4 (*arrow*).

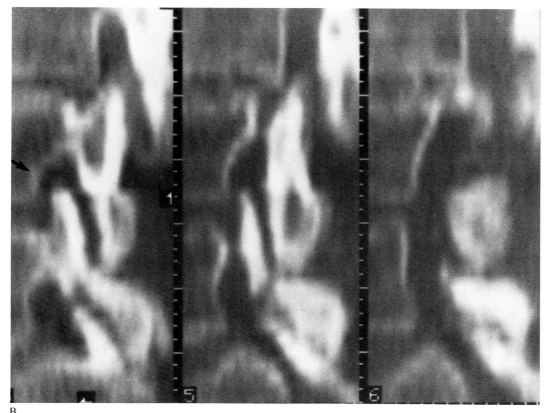

B
FIGURE 8.38 (*cont'd*)

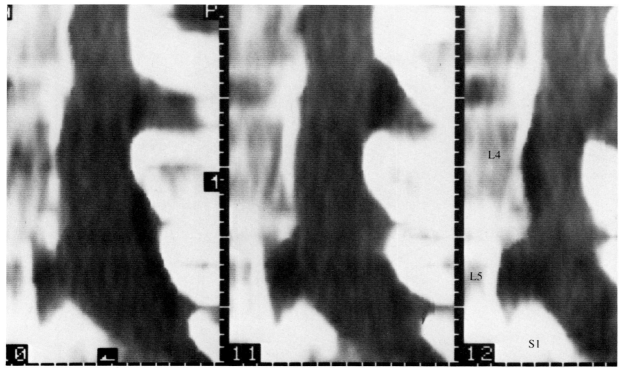

FIGURE 8.39 Retrolisthesis above spondylolisthesis. A series of sagittal reformations reveals that there is 9-mm forward spondylolisthesis of L5 on the sacrum, and 9-mm retrolisthesis of L4 on L5. Note that there is only minimal compression of the spinal canal in this patient.

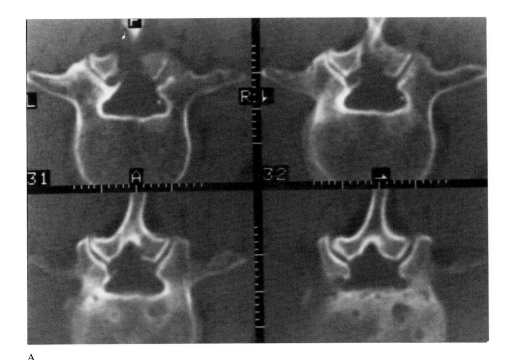

A

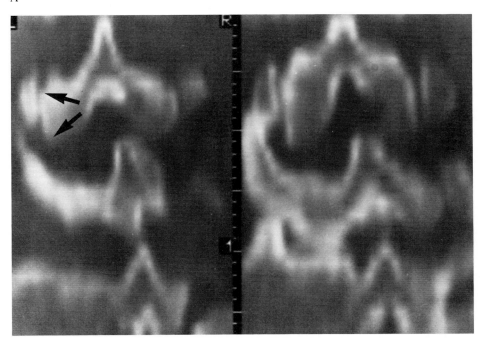

B

FIGURE 8.40 Unilateral rotatory retrolisthesis. **A.** Axial scan demonstrates the normal position of the right articular process but posterior displacement of the inferior facet of L3 with respect to the superior facet of L4 (*arrow*). **B.** Coronal reformation defines downward subluxation of the inferior facet (*arrows*).

suspected. The diagnosis may be very difficult to make in the axial plane. Radiculopathy is likely to be caused by root compression within the neural foramen.

Unilateral rotatory subluxation may also occur in patients with retrolisthesis (Fig. 8.40). On the axial views of this patient, note the relative posterior and inferior displacement of the left inferior articular process of L3, as compared with the superior facet of L4. The downward dislocation of the left inferior facet is best seen on the coronal view.

Iatrogenic Spondylolisthesis

Iatrogenic spondylolisthesis includes two distinctly different types of lesion. The first, known as "spondylolisthesis acquisita", is believed to be a stress fracture of the pars at a level immediately above a spine fusion. Many patients with this lesion have had their fusions because of spondylolisthesis. This suggests an underlying predisposition to pars fracture. The exact mechanism of this fracture is not well understood. It is clear, however, that there usually is abnormal stress above or below spine fusion. This is most obvious in patients with congenital fusion who develop severe degenerative arthritis adjacent to the fused vertebrae. This rare phenomenon was not seen in our series, as spine fusions performed in our geographic area are transverse process and lateral mass fusions, which tend to buttress the pars, protecting them from fracture.

The second disorder in this group is caused by overzealous posterior and posterolateral decompression. This is generally termed "iatrogenic spondylolisthesis." Radical decompression of the spine with facetectomy removes most of the bony support for the posterior elements (Fig. 8.41). We have studied many patients with this disorder. Forward and backward subluxation occur with almost equal frequency. The largest amount of displacement was 13 mm; the smallest was 7 mm. The lack of bony support in these patients accounts for the unusual degree of slippage. It is not clear why some patients with radical decompression subluxate and some do not; it may relate to the anatomy of the remaining facets. Coronally oriented facets seem to resist forward subluxation more successfully than do sagittally oriented facets.

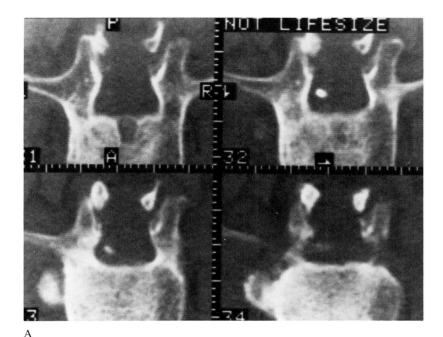

A

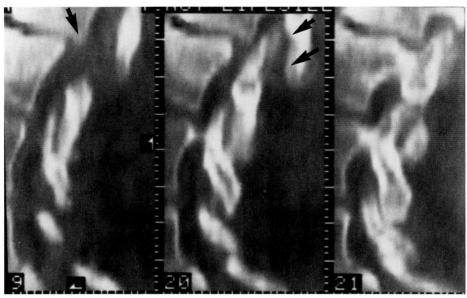

B

FIGURE 8.41 Iatrogenic spondylolisthesis. **A.** Axial scans demonstrate wide bilateral laminectomy and facetectomy in a patient with sagitally oriented facets. **B.** Sagittal views reveal retrolisthesis of L3 on L4, with widening of the joint space (*arrows*).

References

1. Schmorl G, Junghanns H: Besemann EF (ed): The Human Spine in Health and Disease. 2nd American edition. Grune & Stratton, New York, 1971, p. 378
2. Stewart TD: Neural arch defects in Alaskan natives. J Bone Joint Surg 35A:937, 1953
3. Wiltse LL, Widell EH Jr, Jackson DW: Fatigue fracture the basic lesion in isthmic spondylolisthesis. J Bone Joint Surg 57A:17-22, 1975
4. Wiltse LL: Spondylolisthesis: Classification and Etiology. In: American Acadamy of Orthopaedic Surgery Symposium on the Spine. St. Louis, Mosby, 1969, pp. 143-167
5. Wiltse LL: Spondylolisthesis and its treatment. In Ruge D, Wiltse LL (eds): Spinal Disorders. Lea & Febiger, Philadelphia, 1977, pp. 193-217
6. Rothman SLG, Glenn WVG Jr: CT multiplanar reconstruction in 253 cases of lumbar spondylolysis. AJNR 5:81-90, 1984
7. Nathan H: Spondylolysis. J Bone Joint Surg 41A:303, 1959
8. Haughton VM (ed): Spondylolysis in Computed Tomography of the Spine. Churchill Livingstone, New York, 1983, pp. 163-171
9. Sherman FC, Wilkinson RH, Hall JE: The reactive sclerosis of a pedicle and spondylolysis in the lumbar spine. Radiology 124:571, 1977
10. Wiltse LL: The etiology of spondylolisthesis. J Bone Joint Surg 44A:539-569, 1963
11. Briggs H, Keats S: Laminectomy and foramenotomy with chip fusion: operative treatment for the relief of low back pain and sciatic pain associated with spondylolisthesis. J Bone Joint Surg 29A:328-334, 1947
12. Macnab I: The management of spondylolisthesis. Prog Neurol Surg 4:246-276, 1971
13. Rothman SLG, Glenn WV Jr: Spondylolysis and spondylolisthesis. In Newton TH, Potts DE (eds): Computed Tomography of the Spine and Spinal Cord. Clavadel Press, San Anselmo, California, 1983, pp. 267-280
14. Rothman SLG, Glenn WV Jr: Spondylolysis and spondylolisthesis. In Post MJD (ed): Computed Tomography of the Spine. Williams & Wilkins, Baltimore, 1984, pp. 591-615
15. Woolsey RD: The mechanism of neurological symptoms and signs in spondylolisthesis at the fifth lumbar, first sacral level. pp. 67-76
16. Gill GG: Spondylolisthesis and its treatment: excision of loose lamina and decompression. In: Ruge D, Wiltse LL (eds): Spinal Disorders: Diagnosis and Treatment. Lea & Febiger, Philadelphia, 1977, pp. 218-222
17. Johansen JG, Haughton VM: Differentiation of retrosomatic and retroisthmic defects from spondylolysis. Presented at Radiological Society of North America, 69th meeting, Chicago, November 1983
18. Junghanns H: Spondylolisthese, pseudospondylolisthese und wirbelverschiebung nach hinten. Beitr Klin Chir 151:376, 1931
19. Epstein BS, Epstein JA, Jones MD: Degenerative spondylolisthesis with intact neural arch. Radiol Clin North Am 15:275-287, 1977
20. Macnab I: Spondylolisthesis with an intact neural arch—the so-called pseudo-spondylolisthesis. J Bone Joint Surg 32B:325-333, 1950
21. Rosenberg NJ: Degenerative spondylolisthesis: surgical treatment. Clin Orthop 117:112, 1976

The Postoperative Spine

9

The failed back surgery syndrome (FBSS) is one of the most perplexing medical and medicoeconomic problems facing our health system today. In many studies reoperation rates tend to be between 10 and 20%,[1,2] but as many as 20–45%[3] of patients may have persistent back or radicular pain following what was to have been definitive therapy.

The causes for the FBSS are very complex. The Workmen's Compensation system and medicolegal trends toward very high settlements of litigation for injury have provided serious incentive for patients to remain symptomatic. It is difficult to analyze any statistical survey of symptomatic back patients without serious bias from this group of patients.

Others suggest that patients with severe psychological problems, drug abuse, and alcoholism are inappropriately selected as surgical candidates.[4] They believe that careful psychological evaluation of patients minimizes FBSS. Even if all extrinsic factors could be eliminated, the problem of failed back surgery would still be a major one. This chapter is based on a review of 300 postoperative lumbar spine multiplanar CT scans performed over a 15-month period. All patients had a complete set of axial images, with sagittal and coronal reformations photographed twice: optimized once for bone definition and once for soft-tissue contrast resolution.

CT Appearance of the Uncomplicated Postoperative Lumbar Spine

A description of the radiographic findings in the more common surgical procedures facilitates understanding of the abnormal postoperative CT spine scan.

Microsurgical Discectomy

In microsurgical discectomy the entire lamina is left intact. Free disc fragments are removed under the dissecting microscope. The intact anulus is not incised with a scalpel but is probed using a dissector. Most surgeons do not curette the disc space.[5,6]

CT scans of these patients usually reveal no evidence of previous surgical intervention. The laminae and facets are intact. The epidural fat is left intact at surgery, and scarring is very minimal. The only hint of surgery may be asymmetry in the facial planes adjacent to the laminae due to paravertebral fibrosis.

Laminotomy and Discectomy

Simple laminotomy and discectomy through a small incision over one interspace is a common surgical technique.[7,8] The ligamentum flavum beneath the superior lamina is separated, and a small opening is rongeured in the inferior border of the superior lamina. A similar defect is made when necessary in the superior border of the inferior lamina. The amount of bone removed varies with the surgeon and depends to a large extent on adequacy of visualization of the surgical field. The ligamentum flavum is incised. With gentle retraction, the disc space is explored and disc fragments are removed along with the epidural fat. Some surgeons routinely curette the disc space; others do not.

Rongeurs or curettes used to clean out a disc space frequently produce a characteristic bony groove or holes in the vertebral end-plates (Fig. 9.1). This is easily seen in the axial projection (Fig. 9.1A). Compare the vertebral end-plates on the coronal projections in the preoperative and

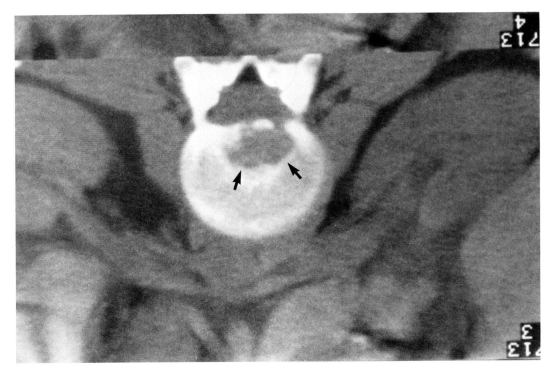

A

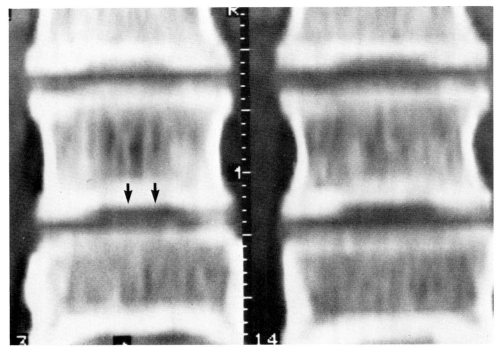

B

FIGURE 9.1 Disc-space curettage. **A.** Axial scan demonstrates a well-defined lucency within the bony end-plate (*arrows*). The margins are smooth and sclerotic. **B.** Normal coronal view, preoperative. Note the subtle concavity of the cartilaginous end-plate (*arrows*). **C.** Postoperative coronal view shows sclerosis and irregularity of the operated end-plate (*arrows*). **D.** Preoperative scan showing no anterior L4–5 osteophytes. **E.** Postoperative scan on the same patient, 2 months later, shows a new anterior osteophyte (*arrows*), which must have been caused by anterior perforation of the anulus and the anterior longitudinal ligament.

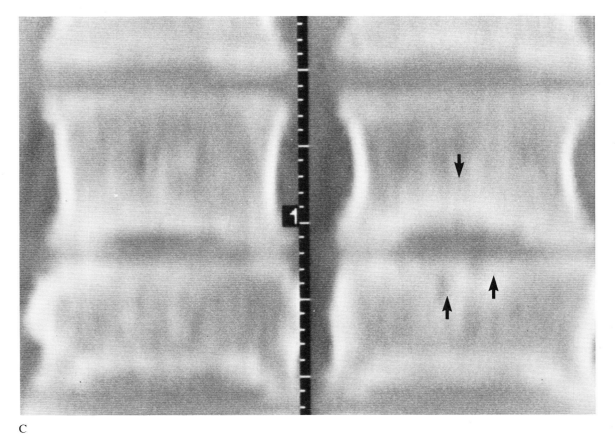

C

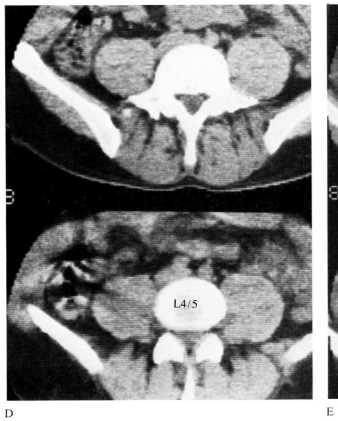

D

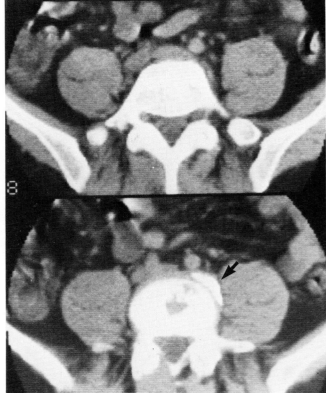

E

postoperative scans. Note the reactive sclerosis and deep-penetrating lucencies. The disc space has also narrowed considerably in the interval (Figs. 9.1B, C). Utmost caution must be exercised by the surgeon when judging the depth of insertion of surgical instruments in a cavity into which he cannot see. The overzealous use of curettes and rongeurs has led to perforation into the retroperitoneal space and even, though rarely, to rupture of the aortic iliac vessels or vena cava, with fatal retroperitoneal hemorrhage.

The postoperative scan in Figures 9.1D, E was per-formed several months after exploration of the L5–S1 and the L4–5 disc spaces. Note the new anterior vertebral osteophyte that has formed at L4–5. This could have occurred only as a response to rupture of the anterior Sharpey's fibers caused by overpenetration with the surgical instruments. The ridge, and therefore the perforation, was just lateral to the iliac artery, fortunately.

In patients with small laminotomy, a CT scan in the axial plane may demonstrate only subtle irregularities in the laminae (Fig.9.2A). Sometimes no laminar defect can be

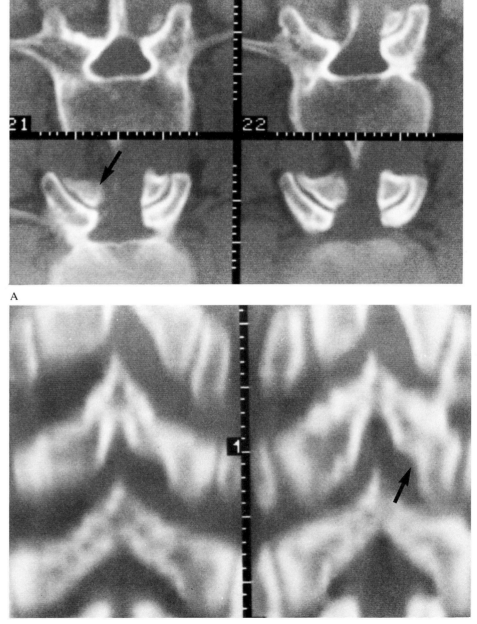

A

B

FIGURE 9.2 Laminotomy. Axial (**A**) and coronal (**B**) views on a patient with a small laminotomy. The inferior margin of the lamina has been removed (*arrows*).

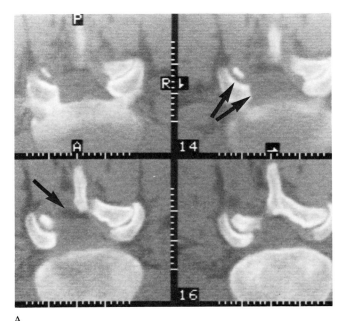

A

FIGURE 9.3 Laminectomy. Axial (**A**) and sagittal (**B**) views demonstrate laminectomy and medial facetectomy. Note on the sagittal view that the articular surface is left intact and the medial and inferior surfaces are removed.

identified. It is important to realize that a minor amount of patient tilt will cause the axial scans to traverse the laminae at a slight angle, thus simulating a laminectomy defect when none is present. Coronally reformatted images (Fig. 9.2B) may demonstrate the minor asymmetry of small laminotomy defects.

Lumbar Decompressive Laminectomy With or Without Foramenotomy

Lumbar decompressive laminectomy is commonly used for chronic disc degeneration or large disc herniations and lateral root entrapment. In the simplest case the bony lamina is removed from the base of the spinous process medially to the medial surface of the pedicle laterally (Fig. 9.3). On the postoperative CT scan this is seen as a clearly defined defect with clean edges. The ligamentum flavum is absent beneath the bone defect. In the ideal condition fat is seen below the bony defect. A small amount of fibrotic scar is usually present at the surgical site. Free-fat grafts have been found to be useful in reducing the amount of postoperative fibrosis.[9,10] It is common practice to purposely replace the epidural fat with extraspinal fat in an attempt to minimize

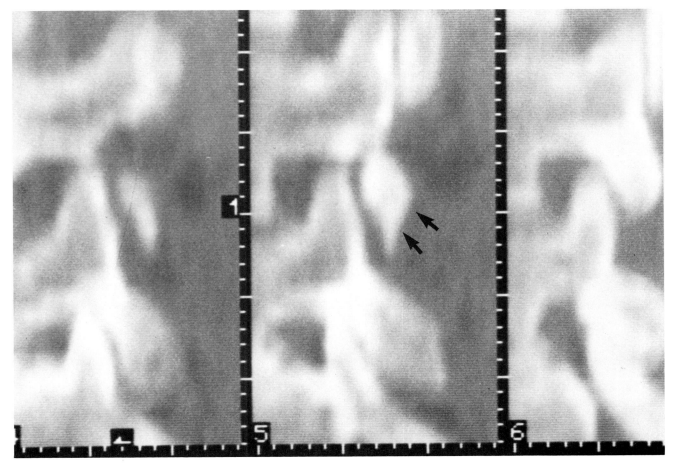

B

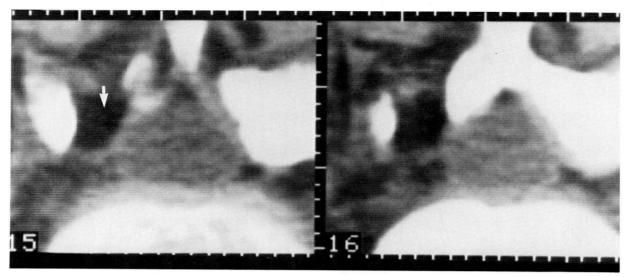

FIGURE 9.4 Fat graft. A pedicle of fat has been placed on the left and has successfully prevented the formation of postsurgical scar.

postoperative intradural scarring. CT scanning often demonstrates a striking amount of lateral fat within the laminectomy defect and an absence of scar in successful cases (Fig. 9.4).

Bilateral laminectomy is frequently performed when central decompression is necessary. The spinous processes and both laminae are then removed at the appropriate levels (Fig. 9.5).

In patients with severe spinal stenosis in whom even more radical decompression is necessary, partial or even total facetectomy may be performed. When possible, the opposing facet surfaces are left in place and the medial extension of the joint is resected (Fig. 9.5D). The spectrum of visible CT changes exactly mirrors the surgical procedure. Minor partial facetectomy usually demonstrates a joint complex with a straight medial edge. As more bone is resected the scans will clearly demonstrate the anatomic decompression. Bilateral laminectomies and facetectomies are occasionally performed at several levels. It is striking that it is often possible to remove the posterior elements without gross spinal instability.

Anatomic Causes of FBSS

The FBSS patients can be grouped into two general categories: (1) patients for whom the indication for surgery was questionable; and (2) patients for whom the surgery was indeed indicated, but the operation did not succeed in alleviating the presenting symptoms.[11]

Inappropriate or Poorly Indicated Surgery

Within the group of patients for whom surgery was inappropriate or poorly indicated fall a large number of individuals who present with back pain either temporily related to trauma or of a chronic nature. Their frequent complaints tend to cause them to undergo clinical and radiologic evaluation without ever having objective neurologic deficits (weakness, reflex changes) or true radiculopathy. Some of these patients have had negative or equivocal myelography. The incidence of failed surgery is extremely high in this group of patients.

The poor presurgical evaluation of these patients was partially due to the inherent limitations of the previously available diagnostic radiographic techniques. It is generally accepted that plain radiographs of the lumbar spine are of very limited value in the diagnosis of disc herniation. Epidural venography has had its proponents over the years, but even at its best it provides secondary information about spinal roots, which is obtained by making inferences about the probable neural compression from apparent venous distortion. Pantopaque myelography is a considerable improvement, but it also provides only inferential information. We are left to assume that one or another defect is due to free-disc-fragment herniation or a hypertrophic spur or ridge. Water-soluble-contrast myelography is still more accurate because it allows better definition of the roots, the root sleeves, and the cauda equina. This too, however, provides information by inference only. We diagnose disc herniation not by seeing the herniation but by noting a particular pattern of extradural deformity. Only high-resolution CT allows us to actually see the cause of theneural compression.

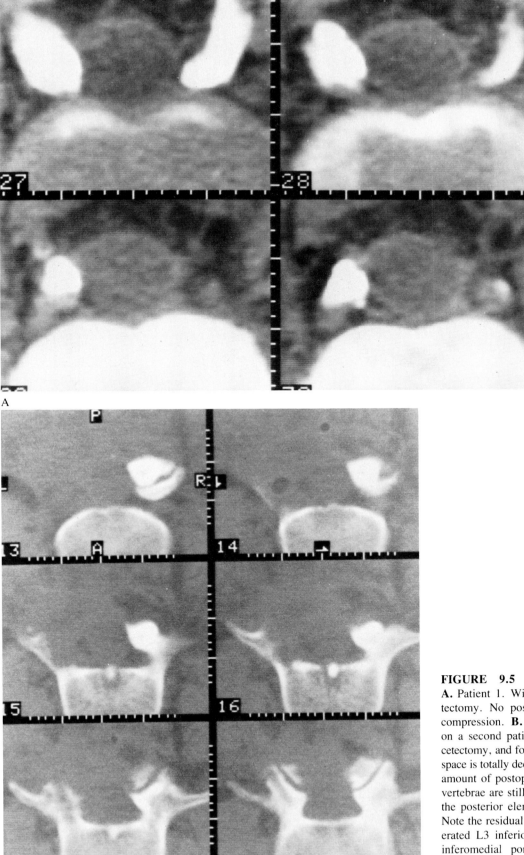

A

B

FIGURE 9.5 Bilateral laminectomy. **A.** Patient 1. Wide laminectomy and facetectomy. No postoperative scar; good decompression. **B.** Axial views respectively, on a second patient with laminectomy, facetectomy, and foraminotomy. The L4–5 disc space is totally decompressed. There is a large amount of postoperative scar. Note that the vertebrae are still well aligned, even though the posterior elements have been removed. Note the residual articular surface of the operated L3 inferior facet (*arrow*). Only the inferomedial portion has been removed. (*Figure continued* on page 262.)

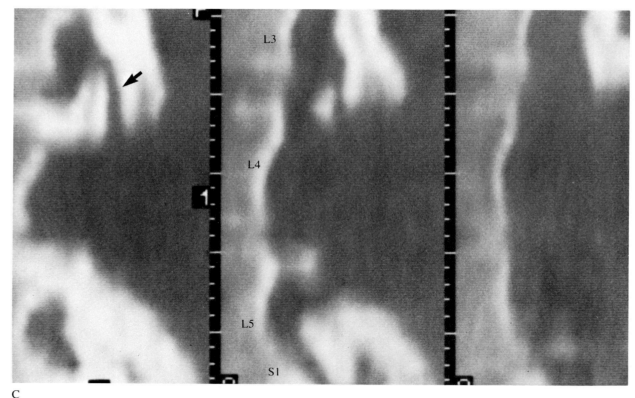

C

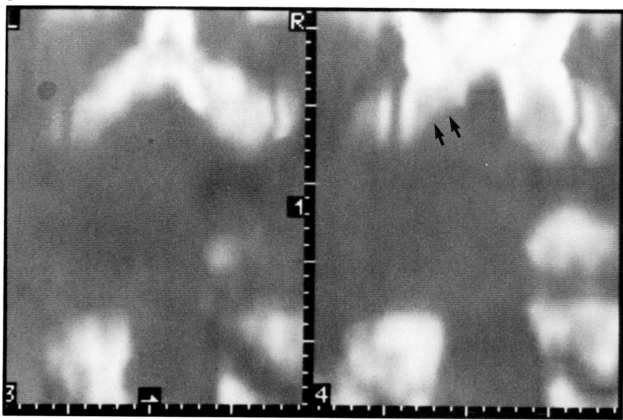

D

FIGURE 9.5 (*cont'd*) **C–D.** Sagittal and coronal views respectively, on a second patient with laminectomy, facetectomy, and foraminotomy. The L4–L5 disc space is totally decompressed. There is a large amount of postoperative scar. Note that the vertebrae are still well aligned, even though the posterior elements have been removed. Note the residual articular surface of the operated L3 inferior facet (*arrow*). Only the inferomedial portion has been removed.

It allows differentiation of disc herniation from facet hypertrophy, lateral recess stenosis, andepidural scarring.

During the past 3 years it has become obvious that the diagnosis of disc herniation can be made by CT.[12–14] The CT distinction between soft-tissue disc herniation and canal stenosis caused by ridges and spurs is also well established.[15,16] It is now possible by careful CT examination to exclude significant extradural compression of the cauda equina or exiting nerve roots before surgery. Although there are those who do not see CT as the primary screening examination for spines,[17] it is difficult to justify any surgical intervention without an objective lesion on CT. Carefully performed high-resolution multiplanar CT scans have very few false-negative results. The one possible exception is the rare patient in whom spine scanning (and prone flexed myelography) fails to define a disc abnormality but extension CT or upright extended myelography reveals a sizable extradural defect.

Before the routine use of high-resolution spine CT the most common source of failed laminectomy and discectomy was reported to be recurrent disc herniation.[1,18] More recent surveys based primarily on CT evaluation demonstrated lateral spinal stenosis to be the source of FBSS in 53% of cases.[16] It is obvious that simple discectomy is not curative in patients with significant bony overgrowth. Even myelography may not be able to differentiate lateral disc herniation from the compression due to lateral bony ridges and spurs.[19] It is now known that there are other causes of back pain and radiculopathy that may mimic disc herniation. The articular facet syndrome has received a great deal of interest in recent years, and therapeutic facet injection and other ablative procedures have become accepted modes of treatment.[5,20–24] It is obvious that disc excision will not relieve facet or other nondiscal pain syndromes.

Indicated Surgery With Poor Technical Results

The category "indicated surgery with poor results" can be conveniently subdivided into two groups: (1) those patients in whom surgery was indicated and properly performed but whose symptoms recurred: and (2) those in whom surgery was indicated but inadequately performed.

Surgery Indicated but Symptoms Recur

The two most important causes of FBSS, in the case of appropriately conceived and properly performed surgery, are recurrent or residual disc-fragment herniation and postoperative fibrosis and scar formation. Their differentiation by CT has caused considerable controversy. There are those who believe that it is important to examine all postoperative spines with dilute intrathecal metrizamide. Others,[25] including the authors, believe that for the most part this is unnecessary. On CT myelograms, metrizamide within the nerve roots is displaced posteriorly by recurrent disc fragment and circumferentially distorted by fibrous scar. This may be helpful in doubtful cases.

The attenuation value of disc material is for the most part significantly higher than that of epidural scar tissue. If one desires to actually measure the attenuation numbers, care must be taken to compare relative values on the same scan because target magnification frequently causes some aberration in the absolute attenuation values. Some authors use the blink mode of the scanner to highlight the attenuation range of disc material.

Intravenous contrast enhancement has also been suggested as an adjuvant to the diagnosis of recurrent disc herniation.[26] Fibrous extradural scar enhances; inert disc does not. In our experience, intravenous contrast media are almost never necessary. Using overlapping axial scans and a complex polynomial reformation algorithm, it is almost always possible to distinguish between scar and disc. We believe that the difference in attenuation is significant enough that it can be appreciated in almost all cases without measurement or blinking dots.

Primary in making this differential diagnosis are the sagittal and coronal views (Fig. 9.6). Herniated discs (free fragments) demonstrate a distinct, clearly defined edge on both coronal and sagittal views. On the sagittal view one can always identify the normal anulus fibrosis extending from one vertebral end-plate to the other. The bulging anulus or herniated disc fragment can be most precisely defined and measured on these views. Scar is best seen on the coronal images. Scar does not have clearly demarcated edges; and one cannot identify a plane between the descending roots and the scar tissue (Fig. 9.7). The coronal view is frequently better than the sagittal view foridentifying the edge of the disc fragment.

Some amount of epidural scar is seen in many patients. In our study the scar tissue was considered to be clinically significant only if it involved the nerve root on the side and at the level of symptoms. Diffuse scar surrounding the theca and causing diffuse myelographic defects has been shown to correlate poorly with the site and level of radiculopathy. Myelographic abnormalities may be seen bilaterally at several levels in patients with unilateral radicular pain; so too with CT. Some patients demonstrate total replacement of epidural fat at several levels with complaints referable to only a single root radiculopathy. It is important, therefore, to carefully correlate the CT abnormalities with the patient's clinical history and physical findings.

There is much controversy regarding the efficacy of reoperation for postoperative scar. Some authors favor microdissection techniques for freeing bound-down roots,[27] whereas others suggest that operations to remove scar are frequently destined to failure because of rapid recurrence of the adhesive fibrosis.[28]

Arachnoiditis means, literally, inflammation of the arachnoid. It is therefore an intradural process and may be totally unrelated to extradural scar. It is sometimes possible to make the diagnosis of intradural adhesions on nonmetrizamide CT scans. This can occur only when there are drop-

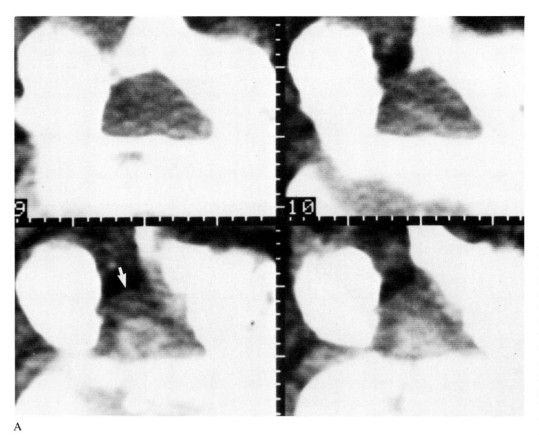

A

FIGURE 9.6 Postoperative recurrent disc herniation. Axial (**A**), sagittal (**B**), and coronal (**C**) views demonstrate a well-circumscribed high-attenuation mass extending posteriorly from the disc space. Note the well-defined edges on the coronal reformation (*arrows*). Note the shadow of the normal anulus at L3 (*arrowheads*).

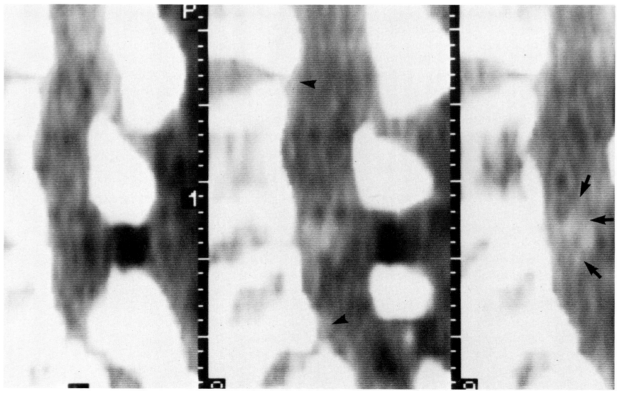

B

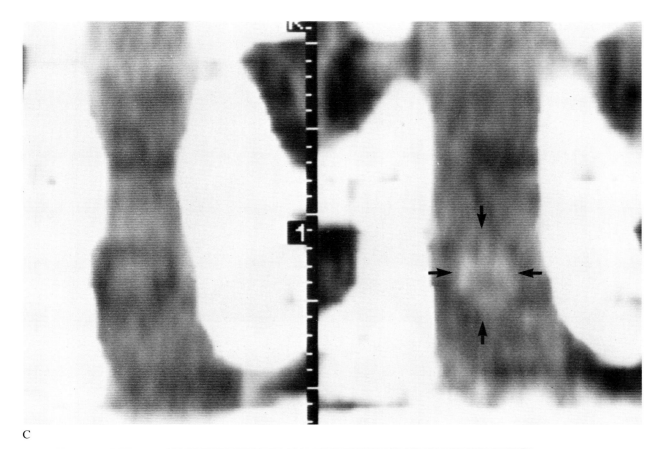

C

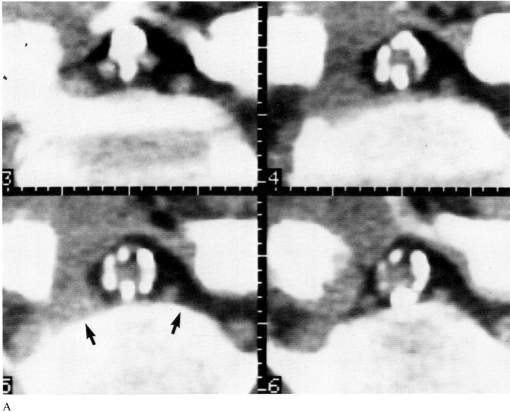

A

FIGURE 9.7 Postoperative scar. **A, B.** Axial and coronal views demonstrate some residual Pantopaque in the subdural space. There is a large amount of scar surrounding both the L5 and the S1 nerve roots. Note the asymmetry of the epidural fat (*arrows*). On the coronal view one can see that the S1 root is surrounded by homogeneous soft tissue, with no clearly defined edges. This is the hallmark of scar. **C.** Coronal view on a second patient. Note the large amount of homogeneous scar surrounding the exiting roots (*arrows*). The epidural fat is missing on the right. (*Figure continued on page 266.*)

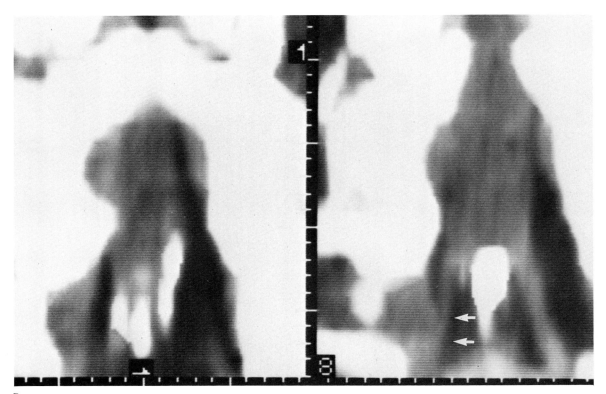

B

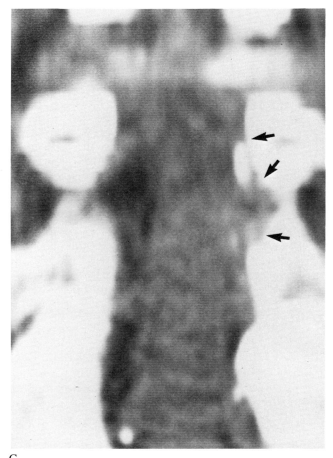

C
FIGURE 9.7 (*cont'd*)   See legend page 265.

lets of residual Pantopaque trapped within the theca. Otherwise the procedure of choice is low-dose metrizamide CT (Fig. 9.8). Because arachnoid adhesions may contraindicate surgery, excluding extradural compression and extradural adhesions without metrizamide in the canal may actually be all that is necessary in the preoperative evaluation of these patients.

There may be those who still favor metrizamide myelography in postoperative patients. We believe that the abnormal postoperative myelogram is the single most difficult neuroradiographic procedure to evaluate. These myelograms are frequently abnormal. The extradural defects are obvious; but the cause of these defects is practically never apparent. We believe that contrast study is necessary only in the minority of patients. Perhaps the demonstration of a single swollen intradural nerve root might be adequate justification for an invasive procedure. This is one of the only objective myelographic findings that is useful in defining the cause of radiculopathy in complex cases.

Other less common causes of FBSS in appropriately conceived surgery include pseudomeningocele formation, postoperative infection, and spinal stenosis due to bony overgrowth and dystrophic calcification and ossification.

Pseudomeningocele is the result of inadvertent, uncorrected laceration of the dura at the time of surgery. On nonenhanced CT there is a well-circumscribed water-density mass within the spinal space (Fig. 9.9). Metrizamide enters the mass and clearly defines its borders.[29] Occasionally in patients with wide bilateral laminectomy, there is posterior displacement of an unusually widened theca. The

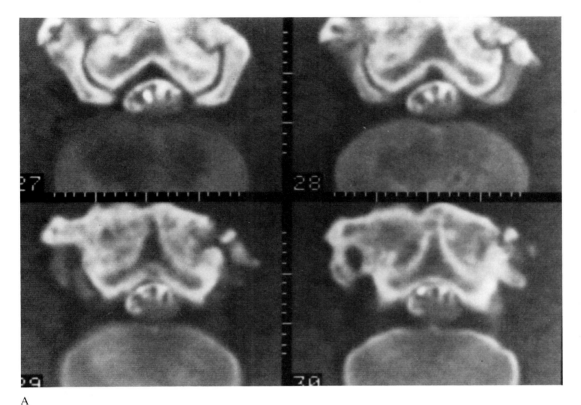

A

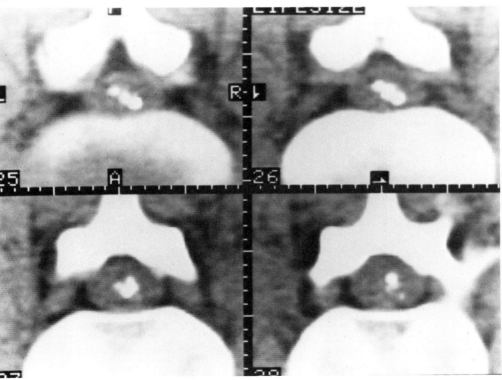

B

FIGURE 9.8 Intradural arachnoid adhesions. **A.** Intradural arachnoid adhesions can be diagnosed only with intrathecal contrast medium in place. The roots are abnormally positioned and attached to each other by irregular fibrous bands, producing a negative filling defect. **B.** Pantopaque adherent to nerve roots does not fall to the most dependent portion of the thecal sac. This is a sign of arachnoiditis.

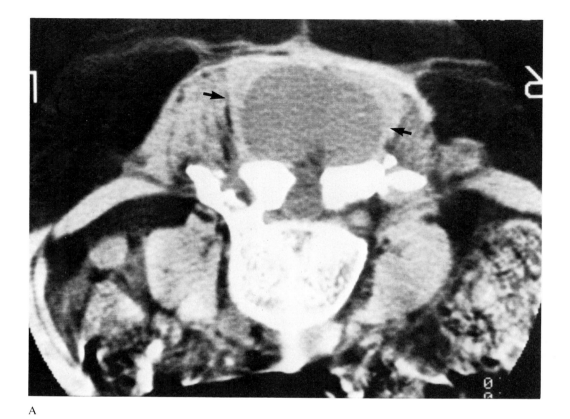

A

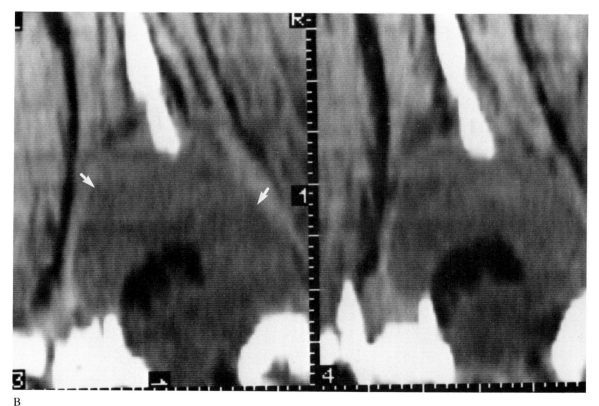

B

FIGURE 9.9   Postoperative pseudomeningocele. Axial (**A**), coronal (**B**), and sagittal (**C**) views. The pseudomeningocele is a very large water-density mass (*arrows*) which is continuous with the subarachnoid space.

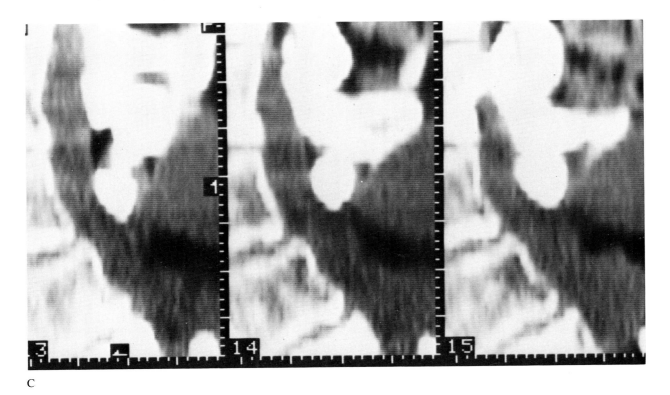

C

clinical significance of these findings is unclear. On occasion it seems that the dura expands to fill the extra space newly allotted to it.

Postoperative infection is usually suggested by its clinical manifestations and provable by appropriate cultures. CT is helpful in the evaluation of extraspinal extension of the infectious process (Fig. 9.8) and occasionally in distinguishing hypertrophic bone sclerosis at a narrow disc space from purulent infection. The patient in Figure 9.10 had marked narrowing and sclerosis of his L4–5 intervertebral disc space. This was at first thought to represent bone reaction to suppuration at the disc space. However, the presence of bubbles of gas within the disc strongly suggest benign bone sclerosis about a narrowed and destroyed but uninfected disc space. Disc-space infection with gas-producing organisms is very rare.

Spinal stenosis after laminectomy may be caused by a variety of pathologic changes. Dystrophic bone may form in the surgical bed, causing recess or lateral canal stenosis. The patient in Figure 9.11 had a right-sided laminectomy and a medial facetectomy. Right-sided radiculopathy recurred. The axial views clearly demonstrate a spikelike projection of bone extending posteriorly from the posterior surface of the vertebral body. This has the appearance of uncorticated dystrophic bone filling the surgical bed. The coronal views clearly define the bony compression of the exiting right L5 root. The descending S1 root may also be compressed and displaced.

Symptomatic bony overgrowth from a laminectomy is rare and was found in only one patient in our series.

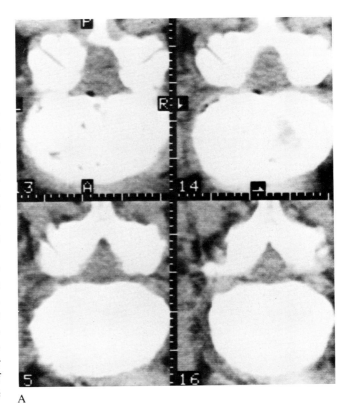

A

FIGURE 9.10 Noninfectious vertebral sclerosis. Axial (**A**), coronal (**B**), and sagittal (**C**) views demonstrate a narrow disc space with marked sclerosis of both vertebral bodies. The presence of gas in the disc space and the absence of paravertebral mass speak strongly against infection (*arrowhead*). (*Figure continued* on page 270.)

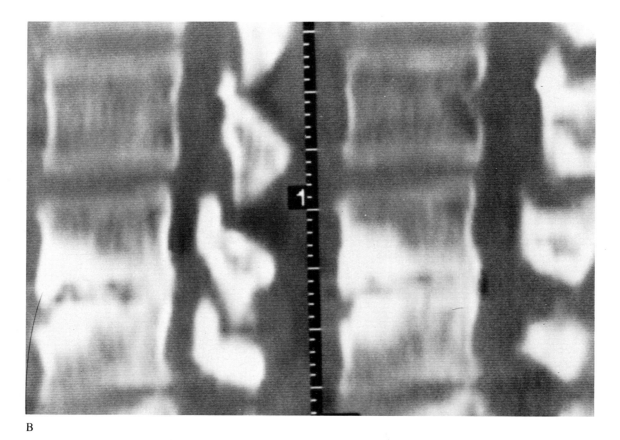

B

C

FIGURE 9.10 (*cont'd*)   See legend page 269.

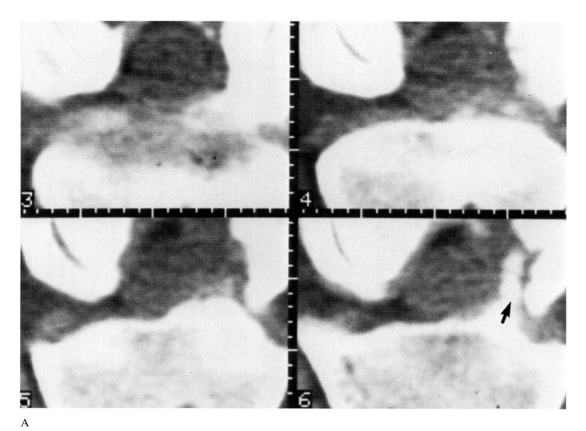

A

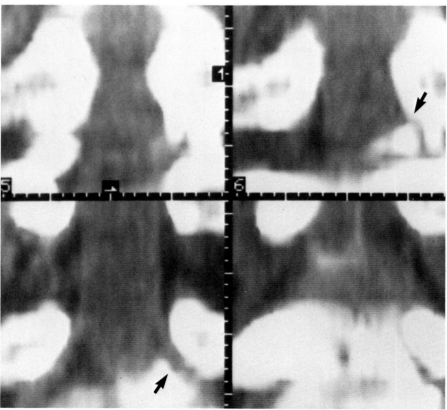

B

FIGURE 9.11 Postoperative recess stenosis. Axial (**A**) and coronal (**B**) views demonstrate a spikelike projection in the right gutter (*arrow*). The coronal view demonstrates bony compression of the exiting L5 root (*arrow*). The sagittal view reveals associated foraminal narrowing (*arrows*). (*Figure continued* on page 272.)

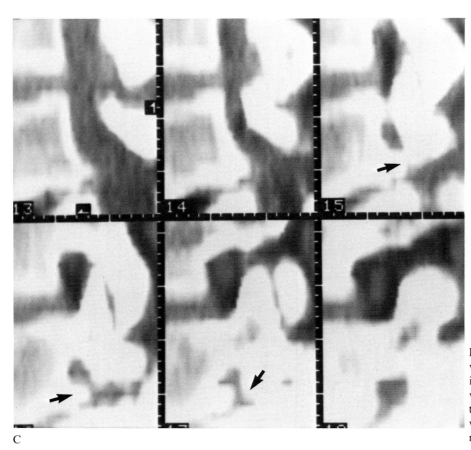

C

FIGURE 9.11 (*cont'd*) (**C**) Coronal views demonstrate a spikelike projection in the right gutter (*arrow*). The coronal view demonstrates bony compression of the exiting L5 root (*arrow*). The sagittal view reveals associated foraminal narrowing (*arrows*).

Hypertrophy and healing of the laminectomy site is clearly the cause of canal compression in the patient in Figure 9.12. The neural ring is narrowed and deformed.

Surgery Indicated But Inadequately Performed

Into the group of patients for whom surgery was indicated but inadequately performed fall a very large number of

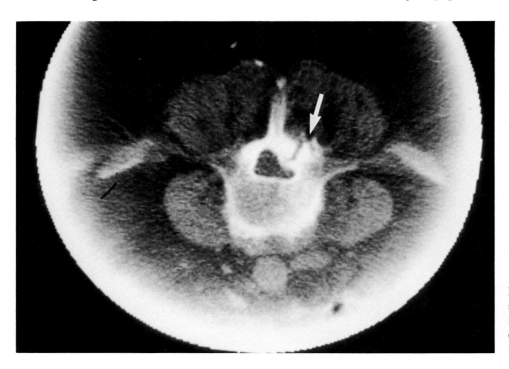

FIGURE 9.12 Postoperative stenosis. Axial scan demonstrating posterior canal compression due to bony overgrowth of a laminectomy defect.

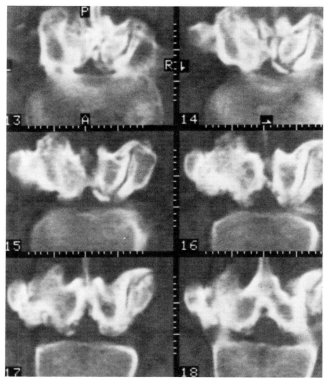

FIGURE 9.13 Postoperative spinal stenosis. Severe spinal stenosis due to massive hypertrophy of the posterior elements. Discectomy and posterior fusion have not relieved the neural compression.

by preoperative screening with high-resolution CT. With CT it is possible for the surgeon to know the precise dimensions of the neural foramina and the lateral recesses as well as the overall surface dimensions of the spinal canal before surgery. The operative approach can then be chosen appropriately and the amount of decompression can be commensurate with the clinical problem.

The patient in Figure 9.13 demonstrates the value of preoperative CT. This patient underwent discectomy and posterior midline spinal fusion. Symptoms recurred after surgery. It is obvious from the scans that a posterior spine fusion only further compromised an already extremely narrow spinal canal. Removal of the disc material does not eliminate bony neural entrapment. Midline fusion completely encircles the dura in a narrow and deformed bony tube. This is perhaps the most flagrant case in this series. Other less obvious abnormalities can cause bony neural compression that requires appropriate decompression.

The patient in Figure 9.14 had bilateral wide laminectomy, and the axial images demonstrate no hint of recurrent disc herniation or postoperative scar. The sagittally reformatted images clearly define severe foraminal stenosis. A prominent bony ridge fills the anterior inferior portion of the foramen. The normal exiting L5 root cannot be defined. There is no surrounding perineural fat. Compare the upper normal foramina to the stenotic L5. Lateral canal stenosis, as described by Burton et al.,[16] may be overlooked during simple discectomy.

The patient in Figure 9.15 underwent laminectomy and disc removal. An overlooked, posterior-projecting osteoarthritic spur caused left-sided lateral recess stenosis as well as indentation on the medial end of the neural foramen. The reason for the residual left radiculopathy is obvious.

patients who have symmetrical prominent bulge of the disc and anulus into a canal that is narrow due to facet-joint enlargement or degenerative hypertrophic spondylitic spurs and ridges. It is this group of patients that are eliminated

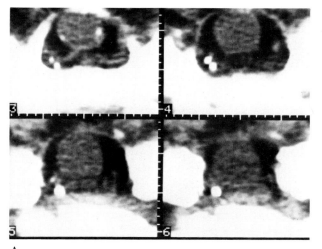

A

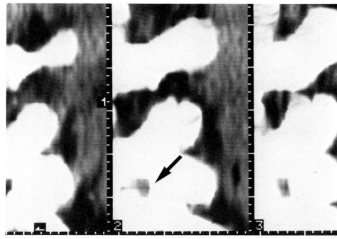

B

FIGURE 9.14 Inadequate decompression. **A.** Axial views demonstrate a wide bilateral laminectomy. The theca is decompressed and there is no postoperative scar. **B.** Sagittal views reveal severe left foraminal stenosis (*arrow*). Decompression of the theca with unrecognized foraminal stenosis is a common cause of surgical failure.

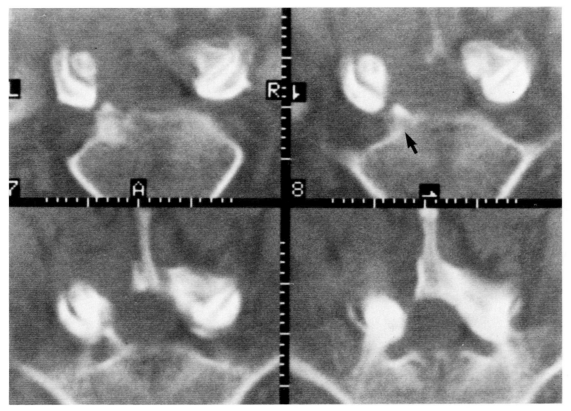

FIGURE 9.15 Postoperative ridging. Although this patient has undergone laminectomy and discectomy, left radiculopathy persisted because of a bony ridge (*arrow*), which was not appreciated at surgery.

Specific Complications of Facetectomy

Certain postoperative complications arise specifically as sequelae to facetectomy. The most obvious is "iatrogenic" spondylolisthesis. There may be some subluxation of the involved vertebral segments as a consequence of massive posterior decompression and facetectomy. Figure 9.16 shows a patient with total left facetectomy at two levels and wide laminectomy on the right with dislocation of eroded coronally oriented facets. The sagittal view defines the extent of the instability. This occurrence is fairly common. Twenty-four of the 500 spondylolisthesis patients in our series demonstrated postoperative spondylolisthesis. Most of these were dislocated posteriorly, but anterior subluxation was seen in approximately 25% of the group.

The usefulness of multiplanar reformation is demonstrated dramatically in Figure 9.17. On axial scan #6 one sees two inferior facets on the same side. On axial scan #12 a fragment of bone is noted filling the lateral recess on the left. The sagittal reformation completely elucidates the very complex postoperative anatomy. There is approximately 5 mm of forward subluxation of L2 on L3, with a "vacuum" disc effect. At L3–4, the level of total facetectomy, there is 3 mm of forward subluxation. There is marked compression of the L5 vertebral body, with sclerosis of the end-plates. The superior facet at L5 is herniated into the lateral recess behind L4, and the inferior facet of L5 overlies the L5–S1 articulation. A vacuum disc effect is also noted at L5–S1.

Surgical correction of this disastrous spine requires all the three-dimensional information that we as radiologists can provide. Even if we are clever enough to accurately untangle the complexities of the axial images, we must be able to display the anatomy to our surgical colleagues in an easily understandable way. The sagittal reformations accomplish this.

One other previously unreported entity has become obvious in the postfacetectomy group. Eight of 50 patients in whom facetectomy was performed demonstrated a peculiar fracture of the inferior facet. In two surgically proven cases the inferior facet was seen to be lying free in the soft tissue. The patient in Figure 9.18 is such a case and is typical of this group. The axial scans demonstrate a wide laminectomy and a partial facetectomy. Subtle malalignment of one facet suggests facet fracture, even in the axial plane. However, definitive diagnosis requires both sagittal and coronal views.

On the sagittal view the inferior facet of L3 is clearly fractured and displaced posteriorly. This is also demonstrable on the coronal view. It is important to note that this is

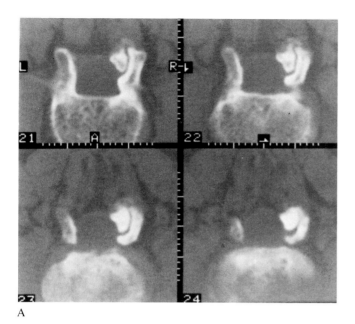

A

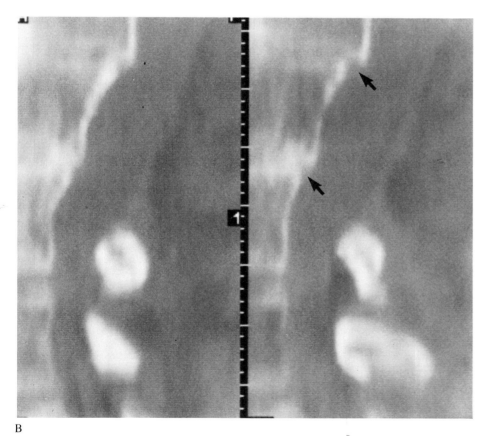

B

FIGURE 9.16 Postoperative spondylolisthesis. In some patients who have undergone decompression and facetectomy, gross dislocation occurs, producing canal recess or foraminal stenosis. Note the dislocation (*arrows*) on the sagittal view (**B**). Spondylolisthesis, especially in the upper lumbar spine, is underestimated in the axial plane (**A**).

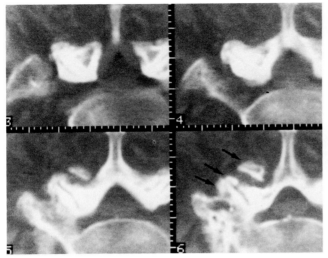

A

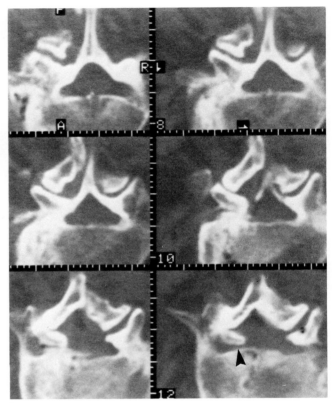

B

FIGURE 9.17 Postoperative degenerative subluxation. **A, B.** Axial scans demonstrate what appears to be three facets at one level (*arrows*). At the next level there is a fragment of bone in the spinal canal (*arrowhead*). **C.** The sagittal view elucidates the deformity to advantage. L2 is subluxated forward on L3, and L3 is subluxated forward on L4, (*arrows*). There is compression of the L5 vertebral body. The superior facet of L5 is dislocated upward and lies in the L4 lateral recess (*arrowheads*).

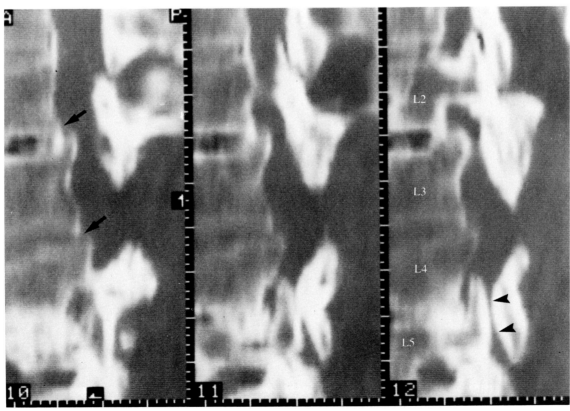

C

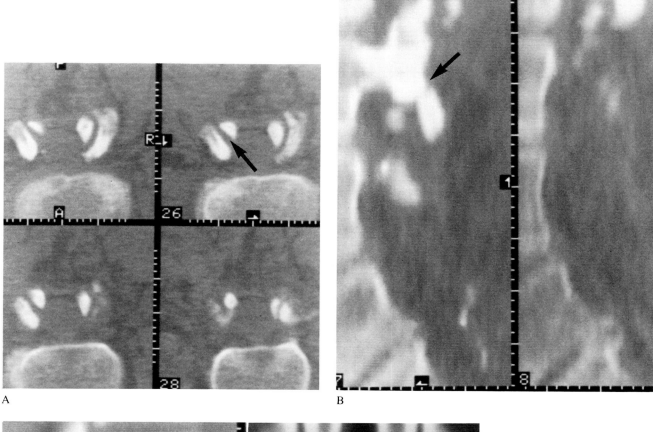

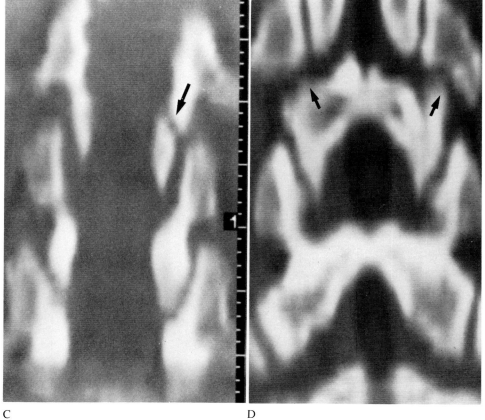

FIGURE 9.18 Postoperative facet fracture. Axial (**A**), sagittal (**B**), and coronal (**C**) views demonstrate the fracture through the base of the inferior facet of L3. In the axial view there is bilateral laminectomy and facetectomy. Slight asymmetrical widening of the joint space is noted (*arrow*). **D.** Coronal view on a patient with bilateral pars interarticularis fractures (*arrows*). Note that pars fractures are higher on the posterior arch than is the postoperative facet fracture.

not a pars interarticularis defect. The fracture in these patients usually occurs within the inferior facet itself and almost always at its base. Compare the coronal views on this patient with the coronal views on a patient with a typical pars interarticular is defect (Fig. 9.18D). The differentiation is obvious in most cases. It is crucial to see the fracture on both sagittal and coronal images. The sloping course of the facet and lamina frequently mimic fractures in the sagittal plane. The lateral surface of the articular process always projects more laterally in the neck of the inferior facet, and therefore on the far lateral reformations it appears to be separate from the rest of the posterior neural arch. Coronal reformations from properly performed CT scans always differentiate the true defect from these pseudofractures. On occasion, curved or warped coronal reformations are useful when the lamina slopes sharply across the coronal plane (Fig. 9.19). At the time of this writing, 25 similar cases have been seen by the authors.

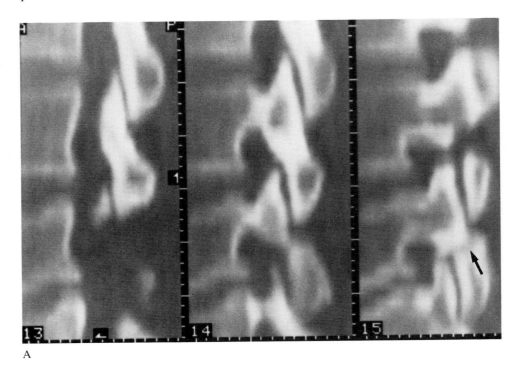

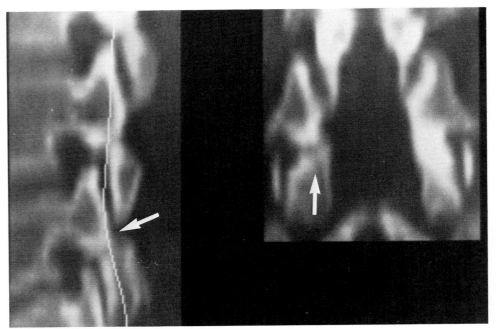

FIGURE 9.19 Facet fracture. Sagittal (**A**) and coronal (**B**) reformations. A typical facet fracture is noted on the sagittal view (*arrow*). Because of the sloping nature of the facet, one should always identify the fracture on two nonaxial perpendicular projections.

Spine Fusion

A wide variety of spine fusion techniques are used to stabilize the spine, prevent abnormal motion at a disc space, or correct scoliosis. CT scanning may be useful in defining postoperative anatomy and some of the causes of FBSS in postfusion patients.

The procedures used most often are posterior or posterolateral fusion of the neural arches, transverse processes, and facets. Of the 72 spine fusion patients reviewed in this study, 61 were approached in this manner; the other 11 patients had interbody spine fusion, the majority performed from the posterior approach using the Cloward technique.[30,31]

It is beyond the scope of this chapter to document all of the possible mechanical devices that are used for spine fusion. Suffice it to say that the presence of large amounts of metal, although causing prominent streak artifact, does not preclude the use of CT. Harrington rods are the most commonly used metallic devices placed posteriorly, and the artifacts they produce tend to lie sufficiently posterior to the vertebral bodies that a significant amount of useful in-

formation is obtainable, especially on sagittal reformations (see Chapter 12).

Central Posterior Fusion

For many years the central posterior approach was the preferred method of spine fusion. After laminectomy and discectomy, bone was laid down between the laminae in an attempt to produce a complete posterior bony wall to the neural canal (Fig. 9.20). Several theoretical problems exist with this approach. Biomechanically, the fusion mass is at the worst possible end of a theoretical lever extending posteriorly through the axis of vertebral flexion and extension. This is possibly the major contributing factor to the relatively high incidence of pseudarthrosis in this group. The very fact that the operation was designed to encapsulate the neural tissue leads to its second theoretical drawback.

In patients with narrow or borderline spinal canals the fusion itself may cause severe spinal stenosis. In Brodsky's large series,[28] spinal stenosis was noted in 106 postsurgical fusion patients. He designated concentric stenosis just above

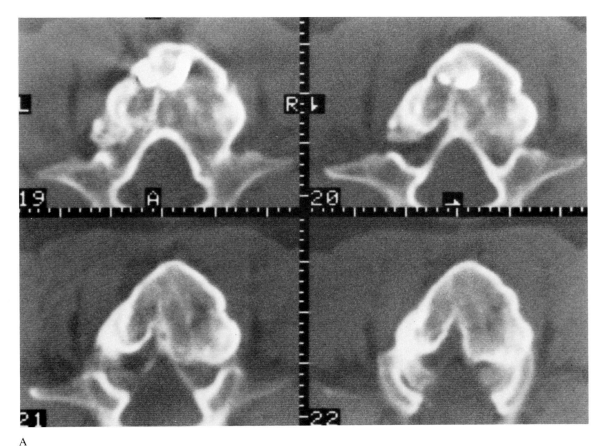

A

FIGURE 9.20 Posterior spine fusion. **A.** Axial views on a patient with an intact posterior spine fusion. There is no question of pseudarthrosis in this patient. The fusion is solid over two levels. (*Figure continued* on page 280.)

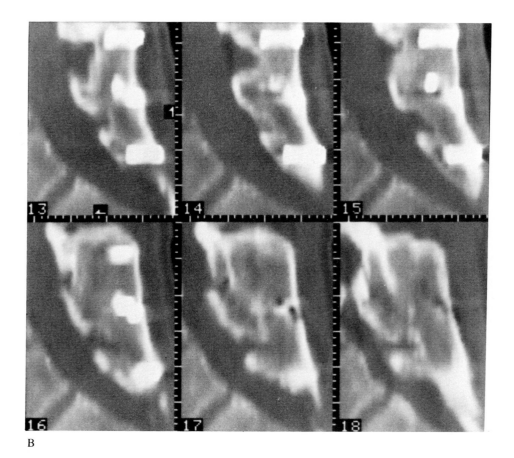

B

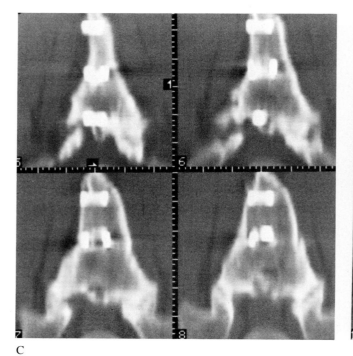

C

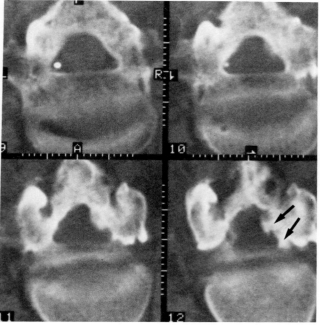

FIGURE 9.20 (*cont'd*)   Sagittal (**B**) and coronal (**C**) views on a patient with an intact posterior spine fusion. There is no question of pseudarthrosis in this patient. The fusion is solid over two levels.

FIGURE 9.21   Posterior spine fusion. Solid posterior spine fusion, with prominent "whiskering" of the lamina and fused right facet (*arrows*) causing spinal stenosis.

the fusion as the most common lesion. These stenoses are caused by a combination of factors, including ligamentum flavumhypertrophy and infolding, degenerative disease of the facet joints with hypertrophic expansion, ventral protrusion of the uppermost border of the fusion mass, and bulging of the disc or anulus.

The axial images in Figure 9.21 demonstrate lateral canalstenosis at the upper level of a posterior spine fusion. Note the severe degenerative arthropathy of both facet joints and the dystrophic bone extending forward from the lamina. This ''whiskering'' of the lamina and the laminar hypertrophy is probably related to stripping of the periosteum from the lamina at the time of surgery.

The patient in Figure 9.22 demonstrates another similar cause of spinal stenosis at the top of a fusion. Careful examination of the soft tissue in axial images 9 and 10 demonstrate partially calcified high-density scar behind the dura. This soft-tissue scar is causing severe posterior cauda equina compression.

Pseudarthrosis is a common postsurgical problem that may be very difficult to diagnose even on good-quality scans. At the time of surgery many small pieces of graft bone are laid down against the host site. It is no wonder that the postoperative scan so frequently demonstrates multiple disconnected islands of bone in the soft tissue (Fig. 9.23). It is the radiologist's responsibility to decide if there is con-

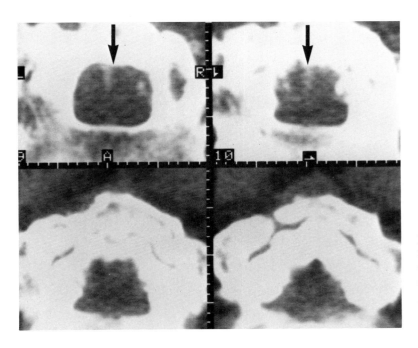

FIGURE 9.22 Posterior spine fusion. A solid posterior fusion is evident. There is a large, partially calcified scar compressing the theca posteriorly (*arrows*). The patient had classic signs of spinal claudication.

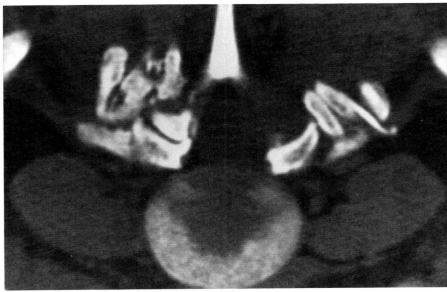

FIGURE 9.23 Fragmented spine fusion. Multiple fragments of bone are noted in the posterior soft tissues.

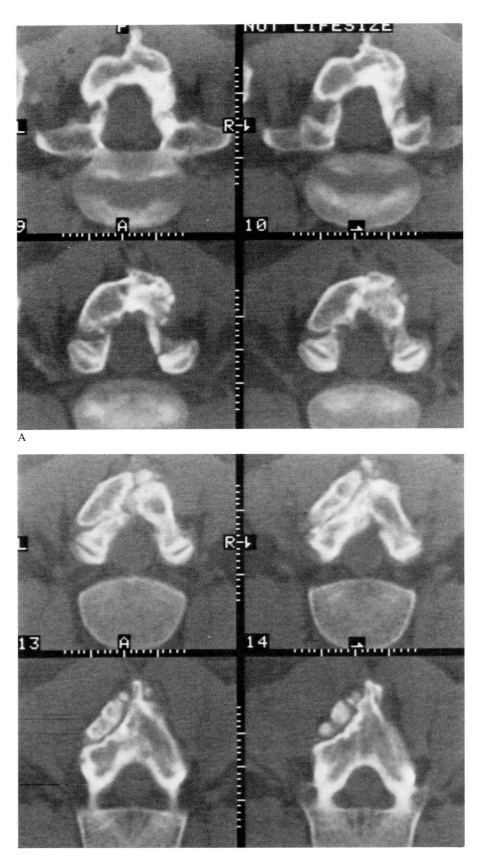

A

B

FIGURE 9.24 Pseudarthrosis. **A, B.** Axial scans demonstrate a large amount of fusion posteriorly. On axial scans 13–15 there is some bone apparently free in the soft tissue. **C, D.** Sagittal and coronal views prove that although most of the fusion bone is fused to L5 there is no intact bony fusion. A cleft is clearly seen between the two irregular segments of the fractured fusion (*arrows*).

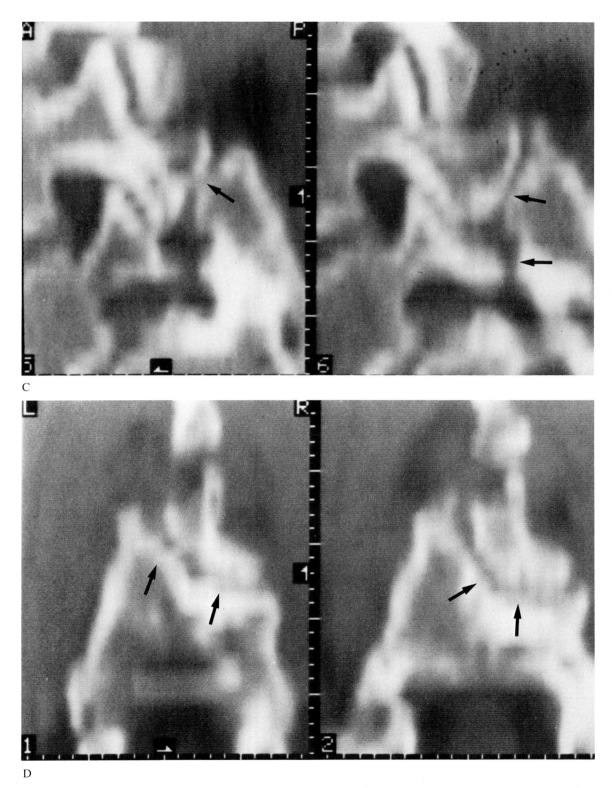

C

D

tinuity between most of the graft bone and the two adjacent host bones. Sagittal and coronal reformations are frequently required to define the anatomy of the abnormal spine fusion.

The patient in Figure 9.24 had a dense posterior spine fusion. An oblique line is noted traversing part of the fu-sion. From the axial views one can only speculate if the vertebrae are actually connected. The coronal and sagittal reformations clearly show them to be separable by a bony cleft running obliquely through the fusion.

Lateral Spine Fusion

When arthrodesis of the spine is contemplated, most sur- geons now favor bilateral lateral fusion.[7,32,33] The incidence of pseudarthrosis is lower because the fusion extends more anteriorly closer to the fulcrum of flexion; hence there is less mechanical stress at the fusion site.

A fusion operation can also be performed on patients with previous laminectomy, and the incidence of postoperative spinal stenosis from overgrowth of the lamina is greatly reduced. Spondylolisthesis aquisita does not occur after this type of procedure, whereas it is fairly common after central laminar fusion.

A brief description of a typical surgical approach is necessary in order to understand the expected radiographic changes (Wiltse's technique)[33]. A midline incision is made over several segments. The muscles are stripped subperiosteally from the spinous processes and laminae. The facets are denuded of their capsules and the transverse processes of their soft tissue. The posterior two thirds of the facets are excised and bone plugs are placed in the grooves. Graft bone is removed via the same excision from one iliac crest and placed in strips over the denuded facets, transverse processes, and laminae.

The patient in Figure 9.25 had an intact posterior lateral L3–4 spine fusion. The dense homogeneous new

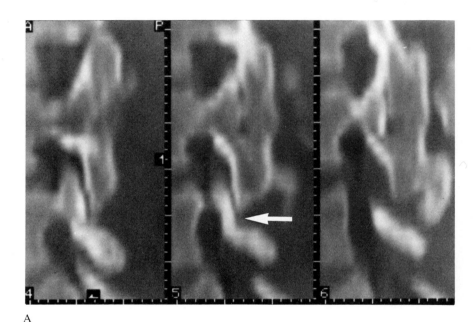

A

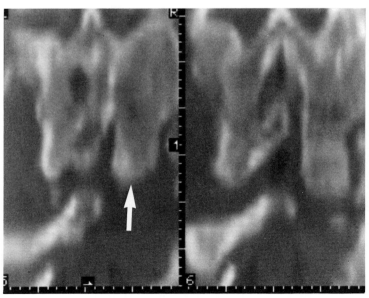

B

FIGURE 9.25 Intact L3–4 fusion; failed L4–5 fusion. Sagittal (**A**) and coronal (**B**) reformations reveal solid posterior bone fusion from L3 to L4. Unfortunately, the inferior portion of the fusion that was to have reached L5 has resorbed (*arrow*).

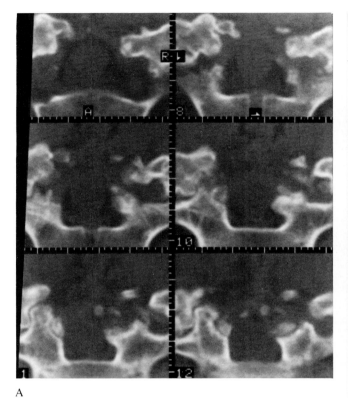

A

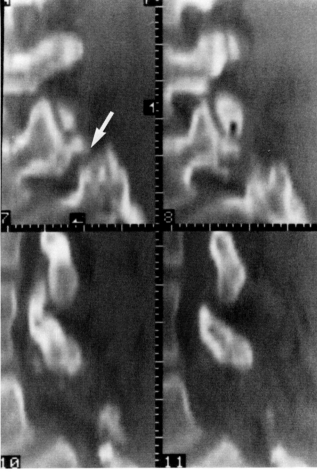

B

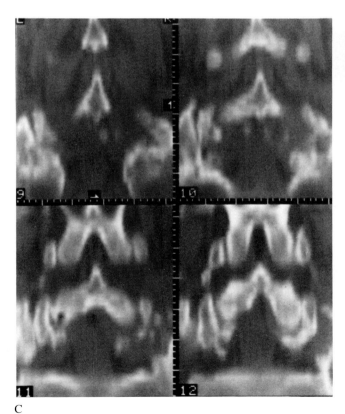

C

FIGURE 9.26 Failed L4–S1 fusion. **A.** Axial scan after attempted fusion for spondylolisthesis. Fragments of bone are noted in the soft tissue. **B, C.** Sagittal and coronal views prove that there is no bone traversing the pars defect (*arrow*).

bone is visible extending from the inferior facet at L3 down to the inferior facet at L4. Unfortunately, L4 is not fused to L5.

Posterior lateral fusions are used frequently in patients with spondylolisthesis. Figure 9.26 demonstrates a failed fusion in one of these patients. On the axial views a wide laminectomy and decompression are obvious, and multiple fragments of fusion bone are identifiable. Both sagittal and coronal images clearly indicate separation of the L5 pars interarticularis from the stump of the attempted fusion. Almost all of the graft bone has resorbed. Of note in this patient is a severe erosive arthropathy in the left inferior facet of L5, with a bubble of gas in the joint surface.

Interbody Fusion Techniques

Because weight-bearing of the lumbar spine is borne primarily by the vertebral bodies and the intervertebral discs, it seems quite logical to fuse an intervertebral motion segment at the disc space rather than posterolaterally. Greater mechanical stability can be accomplished using thick iliac bone struts and the disc space can be widened, thereby relieving compression of the exiting nerve roots. It seems reasonable to assume that because the fusion is performed through the center of rotation pseudarthrosis should be a less common complication.

Interbody fusions may be performed anteriorly via intraperitoneal or retroperitoneal approaches, or posteriorly as described by Cloward.[30,31] The anterior approach described by Raney[34] has the advantage that there is little or no scarring in the area of the neural canal. Disc removal is carried out anteriorly quite similarly to the cervical interbody approach. The great vessels are retracted laterally, exposing the anulus after the intraperitoneal structures are displaced.

In Raney's series, five patients had vascular complications relating to either primary or secondary involvement of one of the major abdominal vessels. Three other patients had thrombophlebitis, possibly related to intra-abdominal vascular compromise. Twenty-seven of his 160 patients had at least one level of pseudarthrosis.

Postoperative reformatted CT clearly demonstrates an intact interbody fusion. Occasionally, metal clips in the retroperitoneum indicate that the anterior approach was used.

Only two anterior interbody fusions were included in our series.

Posterior lumbar interbody fusion (P.L.I.F.) was more commonly seen in our patient population. Eleven patients had postoperative CT scans, mostly because of recurrent or residualback pain or radiculopathy.

According to the Cloward technique,[35] the ligamentum flavum is stripped from the lower margin of the upper lamina. A transverse incision is made in the upper lamina, and bone is removed laterally to include the lower one third of the inferior facet. The inner portion of the laminar bone is shaved to widen the anteroposterior diameter of the spinal canal. The medial half of the superior facet is also removed, further decompressing the lateral surface of the canal. The dura and its contents are retracted, exposing the disc space. The primary goal of this procedure is total removal of the disc and replacement of this material by as much bone as possible. Four or more struts of bone are inserted, and an attempt is made to widen maximally the disc space. By this method the entire disc is removed, the lateral recess and foraminal stenosis is reduced, and fusion is accomplished. Cloward reported greater than 96% success in more than 2,000 such procedures.

The appearance of the lumbar spine after successful P.L.I.F. is shown in Figure 9.27. The surgical approach in this case is somewhat different from the one described above

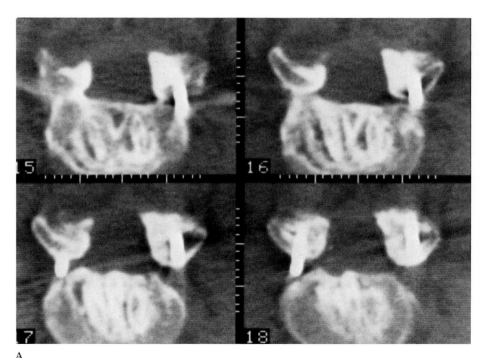

A

FIGURE 9.27 Intact interbody fusion. Axial (**A**), sagittal (**B**), and coronal (**C**) views on a patient with an intact interbody fusion. Iliac bone grafts are noted between each pair of vertebral bodies. In the axial and coronal views one is able to identify the cortical and medullary layers of graft when they are healthy (*arrows*). Screws through the facets (unusual in interbody surgery) are seen posteriorly.

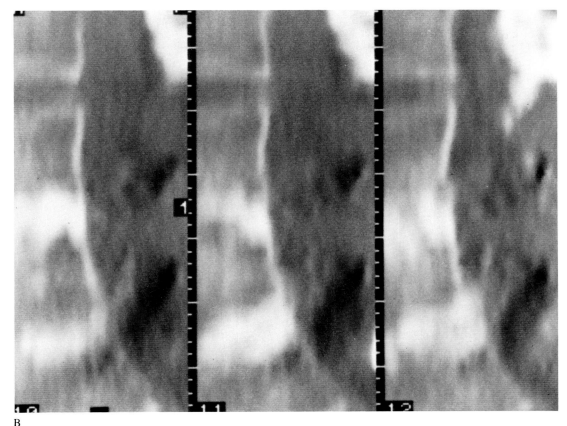

B

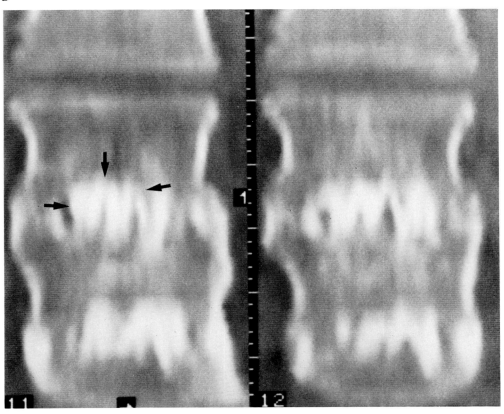

C

in that a laminectomy has also been performed and screws are seen through the facet joints. The sagittal and coronal reformations clearly testify to the fact that the fusions are intact. There is, of course, no recurrent disc herniation.

The patient in Figure 9.28 had had a previous interbody fusion operation. He was scanned because of severe back pain. The fusion was thought to be intact on routine radiographs, and no motion was noted on flexion/extension films. However, the CT clearly indicated pseudarthrosis with dissolution of the fusion mass. Curved coronal reformations demonstrated not only the pseudarthrosis but significant lateral offset at L4 on L5.

In our series, five patients were shown to have incontrovertible evidence of failure of fusion after P.L.I.F. procedures. Figures 9.29 and 9.30 are two such cases. Note the amorphous nature of the sclerotic graft material. There

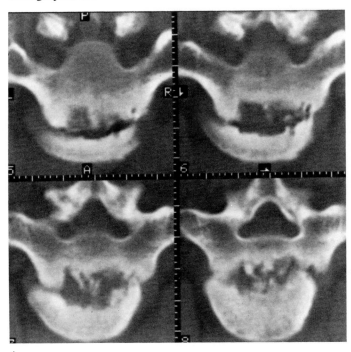

A

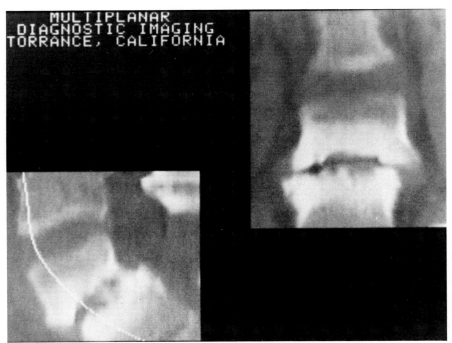

B

FIGURE 9.28 Failed interbody fusion. Axial (**A**) and sagittal and coronal (**B**) views demonstrate no hint of bone between the vertebral bodies. L5 is dislocated forward and to the right. The scan provides incontrovertible evidence of pseudarthrosis.

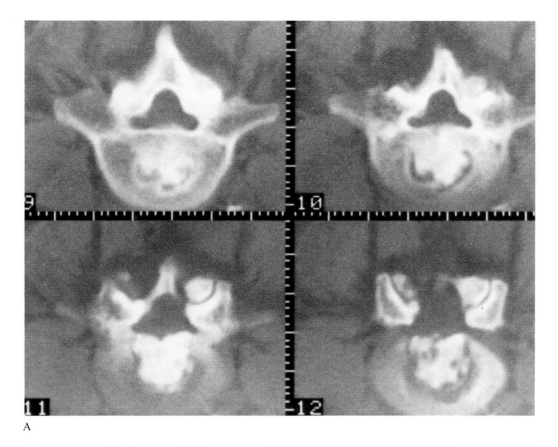

A

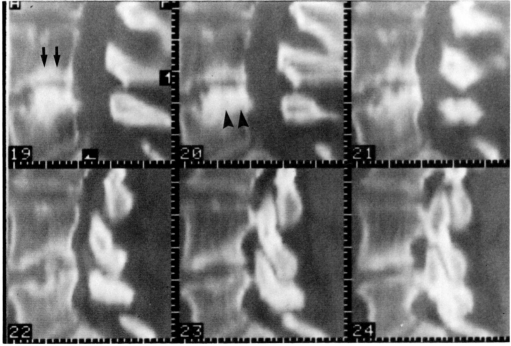

B

FIGURE 9.29 Failed interbody fusion. **A.** Axial scans reveal amorphous sclerotic graft bone. This strongly suggests that the graft is not healthy. **B.** Sagittal views reveal that the amorphous graft is fused inferiorly (*arrowheads*) but not superiorly (*arrows*); hence this is a pseudarthrosis. (*Figure continued* on page 290.)

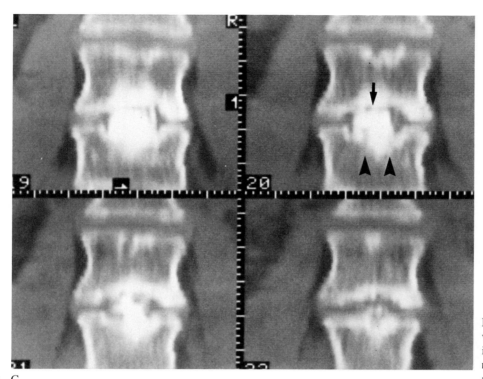

C

FIGURE 9.29 (*cont'd*) **C.** Coronal views reveal that the amorphous graft is fused inferiorly (*arrowheads*) but not superiorly (*arrows*); hence this is a pseudarthrosis.

is definite bone continuity between the inferior portion of the graft and L5 in Figure 9.29 but total absence of fusion between the top of the graft and L4. The patient in Figure 9.30 had a two-level interbody fusion. The lower level is intact. On the coronal views one can recognize the parallel cortical and medullary portions of the healed graft. Bone traverses the graft. At L4–5, however, the graft is fused to L4, but it is definitely not fused to L5.

A rare complication of P.L.I.F. surgery was seen in the patient in Figure 9.31. After surgery he had severe pain and symptoms of radiculopathy. Obvious posterior extrusion of one of the bone plugs is clearly noted on the scans. The right recess is almost totally occluded.

Properly performed high-resolution multiformatted spine CT is extremely useful in the evaluation of almost all forms of spinal surgery. It is used as a preoperative screen-

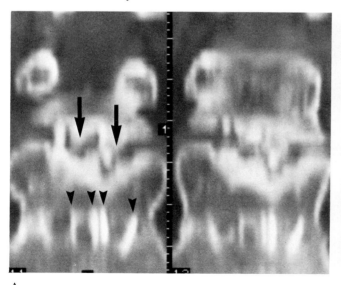

A

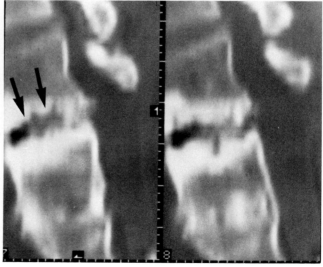

B

FIGURE 9.30 Failed interbody fusion. Axial (**A**) and coronal (**B**) views on a patient with a two-level interbody fusion. The upper level is definitely failed (*arrows*); the graft is fused superiorly and dissolved inferiorly. The lower level is definitely fused. Note the cortical and medullary bone (*arrowheads*).

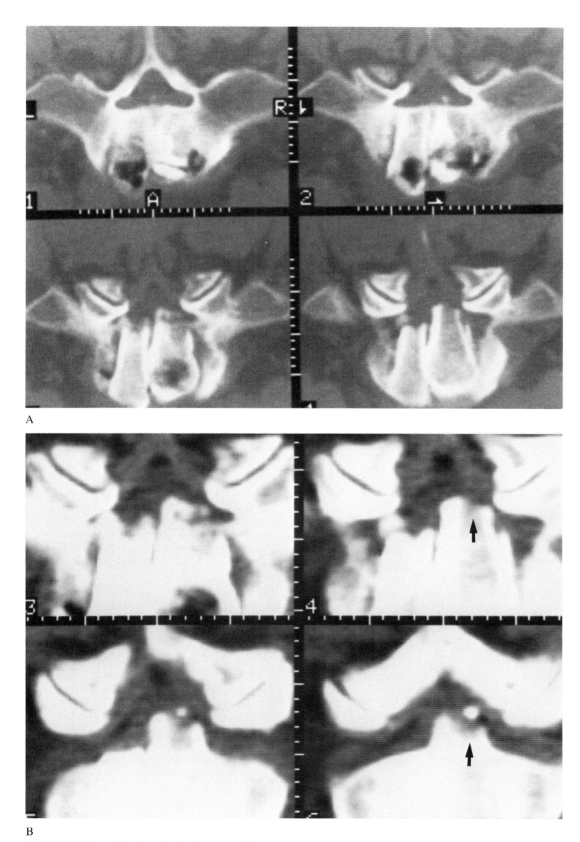

A

B

FIGURE 9.31 Failed interbody fusion. Axial scan performed 2 weeks after attempted interbody fusion reveals that one of the plugs has slipped posteriorly (*arrows*). **A.** Bone-window view. **B.** Soft-tissue view.

ing procedure to evaluate the anatomy of the canal, foramina, and recesses to prevent inadequate surgery. There should be objective evidence of disc herniation or bone encroachment before surgical exploration. With adequate preoperative information, the appropriate surgical approach and design will eliminate the majority of surgical failures. Should the patient remain symptomatic or should symptoms recur despite adequate surgery, the postoperative CT can of itself, without intrathecal contrast injection, provide useful information for excluding surgically remediable causes of failure. We believe that many of the key observations that are surgically important can best be made on the multiplanar reformatted images. In order for these images to be clinically useful they must be computed from high-quality closely spaced axial scans. As in any radiographic procedure, exquisite attention to technical detail, mechanical and x-ray calibration, and patient comfort greatly enhance the diagnostic usefulness of the CT examination.

References

1. Frymoyer JW, Hanley E, Howe J, et al: Disc excision and spine fusion in management of lumbar disc disease. Spine 3:1–6, 1978
2. Weir BKH, Jacobs GA: Reoperation rate following lumbar discectomy: an analysis of 662 lumbar discectomies. Spine 5:366–370, 1980
3. Sprangfort EV: The lumbar disc herniation: a computer aided analysis of 2504 operations. Acta Orthop Scand [Suppl] 142, 1972
4. Spengler DM, Freeman C, Westbrook R, Miller JW: Low back pain following multiple lumbar spine procedures. failure of initial selection? Spine 5:356–360, 1980
5. Shealy CN: Facet denervation in management of back and sciatic pain. Clin Orthop 115:157–164, 1976
6. Williams R: Cited in Finneson
7. Rothman RH, Simeone FA: The Spine, Vol. II. Saunders, Philadelphia, 1975, pp. 485–503
8. Finneson BE: Low Back Pain. Lippincott, Philadelphia, 1980, pp. 331–338
9. Yong-Hing K, Reilly J, de Korompay V, Kirkaldy-Willis WH: Prevention of nerve root adhesion after laminectomy. Spine 5:59–64, 1980
10. Jacobs RR, McClain O, Neff J: Control of postlaminectomy scar formation. an experimental and clinical study. Spine 5:223–229, 1980
11. Fager CH, Freidberg SR: Analysis of failures and poor results of lumbar spine surgery. Spine 5:87–94, 1980
12. Meyer GA, Haughton VM, Williams AL: Diagnosis of herniated lumbar disk with computed tomography. N Engl J Med 301:1166, 1979
13. Williams AL, Haughton VM, Syversten A: Computed tomography in the diagnosis of herniated nucleus pulposus. Radiology 135:95, 1980
14. Haughton VM, Elderik OP, Magnass B, Amundsen P: A prospective comparison of computed tomography and myelography in the diagnosis of herniated lumbar disks. Radiology 142:103, 1982
15. Sheldon JJ, Sersland T, Leborgne J: Computed tomography of the lower lumbar vertebral column. normal anatomy and the stenotic canal. Radiology 124:113, 1977
16. Burton CV, Kirkaldy-Willis WH, Yong-Hing K, Heithoff KB: Causes of failure of surgery on the lumbar spine. Clin Orthop 157:191, 1981
17. Cacayorin EO, Kieffer SA: Applications and limitations of computed tomography of the spine. Radiol Clin North Am 10:185–206, 1982
18. DePalma AF, Rothman RH: Surgery of the lumbar spine. Clin Orthop 63:162–170, 1969
19. Mall JC, Kaiser JA: Computed tomography of the postoperative spine. In Genant HK, Chafetz N, Helms CA (eds): Computed Tomography of the Lumbar Spine. University of California Printing Department, San Francisco, 1982, pp. 245–252
20. Ghormley RK: Low back pain with special reference to the articular facets, with presentation of an operative procedure. JAMA 101:1773, 1933
21. Badgley CE: Articular facets in relation to low back pain and sciatic radiation. J Bone Joint Surg 23A:481, 1941
22. Mooney V, Robertson J: The facet syndrome. Clin Orthop 115:149, 1976
23. Carrera GF: Computed tomography and facet injection in the evaluation of lumbar facet arthropathy. In Genant HK, Chafetz N, Helms CA (eds): Computed Tomography of the Lumbar Spine. University of California Printing Department, San Francisco, 1982, pp. 253–260
24. Carrera GF: Lumbar facet joint injection in low back pain and sciatica, Part I and II. Radiology 137:661, 1980
25. Heithoff KB: High-resolution computed tomography in the differential diagnosis of soft-tissue pathology of the lumbar spine. In Genant HK, Chafetz H, Helms CA (eds): Computed Tomography of the Lumber Spine. University of California Printing Department, San Francisco, 1982, pp. 147–171
26. Schubiger O, Valavani S: CT differentiation between recurrent disc herniation and postoperative scar formation: the value of contrast enhancement. Neuroradiology 22:251–254, 1982
27. Hoppenstein R: A new approach to the failed, failed back syndrome. Spine 5:371–379, 1980
28. Brodsky AE: Cauda equina arachnoiditis: correlative clinical and roentgenologic study. Spine 3:51–60, 1978
29. Patronss NJ, Jafar J, Brown F: Pseudomeningoceles diagnosed by metrizamide myelography and computed tomography. Surg Neurol 16:188, 1981
30. Cloward RB: The Cloward technique. In Finneson BE: Low Back Pain, ed. 2. Lippincott, Philadelphia, 1980, pp. 395–413
31. Cloward RB: The treatment of ruptured lumbar intervertebral discs by vertebral body fusion. I. Indications, operative techniques, and aftercare. J Neurosurg 10:154–165, 1953
32. DePalma A, Rothman R: The Intevertebral Disc. Saunders, Philadelphia, 1970
33. Wiltse LL: Lumbar spinal fusion. In Ruge D, Wiltse LL (eds): Spinal Disorders: Diagnosis and Treatment. Lea & Febiger, Philadelphia, 1977, pp. 142–153
34. Raney FL Jr: Anterior lumbar interbody fusion. In Ruge D, Wiltse LL (eds): Spinal Disorders: Diagnosis and Treatment. Lea & Febiger, Philadelphia, 1977, pp. 162–167
35. Cloward RB: Posterior Lumbar Interbody Fusion Surgical Techniques. Codman and Shurtlett, Randolph, Massachusetts, 1982

Planning and Performing Spine Surgery with CT/MPR: A Primer for Radiologists

Perry Camp
Charles W. Kerber

10

Few things are more discouraging to a surgeon than the patient who has continued bitter complaints after spine surgery. We often show our discouragement by refusing even to name these patients; instead we depersonalize them, calling them ''failed backs.''

The most common cause of the failed-back syndrome is probably an error in the original decision to operate. Many patients have unsolved psychosocial problems that the surgeon may not recognize. Even though we are critical of this lapse in surgical judgment, the most experienced and cautious physician occasionally makes these mistakes.

Not all failed backs are psychosocial in origin. The advent of computerized tomography with multiplanar reconstruction (CT/MPR) has demonstrated several large and important subsets of patients whose operation has failed not for psychosocial reasons but for a lack of appreciation of unrecognized pathology. In a small minority of cases, the surgeon has operated on the wrong interspace. In most, though, important pathology was overlooked and not operated on because the technology to see it was unavailable.

In order that the radiologist can better understand the problems encountered by the surgeon, we now review the most common of these problems and outline how specific abnormalities are diagnosed and treated. The evaluation of back disease is a complex undertaking, and the partnership between radiologist and surgeon is an essential one.

Soft Posteromedial Disc Rupture

Posteromedial disc herniations are the most common lower back problem and at present are the most well managed surgically. R.J., a 54 year-old man, came to the office with low back pain and leg pain along the lateral aspect of his thigh and left small toe. On examination he had numbness in the small toe and an absent ankle jerk. Clinically, we suspected a posteromedial disc herniation at his left L5–S1 interspace, with resulting irritation of his left S1 root.

In R.J.'s CT scan (Fig. 10.1A) note how the disc protrusion (closed arrows) has pushed back (dorsally) the S1 root (open arrow). The L5 root has already left the canal and has escaped this irritation and lies laterally in the foramen (open arrowheads). The coronal view (Fig. 10.1B) shows the lesion again and demonstrates that the herniation has caused swelling of the S1 root in the canal (open arrowheads).

This lesion is approached surgically through a vertical incision just to the left side of the midline, along the spinous processes, and then continued down to the laminae. Retractors are placed on the muscles, which are displaced laterally. The laminae now come into view (Figs. 10.2A,B). The ligamentum flavum, which lies between the laminae, is removed; then, using a biting instrument called a rongeur, a small amount of the lamina is removed.

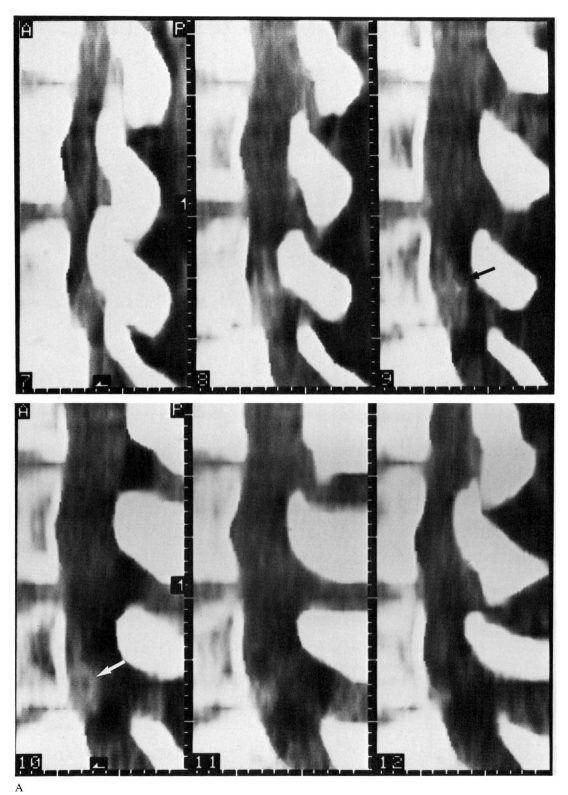

A

FIGURE 10.1 Lateral views of a CT/MPR examination. **A.** A large posterolateral soft disc herniation at the L5–S1 interspace is evident (*arrow*). **B.** The coronal views demonstrate the dense herniation (*arrows*) and its relationship to the caudal sac and S1 roots. Not surprisingly, the patient had a left S1 radiculopathy. (*Figure continued* on page 295.)

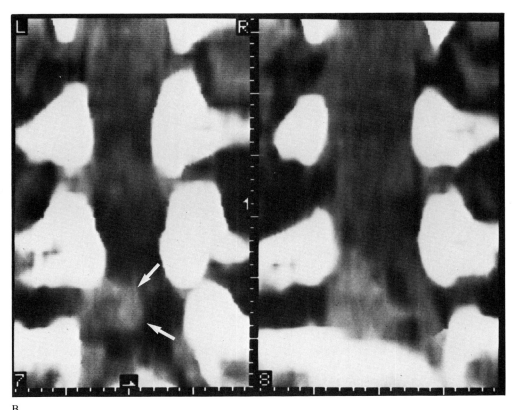

B

FIGURE 10.1 (*cont'd*) **B.** The coronal views demonstrate the dense herniation (*arrows*) and its relationship to the caudal sac and S1 roots. Not surprisingly, the patient had a left S1 radiculopathy.

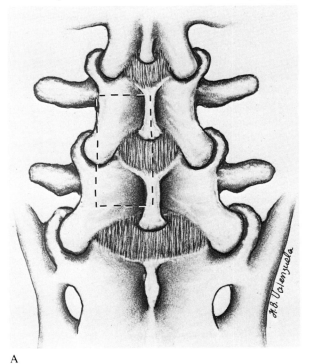

A

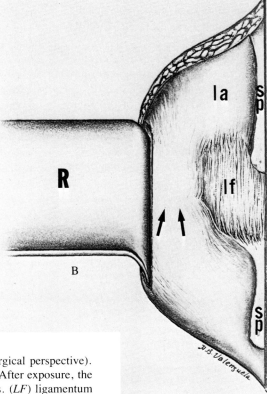

FIGURE 10.2 Normal lumbar spine bony relationships from behind (the surgical perspective). **A.** The dotted line shows the area exposed during microsurgical dissection. **B.** After exposure, the retractor (*R*) displaces the fat, skin, and muscle laterally. (*SP*) spinous process. (*LF*) ligamentum flavum. (*LA*) lamina. The bulge of the apophyseal joint is visible (*arrows*).

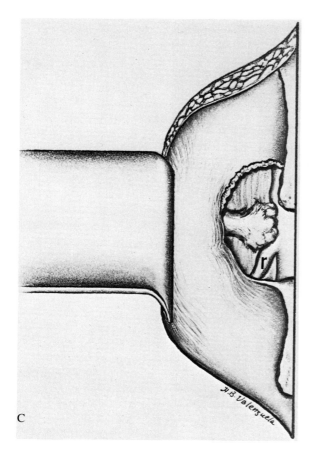

C

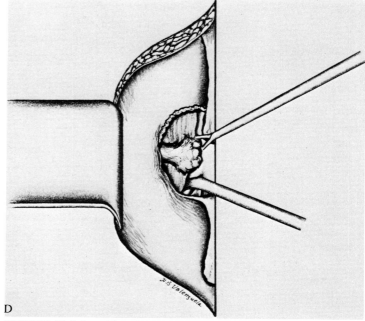

D

FIGURE 10.2 (*cont'd*)   **C.** The ligamentum flavum has been excised, and a small amount of the lamina has been removed (laminotomy). The caudal sac, roots, and a herniated disc come into view. Note the displacement of the root (*r*) by the disc fragment. **D.** Gentle medial retraction of the root exposes the herniation better. Disc material is then lifted out using a small rongeur.

The lateral portion of the caudal sac now comes into view. Note how the protruding disc fragment has pushed the irritated nerve root toward us. We move the nerve gently to the side to prevent damaging it and then grab the disc herniation with a small rongeur and remove it (Figs. 10.2C,D). The dissection is usually carried down into the interspace to remove additional disc material, although some surgeons omit this part of the operation. At this point experienced surgeons often do a routine foraminotomy; this maneuver (Fig. 10.3A) has been found through experience to improve results, but it leads to weakening of the facet joint (Figs. 10.3B–D) and may contribute to postoperative facet fractures (Fig. 10.4).

Although soft discs may recur, these patients generally do well and awaken in the recovery room free of radicular pain. Recovery time is short and many patients walk within hours, especially those who have had only microdissection and discectomy.

Posterolateral Herniation

Sometimes the direction of disc herniation is posterolateral rather than posteromedial. Before CT scanning, these patients presented with radicular syndromes but had generally normal myelograms. The surgeon who operated at the tra-

ditional level missed the herniation. If the patient presented with an L4 radiculopathy, for instance, the surgeon would operate at the level above, L3–4, and would of course miss the abnormality. Even worse, because that is the site of normal bulging of disc in most of us, he would remove the bulge and think he had done the patient some good. Unfortunately many patients improve after surgery no matter what is done and everyone feels satisfied for a time. Then, more unfortunately, the symptoms recur and the patient is considered a ''failed back.''

Figure 10.5A is an axial view of a patient with such a problem. Note the high-density lesion filling the neural canal far laterally. This extends even beyond the foramen. Coronal views (Fig. 10.5B) show this type of herniation even better. The high-denisty lesion completely fills the foramen (arrow). Compare this side with the other side and with the levels below, where there are normal nerves surrounded by fat.

The myelogram of the same patient was interpreted as normal (Fig. 10.5C). When this patient came into the office he had an electromyelogram that was abnormal in the L3 distribution. If he had not had the CT scan he might have been operated at the wrong interspace.

Let us assume that we had no CT scan to show us where the actual pathology was—far lateral in and beyond the neural foramen—and we had explored at the wrong (i.e., higher) level. Most surgeons would realize the mis-

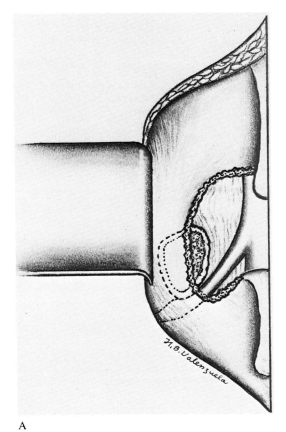

A

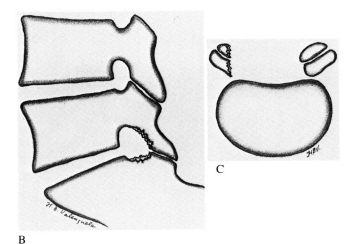

B

C

FIGURE 10.3 **A.** Before CT scanning it was easy to misdiagnose lateral nerve-root impingement by bony foraminal stenosis or far lateral disc herniation. When a standard laminotomy failed to find the expected disc herniation, the surgeon was forced to remove more bone, following the root inferiorly and laterally. This extra removal decompressed the root but frequently removed so much bone that the apophyseal joint was nearly destroyed, with possible subsequent spinal instability the result. **B.** The lateral view shows the patency of the foramen after the standard foraminotomy. **C.** The axial view shows how much of the apophyseal joint has been removed. **D.** Axial CT scan of such a patient. Little apophyseal joint remains (*arrows*).

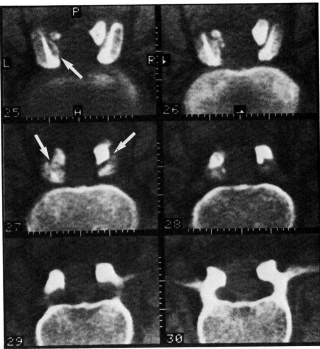

D

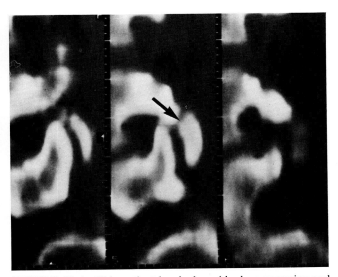

take during the procedure and then would start to remove bone laterally, following the nerve root well out into the foramen, wondering if some foraminal disease had been missed. In doing so, that apophyseal joint would be ruined,

FIGURE 10.4 This patient has had a wide decompression and developed another complication of classic foraminotomy. A facet stress fracture (*arrow*) is now the cause of his recurrent back pain.

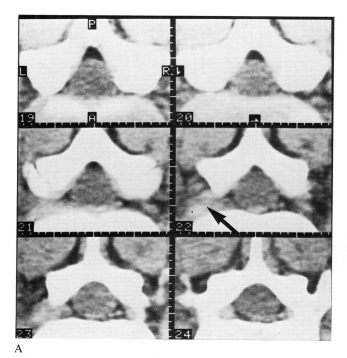

A

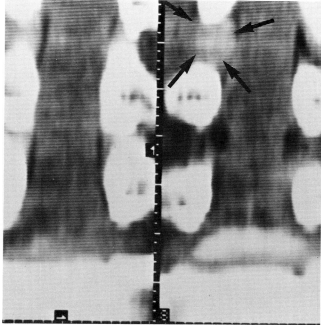

B

FIGURE 10.5 A. Far lateral disc herniations (axial views) demonstrate dense soft tissue (*arrows*) lateral to the foramen. **B.** The disc herniation is even more noticeable on the coronal (frontal) views. The extra density (*arrow*) has obliterated the foraminal fat. Compare this to the opposite foramen. **C.** His myelogram was normal, as expected.

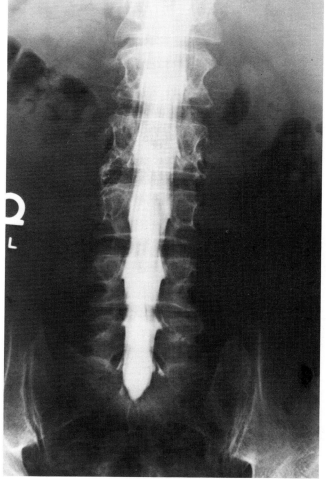

C

probably leading to some back instability that could worsen as the patient grows older. Even with all the extra bone removed, the far lateral disc herniation could have been difficult to see.

With the CT scan we know where the pathology is. Let us now make an approach at the "wrong" level, the level below which textbooks tell us to explore for this radiculopathy. We begin as before and carry our incision down to the laminae and remove the ligamentum flavum using sharp dissection (Fig. 10.6A). We then remove a small amount of facet joint, as before. At this point, the operation differs from the first. Let us make a small incision into the posterior longitudinal ligament over the disc, then scrape out enough of the disc material on that side to make a cavity.

Through that cavity one can reach far laterally with a hyperextended curette and deliver the herniated disc fragment down to the newly created cavity (Figs. 10.6B–D). From that cavity in the interspace it is easy to remove the disc material using a small rongeur. Because we know the position of the nerve root, we can make this removal without damaging it. Note how little bone has been removed to get this far-lateral disc fragment out. This patient's back has not been destabilized.

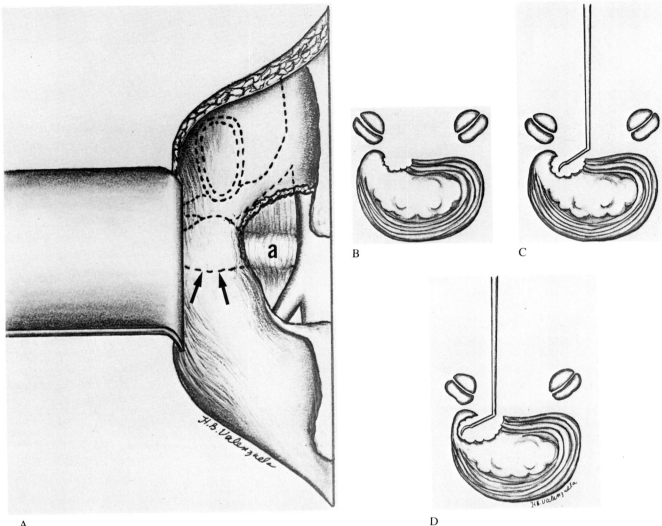

A

FIGURE 10.6   A. A surgical approach to this lesion is now performed at the "wrong" level. (An L3 radiculopathy would ordinarily be caused by an L2–3 herniation.) With the information from the CT scan, the surgeon will expose the L3–4 interspace. The standard laminotomy shows normal structures as the herniation is out of sight under the joint (*arrow*). The problem is to remove the disc without destroying the joint. First, an incision is made into the anulus (**a**) and as much disc material is removed as is possible. **B–D.** The axial views show the next stages. The lateral disc material is then teased down into the newly created interspace cavity by using a recurved curette and then is removed from that cavity using a small rongeur. This technique does not disrupt the apophyseal joint.

Central Disc Herniations

Central disc herniations are well shown by both myelography and CT, and for obvious reasons patients prefer the CT scan. Patients usually present with a cauda equina syndrome, which may include saddle anesthesia around the rectum as well as bowel and bladder dysfunction. This le-

sion can be removed in the same manner as a far-lateral disc, but instead of reaching far to the side we first create the cavity and then reach forward and to the midline, under the dural sac. As before, we create a posterolateral cavity in the interspace and then, using the hyperextended curette, push and tease the fragment down into that cavity, where it will be removed without damaging the nerves or the sac within it. Again, little bone is removed, and so the spine is not destabilized.

Spinal Stenosis and the Lateral Recess Syndrome

Physicians have only recently accepted the lateral recess syndrome as a real clinical entity (see Chapter 7). It was described by Verbiest first in 1950[1] and then again in 1954.[2] The patients generally present with bilateral lower-extremity pain and loss of function. Their difficulty is increased

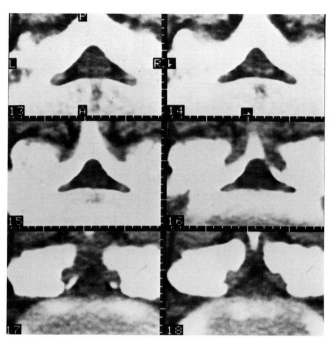

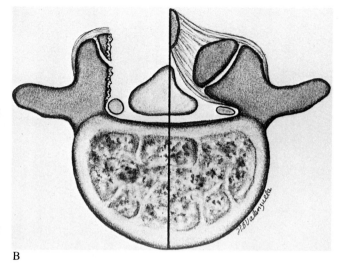

B

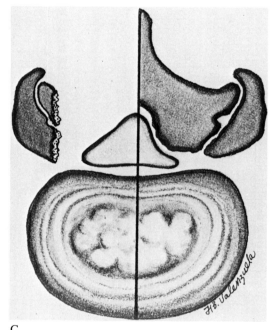

C

FIGURE 10.7 Spinal stenosis. This series of axial slices shows bony narrowing of the lateral recesses—a typical lateral recess stenosis. Note the relationship of the stenosis to the pedicle above the interspace.

by exercise and hyperextension of the back. Rest usually relieves the pain, at least in part. The neurologic findings vary considerably; in fact, when examined, the patient may appear completely normal.

Although there are many pathologic entities that cause this syndrome, in addition to the one originally described by Verbiest, the CT scanner allows us to understand the altered anatomy precisely. Thus the correct operative approach may be planned. The patient shown in Figure 10.7 has a lateral recess stenosis caused by bony overgrowth of the laminae between the apophyseal joints. This bony overgrowth extends a considerable distance cranially from the interspace. To perform this operation one must begin with a slightly larger exposure and then remove the lamina as shown in Figure 10.8. After this extensive bone removal,

FIGURE 10.8   A. Posterior/anterior (operative) view of a two-level spinal stenosis operation. The left side shows the extent of bone removed. Note that the lamina above the interspace must be removed in order to decompress the root adequately. **B.** An axial view through the foramen shows the bone removed (left side). On the right is the appearance of the stenosis before treatment. (See **A** for the level.) **C.** This axial view is drawn through the pedicle. (See **A** for the level.)

the nerve root may travel freely from its exit point from the caudal sac down to the foramen without being squeezed by the bony overgrowth. This procedure was well described by Ciric et al. in 1980.[3]

We should emphasize that a considerable amount of bone must be removed for good relief of symptoms. Figure 10.9 shows a patient with spinal stenosis who was treated by Ciric's method.

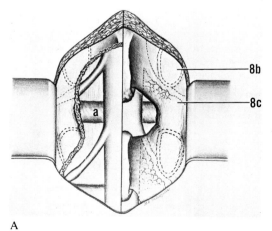

—8b

—8c

a

A

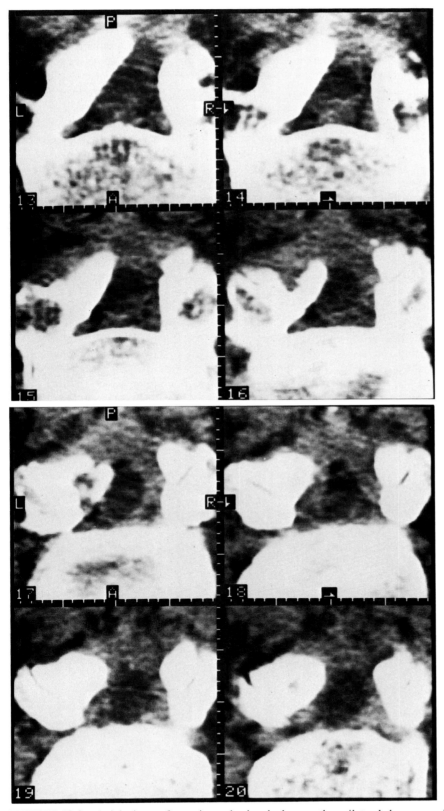

FIGURE 10.9 Axial views of a patient who has had a mostly unilateral decompression. (His symptoms were unilateral.) Note that the decompression extends superiorly from the interspace well up along the pedicle.

Stenosis of the Neural Foramen

Failure to appreciate significant disease in the neural foramina probably accounts for more failed backs than does any other cause. Foraminal stenosis may be caused by two basic processes: narrowing caused by overgrowth of the articular facets, generally the superior, and narrowing caused by overgrowth of vertebral body end-plates. Mixtures of the two processes are the rule, of course, but for learning purposes we may divide them into pure forms.

Let us first look at a patient with almost pure superior articular facet hypertrophy (Fig. 10.10). Note on the lateral reconstructions how severe the foraminal stenosis appears. The bone windows slightly undercall the stenosis; but even so, note how complete is the obliteration of the foramen. The foramen should look as it does at the level above an inverted teardrop.

Traditionally, this lesion is treated by removing bone 90 degrees away from the pathology. This is only logical, as that is the surgeon's visual orientation. The back is viewed from above, and the tendency is to remove disease that can be readily visualized. The surgeon begins removing bone where the nerve exits from the caudal sac and follows it out laterally. This certainly opens up the foramen—but at the cost of removing the apophyseal joint. This may destabilize the spine, especially in younger individuals. Current spine surgery dogma states that one-third of the triple-joint complex (one of the apophyseal joints) can be removed

with impunity without such destabilization, but we are slowly learning that not all patients tolerate this removal.

There is another aspect to this problem. It is surprising how many patients who have had operative reports describing wide foraminotomy still have persistent foraminal stenosis when a follow-up CT scan is performed. One can only speculate about this failure to remove bone adequately, but in fairness to the surgeon the operation is performed with the patient in the slightly flexed position and this tends to open the neural foramina.

One may use an alternative approach that spares a major part of the apophyseal joint. The CT scan allows us to measure the facets on the lateral view to determine exactly how far superiorly we must carry an excision (Fig. 10.11A). At the operating table a measurement is made up from the superior vertebral body end-plate (Fig. 10.11B). An angled Kerrison rongeur is used to remove bone *under* the superior articular facet, where the actual pathology lies, rather than at right angles to it (Fig. 10.11C–F). Because of the limitations of the deep surgical hole, we are not exactly parallel to the bony overgrowth, but it is nontheless an improvement over the older technique. The facet removal is planned using CT. The surgeon continues to remove bone until the small superior fragment is delivered into the cavity, much as one would remove a fragment of tooth (Fig. 10.11H).

The drawing in Figure 10.11I is of a postoperation CT scan and shows the wide opening of the neural

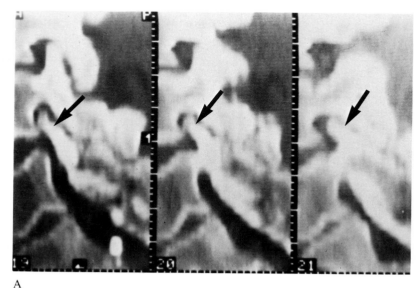

A

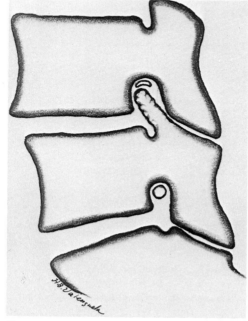

B

FIGURE 10.10   A. Lateral (sagittal) reconstruction of a patient who has superior articular facet hypertrophy (*arrows*). The bone-window setting tends to underestimate the severity of the stenosis, in part because it does not show the attendant soft-tissue hypertrophy. Note the normal level above for comparison. **B.** This diagram corresponds to the changes seen on the scan in **A.**

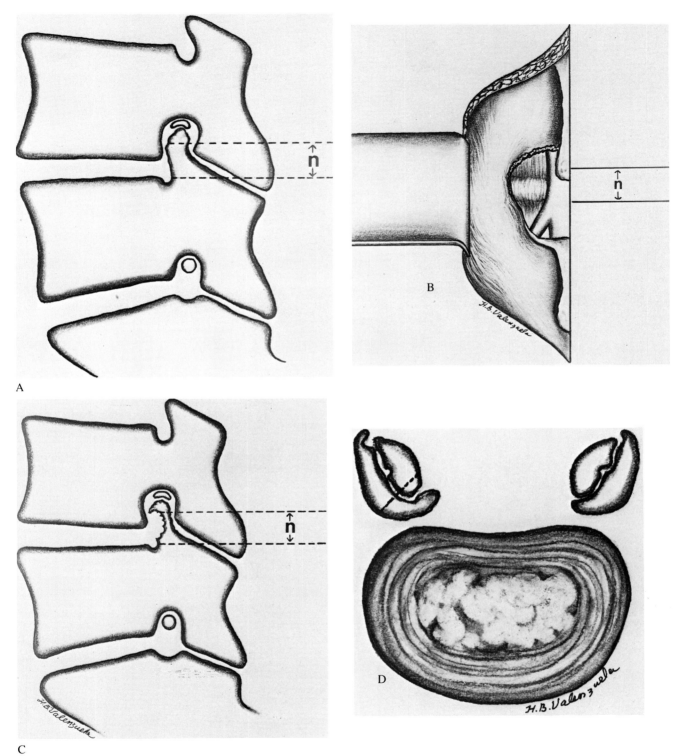

A

C

B

D

FIGURE 10.11 **A.** One may measure directly from life-size CT scans and transpose these measurements to the patient. The vertebral-body superior end-plate and the superior articular facet are part of the same structure; the end-plate can be seen by the standard operative exposure; the superior articular facet cannot. The surgeon then chooses a distance (n) up (cranially) from the end-plate that allows him to nibble away at the extra bone but provide enough safety margin to avoid damaging the nerve. **B.** This is the view the surgeon sees after measuring from the film. He then places the instrument along and parallel to the upper line. **C.** This is the appearance laterally after some of the bone has been removed. At no time must the instrument be allowed to dissect more cranially. **D.** The more classic foraminotomy (Fig. 10.3) removed bone at right angles to the foramen; this approach more directly removes the spur. The dotted line shows the expected path of removal. (*Figure continued* on page 304.)

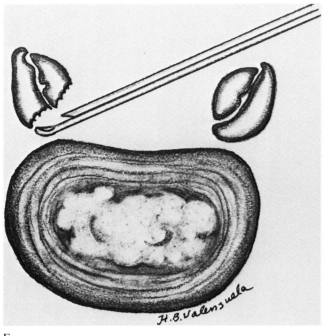

E

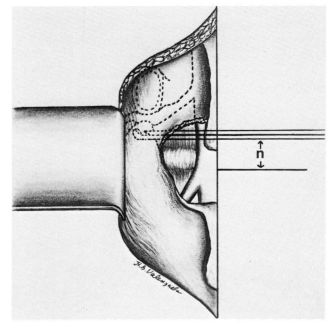

F

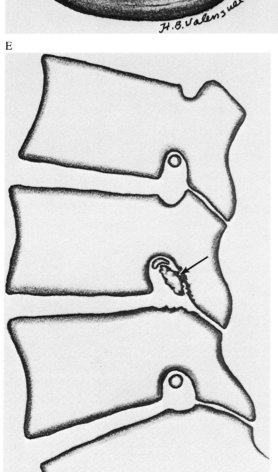

G

FIGURE 10.11 (*cont'd*)   **E.** Spur removal is now nearly complete. This axial view closely corresponds to lateral views **C** and **F**. **F.** The surgeon's view of a nearly complete spur removal. **G.** When the angled Kerrason bites through the spur, a small piece remains cranially (*arrow*). This piece is gently teased caudally into the opening and then removed. **H.** Here the instrument is delivering that last piece out of the foramen. **I.** The lateral view now has this appearance (compare to **A**).

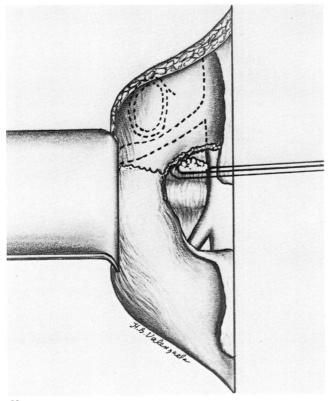

H

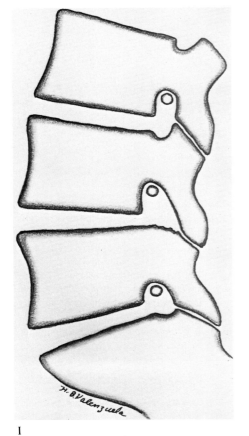

I

foramen and preservation of a majority of the apophyseal joint. Although this is a relatively new technique, this approach should not lead to later spine instability.

End-Plate Hypertrophy

Foraminal stenosis caused by end-plate hypertrophy has been largely ignored by the surgical community. Note on the lateral view of the CT/MPR films (Figs. 10.12A–C) that such a disease process not only exists but in this patient has led to a failed-back syndrome. This 55-year-old man had persistent L5 radiculopathy after decompression by standard foraminal operation at the L4–5 level. His persistent signs and symptoms had led to this complete evaluation. The soft-tissue windows demonstrate the remarkable narrowing (Fig. 10.12B); and the end-plate hypertrophy, the cause of the narrowing, is well appreciated on the bone window views (Fig. 10.12C).

Surgery for this lesion is much the same as for a far-lateral herniated disc, but the surgeon must take out bone rather than disc material. Again, sharp dissection is used to expose the lamina and remove a minimal amount of that lamina. Then an incision into the posterior longitudinal ligament and anulus fibers allows creation of a cavity in the interspace, as for removal of the far-lateral disc. Note how

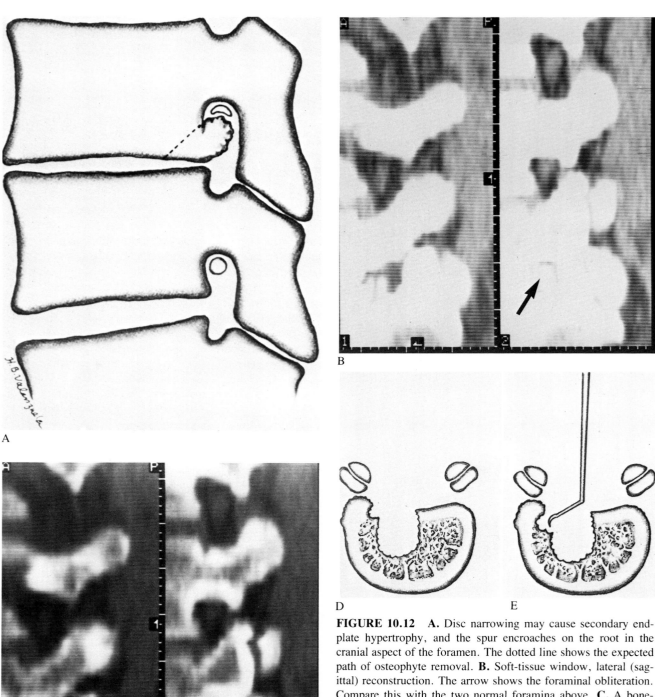

A

B

C

D   E

FIGURE 10.12   A. Disc narrowing may cause secondary end-plate hypertrophy, and the spur encroaches on the root in the cranial aspect of the foramen. The dotted line shows the expected path of osteophyte removal. **B.** Soft-tissue window, lateral (sagittal) reconstruction. The arrow shows the foraminal obliteration. Compare this with the two normal foramina above. **C.** A bone-window view of the same patient shows the large osteophyte (*arrows*) causing the stenosis. **D–F.** Surgery for removal of an end-plate osteophyte is done much as that for far lateral disc removal. First, a cavity is created in the interspace, and then the osteophyte is undermined slowly with a hyperextended curette. When the undermining is complete, the remaining fragment is fractured off and delivered into the interspace using the tip of a Frasier dural elevator. Care is taken to avoid the nerve root during the undermining, as during removal of a superior articular spur. **G.** This patient's L4–5 osteophye has been removed. Note the beveled appearance and patency of the superior portion of the foramen (*arrows*).

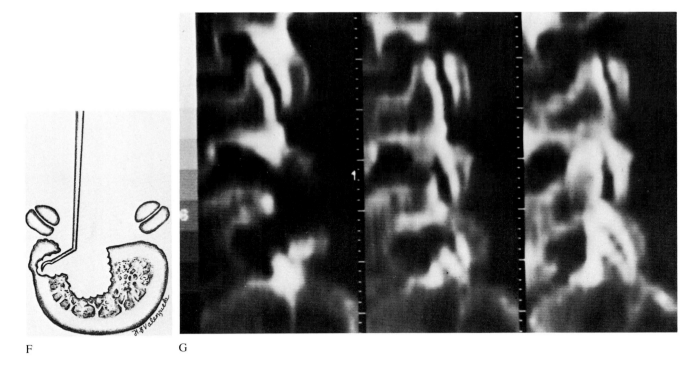

F   G

creation of the cavity gives the surgeon a work space and allows him to curette progressively laterally and remove the osteophyte (Figs. 10.12D–F). Here the hyperextended curette is shown removing the underside of the osteophyte from within the interspace. The fragments of bone delivered into the cavity may be removed with another instrument, a small rongeur. It is never necessary to place an instrument into the tight foramen, thus protecting the nerve root. Bit by bit the osteophyte is undermined, and finally a chunk of bone falls into the cavity. The bone window, lateral view (Fig. 10.12G), shows the results of such an operation. Note the large amount of space remaining for the nerve root to pass through, as well as the large amount of apophyseal joint that remains. A similar procedure is used if the osteophyte arises from the end-plate of the more inferior vertebral body. Combinations of disease may exist in this area, in which case the operations are simply combined.

Summary

The information available to back surgeons and radiologists allows more complete and accurate assessment of the altered anatomy and pathophysiology of this complex and important part of the body. With that knowledge, the appropriate operation may be planned and carried out. We know that some of the operative approaches described here are new and have been tested for only a short time. Short-term follow-up, however, has proved them worthwhile and encourages us to continue. The procedures described above remove a minimal amount of normal apophyseal joint and should not lead to subsequent destabilization of the spine.

The smaller exposure and diminished exploration damage less tissue and certainly decrease the postoperative discomfort felt by the patient. Just as important, a postoperative scan is invaluable to the surgeon for assessing the results of surgery.

Finally, we stress again that the leading cause of failed backs is not a misunderstanding of alternate anatomy, nor is it poor surgical technique—it is a misunderstanding of the emotional/psychosocial milieu in which the patient lives. Bulging discs rarely cause symptoms, except in combination with severe degenerative apophyseal disease, and are found in asymptomatic patients over the age of 40 in more than 50% of cases. That these bulging discs are more easily visualized on CT scans than on myelography could lead an unwary surgeon to the operating room, to the detriment of all involved. We are now using the most powerful diagnostic tool in the history of man. Anatomy is displayed with a clarity only dreamed of a few years ago. This direct visualization of the anatomy allows an understanding of the altered biomechanics. This new information, coupled with sound surgical judgment, can lead to more effective and less expensive patient care.

References

1. Verbiest H: Primaire Stenose Can Het Lumbale Wervelkanaal Bej Volwassenen. Ned Tijdschr Geneeskd 94:2415–2433, 1950
2. Verbiest H: A radicular syndrome from developmental narrowing of the lumbar vertebral canal. J Bone Joint Surg [Br] 36:230–237, 1954
3. Ciric I, Mikhael M, Tarkington JA, Vick NA: The lateral recess syndrome. J Neurosurg 53:433–443, 1980

Spinal Neoplasia and Its Differential Diagnosis

11

The radiographic assessment of neoplastic lesions affecting the spine is undergoing radical change even as this chapter is being written. The high-magnetic-field nuclear magnetic resonance (NMR) systems have begun to show remarkable images of spinal and paraspinal abnormalities. By the end of the decade, NMR will quite likely change the way we diagnose these lesions.

For practical purposes, the best screening examination for osseous spinal neoplasms is still the radionuclide bone scan. This method allows total osseous examination at a low radiation dose and for relatively low cost. For the most part, bone scanning is more sensitive than plain films for detecting subtle secondary bone lesions, which are the type encountered most often in clinical practice. CT, by its very nature, is a zonal examination. It must be limited to an anatomic area where the index of suspicion for finding a tumor is high. This is its one major weakness. CT is an extraordinary tool for answering specific diagnostic/anatomic questions, but it is a poor screening device for the spine.[1]

This chapter is limited to the description of basic principles of multiplanar CT as related to neoplastic disorders of the spine and to those lesions that at times are included in the differential diagnosis. For the most part, the discussion centers on lesions that may be evaluated without intrathecal contrast medium. It is in this large group of patients that CT affords the greatest benefit—the avoidance of myelography and its potential discomfort.

Neoplastic lesions of the spine are conveniently divided into three classes: extradural, intradural extramedullary, and intramedullary. Primary lesions of the spinal cord are relatively rare and include astrocytomas and ependymomas. Most intradural extramedullary lesions are meningiomas or neurofibromas. Extradural tumors usually arise either primarily or secondarily in bone and are far and away the most common spinal neoplasm. It is for this reason that the discussion begins with the evaluation of metastases.

Extradural Lesions

The assessment of the spine for metastases occurs most frequently in three clinical settings. In the first, a primary tumor is found somewhere in the body, and as part of a diagnostic evaluation for definitive therapy the presence of bony metastases is sought. These patients are usually asymptomatic, and bone screening is primarily done by radionuclide scan or radiography. In the second setting, a person with known cancer is being evaluated because of symptoms relating to the spine (bone pain) or spinal cord and nerve roots (myelopathy or radiculopathy). In these instances the symptoms may allow localization without a screening examination, but in many cases bone scanning may still be indicated. In the third clinical setting there is no known tumor, but some benign process, e.g., disc prolapse or herniation, is suspected.

We have found the best evaluation of a known osseous lesion to be a complete series of 5 mm thick scans every 3 mm or, if possible, 3–mm scans every 3 mm, with multiplanar reformatting. These data are viewed in at least two nonaxial planes for both soft-tissue and bone detail. The examination includes at least one vertebral segment below and one above the suspected metastasis, as the epidural component of tumors may extend some distance from the site of bone involvement. The key diagnostic information in these cases is assessment of the full extent of the tumor, which is usually best seen on the sagittal and axial views. Only then can appropriate surgical or radiotherapeutic planning be done.

The majority of osseous metastases occur within the vertebral bodies and are lytic on x-ray and lucent on CT examination (Fig. 11.1). They most commonly come from primary tumors in the breast, prostate, lung, and kidney. Carcinoma of the breast and prostate commonly cause either sclerotic or mixed sclerotic and lytic lesions (Fig. 11.2).

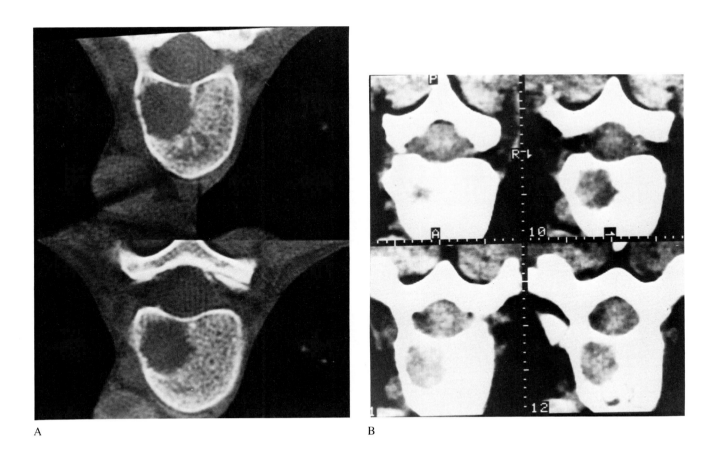

A

B

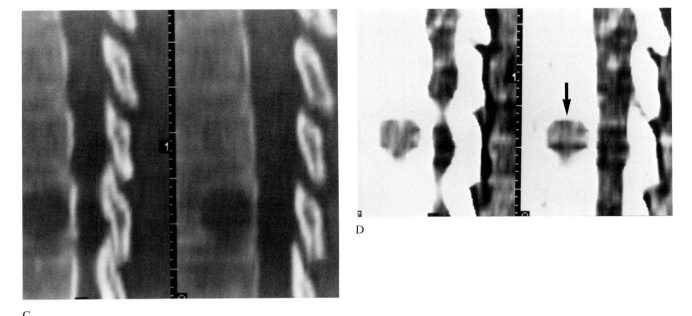

C

D

FIGURE 11.1 Localized osseous metastasis from carcinoma of the breast. Axial bone-window (**A**) and soft-tissue (**B**) views. Sagittal bone-window (**C**) and soft-tissue (**D**) views demonstrate a bone-destroying lytic lesion with poor borders (*arrows*). The vertebral end-plates and outer edges are preserved. There is no epidural tumor.

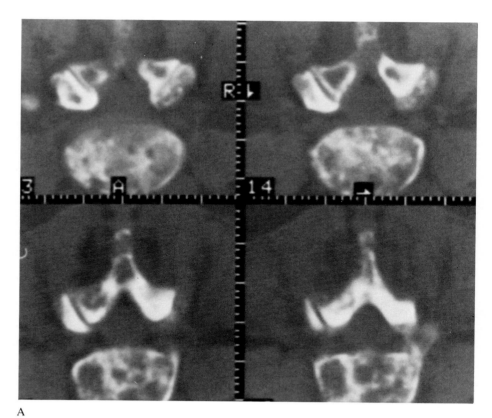

A

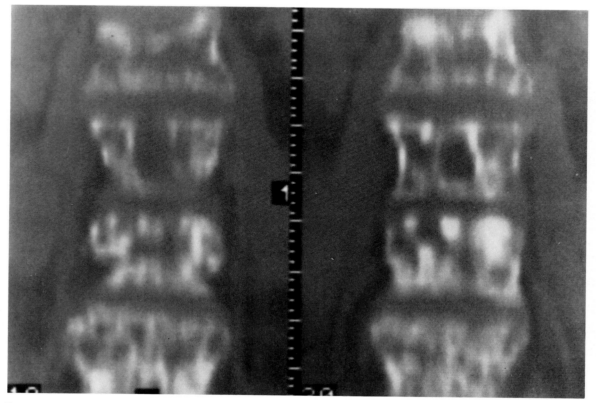

B

FIGURE 11.2 Diffuse metastatic prostatic cancer. Axial (**A**), coronal (**B**), and sagittal (**C**) images. The bones of the lumbar spine are diffusely abnormal. Virtually no bone is spared. There is, however, no hint of epidural tumor.

(*Figure continued* on page 311.)

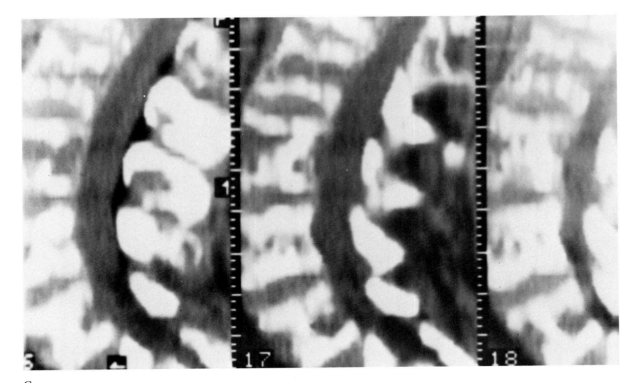

C

FIGURE 11.2 (*cont'd*)

CT is far more sensitive than is routine radiography in assessing these lesions. Extraspinal, spinal, and epidural components can be evaluated without intravenous or intrathecal contrast enhancement.

The patient in Figure 11.3 was evaluated because of an S1 radiculopathy. Routine radiographs and the digital ScoutView that was performed as part of the CT scan were interpreted as normal. Clinincally, the patient was thought

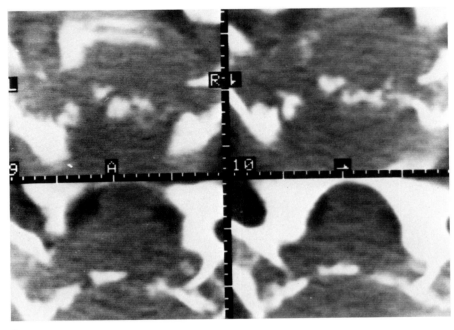

A

FIGURE 11.3 Carcinoma of the breast. **A.** Axial views define a vertebral-body metastasis, with a small intraspinal component compressing roots but not totally obstructing the spinal canal. (*Figure continued* on page 312.)

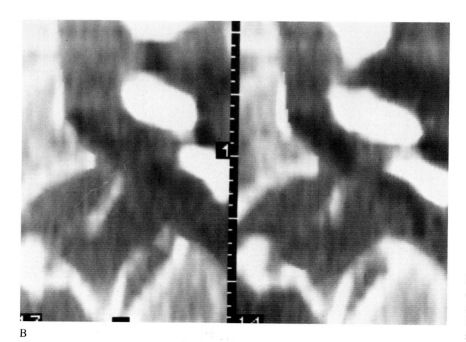

B

FIGURE 11.3 (*cont'd*) **B.** Sagittal views define a vertebral-body metastasis, with a small intraspinal component compressing roots but not totally obstructing the spinal canal.

to have a herniated L5–S1 disc. Axial and sagittal CT defined a partially destroyed vertebral body with extradural soft-tissue mass. In this case the vertebral height was maintained, and the end-plates were partially intact. The sagittal view allowed very precise assessment of the extradural mass. The neural canal was narrowed by less than 25%. This patient is therefore in no imminent danger of acute spinal root compression. Note that the entire volume of the tumor can be assessed from the CT scan.

Another unsuspected metastasis in a patient being evaluated for disc disease is shown in Figure 11.4. Plain films were negative. Note the active destruction of the lam-

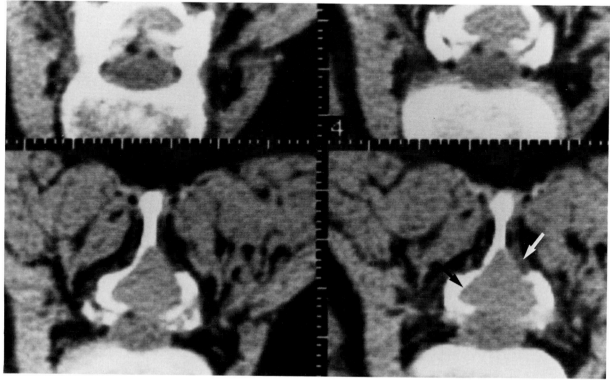

A

FIGURE 11.4   Solitary metastasis to the lamina. Axial view. (*Figure continued* on page 313.)

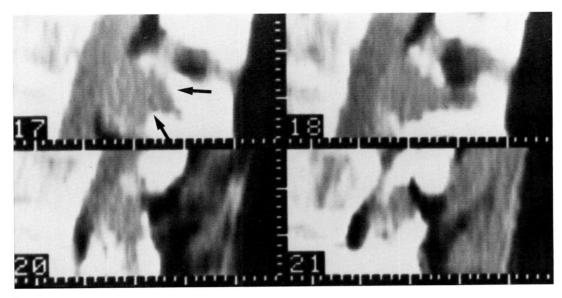

B

FIGURE 11.4 (*cont'd*)   Solitary metastasis to the lamina. Axial (**A**) and sagittal (**B**) views. The lamina is expanded and destroyed. The tumor extends forward into the spinal canal (*arrows*) but causes only minor thecal indentation.

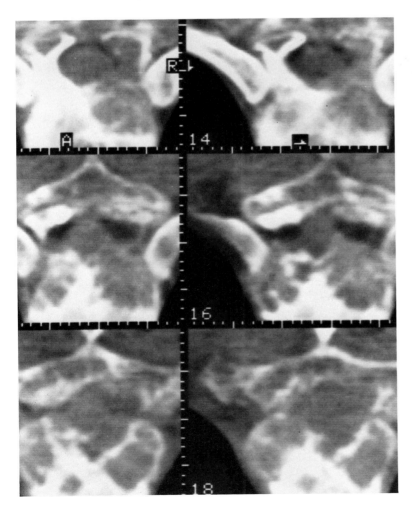

FIGURE 11.5 Vertebral-body metastasis. A large, extradural tumor mass extends into the spinal canal on the right; a smaller mass is seen on the left.

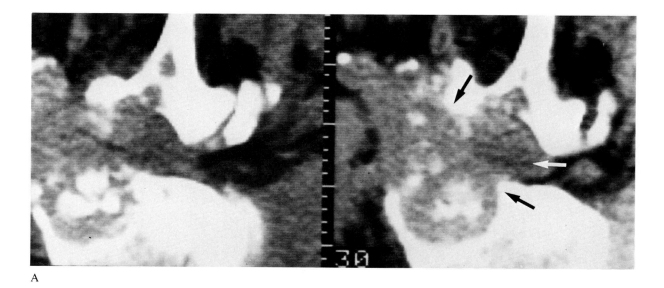

A

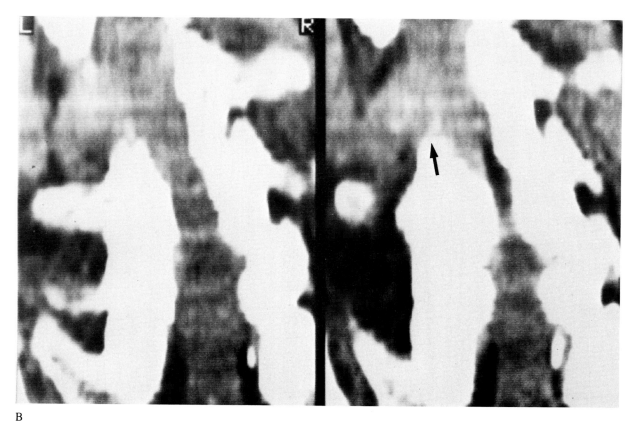

B

FIGURE 11.6 Solitary metastasis to the vertebral body and pedicle. Note the extensive mass (*arrows*) on both the axial (**A**) and coronal (**B**) views.

ina and spinous process. The tumor mass is convex into the spinal canal but only slightly distorts the theca posteriorly.

The two patients in Figures 11.5 and 11.6, on the other hand, demonstrate bony metastases—one to the vertebral body and one to the body and pedicle. These differ from those lesions previously described in that the soft-tissue component of the lesion is large and causes consid-

erable spinal canal compression. These must be treated quickly and definitively because of the imminent danger of cauda equina compression with irreversible bowel and bladder dysfunction and paralysis.

The most important point to be made by these two cases is that the nonenhanced, nonmetrizamide CT, when reformatted, accurately defines the entire tumor. Even those

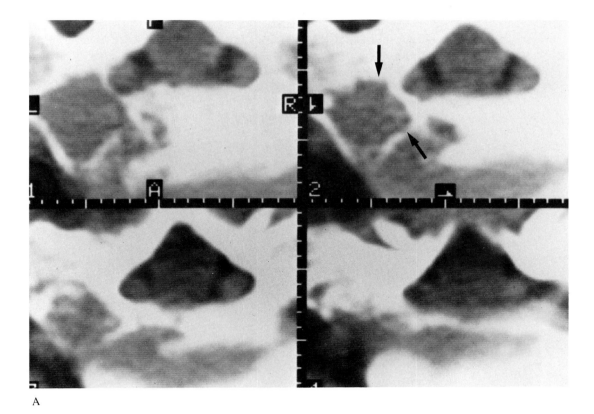

A

B

FIGURE 11.7 Localized metastasis to the left pedicle of the sacrum. Sagittal (**A**) and coronal (**B**) images demonstrate a small localized bone lesion immediately below the exiting L5 nerve root (*arrows*).

cases that clinically demonstrate a total spinal blockage frequently do not need myelography for assessment of the mass. Remember, patients with metastatic block are some of the sickest and most miserable human beings. Bending and turning may be extremely painful to them. During the pre-CT era, or in those cases where reformation does not outline the extent of the mass, two myelographic injections are usually required—one below and one above the mass—in order to define the full extent of the disease for the surgeon or the radiation oncologist.

Small localized metastases may also be distinguished by CT/MPR. Figure 11.7 demonstrates a localized lesion in the pedicle of the sacrum in a patient with an S1 radiculopathy. Figure 11.8 demonstrates a localized lesion in the inferior articular process and lamina.

It is important when performing spine CT to include the retroperitoneum and as much of the abdomen as possible. Many centers overly target the reconstruction to produce lovely magnified views of the spine. By their very nature, these studies fail to include the retroperitoneum.

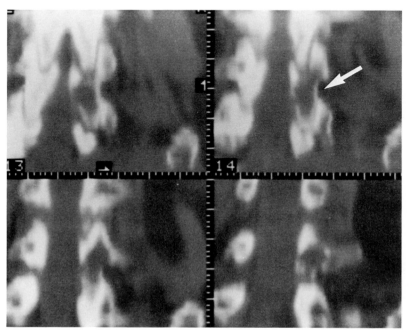

A

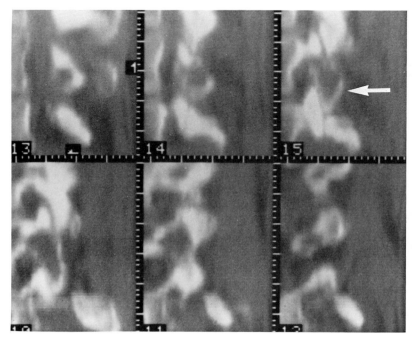

B

FIGURE 11.8 Localized metastasis to the right inferior articular process and lamina. Coronal (**A**) and sagittal (**B**) views demonstrate a lytic lesion (*arrows*) confined to the inferior facet and lamina. There was no significant intraspinal soft-tissue component to the lesion on the narrow-window views.

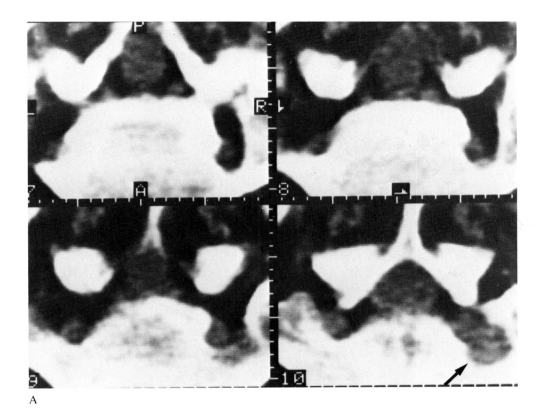

A

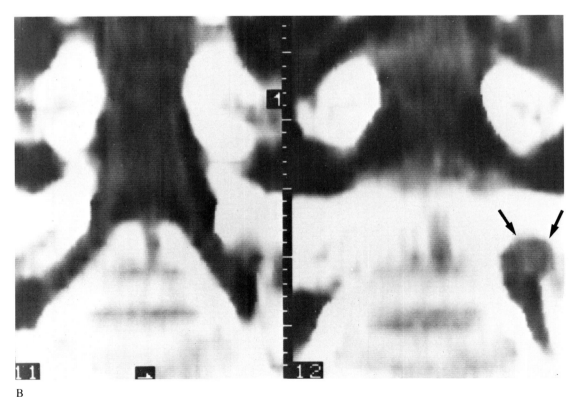

B

FIGURE 11.9 Diffuse metastases. **A.** Targeted cone-down scan easily misinterpreted as normal. **B.** Coronal reformation at the time of diagnosis and 6 months before. Note the new lesion adjacent to the S2 nerve root on the right (*arrows*). (*Figure continued* on page 318.)

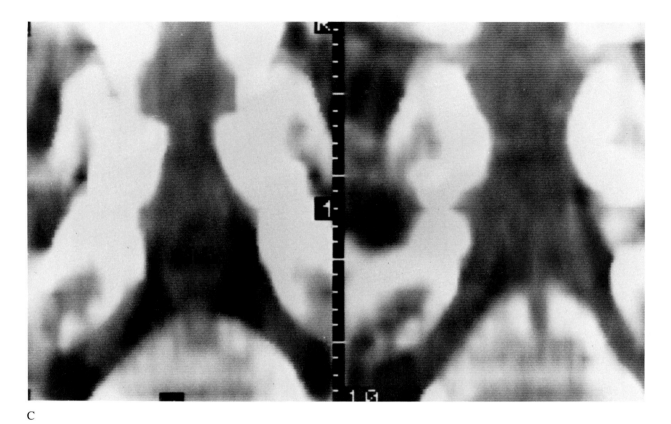

C

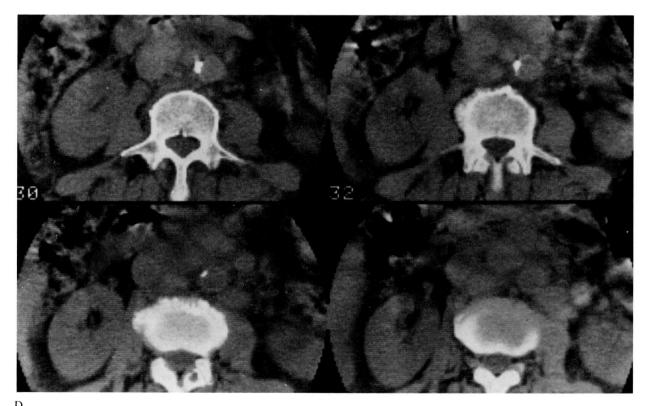

D

FIGURE 11.9 (*cont'd*) **C.** Coronal reformation at the time of diagnosis and 6 months before. Note the new lesion adjacent to the S2 nerve root on the right (*arrows*). **D.** Nontargeted scan demonstrates diffuse retroperitoneal lymph-node metastases and the normal scan 6 months before.

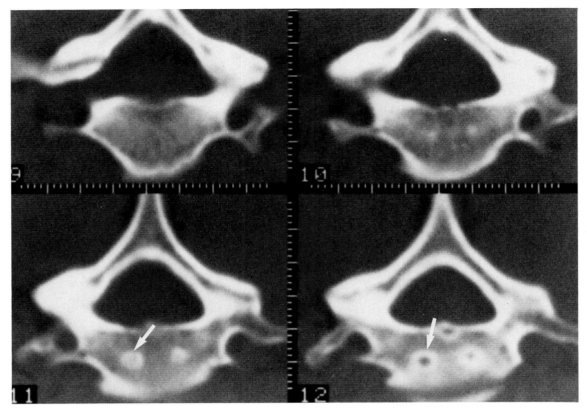

FIGURE 11.10 Cervical Schmorl's nodes. Axial scan demonstrates the typical CT appearance of small areas of intrabody disc herniation (*arrows*). Note the localized areas of surrounding sclerosis.

The patient in Figure 11.9 was scanned twice within the same year. The first scan was normal even in retrospect. The second scan finally revealed the cause of the patient's right radiculopathy. A small localized right-sided bone lesion is clearly evident on the coronal view. During the interim, however, the patient had developed diffuse retroperitoneal adenopathy, which would be missed by overly targeting the scanning field.

Small single or multiple lytic defects are frequently seen within the vertebral end-plates. These represent areas of interbody disc herniation (Schmorl's nodes). Their characteristic location within the end-plates and their sclerotic borders are usually sufficient to preclude misdiagnosing them as neoplasm (Fig. 11.10). Occasionally they reach remarkable size. When this occurs there is always smooth bony sclerosis surrounding the lesion. The key in differentiating these giant vertebral holes of discal origin is the unequivocal demonstration of continuity of the defect with the vertebral end-plate (Fig. 11.11). This should not be confused with the much more irregular end-plate deformity found in patients with osteomyelitis and discitis or in those with neoplastic destruction (Fig. 11.12). The latter defects typically display irregular, ragged walls with bone spiculation. Even if infection extends from the disc spaces into the vertebral body, the differential diagnosis should not be

difficult. Infections of the spine are nearly always grossly bone-destroying. They are frequently associated with moderate or even large paravertebral or psoas abscess (Fig. 11.13).

Sclerotic-bone-producing metastases may or may not cause spinal compression. The full extent of bony expansion is best visualized on the sagittal reformation (Fig. 11.14). It is, of course, impossible to distinguish the cell type of a metastatic lesion from the CT appearance. Common lesions, e.g., breast metastases, may look exactly like the more rare sclerotic lesions from Hodgkin's disease and carcinoid and other tumors.

Multiple myeloma and other diffuse myeloproliferative infiltrating tumors typically distort the internal architecture of the vertebral body[2] (Fig. 11.15). The regular cortical pattern is disrupted by prominent abnormal marrow spaces. The residual bone trabeculae tend to be abnormally prominent. The key differential must be made between myeloma and generalized benign osteoporosis. The diagnosis is easiest when there is cortical destruction.

Superficially, vertebral body hemangioma may simulate myeloma in that the individual bone trabeculae are fewer in number and disorganized. They are, however, denser than normal. The medullary spaces appear unusually prominent when surrounded by the thickened, coarse tra-

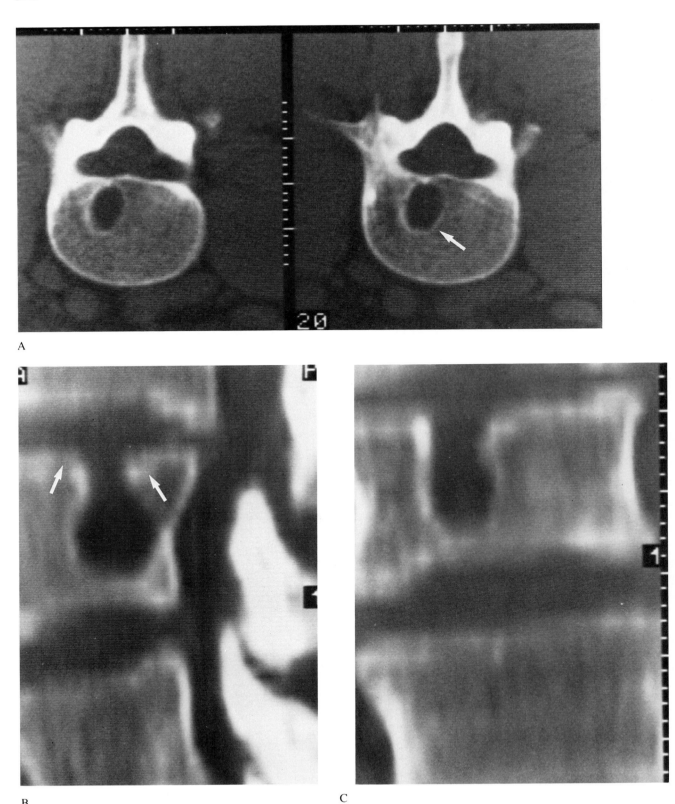

A

B   C

FIGURE 11.11 Giant Schmorl's node. Axial (**A**), sagittal (**B**), and coronal (**C**) CT on a patient with a large, well-circumscribed, lucent defect (*arrows*) that extends into the vertebral body through the cartilaginous end-plate.

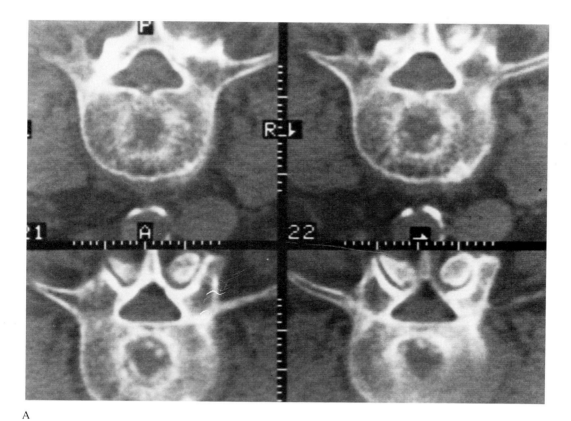

A

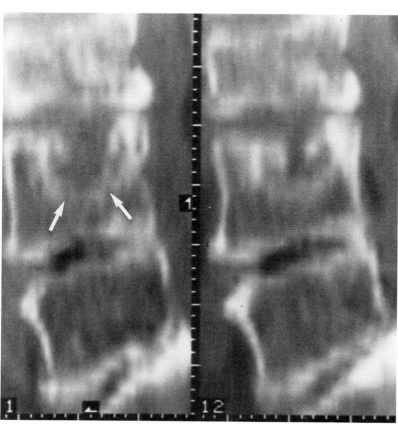

B

FIGURE 11.12 Multiple myeloma, producing end-plate defect. Axial (**A**) and sagittal (**B**) views demonstrate an irregular lucent defect extending downward from the vertebral end-plate into the body (*arrows*). The walls are ragged and fragmented. (*Figure continued* on page 322.)

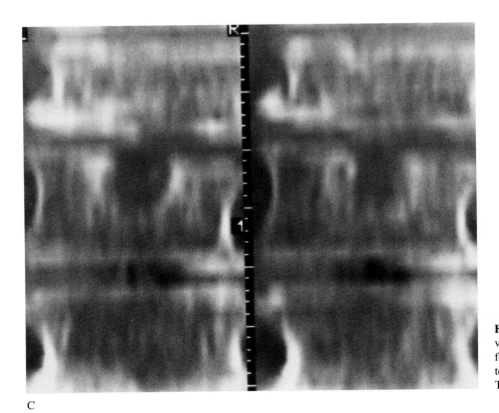

C

FIGURE 11.12 (*cont'd*) **C.** Coronal views demonstrate an irregular lucent defect extending downward from the vertebral end-plate into the body (*arrows*). The walls are ragged and fragmented.

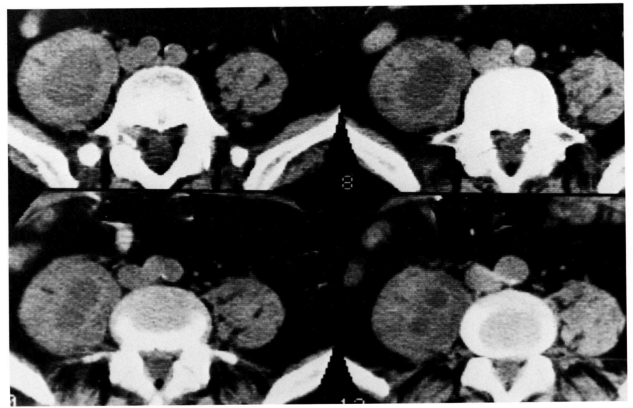

A

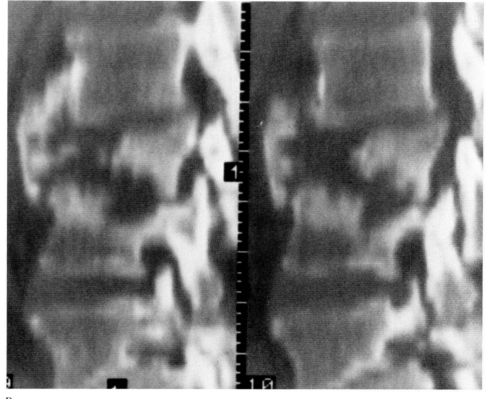

B

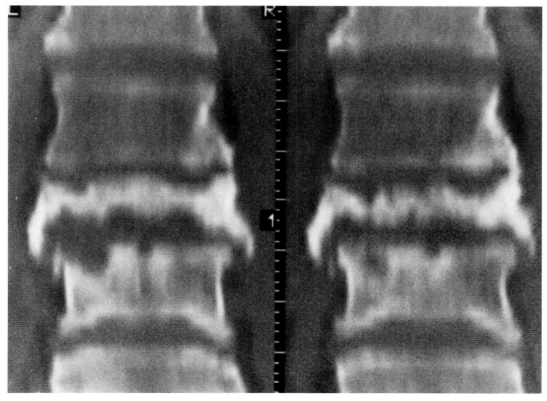

FIGURE 11.13 Spinal discitis and osteomyelitis. Axial (**A**), sagittal (**B**), and coronal (**C**) views on a diabetic patient who was treated medically for a psoas abscess (*arrow*). Within a month, disc space and vertebral infection have become obvious. Note the bone destruction and associated paravertebral mass. C

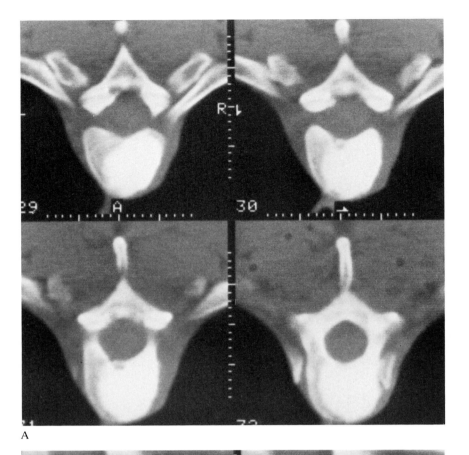

A

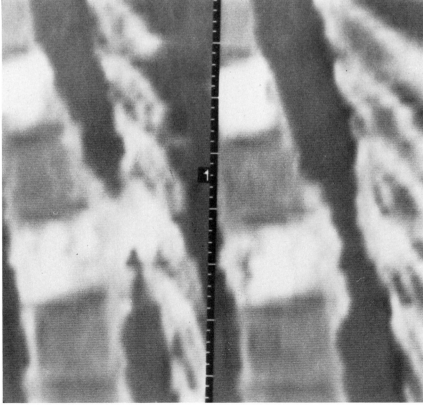

B

FIGURE 11.14 Multiple sclerotic metastases. Axial (**A**) and sagittal (**B**) views on a patient with two large sclerotic metastases. On the sagittal view, one can identify a plaque of hyperostotic tumorous bone invading the spinal canal.

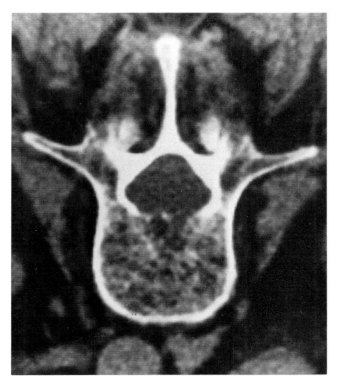

FIGURE 11.15 Multiple myeloma. Axial scan demonstrates diffuse patchy infiltrate of the vertebra. The subtle intravertebral architecture is disrupted. In this case, the diagnosis is more difficult because the cortical margins are intact.

beculae. In fact, differentiating the lesions is easy on reformations because the involved bone displaces the typical coarse pattern and is actually hyperostotic. Vertebral hemangiomas may be small and insignificant, being confined to all or a portion of the vertebral body (Fig. 11.16). Rarely, however, when the hemangioma extends into the neural arches, symptomatic neurocompressive symptoms occur because of vascular encroachment on the spinal cord or roots.

Another common condition that may be confused with myeloma and hemangioma on axial CT is Paget's disease. In the sclerotic phase of the disorder, the bone trabeculae are thickened and abnormally prominent. Unlike hemangioma, the medullary spaces do not appear unusually prominent. The internal architecture is disorganized, but there seem to be too many rather than too few trabeculae. Most importantly, bones involved with Paget's disease are usually enlarged. This enlargement may be difficult or impossible to detect on axial views because there is no way of directly comparing individual levels. Figure 11.17 is a typical example of a patient with vertebral Paget's disease. The vertebra is larger than normal and hyperdense. The individual trabeculae are abnormally prominent.

Fibrous dysplasia is occasionally confused with Paget's disease. The disorder tends not to involve vertebral bodies primarily and to be asymmetrical and unilateral.

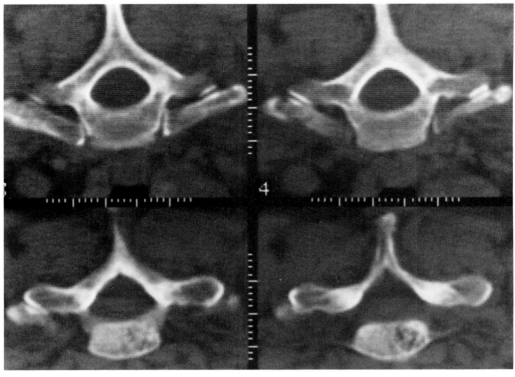

FIGURE 11.16 Vertebral hemangioma. **A.** A small hemangioma of T1. Thickened vertical trabeculae appear as sclerotic dots surrounded by a lucent matrix. (*Figure continued on page 326.*)

A

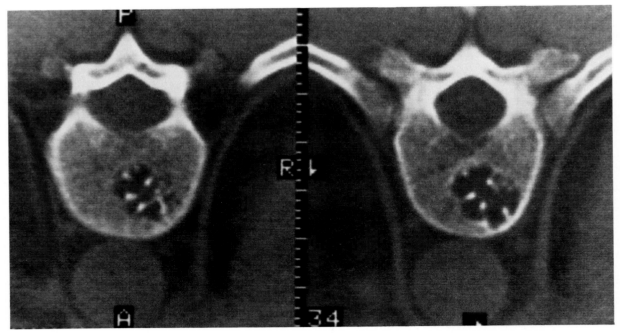

B

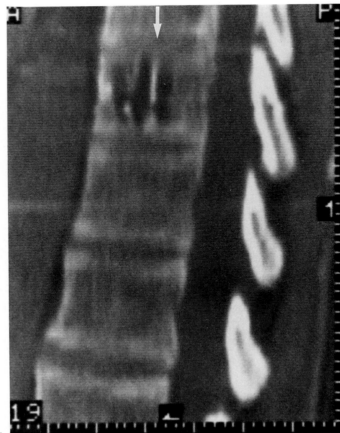

FIGURE 11.16 (*cont'd*)   **B, C.** Large, mostly lucent hemangioma, with dense internal trabeculae (*arrow*).

C

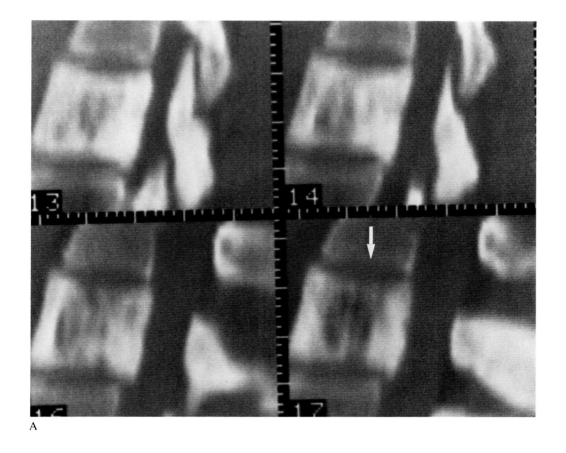

A

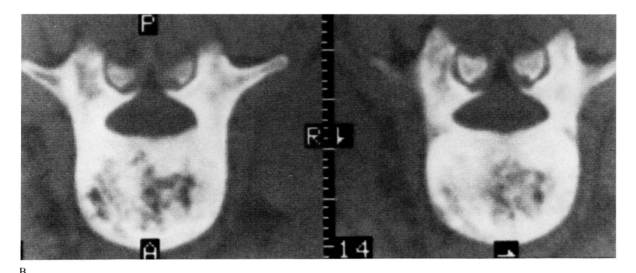

B

FIGURE 11.17 Paget's disease. Axial scans (**A**) and sagittal (**B**) reformations demonstrate an expanded, hyperdense vertebral body, with thickened individual trabeculae (*arrow*).

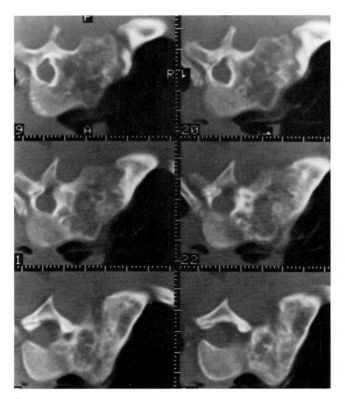

A

Bubbly hyperostosis may be deforming, as in the patient in Figure 11.18. there is a large expansile process involving the lateral surface of the vertebral body, the neural arch, and the attached rib. The abnormal bony overgrowth has produced secondary kyphoscoliosis. It is doubtful that one can make a specific diagnosis based on the CT appearance of the abnormal bone. One needs to evaluate the overall spinal and paraspinal involvement to differentiate this from other bone-producing lesions. The patient's age should be noted, because fibrous dysplasia is a disease of young adults.

Solitary sclerotic bone lesions are frequently benign. They are usually nothing more than solitary bone islands (Fig. 11.19). These are small nonexpansile sclerotic areas in otherwise normal bones. Their existence is usually unrelated to clinical signs and symptoms. When performed, radionuclide bone scans are negative. Bone islands must be differentiated from osteoid osteomas and benign osteoblastomas. Osteoid osteoma and benign osteoblastoma may be considered as one entity. Together they account for approximately 6% of benign spinal bone tumors.[3] They frequently arise in the neural arches and tend to expand the involved bone. These lesions are most commonly found in males in the teenage years. Patients usually present with localized back or neck pain that is worse at night and is relieved by aspirin. Radionuclear bone scans are usually abnormal. Occasionally a radiolucent nidus is visualized

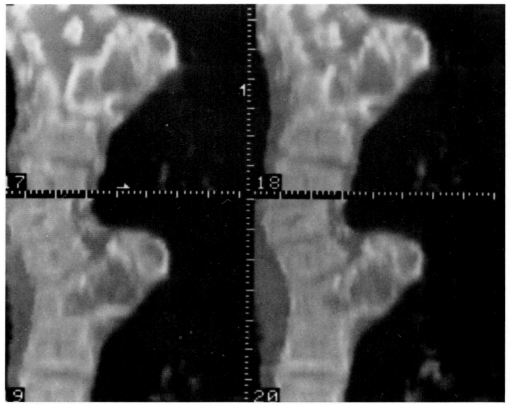

B

FIGURE 11.18 Fibrous dysplasia. Axial (**A**) and coronal (**B**) views reveal marked vertebral and costal hyperostosis. Enlargement and deformity producing severe kyphoscoliosis.

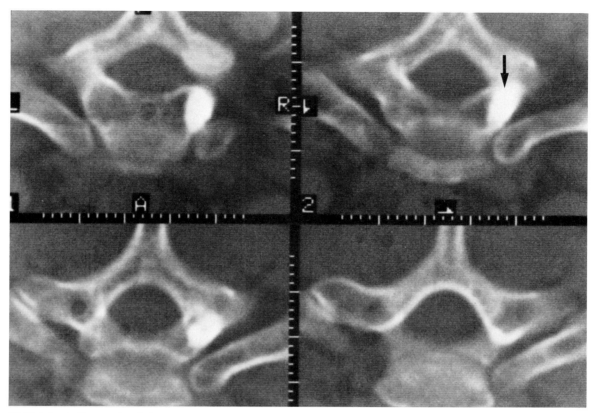

FIGURE 11.19 Benign solitary bone island. Note the presence of a small sclerotic area (*arrow*) with the otherwise normal vertebrae.

within the expanded bone; however, it may be densely sclerotic and impossible to localize. CT is most useful in localizing the lesion and defining the full bony and soft-tissue extent of the tumors (Fig. 11.20). Occasionally, cer-tain congenital abnormalitites of the neural arches are mis-taken for these lesions,[4] the most common of which is the sclerotic lamina on the contralateral side of a unilateral pars interarticularis defect (see Fig. 8.16).

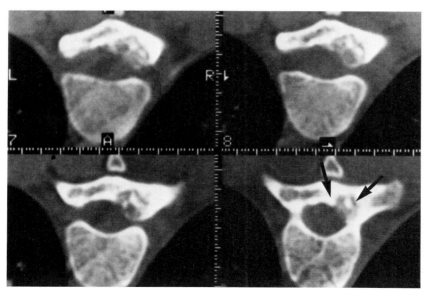

A

FIGURE 11.20 Benign osteoblastoma. **A.** Axial views, note the expansion of the right lamina, as well as the low-attenuation bubbly nidus extending slightly into the spinal canal. (*Figure continued* on page 330.)

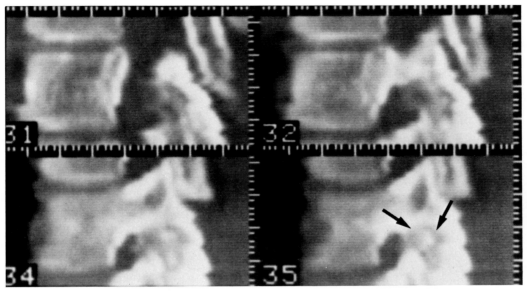

B

FIGURE 11.20 (*cont'd*) **B.** Sagittal views, note the expansion of the right lamina, as well as the low-attenuation bubbly nidus extending slightly into the spinal canal.

Intraspinal Lesions

Intradural Extramedullary

The most common intraspinal lesions are meningiomas and schwannomas. Examples of each lesion are shown in Figures 14.26 and 14.27. These tumors tend to enhance after intravenous infusion of contrast medium. Although many authors still suggest myelography for their evaluation,[5] it seems that when an enhancing mass is located by CT/MPR little or no information is lacking—the entire tumor is outlined, and appropriate resection can be planned.

Meningiomas and neurinomas present intradurally, extradurally, or straddling both compartments. When there is significant extradural component, the mass may extend extraspinally through the neural foramina, causing either subtle or gross smooth expansion of the involved foramen. Figure 11.21 depicts subtle foraminal expansion. The axial soft-tissue views define a small high-attenuation mass in

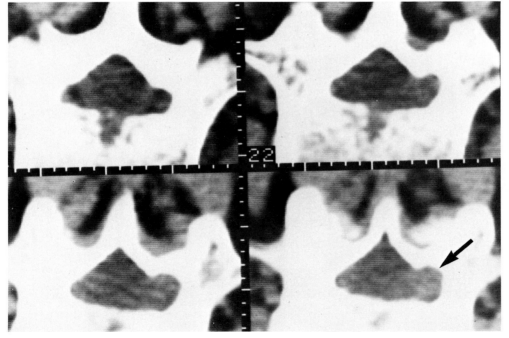

A

FIGURE 11.21 Small extramedullary mass. Axial (**A**) and coronal (**B**) views demonstrate a slightly high attenuation mass in the lateral recess (*arrow*), and modeling and erosion of the medial surface of the pedicle. (*Figure continued* on page 331.)

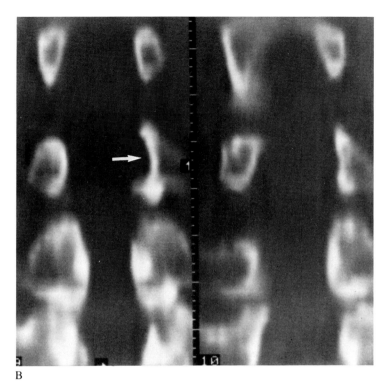

B

FIGURE 11.21 (*cont'd*)

the right lateral recess. The coronal bone-windowed view defines a smoothly molded thinned right pedicle indicative of a longstanding mass.

Similar findings are noted on the metrizamide CT scan in Figure 11.22. The axial view demonstrates subtle erosion of the left lamina and a minimal widening of the neural foramen. The coronal metrizamide view demonstrates the classic finding of intradural extramedullary mass. The spinal cord is displaced to the right, and the contrast medium column is widened on the side of the lesion. There

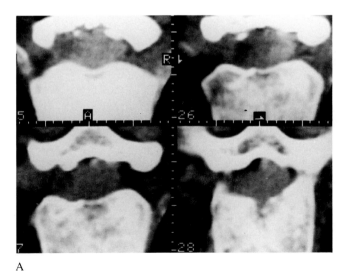

A

FIGURE 11.22 Dumbbell neurinoma. Axial (**A**) and coronal (**B**) metrizamide-enhanced views show a typical intradural but extramedullary mass. The spinal cord is displaced away from the mass (*arrow*). There is subtle undercutting of the pedicle and CT evidence of an extradural component extending through the neural foramen.

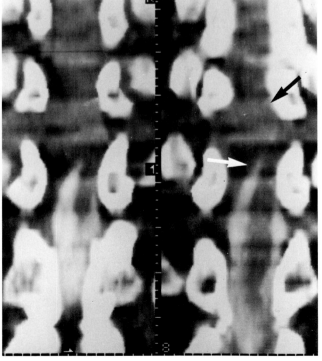

B

is considerable extradural component to this lesion, accounting for the displacement of the arachnoid away from the left pedicle.

The young woman in Figure 11.23 was thought, before CT scan, to have typical lumbar disc symptoms. Unlike the previous two patients, she demonstrates a very large tumor, arising within the spinal canal but extending through the neural foramen and producing a very large paraspinal mass. The lateral recess and the neural foramen were profoundly enlarged. These findings were not appreciated on routine radiographs. The coronal reformation shows the exiting L5 roots arising normally from the thecal sac. The tumor origin is clearly visible approximately 1 cm from the origin of this nerve.

Other rare extramedullary masses can be diagnosed by CT, although it is impossible to distinguish them from the other more common lesions. After an obviously abnormal myelogram that was thought to be atypical for a disc herniation, CT/MPR was performed on the patient in Figure 11.24. An obvious mass of high attenuation arises from the posterior aspect of the spinal canal along the medial edge of the right lamina. This is clearly not a calcified disc fragment, as its broadest base lies along the posterior portion of the canal and only its anterior tip abuts the disc space. It was clear from these scans that we were dealing with a

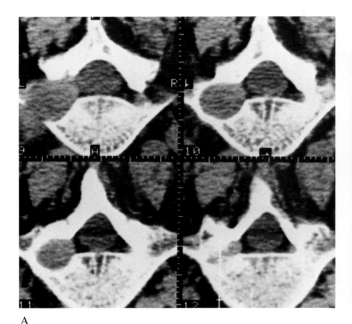

A

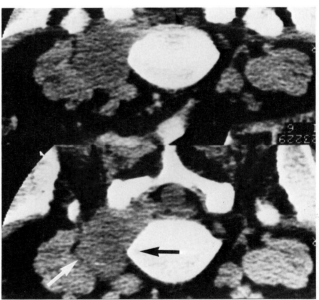

B

FIGURE 11.23 Neurinoma of L5. **A.** Axial composite group demonstrates bulbous enlargement of the left L5 root. The lamina and vertebral body have molded around the slow-growing tumor. **B.** Axial scans lower down reveal that there is a large paravertebral extension of this tumor (*arrows*). Note that it is nearly the same density as the psoas muscle. **C.** Sagittal views define the mass within the neural foramen. **D.** The coronal view is most informative because it shows a normal origin of the L5 roots bilaterally. The tumor mass begins approximately 1 cm from the dural origin of the nerve.

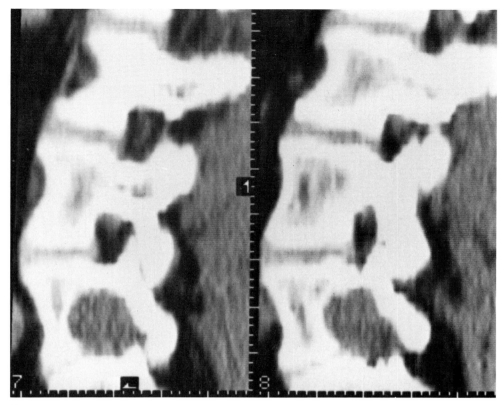

C

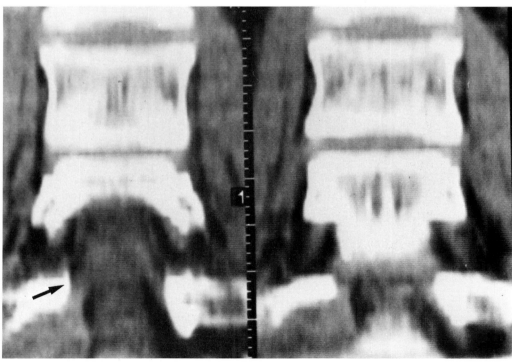

D

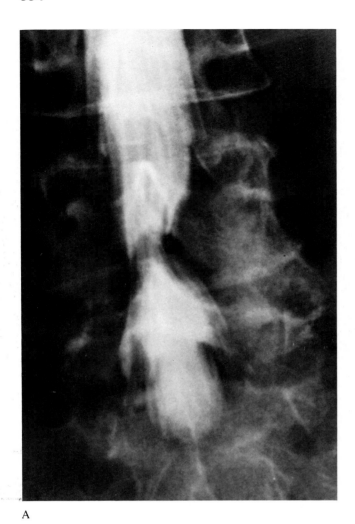

A

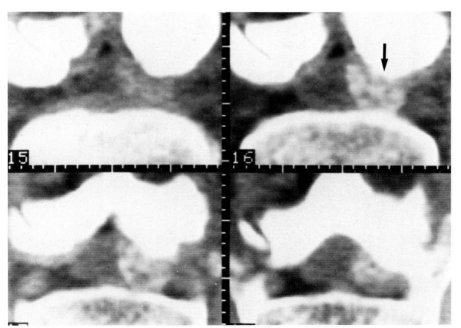

B

FIGURE 11.24 Intraspinal hemangioma. **A.** A frontal metrizamide myelogram demonstrates a long, lateral, extradural defect, atypical for disc herniation. **B, C.** Axial and coronal views demonstrate a partially calcified mass, with its base along the lamina (*arrow*). (*Figure continued* on page 335.)

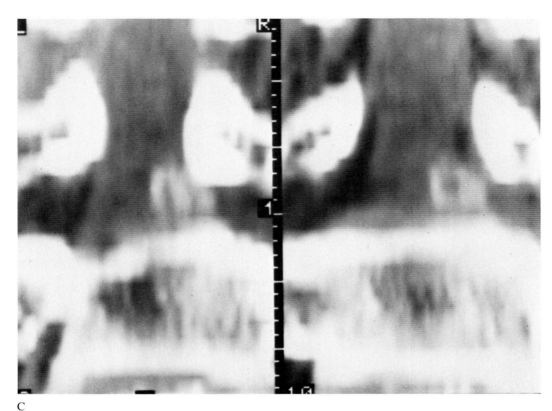

C

FIGURE 11.24 (*cont'd*)

neoplastic process of unknown cell type. Because of this preoperative diagnosis, a wide laminectomy was performed. Biopsy produced extraordinary bleeding, which was stopped with great difficulty. The pathologist diagnosed hemangioma.

Another large noncalcified extra-axial mass is shown in Figure 11.25. The lesion is causing extraordinary canal compression but is not producing bone destruction or erosion. The entire mass is outlined on the coronal reformation, even without intravenous enhancement. It is a synovial cyst, which may masquerade as a tumor, and in fact looks very similar to the previously described lesions. These lesions may become quite large (Fig. 11.26), and they frequently calcify about their rim. Most important, they arise from the facet joints and project medially into the spinal canal. The joint surfaces may be eroded and irregular. Would myelography add any significant information?

Surgeons trained during the myelography-only era are comfortable with myelograms, and so they tend to order them even when they are not objectively necessary. Radiologists must be aware of this need for reassurance in the operating room and provide the best pictorial display of the lesion and surrounding normal structures. It is the obligation of the radiologist when performing noninvasive CT to display the information in a manner that the referring surgeon can relate to. This is the underlying thrust of the CT/MPR format—to produce "familiar" images (images that look like myelogram images).

Intraspinal Lipoma

Lipomas are unique among intradural lesions because they are easily diagnosed by nonmetrizamide-enchanced CT. They show as partially encapsulated, well-circumscribed collections of fat, usually with some connection to the meninges or spinal cord. Although they are probably developmental in origin, they are considered here with the description of other mass lesions. They have been grouped into two broad categories.[6] "Intradural" lipomas remain nearly completely within either a normal or an only midly dysraphic spine, and they are not associated with major cutaneous or subcutaneous lesions. Lipomeningoceles are attached to the cord, which herniates extraspinally through major neural arch defects. The latter are usually associated with some dermal abnormality, ranging from a small skin dimple to huge meningomyoceles. Both probably represent varying manifestations of a similar process.

Thoracic and cervical lipomas may present as slowly progressive myelopathic lesions. Lumbosacral lesions present with leg weakness and bladder dysfunction, or they may be

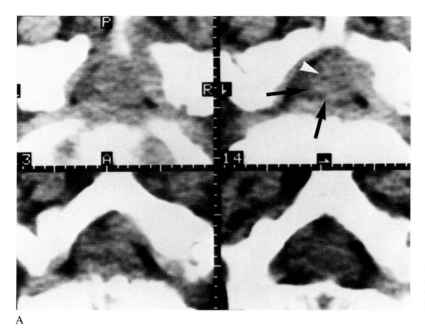

A

FIGURE 11.25 Noncalcified intraspinal mass. Axial (**A**) and coronal (**B**) views demonstrate the entire extra-axial mass (*arrows*). No bone deformity or destruction is shown.

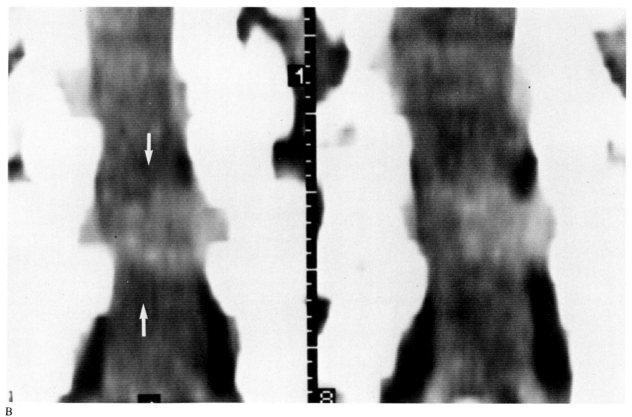

B

asymptomatic. CT has allowed us to see small collections of fat that should probably be characterized as the normal end of the lipoma spectrum (Fig. 11.27). These small string-like fat collections are occasionally seen when evaluating patients for radicular or back pain syndromes. Pain is not usually associated with lipoma, and hence one must pre-sume that these fat collections are chance findings. None of our dozen similar cases has had intradural surgery, so the clinical significance is a matter of speculation. The patient in Figure 11.28 has a larger fat collection, and it appears to surround the filum terminale. Note that the bony spinal canal is normal in both of these cases.

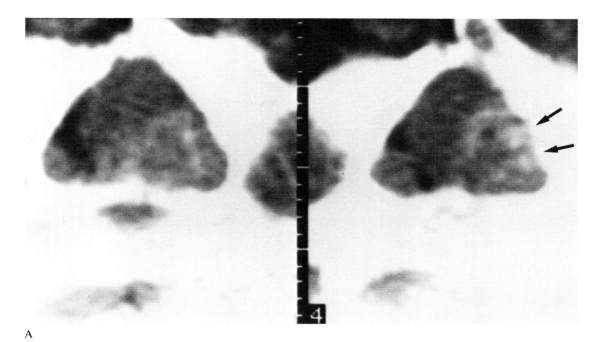

A

B

FIGURE 11.26 Synovial cyst. Axial (**A**) and (**B**) views demonstrate a large, partially calcified extradural mass (*arrows*). The calcifications are rounder and larger than the tumor in Figure 11.24.

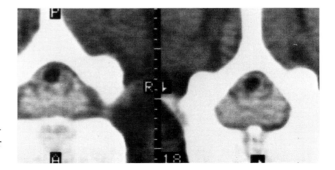

FIGURE 11.27 Small intradural fat collection. Axial view depicts a 1- to 2-mm cylindrical collection of fat that extends over at least one vertebral segment.

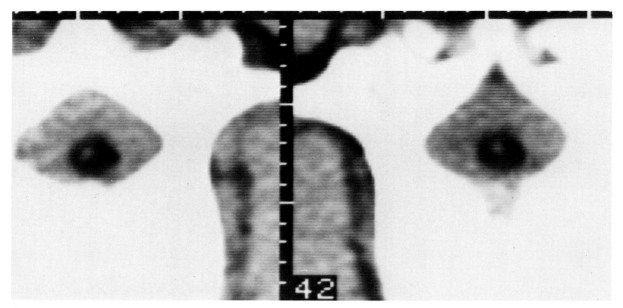

A

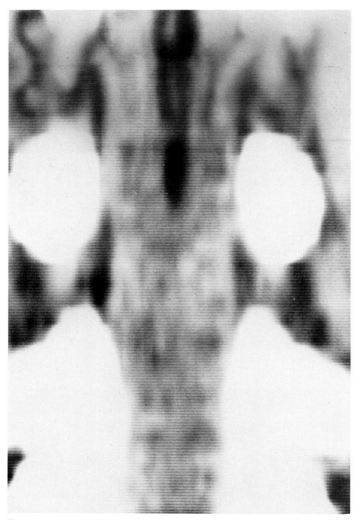

B

FIGURE 11.28 Intradural lipomas. Axial (**A**) and coronal (**B**) views demonstrate a fat collection surrounding a small soft-tissue density thought to be filum terminale.

Lipomyelomeningoceles are commonly associated with occult spinal dysraphism. Patients usually present with visible lumbosacral masses, dimples, or clefts, and often develop sensory signs, e.g., bladder dysfunction, extremity paralysis, and deformities of the feet. These lesions are almost uniformly associated with bifid spines. The spinal cord is low in position, with the conus tethered by the lipoma in the posterior neural arch defect (Fig. 11.29). The ventral nerve roots exit more horizontally than is normal and are frequently stretched over long distances from their

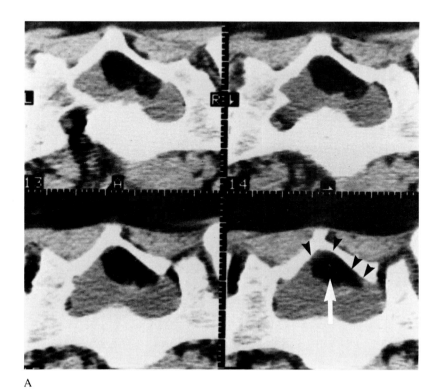

A

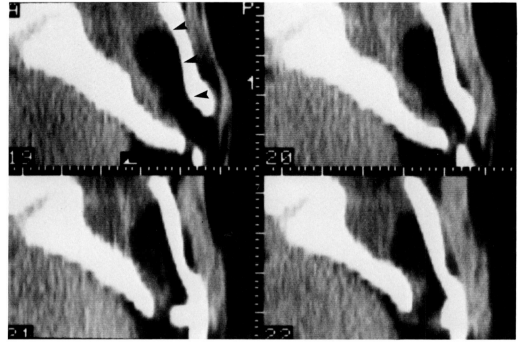

B

FIGURE 11.29 Small lipomeningocele. Nonmetrizamide-enhanced CT; axial (**A**), sagittal (**B**), and coronal (**C**) views. Note the tethered cord (*arrow*), the lipoma (*arrowheads*), and the bony laminar defect. (*Figure continued* on page 340.)

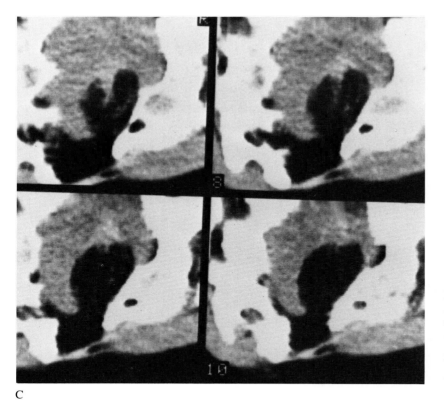

C

FIGURE 11.29 (*cont'd*)   Small lipomeningocele. Nonmetrizamide-enhanced
CT; axial (**A**), sagittal (**B**), and coronal
(**C**) views. Note the tethered cord (*arrow*), the lipoma (*arrowheads*), and the
bony laminar defect. Compare with figures **A** and **B** on page 339.

abnormal posterior origin through the neural foramina (Fig.
11.30). Kaiser et al.[7] described an easy technique for direct
coronal scanning for the evaluation of these lesions in children and neonates. Adults almost always require at least
sagittal and curved coronal reformations for complete assessment of the size, position, and anatomic relationships

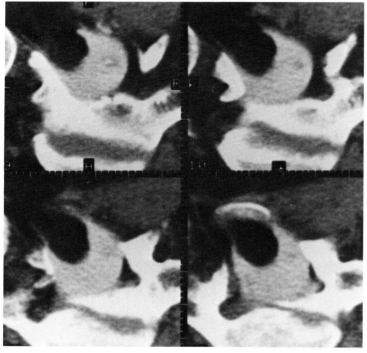

A

FIGURE 11.30   Lipomeningocele. Axial (**A**), sagittal
(**B**), and coronal (**C**) views. When surrounded by dilute
metrizamide, the exiting roots can often be seen. This
adds little to the surgical management of the case because
the cord and the mass are easily evaluated without metrizamide, and these roots, which are seen lying free, are
not entrapped by the mass.

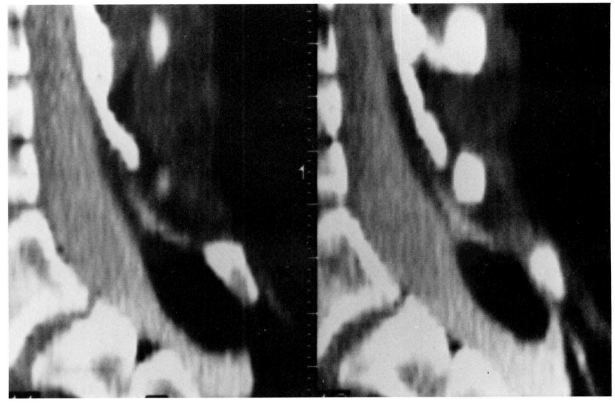

B

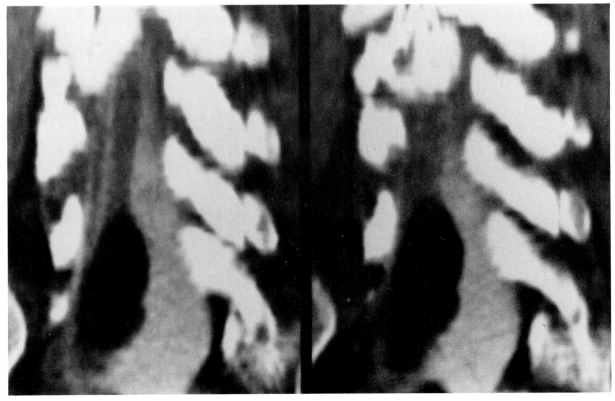

C

of the mass and the tethered cord. In most cases this type of study provides the information needed for surgical planning. It is possible, therefore, to repair many of these defects without resorting to myelography.

Although frequently associated with lipomas, tethering of the spinal cord may also occur without intradural fatty mass. Patients frequently present with weakness in the lower extremities as well as bowel and bladder dysfunction. Radiculopathy is occasionally present and may mimic disc herniation. On high-quality CT it is possible to make the diagnosis of tethered spinal cord even without metrizamide enhancement, although the anatomic abnormality produces very subtle radiographic changes. Figure 11.31 demonstrates a pair of axial scans at the L3–4 level in which a

tethered, split spinal cord is seen as a faint shadow, somewhat higher in attenuation than the surrounding cerebospinal fluid (CSF). The normal conus medullaris ends at L1 or above. This is therefore definitely abnormal.

The patient in Figure 11.32 also has a tethered spinal cord without a lipoma. She sought medical attention because of back and leg pain. Routine radiographs demonstrated a spina bifida and some asymmetry of the posterior elements. The CT revealed a large bony crest traversing the thecal sac. Diastematomyelia, unusual at the lumbosacral junction, was a surprise. Clinically of note is the fact that the sagittal and coronal reformations, without metrizamide, clearly define tethering of a split spinal cord. It is unlikely that myelography will add objective information in this case.

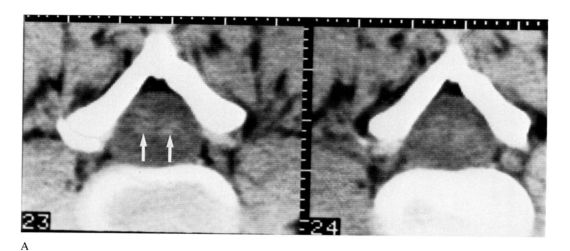

A

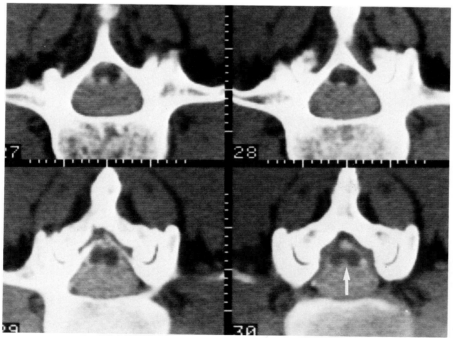

B

FIGURE 11.31 Tethered spinal cord. **A.** Axial scans without intrathecal metrizamide reveal a subtle shadow of high attenuation (*arrows*) within the CSF at the L3–4 level. Note the bilobed configuration of the spinal cord. **B.** Metrizamide CT on a similar case, for comparison.

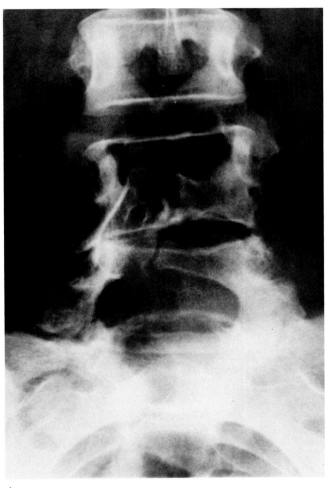

A

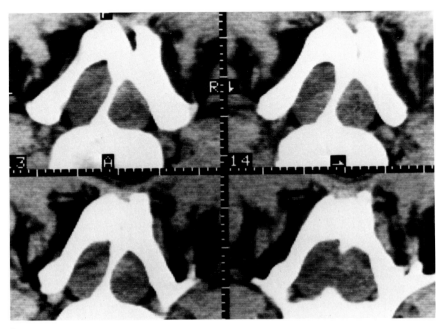

B

FIGURE 11.32 Diastematomyelia, with tethered cord. **A.** Frontal radiograph shows a dysraphic spine. **B.** Axial views reveal a thick, bony septum extending from the vertebral body to the neural arch. **C.** Sagittal reformations show the bony bridge and the cord extending down to the spur (*arrows*). **D.** Coronal reformations outline the entire length of the split, tethered cord. Note the linear lucency extending down to the spur (*arrowheads*). (*Figure continued* on page 344.)

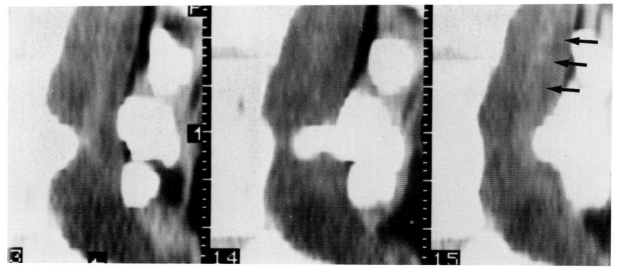

C

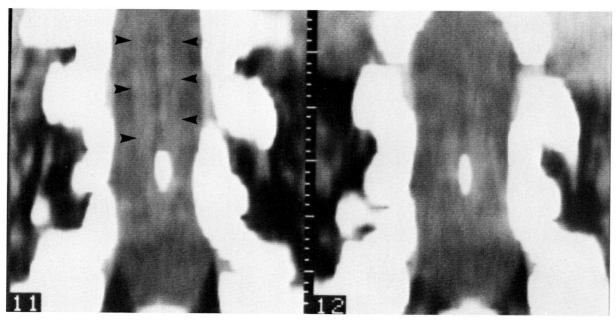

D

FIGURE 11.32 (*cont'd*)   Legend on page 343.

Intramedullary Masses

Intramedullary lesions almost always require intrathecal metrizamide for adequate evaluation. Because they usually extend over many segments, they should be evaluated by routine metrizamide myelography. CT may provide useful information as an adjunct to routine myelography, but otherwise CT is of limited value (Fig. 11.33). When the lesions are small and do not occupy the entire spinal canal, they may expand the spinal cord and be seen even without metrizamide enhancement. However, when the lesions fill the canal, they are usually impossible to identify, especially in the lumbar region. They are almost always homogeneous and therefore cannot be distinguished from the normal CSF density. There are those who deny the usefulness of routine spine CT without myelography because of the possibility of missing these lesions. One very important rule must be followed: whenever a patient has objective neurologic deficit and a negative CT, one must perform total myelography in order to include any and all areas of potential neural involvement.

The most important lesion to differentiate from intramedullary tumor is benign cord expansion due to syringomyelia. Syringomyelia, or hydromyelia, is frequently associated with the Arnold-Chiari malformation,[8,9] cervical trauma, and surgery. Posttraumatic or postoperative cysts

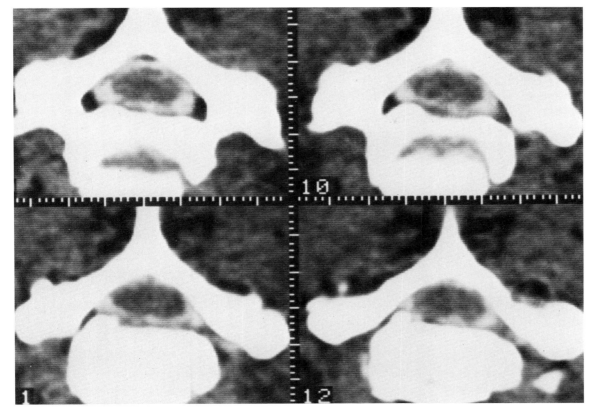

A

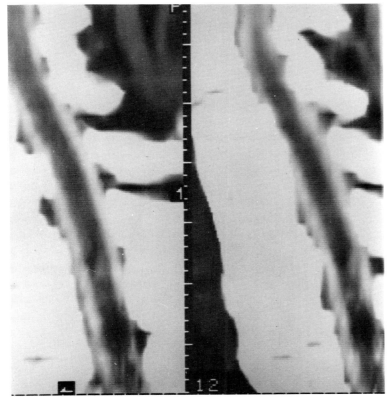

B

FIGURE 11.33 Metrizamide CT. **A.** Normal cervical spinal cord and roots. **B.** Sagittal view of normal cervical cord. (*Figure continued* on page 346.)

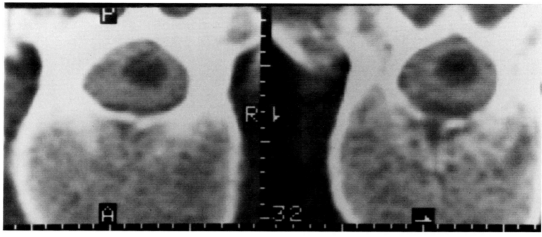

C

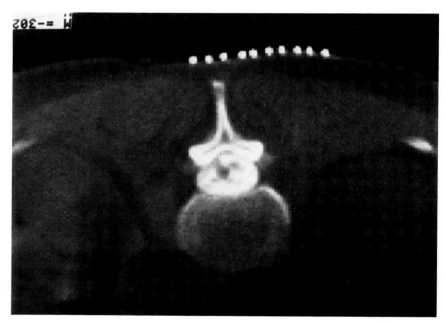

FIGURE 11.33 (*cont'd*) **C.** Normal midthoracic cord. **D.** Normal conus medullaris. **E.** Normal cauda equina. **F.** Intramedullary tumor that expands the upper cervical spinal cord.

D

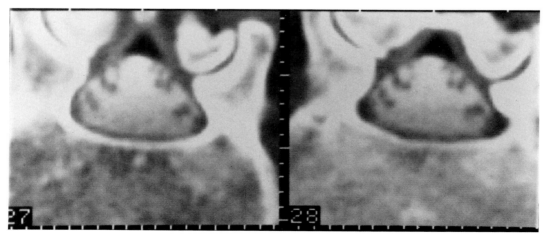

E

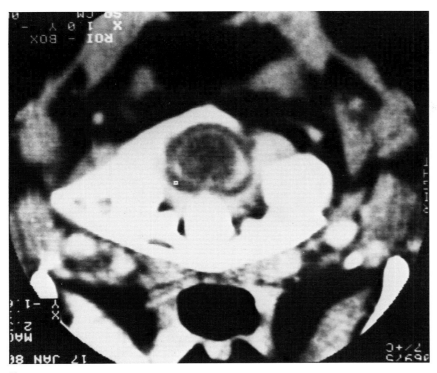

F

tend to be small and impossible to diagnosis without me-trizamide in the thecal sac. In the Arnold-Chiari group the cysts tend to be very large and easily seen on noncontrast examination. Reformations are very useful in differentiating random low-density areas due to artifacts from true longi-tudinal intramedullary fluid collections. It is also not nec-essary to instill intrathecal metrizamide to diagnose low-lying tonsils. If the chin is elevated in order to project the teeth above the plane of the craniocervical junction, routine reformations demonstrate tonsillar malposition most ade-quately (see Figs. 14.21, 14.22).

When clinical suspicion is very high, especially in postoperative or posttrauma patients, CT is performed 4–6 hr after intrathecal installation of water-soluble contrast me-dium. We have successfully used doses as low as 5 cc metrizamide (85 mg/100 cc) to fill the intramedullary cav-ities. It is thought that the contrast medium reaches the cysts by diffusion through either an abnormal spinal cord or small pores leading directly to the cyst. In some cases the cyst does not fill, but the contour of the cervical cord is concave or peculiarly flattened.[10] This is true in many patients in whom the cysts have been surgically drained or shunted

Dural ectasia may also simulate mass because it pro-duces diffuse expansion of the spinal canal. A not uncom-mon cause of dural ectasia is ankylosing spondylitis. The patient in Figure 11.34 has peculiar asymmetrical expansion of the spinal canal. The lamina is irregular and appears eroded. In the appropriate clinical setting, one must pre-sume the diagnosis of dural ectasia. It can be proved, of course, with myelography.

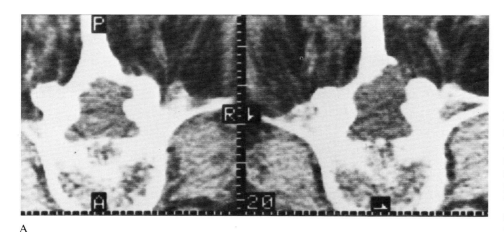

A

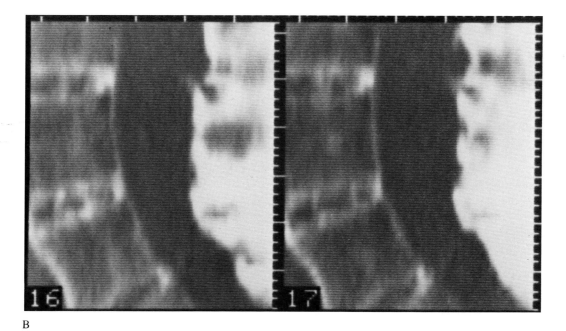

B

FIGURE 11.34 Ankylosing spondylitis and dural ectasia. **A.** Axial views demonstrate irregular erosion of the left lamina, with a "soft-tissue mass" extending beyond the confines of the canal. This is typical of the pattern of dural ectasia in these patients. **B.** Sagittal view.

References

1. Roub LW, Drayer BP: Spinal computed tomography: limitations and applications. AJR 133:267–273, 1979

2. Dorward RH, LaMasters DL, Watanabe TJ: Tumors. In Newton TH, Potts DG (eds): Computed Tomography of the Spine and Spinal Cord. Clavadel Press, San Anselmo, California, 1983, pp. 115–147

3. Dahlin DC: Bone Tumors: General Aspects and Data on 6,221 Cases, ed. 3. Charles C Thomas, Springfield, Illinois, 1978

4. Wedge JH, Tchang S, MacFadyen DJ: Computed tomography in localization of spinal osteoid osteoma. Spine 6:423–427, 1981

5. Aubin ML, Jardin C, Bar D, Vignaud J: Computerised tomography in 32 cases of intraspinal tumor. J Neuroradiol 6:81–92, 1979

6. Naidich TP, McLone DG, Harwood-Nash DC: Spinal dysraphism. In Newton TH, Potts DG (eds): Computed Tomograhy of the Spine and Spinal Cord. Clavadel Press, San Anselmo, California, 1983, pp. 299–353

7. Kaiser MC, Pettersson H, Harwood-Nash DC, et al: Direct coronal CT of the spine in infants and children. AJNR 2:465–466, 1981

8. MacKenzie NG, Emery JL: Deformities of the cervical cord in children with neurospinal dysraphism. Dev Med Child Neurol [Suppl. 25] 13:58–67, 1971

9. Naidich TP, McLone DG, Harwood-Nash DC: Malformation of the craniocervical junction. In Newton TH, Potts DG (eds): Computed Tomography of the Spine and Spinal Cord. Clavadel Press, San Anselmo, California, 1983, pp. 355–366

10. Grogan JP: Congenital spine anomalies. In Haughton VM (ed): Computed Tomography of the Spine. Churchill Livingstone, New York, 1983, pp. 150–151

Trauma

12

Fractures of the thoracic and lumbar spine are distressingly common lesions which are becoming even more prevalent because of the increasing incidence of vehicular accidents. The severity of the fractures—and the chance of paraplegia—argue well for greater observance and enforcement of the 55–mph speed limit in the United States. The public health cost of this trauma is high because most victims are less than 40 years of age and the incidence of permanent neurologic deficit approaches 40%.

Complete radiographic diagnosis is essential in guiding management of these fragile individuals. After stabilizing the patient, ensuring an adequate airway, establishing intravenous lines, and controlling bleeding, high-quality emergency-room films should be provided. Bony integrity and vertebral alignment must be assessed and a preliminary diagnosis made. If the patient is a surgical candidate or if further diagnostic information is deemed necessary, CT is considered as the next radiographic procedure. Conventional radiographs frequently underestimate the extent and severity of the injury. They certainly afford no direct information about the exiting nerve roots and the spinal cord.

The vertebral column performs several functions: It supports the weight of the head and upper body; it allows controlled flexibility, rotation, tilting, and bending; and it affords bony protection to the spinal cord. Appropriate diagnostic evaluation must assess the spine's ability to perform each of its tasks. Vertebral-body and vertebral-joint integrity are the primary factors in weight bearing, vertebral-joint stability and longitudinal-ligament integrity are the primary factors limiting flexibility; and a stable bony neural ring is the primary factor in protecting the spinal cord.

Stability and vertebral integrity are most easily evaluated by conventional radiographs, whereas vertebral-ring integrity is best studied in the axial plane by CT. This is obvious because the bony neural tube is oriented axially in the patient. This is CT's primary advantage over other tomographic diagnostic procedures. It is not, however, its only advantage. It is crucial that patients with spinal injury be moved as little as possible. This often precludes oblique filming and pleuridirectional lateral tomography. CT can always be performed with the patient supine. When necessary, the patient may be secured in traction within the scanner to maintain stability. Using any of the currently available reformation programs, images of the spine can be created in any plane without moving the patient, thus reducing the possibility of increasing the neurologic deficit by excessive patient handling.

If neurologic deficit is present, it is generally easy to instill water-soluble contrast agents to delineate the integrity of the subarachnoid space, the cord, and the nerve roots. This can be accomplished by lateral cervical C1–2 puncture without turning the patient from the supine position. CT does have some limitations in these patients, the most important being the sensitivity of the reformatted CT examination to patient motion. This is of only minor importance when evaluating the neural ring but may critically flaw a study when the fracture is oriented along the plane of the CT slice, as in fractures of the base of the dens and the lumbar articular processes. Motion artifact can be reduced by rapid scanning and good clinical management of the patient, but it may be impossible to eliminate totally.

One should optimize the CT scan for bone or, rarely, for bone and soft tissue. This can be accomplished by re-

349

constructing the axial data twice: filtered once for high-contrast resolution and once for low-contrast resolution. This is not actually necessary in most instances. As indicated in Chapter 14, it is important when evaluating cervical fractures to scan the patients using the thinnest possible slices—ideally 1.5–2 mm. This affords maximal geometric resolution and the best reformations. When time does not permit or when the patient is moving uncontrollably, one may have to be satisfied with slices of 3– or 5–mm thickness. It is of doubtful necessity to produce 1.5–mm sections in the thoracic and lumbar areas because the vertebrae are relatively large and the amount of volume averaging is relatively small.

We are not alone in our strong feelings about the value of reformation, at least not in this group of patients.[1–5] Brant-Zawadzki and Minagi summarized their thinking on the subject succinctly[3]:

> The ability to image the spine in multiple planes is a distinct advantage of computed tomography. On first thought, it may appear that since image reformation only manipulates the information present on axial slices, no additional information can be obtained. However, the relationship of adjacent vertebrae is vertically oriented, and disturbances in this relationship are difficult to appreciate on axial images. Subluxation of the vertebral bodies or the facets is much easier to detect on sagittal reformations and, indeed, may be missed without use of such reformations.

CT may be a useful procedure in the postoperative evaluation of spine fractures as well. Indeed, the author's experience is larger with this group of patients. One can easily assess the extent of decompressive surgery, adequacy of fusion stabilization, presence of bone fragments within the spinal canal or neural foramina, concomitant disc herniation, and many other abnormalities.

Vertebral Compression

The most common type of fracture in the thoracic or lumbar areas is vertebral-body compression, as almost all trauma carries with it some downward compressive force vector. In the simplest case, a direct fall on the feet, the noncompressible nucleus pulposus may act as the focal point of a fracture of the vertebral end-plates.[6] This is most commonly seen in patients with osteoporosis and produces typical "fishmouth deformity" of the vertebral end-plates on routine radiographs. On axial CT this usually appears as an area of ill-defined, low attenuation with the vertebral body. It is frequently misinterpreted as normal because of partial-volume averaging. Reformations clearly define the deformity of the end-plates and a relatively normal-appearing disc space (Fig. 12.1). A similar appearance of the vertebral

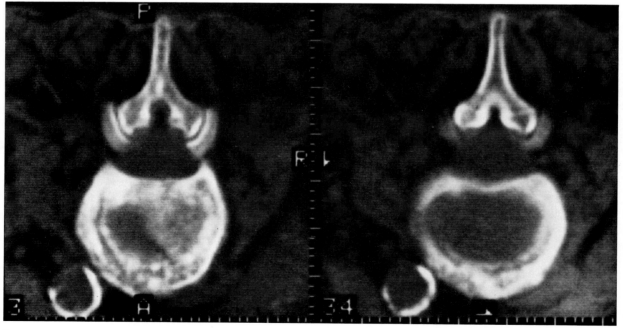

A

FIGURE 12.1   Vertebral end-plate fracture. Axial (**A**), sagittal (**B**), and coronal (**C**) views demonstrate a typical "fishmouth" deformity of the vertebral end-plates (*arrows*). There is no soft-tissue mass indicative of tumor. The disc-space height is maintained.

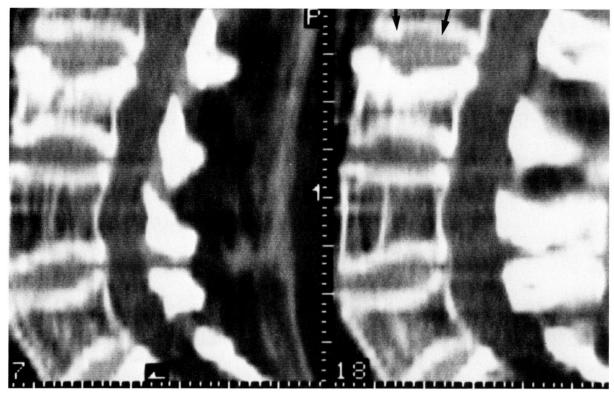

B

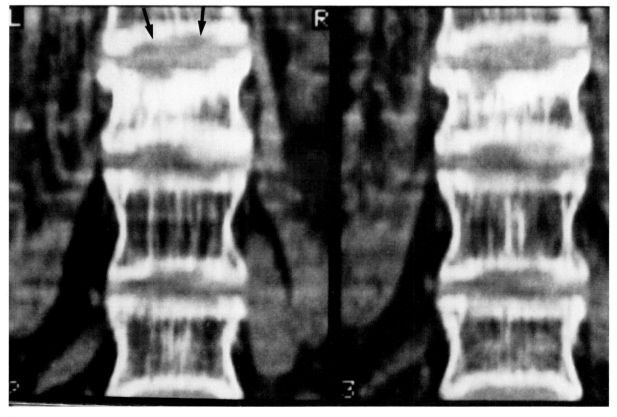

C

end-plates occurs with vertebral compression in a diseased vertebral body (Fig. 12.2). Minor trauma may propel the noncompressible nucleus through the end-plate and fracture bone infiltrated by tumor (Fig. 12.3). The challenge is to differentiate between the two. In patients with infiltrating neoplasm one can often define abnormal osseous architecture and epidural or paraspinal soft-tissue mass. Occasionally the differentiation is impossible.

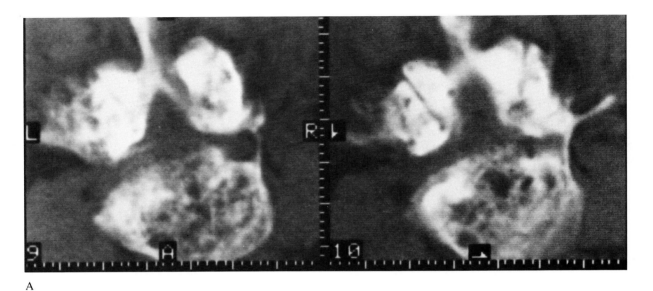

A

B

FIGURE 12.2 Compression fractures through pagetoid bone. Axial scans (**A**) demonstrate thickened, sclerotic, abnormal bone trabeculae typical of Paget's disease. The end-plate compression is difficult to diagnose because of volume-averaging artifact (**B, C**). Sagittal and coronal reformations define the extent of vertebral fracture. Note the normal height of the disc spaces and loss of height of the abnormal vertebral bodies.

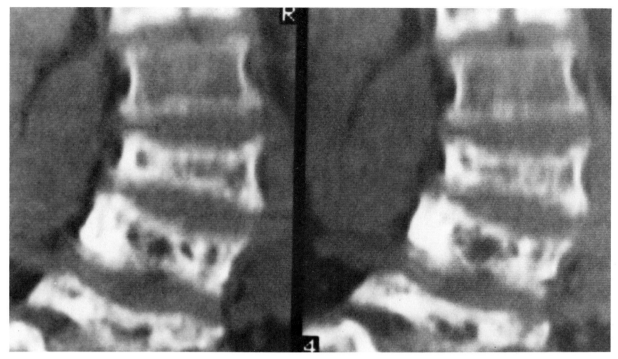

C

Vertebral Compression with Flexion

The mechanism of bony disruption in the thoracic, thoracolumbar, and lumbar areas is frequently complex, as a rotational component acts together with an acute flexion force[7] (Fig. 12.4). Pure compressive fractures are unusual in the upper and midthoracic areas. Most often these vertebrae are anteriorly wedged, indicating a significant forward flexion force vector. The normal thoracic kyphos transmits compressive forces anteriorly. The rib cage and the costovertebral joints tend to add further stability to this area and to diffuse much of the compressive force. The posterior bony elements, ligaments, and soft tissues tend to be preserved (Fig. 12.5).

The wider use of lap-type seat belts has dramatically changed the force vectors applied to the lower thoracic and thoracolumbar areas. When sudden deceleration occurs in a motor vehicle and the patient is wearing a lap seat belt, the fulcrum of the flexion force is displaced forward toward the point of contact of the belt to the abdominal wall, thereby producing a significant distraction force. The higher the belt, the more focal the rotation point; then the force is borne primarily by a single body and its pedicles and liga-

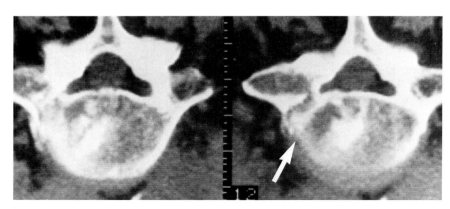

A

FIGURE 12.3 Compression fracture due to bony metastasis. Axial scan (**A**) demonstrates a small left-sided zone of lucency in the vertebral body (*arrow*), which is difficult to diagnose as a metastasis. (*Figure continued* on page 354.)

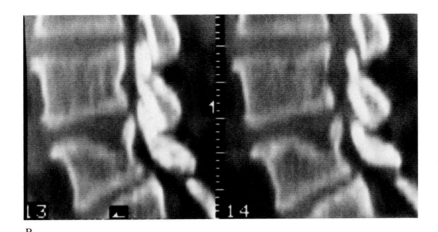

B

FIGURE 12.3 (*cont'd*) Sagittal (**B**) and coronal (**C**) reformations define asymmetrical left-sided endplate collapse with loss of vertebral height. On the soft-tissue-window views a subtle epidural mass was noted behind the body of L4 (not shown).

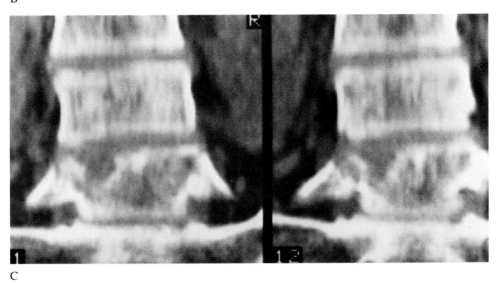

C

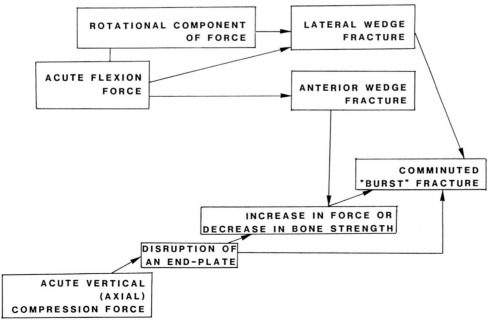

FIGURE 12.4 Mechanisms of thoracolumbar vertebral-body fracture (Redrawn from Smith et al.[6])

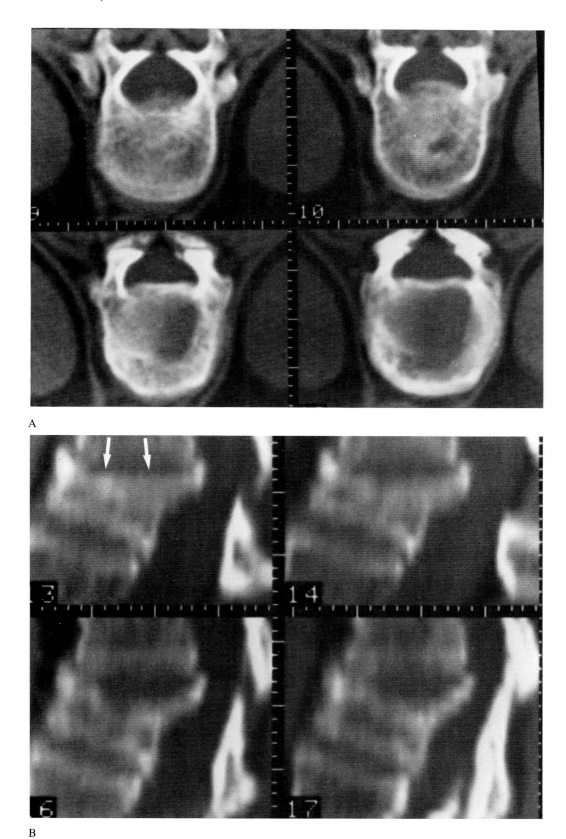

A

B

FIGURE 12.5 Lumbar vertebral-body compression fracture. Axial (**A**) and sagittal (**B**) reformations demonstrate an anterior wedge deformity (*arrows*) with intact neural arch.

ments, and the typical "seat-belt" or "Chance" fracture may occur[8,9] (Fig. 12.6). If the rotational center overlies a disc space, the distraction forces apply primarily to the disc and ligamentous structures. Vertebral body compression is likely to be minimal, but the facet joints may be subluxated or even dislocated. This has been described radiographically as the "naked facets."[10]

Axial CT images show only one pair of facets at a time, as the superior facets have been upwardly displaced away from their inferior mates. Reformations are necessary to fully evaluate the abnormal relationship of the facets. The facets may be simply distracted and spine fusion or conservative therapy may be appropriate; or they may be distracted and abnormally locked and require reduction before fusion (Fig. 12.7).

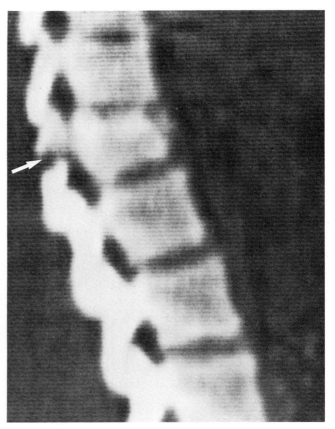

B

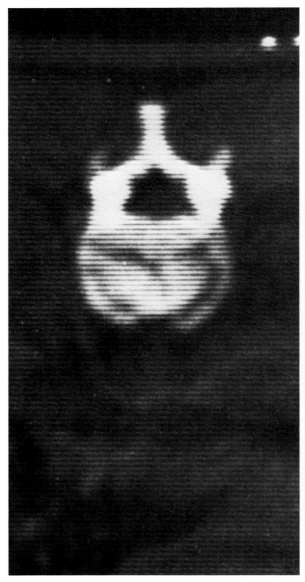

A

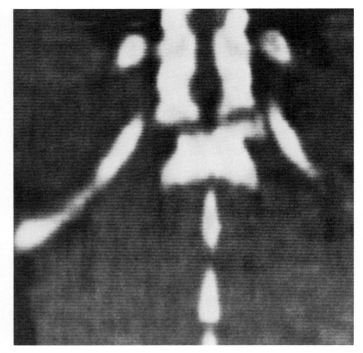

C

FIGURE 12.6 Chance fracture of the vertebra. **A.** Axial scan. **B, C.** Sagittal and coronal views demonstrate a horizontal fracture through the vertebral body and posterior elements. (Reprinted with permission from O'Callaghan et al.[10])

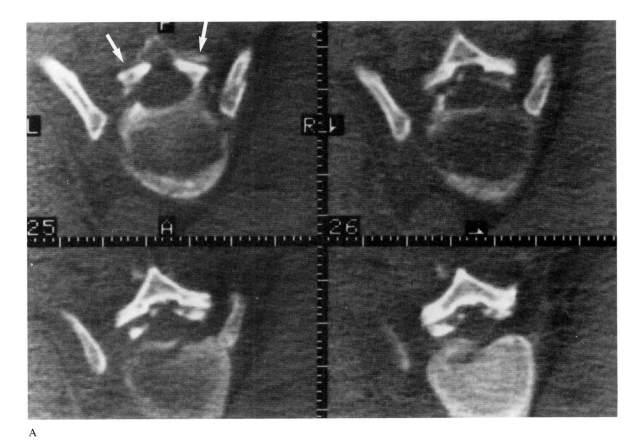

A

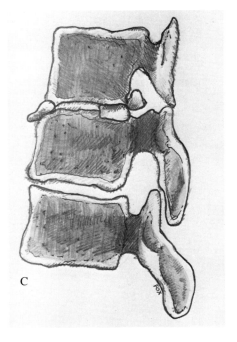

B

C

FIGURE 12.7 Fractured dislocation. **A.** Naked facet sign on axial scan 25. The superior facets are seen without any inferior facets. On axial scan 26 the inferior facets are seen 3-mm higher, without their mates. **B.** Sagittal views on the left reveal dislocation and locking of the inferior facet (*arrow*). The large fragment of bone sitting within the neural foramen is a fragmented superior facet (*arrowheads*). **C.** Diagram of B.

Not all wedged vertebral bodies are due to trauma. Congenital hemivertebrae may be mistaken for traumatic lesions. Figure 12.8 demonstrates a peculiar posterior flattening of both the superior and inferior end-plates of L4. The axial and coronal scans reveal a sclerotic midline cortical line at the plane of prenatal fusion, indicating an anomalous vertebra. This form of the anomaly usually involves the medial ends of both end-plates; the curvilinear appearance on the coronal reformation is pathognomonic.

Severe compressive injuries are usually sustained as a result of falling great distances. These burst fractures can produce severe comminution and fragmentation of the vertebral bodies. Surprisingly, the posterior elements may be preserved. Disc herniation may further complicate this condition. Routine radiographs characteristically underestimate the bony canal compression, often missing small but important bone fragments.[11,12]

CT is essential in evaluating the extent of bony

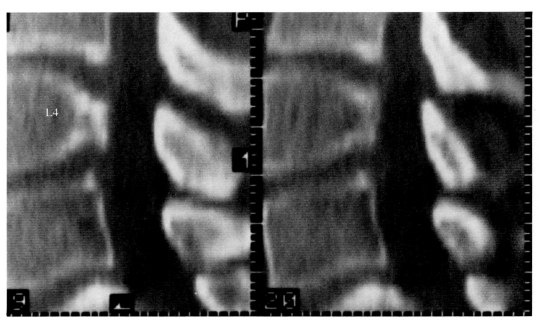

A

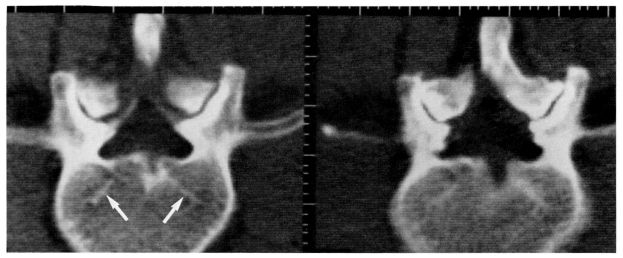

B

FIGURE 12.8 Fusion anomaly. **A.** Sagittal reformation demonstrates loss of height of the posterior portion of the L4 vertebral body. **B.** On the axial view there are sclerotic remnants of the fusion planes between the fetal ossification centers (*arrows*). **C.** Coronal reformation defines the unique appearance of the sclerotic midline fusion plane and the localized deformity of the back of the vertebral end-plates (*arrows*).

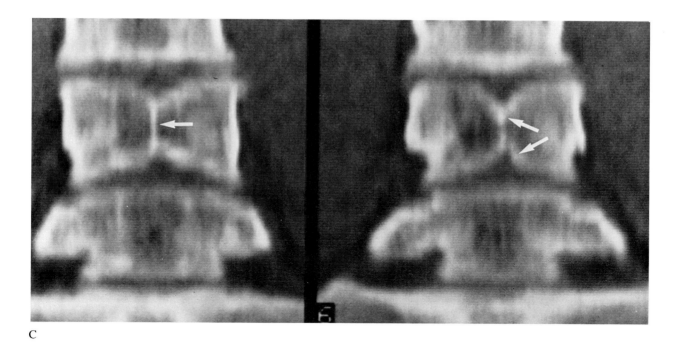

C

compression of the thecal sac (Fig. 12.9). Axial and sagittal views are the most important in depicting the position of bone fragments and their point of origin.[13–15] Sagittal views are crucial for estimating soft disc herniation, as the anatomy is distorted on axial views because of fragmentation (Fig. 12.10).

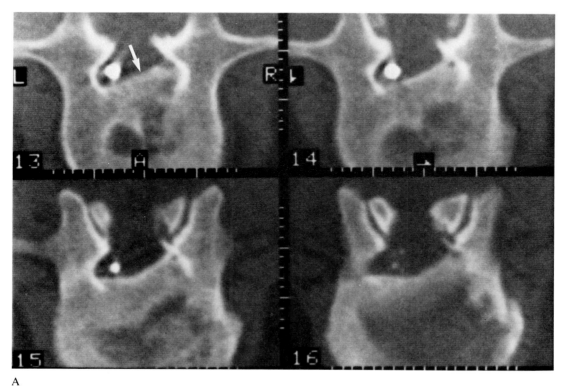

A

FIGURE 12.9 Bursting fracture of the vertebral body. **A.** Axial scans demonstrate a large fragment in the spinal canal (*arrow*). (*Figure continued* on page 360.)

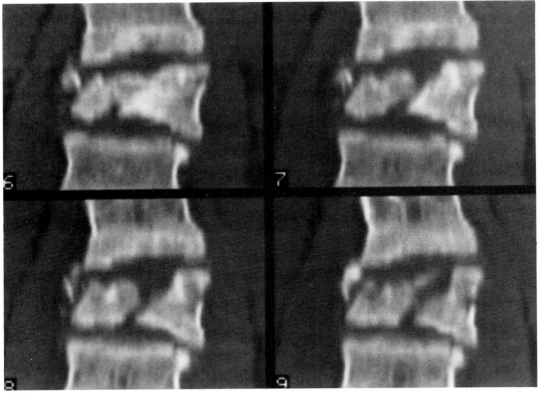

B

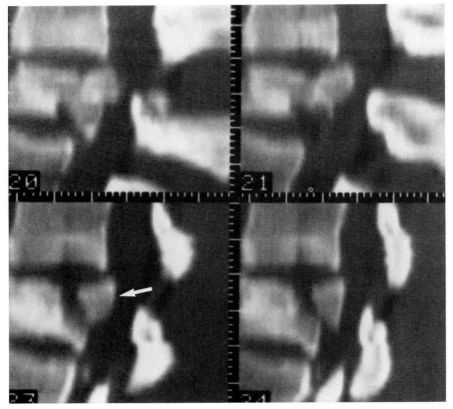

C

FIGURE 12.9 (*cont'd*) **B, C.** Coronal and sagittal views on another patient. There are large bone fragments extruded into the spinal canal (*arrow*).

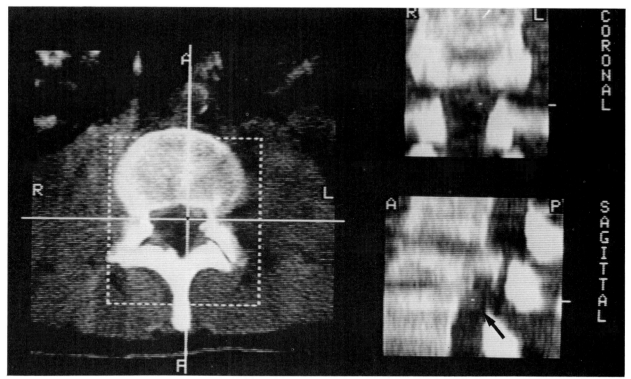

FIGURE 12.10 Traumatic disc herniation. Second-generation CT scan demonstrating vertebral fracture. No disc herniation was diagnosed in the axial projection. Sagittal reformation clearly defines a disc herniation at the lower disc space (*arrow*).

Congenital vertebral malformations may be mistaken for anteriorly wedged bursting fractures. The patient in Figure 12.11 was scanned several days after a fall from a ladder. Routine radiographs revealed marked anterior wedging and some widening of the vertebral body. A fracture was suspected. CT of the involved vertebral segment demonstrated anterior wedging of the vertebra, but the bone texture and cortical margins were all normal. The coronal view is diagnostic for hemivertebrae. There is a clearly definable cortical margin of each vertebral half. The lucent central defect is a remnant of the failed fused vertebral segments. An important diagnostic point: The lateral diameter of the vertebra is increased in this disorder but the anteroposterior diameter is usually reduced.

Thus far we have discussed only stable fractures, those with a low likelihood of causing progressive neurologic deficit. The unstable thoracolumbar fracture poses a much greater diagnostic and therapeutic challenge.

Spinal fractures have classically been considered stable when the posterior elements are intact but are unstable when these elements are either fractured or dislocated or when there is obvious posterior ligamentous rupture or laxity.

Recently McAfee et al. proposed a broad definition of instability of the thoracolumbar spine which includes: (1) progressive neurologic deficit; (2) posterior element disruption; (3) progressive kyphosis of more than 20 degrees in the presence of a neurologic deficit; (4) greater than 50% loss of vertebral height with facet subluxation, and (5) CT demonstration of bone fragments in a compromised spinal canal.[16]

This change in attitude has been prompted because patients with burst fractures often develop increased neurologic deficit, spinal deformity, or mechanical back pain later in life. For example, progressive neurologic loss may follow healing of a burst fracture. Increasing kyphosis occurs secondary to increasing ligamentous laxity; the cauda equina becomes stretched over the anterior bony structures.

Although the posterior element fractures are frequently visible on axial scans, the coronal view is useful, especially for evaluating horizontal laminar or facet fractures. The articular processes and pars interarticularis defects are best studied in the sagittal plane (Fig. 12.12). One must document posterior element fractures because these patients require especially delicate handling. The CT is important when deciding which patients need decompressive surgery and which require decompression and fusion.

There is a great deal of controversy regarding the appropriate therapy for unstable spinal fractures. Some surgeons rely solely on prolonged bed rest with body casting.

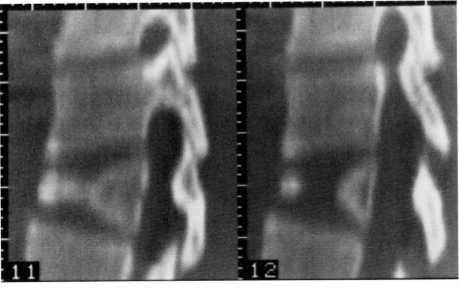

A

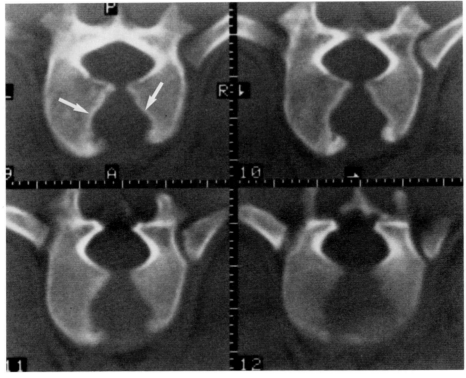

B

FIGURE 12.11 Congenital butterfly vertebra. Sagittal (**A**), axial (**B**), and coronal (**C**) views demonstrate an anteriorly wedged vertebral body with a central lucency (*arrows*). The medial borders of the vertebral-body halves are normally corticated. This is characteristic of congenital hemivertebrae.

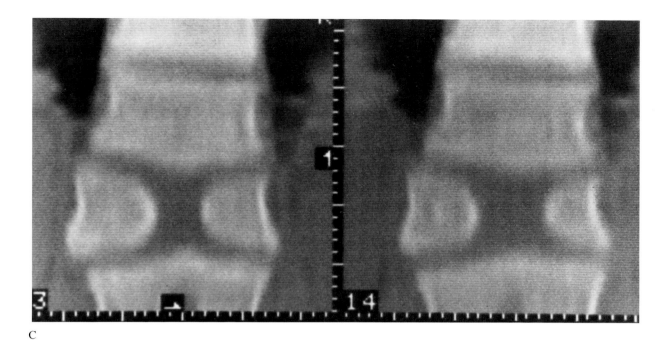

C

A

FIGURE 12.12 Unstable lumbar fracture. **A.** Axial scans demonstrate marked comminution of the vertebral body and fracture of the neural arch (*arrows*). (*Figure continued* on page 364.)

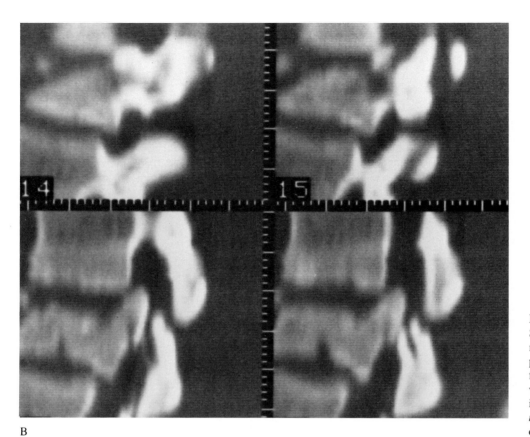

B

FIGURE 12.12 (*cont'd*) **B.** Sagittal view defines bone fragments from the vertebral body displaced into the lateral recess, and fracture of the pedicle. **C.** Coronal view reveals fracture of the lamina, with lateral dislocation (*arrow*). The facet-joint space is opened (*arrowheads*).

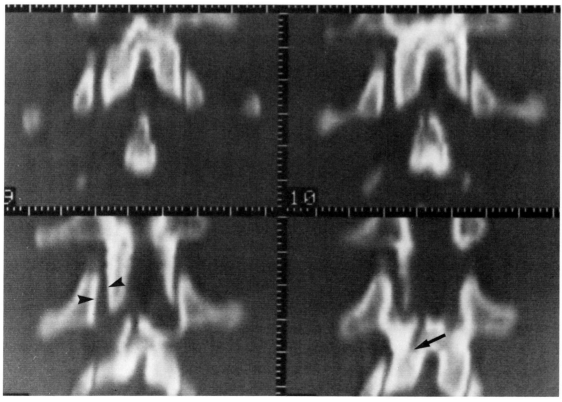

C

Others prefer internal fixation with Harrington rods or some other metallic device. Fixation tends to allow patients to ambulate earlier and permits more rapid rehabilitation.

Recently, surgical approaches that combine laminectomy, decompression, and internal fixation have been proposed in an attempt to treat early instability (bone fragmentation and subluxation) as well as to prevent late instability (increased neurologic deficit or kyphosis).[17,18]

CT plays a key role in treatment planning in that it allows the surgeon to direct his decompression to the side where the posterior elements are most abnormal. The destabilizing effect of surgery can be minimized if the decompression is on the side opposite a nonfractured pedicle or facet.

A specific CT pattern of thoracolumbar fracture was recently described which includes: (1) superior disc injury; (2) bursting or crush fracture through the upper half of the vertebral body; (3) sagittal cleavage fracture of the lower half of the vertebral body; (4) bone fragments in the spinal canal; and (5) laminar fracture. Lindahl et al. termed these crush-cleavage fractures.[18] In each of these cases the frontal and sagittal diameters of the vertebral body are lengthened, the vertebral height is reduced, and the spinal canal is narrowed by retropulsed bone fragments (Fig. 12.13).

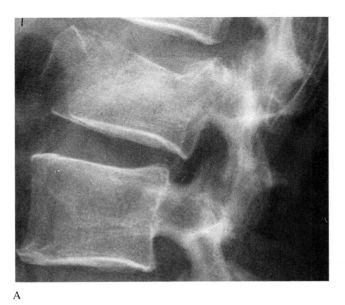

A

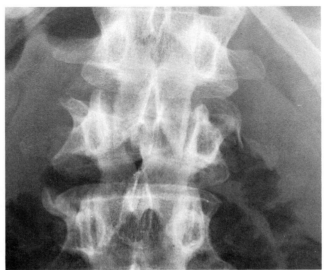

B

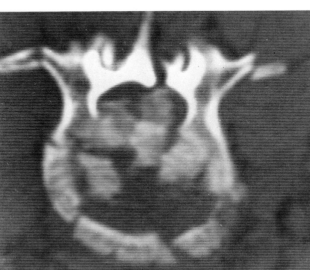

C

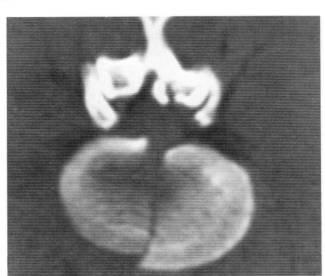

D

FIGURE 12.13 Crush-cleavage fracture. **A, B.** Frontal and lateral radiographs demonstrate wedging and fragmentation of the vertebral body. **C.** Axial scan through the upper half of the vertebral body reveals marked comminution and fragmentation. **D.** Axial scan through the lower half of the vertebra demonstrates a linear cleavage. (Reprinted with permission from Lindahl et al.[18]).

The patient in Figure 12.14, by the aforementioned criteria, is an example of an unstable fracture. He has developed increasing neurologic deficit and pain. The verte- bral body had continued to collapse and is now markedly wedged to the right. The posterior portion of the vertebral body has been displaced into the canal, causing marked

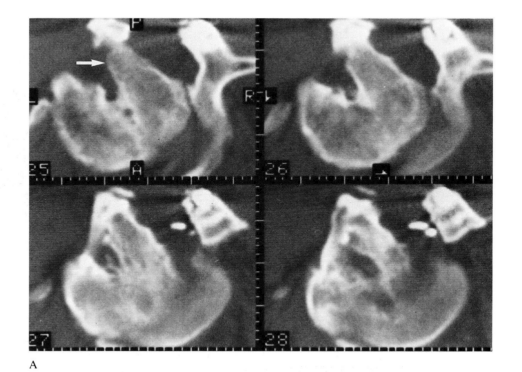

A

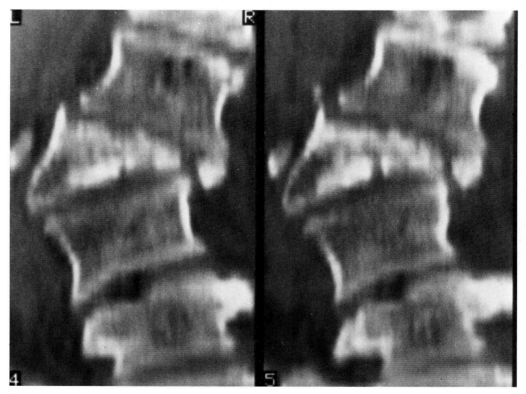

B

FIGURE 12.14 Unstable burst fracture. **A.** Axial views demonstrate a healed vertebral body fracture, with marked rotation of the involved vertebrae. An extruded bone fragment is touching the left facet. **B.** Coronal view reveals collapse of the right side of the vertebral body. **C.** Sagittal view shows marked kyphosis and posterior displacement of the entire fractured vertebral body (*arrows*).

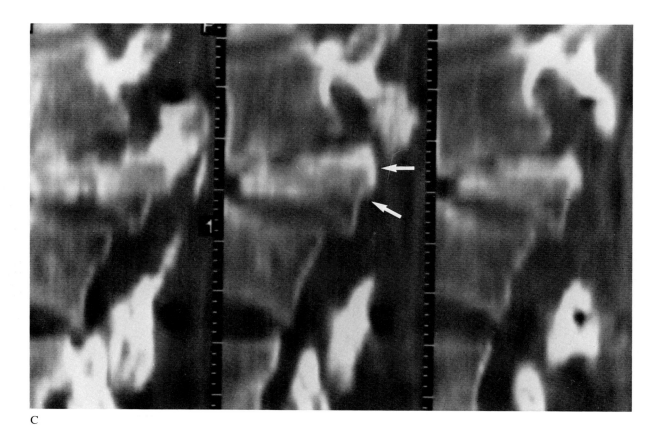

C

stenosis. The neural foramen on the left is also narrowed. A combination of all three right-angled views is necessary for proper anatomic understanding of this case.

The patient in Figure 12.15 was scanned because of radiculopathy after a successful posterior spine fusion for

fracture stabilization. Although the fusion is well healed and the fracture is indeed stable, the sagittal reformation reveals a large bone fragment within the affected neural foramen.

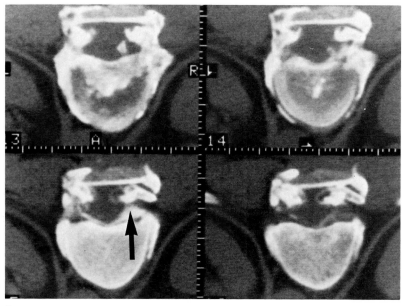

A

FIGURE 12.15 Posteroperative foraminal stenosis. **A.** Axial views reveal a successful posterior spine fusion for fracture. Note the bone fragments extending into the lateral recess and foramen (*arrows*). (*Figure continued* on page 368.)

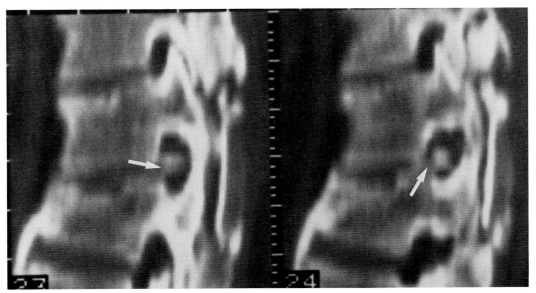

B

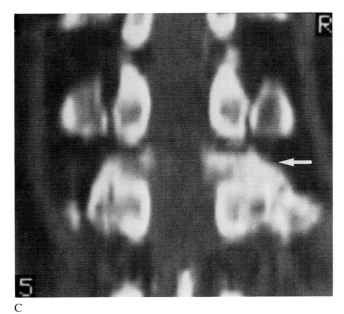

C

FIGURE 12.15 (*cont'd*)   Sagittal (**B**) and coronal (**C**) views reveal a successful posterior spine fusion for fracture. Note the bone fragments extending into the lateral recess and foramen (*arrows*).

Vertebral Compression with Flexion and Rotation

The most disruptive forces affecting the thoracolumbar region occur during rotation. The posterior ligaments are strong and resist a great deal of flexion deformity without rupturing. They readily fail, with disastrous consequences, however, if severely rotated. As a general rule, fractures caused by flexion and rotational forces are frequently unstable because of posterior ligamentous rupture and vertebral-body

collapse. The spine is free to rotate and flex with total lack of support, and neurologic deficit may be very severe.

The patient in Figure 12.16 has such an injury. On the coronal reformation a spiral oblique fracture is noted extending through three vertebral bodies and two disc spaces. The axial views demonstrate marked comminution and fragmentation. Sagittal views display the abnormal spinal angulation and the relative positions of the fractured vertebral bodies.

Metallic foreign material within the body causes marked streaking on the CT scan. This is because of the relative lack of signal from those rays that traverse the metal. Harrington rods therefore pose a special problem in the evaluation of the postoperative traumatized spine. The two parallel dense rods create a remarkable posterior spinal artifact. There is total absence of information in a band extending across the scan through the plane of the two rods. Other streaks radiate out from the two rods in a random distribution, severely degrading the image.

It is quite remarkable, however, how much information can be retrieved even from severely degraded scans. The patient in Figure 12.17 had an unstable fracture dislocation treated by decompressive laminectomy and Harrington rod internal fixation. The postoperative scan, even with the streaks, clearly demonstrates retropulsion of a large bony fragment. Note the posterior black artifact on the sagittal view. Absence of signal has produced a negative cast of the metallic rod. The image is degraded, but the crucial information is still present. It may be impossible to diagnose small soft-tissue disc lesions or blood clots because of the artifact. Even with this drawback, we still feel that reformatted CT is useful in many cases with metallic rods in place. Even though the pictures may not be esthetically pleasing, enough valuable information is obtained to justify the study.

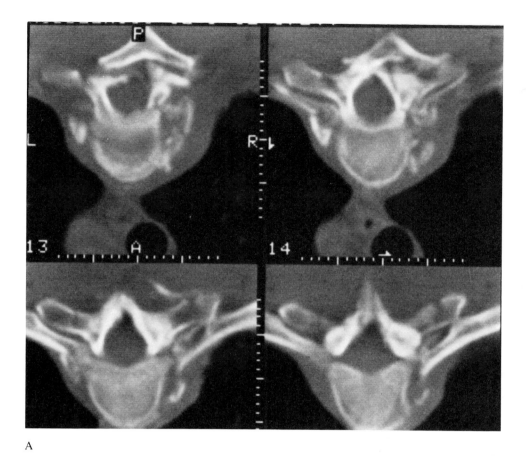

A

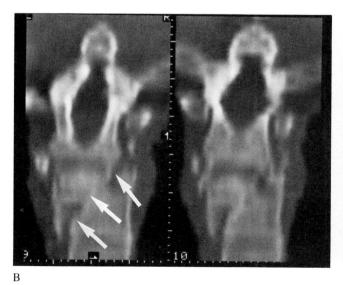

B

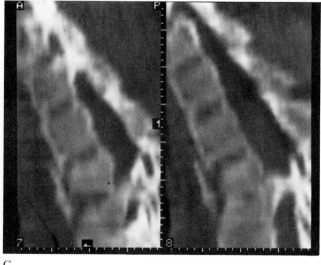

C

FIGURE 12.16 Vertebral flexion and rotation. **A.** Axial scans demonstrate severe shearing and disruption of the vertebral body. There is fracture of the right pedicle and transverse process, and disorganization of the left L4 facet-joint complex. **B, C.** Coronal and sagittal views define the spiral rotatory nature of the fracture, which extends through three vertebral bodies (*arrows*).

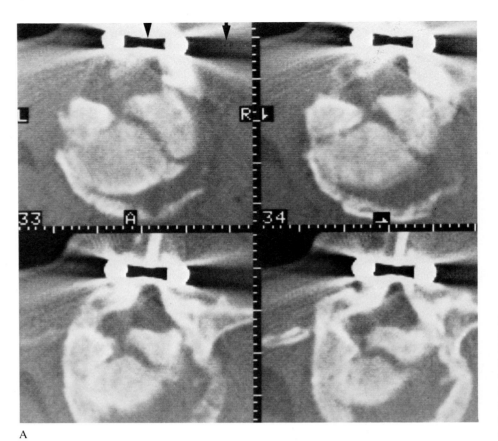

A

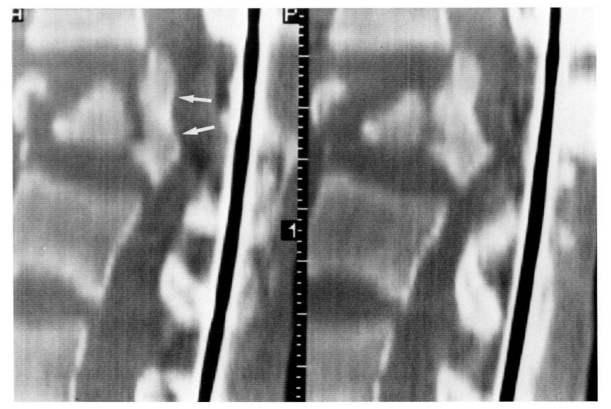

B

FIGURE 12.17 Bursting fracture treated with Harrington rod fusion. Note the streak artifacts (*arrows*) between the two rods on the axial view (**A**). On the sagittal reformation (**B**) one can still identify a large displaced bone fragment (*arrows*), even though the scan is not esthetically pleasing.

Fatigue Fractures

Fractures unrelated to major trauma may occur in the spine. Several of these have been dealt with in detail elsewhere in this book but are mentioned here for completeness.

Spondylolysis

Fractures of the pars interarticularis most frequently occur in children between the ages of 6 and 15. Radionuclide scans are frequently positive in the acute phase. Figure 12.18 shows a young patient who had been experiencing back pain for a month. Sagittal reformation demonstrates a thin fracture line traversing one pars interarticularis. This appearance is atypical for chronic pars defects, as there is no clearly defined corticated cleavage plane typical of adult spondylolysis. This is an acute pars fracture. It is important to conceptualize spondylolysis as a fracture in order to understand the important deformities that occur and produce pain. A complete discussion is found in Chapter 8.

Another unusual fatigue fracture is found in the patient in Figure 12.19. This teenage gymnast was exercising

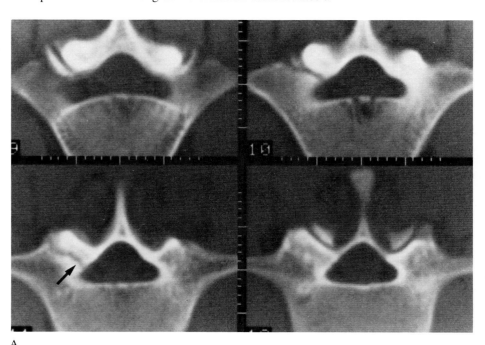
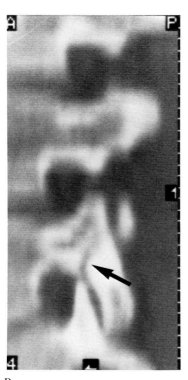

A B

FIGURE 12.18   Acute spondylolysis. Axial (**A**) and sagittal (**B**) views reveal a thin lytic defect in the pars interarticularis (*arrows*). This deficit is different from most chronic spondylolytic defects in that it is not well corticated and there is no clear space filled with fibrous tissue.

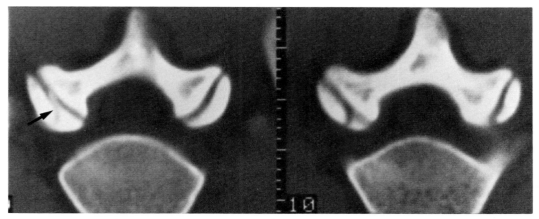

FIGURE 12.19   Stress fracture of the left articular process. Axial scan reveals a small, slightly displaced fracture of the superior S1 facet (*arrow*).

on the parallel rings, and during the performance of an abrupt flexion swing of his legs he allowed his low back muscles to momentarily become lax. With a violent downward extension of the legs, he tightened his back muscles and immediately felt sharp left-sided back pain. This CT scan, performed several weeks after that episode, reveals a displaced crack through the superior facet of the sacrum. As our diagnostic procedures and acumen improve, it is almost certain that we will begin to see more such abnormalities in our athletes.

Postoperative Stress Fractures

In a recent review of postoperative CT spine scans done on patients with laminectomy and at least partial facetectomy, we found 25 patients with a unique fracture through the base of the inferior facet.[19] We believe that this is due to normal stresses placed on an abnormally thinned, surgically weakened inferior facet. To our knowledge, this fracture has never been reported on axial-only CT. Because of its compound curves and sloping nature, the facet should be demonstrated on at least two nonaxial projections (Fig. 12.20). These fractures are not insignificant lesions—for-

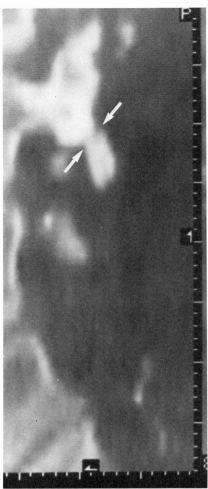

B

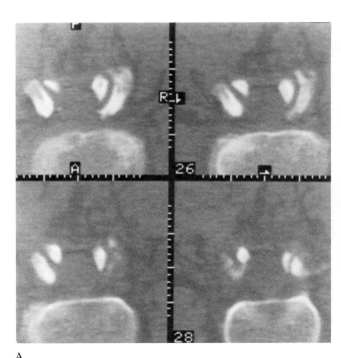

A

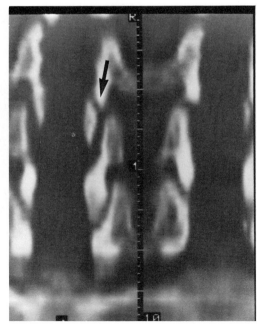

C

FIGURE 12.20 Postoperative stress fracture. Axial scan (**A**) demonstrates laminectomy and facetectomy. There is no evidence of fracture. Sagittal (**B**) and coronal (**C**) reformations demonstrate a specific fracture (*arrows*) through the base of the inferior facet (not the pars interarticularis).

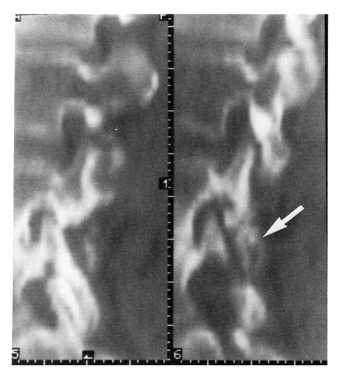

A

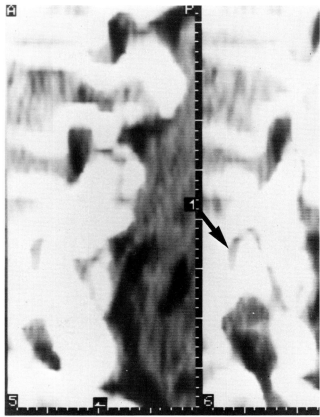

B

FIGURE 12.21 Postoperative stress fracture, with foraminal stenosis. **A, B.** Sagittal reformation demonstrates fracture through the base of the inferior facet (*arrows*). The L4–5 normal foramen is narrow because of rotatory retrolisthesis. **C.** Coronal reformation demonstrates dislocation of the fractured facet (*arrows*).

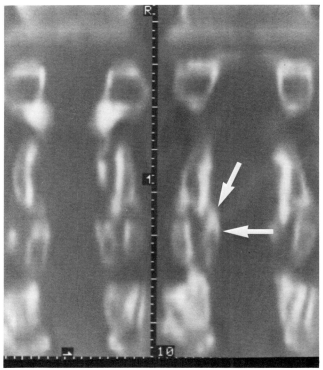

C

ward or backward subluxation may occur at the level of the facet fracture and cause profound foraminal stenosis (Fig. 12.21).

Fractures of the Transverse Process

Stress fractures of the transverse processes may occur because of powerful muscular pull on them. Although uncommon, they do cause back pain. The patient in Figure 12.22 awoke one morning with localized pain in the left side of the back. Radiographs were interpreted as normal. He did not report any significant trauma, but he regularly performed heavy manual labor. Because the pain persisted, a radionuclide bone scan was performed; it showed a hot spot in the area of the transverse process. A CT scan was then performed, which demonstrated a partially healed fracture. The cortex of the transverse process was normal, and there was no mass associated with the fracture (Fig. 12.22B). This benign fracture must be differentiated from more ominous lesions, such as the one in Figure 12.22C in which the bone is abnormal; the cortex of the vertebral body and transverse process is irregular. Metastasis has infiltrated the bone.

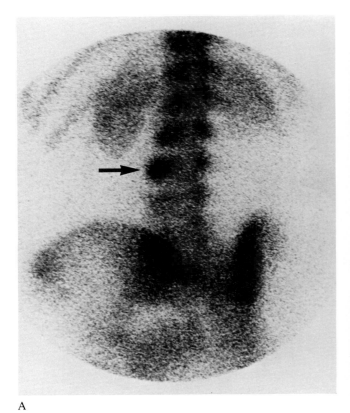

A

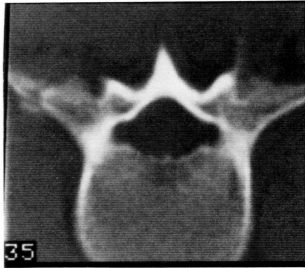

35

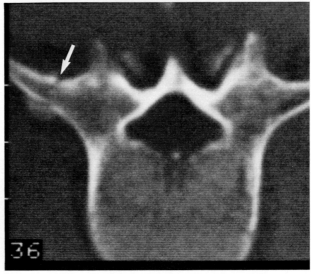

36

B

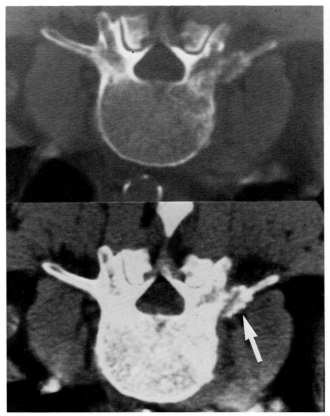

C

FIGURE 12.22 Transverse process fracture. **A.** Positive radio-nuclide bone scan taken approximately 30 days after onset of localized back pain, with no known trauma. **B.** Axial CT showing the fracture. Note a small amount of surrounding callus (*arrow*). The cortical bone is normal. **C.** Another patient, for comparison, with a permeative metastatic lesion involving the transverse process. Note the loss of normal cortical bone (*arrow*).

Spinous Process Avulsion

Spinous process avulsion is a specific lesion of the lower cervical spine and the highest thoracic segments. Because it was commonly encountered in clay shovelers, it has carried that name. It is produced by strong traction forces on the spinous processes due to hyperextension-rotation motions of the upper arms and shoulders. It is a stable lesion that is easily diagnosed in the axial projection (Fig. 12.23).

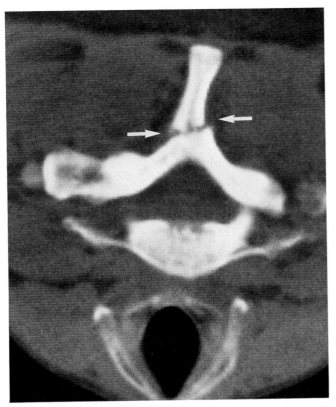

FIGURE 12.23 Avulsion fracture of the spinous process (*arrows*).

Evaluation of Traumatic Soft-Tissue Spinal Abnormalities

Thus far only the bony and ligamentous injuries that occur with spine trauma have been discussed. Let us now consider evaluation of cord and nerves. In patients without neurologic deficit, nonenhanced CT is almost always adequate. However, the CT evaluation of patients with acute neurologic deficit often requires CT myelography, either alone or in conjunction with routine film myelography. These techniques make it possible to delineate major traumatic lesions and to plan intraspinal surgery.

Almost immediately after severe spinal injury with neurologic deficit, the spinal cord may swell because of either hemorrhage or edema, or both (Fig. 12.24).[20] Cord swelling can be diagnosed by seeing diffuse expansion of the spinal cord shadow surrounded by a rim of contrast material.[21] Acute hematomyelia may actually be easier to identify without intrathecal contrast medium—the intraspinal blood appears hyperdense relative to the spinal cord shadow. This subtle attenuation difference of small blood collections may be hidden because of the wide window usually used when photographing metrizamide CT scans (Fig. 12.25). When present, hematomyelia is generally believed to contraindicate surgical intervention. Even more severe cord injury, cord maceration, fissuring, or transection are likewise not considered surgically remediable lesions and must be differentiated from extrinsic compressive

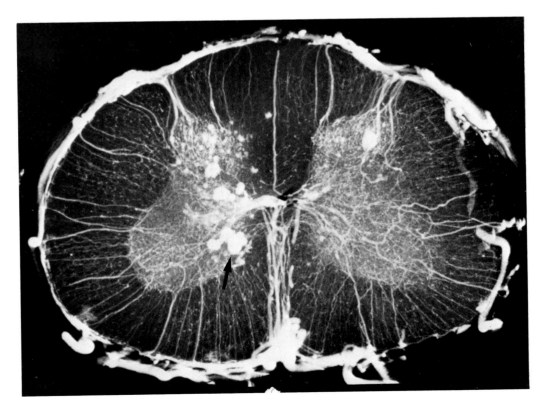

FIGURE 12.24 Cross-sectional microradiograph of the spinal cord of a traumatized cat. Micro-opaque barium injected posttrauma outlines leakage of contrast medium into a central cord hemorrhage (*arrow*). (Reprinted with permission from Allen et al.[20]).

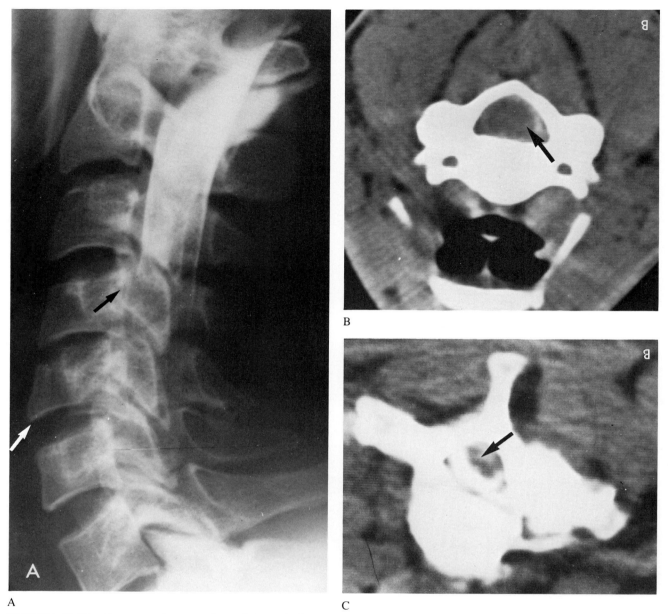

A   C

FIGURE 12.25 Posttraumatic expansion of the spinal cord. **A.** Metrizamide myelogram. **B.** Metrizamide CT showing diffuse cord swelling above the level of a fracture (*arrow*). (Reprinted with permission from Post MJD: Computed tomography of spinal trauma. In Post MJD (ed): Computed Tomography of the Spine. Williams & Wilkins, Baltimore, 1984, pp. 765–808.) **C.** Axial CT demonstrating a high-density blood clot (*arrow*) within the spinal cord. (Reprinted with permission from Post et al.[21])

bony or soft-tissue lesions, which are amenable to surgical correction.

Spinal epidural hemorrhage is a focal collection of blood that may cause severe acute neurocompressive symptoms requiring immediate surgical intervention.[5,22] Patients commonly present with sudden onset of neck or back pain which may rapidly progress to paresis, bladder dysfunction, and even death. Trauma is typically minor; minimal stress

from coughing or twisting has produced the hemorrhage. Iatrogenic hemorrhage from diagnostic lumbar puncture or spinal anesthesia, especially in patients with clotting disorders, is well documented[22,23] (Fig. 12.26).

Dural tears and nerve-root avulsion are seen more easily on metrizamide-enhanced CT than on conventional metrizamide myelography. Avulsion is more common in the cervical area than in the lumbar area. The diagnosis

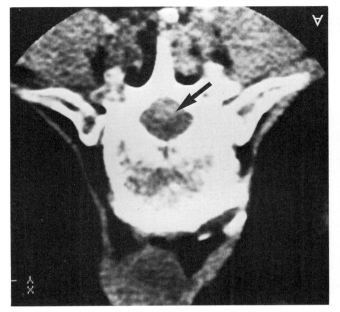

A

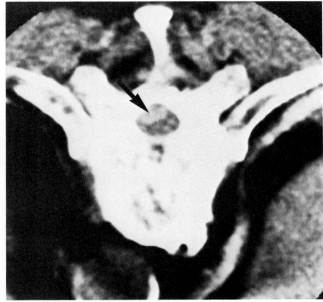

B

C

FIGURE 12.26 Spinal epidural hematoma. **A, B.** Nonmetrizamide CT showing a prominent posterior hyperdense mass (*arrow*), which is an epidural hematoma. **C.** Metrizamide CT proves the extradural nature of the mass (*arrow*) and shows the cord displaced forward. (Reprinted with permission from Post et al.[22])

may be obvious clinically or highly suspected by the history and physical examination. On the axial view the axillary pouch is unusually widened and elongated, extending well out into the neural foramen or beyond (Fig. 12.27). Because the severed roots tend to retract, these dilated sheaths seem empty. In severe injuries there may be associated dural laceration with leakage of metrizamide from the subarachnoid space.

Severe thoracolumbar rotatory unstable fractures with neurologic defects frequently demonstrate dural laceration. These lacerations are best viewed in the axial projection (Fig. 12.28). Gunshot wounds may also cause dural lac-

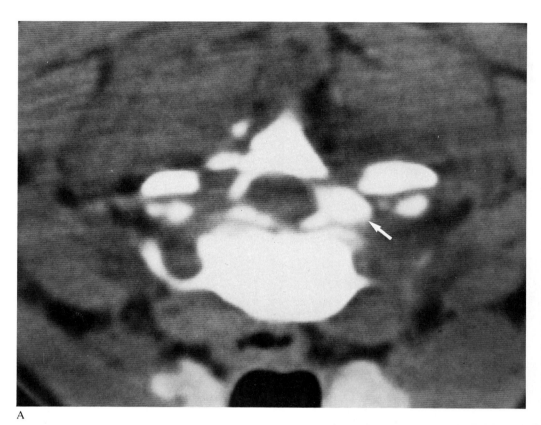

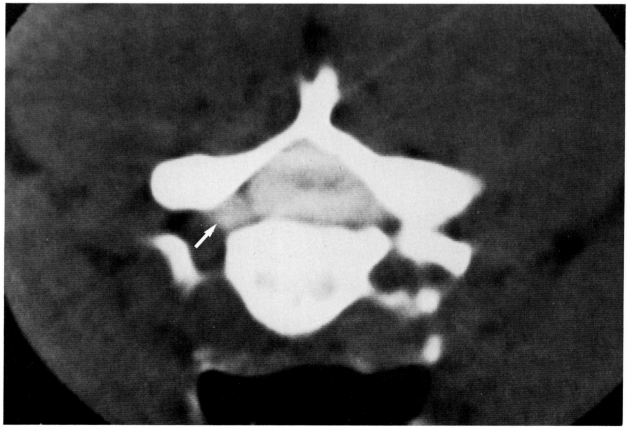

A

B

FIGURE 12.27 Nerve-root avulsion caused by cervical fracture subluxation in two patients. Metrizamide CT demonstrates a contrast-medium-filled dilated root sheath extending into the neural foramen (*arrows*). (Reprinted with permission from: **A:** Post et al.[21] **B:** Brant-Zawadzki and Post.[4])

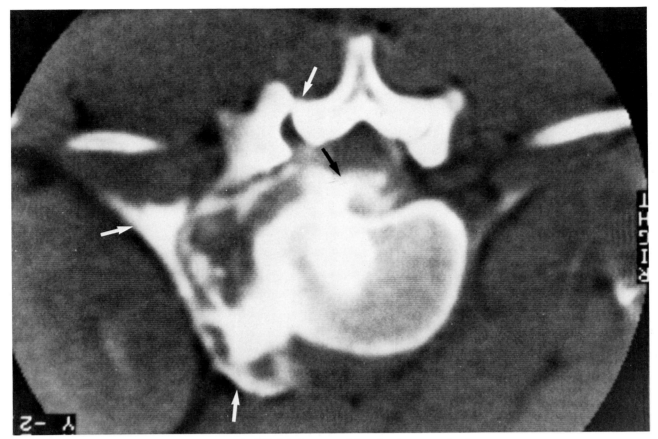

FIGURE 12.28 Dural laceration. A traumatic T12–L1 fracture subluxation has caused a large dural leak. The source of the leak is indicated by arrows. The contrast medium has infiltrated well out into the paravertebral soft tissues. (Reprinted with permission from Brant-Zawadzki and Post.[4])

eration, as well as metal and bone fragmentation, all of which are well visualized on CT (Fig. 12.29). The patient in Figure 12.30 developed sciatica while recovering from a thoracic bullet wound. Noncontrast CT revealed that the bullet had fallen down to the lumbosacral area and had become wedged in the sacral spinal canal. Note that there is artifact from the lead bullet but that it does not significantly detract from the diagnostic value of the examination.

Severe spinal injury may cause delayed spinal cord atrophy. Although cord thinning may be localized, it is likely to be more extensive than the bony fracture. Various

authors demonstrate flattening and thinning of the cord through the affected area on metrizamide-enhanced scans.[5] It is quite simple, however, to evaluate the chronically disabled person without intrathecal contrast injection. The patient in Figure 12.31 was severely injured as a child, and a wide posterior laminectomy was performed. As is typical in children, considerable thoracocervical deformity ensued, requiring spinal fusion. At the time of the present scan, she was paretic below the level of C7. Coronal reformation demonstrates a cord of adequate size. Note the central shadow surrounded symmetrically by cerebrospinal fluid. On the

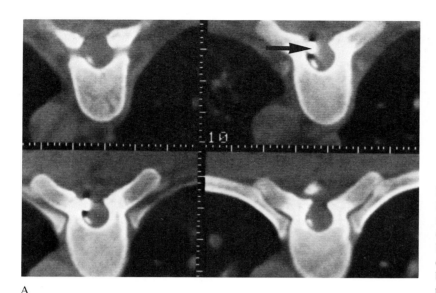

A

FIGURE 12.29 Thoracic bullet wound. Axial (**A**) and sagittal (**B**) views demonstrate a small-caliber bullet in the spinal canal (*arrow*). There has been previous laminectomy.

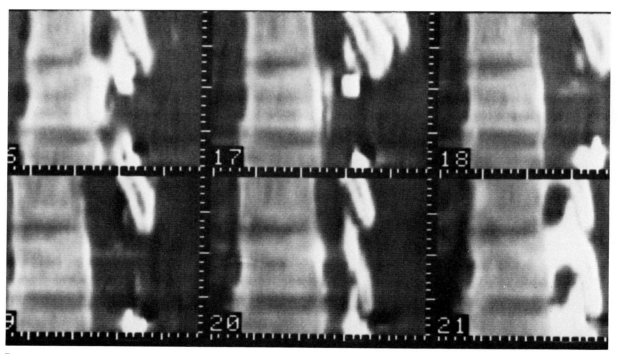

B

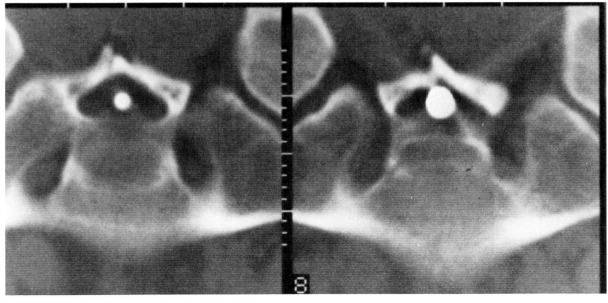

A

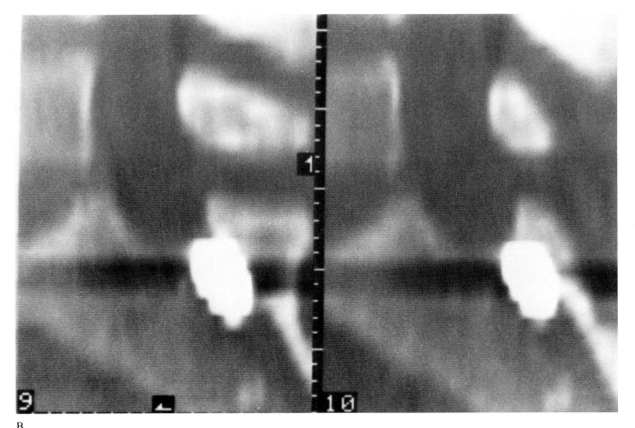

B

FIGURE 12.30 Intraspinal bullet. Axial (**A**) and sagittal (**B**) views. A migrating bullet is wedged in the sacral canal, causing radiculopathy.

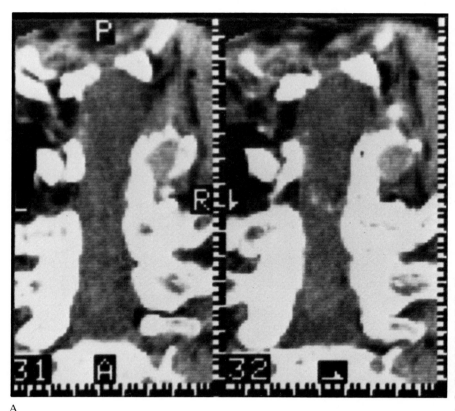

A

FIGURE 12.31 Posttraumatic cord atrophy. **A.** Coronal view of the cervical cord reveals an almost normal size spinal cord. **B, C.** Sagittal reformation for soft tissue and bone detail demonstrate a marked hockey-stick deformity of the thoracocervical junction. A wide posterior laminectomy and anterior intrathoracic fusion procedure has been performed. There is remarkable thinning of the cord (*arrows*).

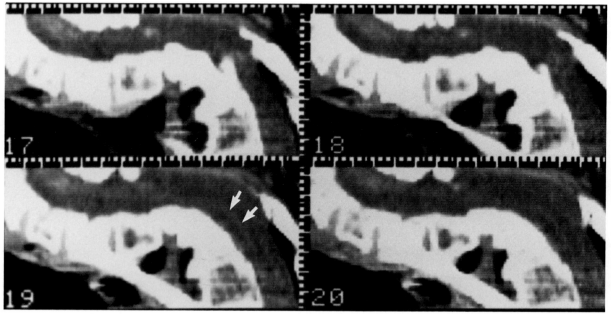

B

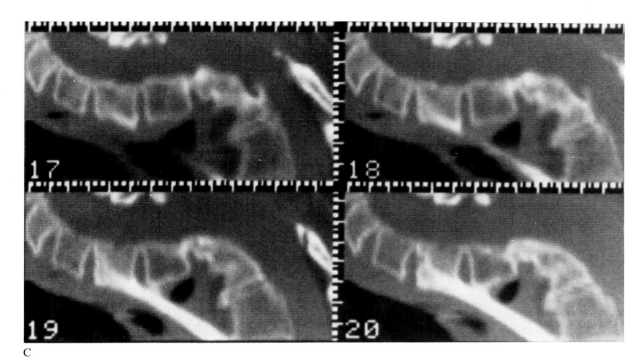

C

sagittal view, however, the cord is a thin ribbon in the center of the canal. This ribbon shape is quite characteristic of atrophy. On occasion, no cord shadow is visible at all, presumably because of complete cord transection. Intrathecal metrizamide is usually necessary to fill small posttraumatic cysts.

References

1. Brant-Zawadzki M, Jeffery RB Jr, Minagi H, Potts LH: High-resolution CT of thoracolumbar fractures. AJNR 3:69–74, 1982

2. Brant-Zawadzki M, Miller EM, Federle MP: CT in the evaluation of spine trauma. AJR 136:369–375, 1981

3. Brant-Zawadzki M, Minagi H: CT in the evaluation of spine trauma. In Federle MP, Brant-Zawadzki M (eds): Computed Tomography in the Evaluation of Trauma. William & Wilkinson, Baltimore, 1982, pp. 106–152

4. Brant-Zawadzki M, Post MJD: Trauma. In Newton TH, Potts DG (eds): The Spine and Spinal Cord. Clavadel Press, San Francisco, California, 1983, pp. 149–186

5. Post MJD, Green BA: The use of computed tomography in spine trauma. Radiol Clin North Am 21:327–375, 1983

6. Smith GR, Northrop CH, Loop JW: Jumpers' fractures: patterns of thoracolumbar spine injuries associated with vertical plunges; a review of 38 cases. Radiology 122:657–663, 1977

7. Roaf R: A study of the mechanics of spine injuries. J Bone Joint Surg 42B:810–823, 1960

8. Chance GQ: Note on a type of flexion fracture of the spine. Br J Radiol 21:452–453, 1948

9. Rogers LF: The roentgenographic appearance of transverse or Chance fractures of the spine: the seat belt fracture. AJR 111:844–849, 1971

10. O'Callaghan JP, Ullrich CG, Yuan HA, Kieffer SA: CT of facet distraction in flexion injuries of the thoracolumbar spine: the "naked" facet. AJNR 1:97–102, 1980

11. Colley DP, Dunsker SB: Traumatic narrowing of the dorsolumbar spinal canal demonstrated by computed tomography. Radiology 129:95–98, 1978

12. Keene JS, Goletz TH, Lilleas F, et al: JF: Diagnosis of vertebral fractures: a comparison of conventional radiography, conventional tomography, and computed axial tomography. J Bone Joint Surg 64A:586–595, 1982

13. Ghoshhajra K, Krisha CVG: CT in spinal trauma. J Comput Tomogr 4:309–318, 1980

14. Jacobs RR, Asher MA, Snider RK: Thoracolumbar spinal injuries. a comparative study of recumbent and operative treatment in 100 patients. Spine 5:463–477, 1980

15. Nykamp PW, Levy JM, Christensen F: Computed tomography for a bursting fracture of the lumbar spine. J Bone Joint Surg 60A:1168–1169, 1978

16. McAfee PC, Yuan HA, Lasda NA: The unstable burst fracture. Spine 7:365–373, 1982

17. LaRocca H: Diagnosis and treatment of unstable fractures of the thoracolumbar junction of the spine. In Post MJD (ed): Radiographic Evaluation of the Spine: Current Advances with Emphasis on Computed Tomography. Masson, New York, 1980, pp. 705–716

18. Lindahl S, Willen J, Nordwall A, Irstam L: The crush-cleavage fracture: a "new" thoracolumbar unstable fracture. Spine 8:559–569, 1983

19. Rothman SLG, Glenn WV: CT in the diagnosis of postoperative stress fractures. Presented at the Radiological Society of North America annual meeting, Chicago, 1983

20. Allen WE III, D'Angelo CM, Kier EL: Correlation of microangiographic and electrophysiologic changes in experimental spinal cord trauma. Radiology 111:107–115, 1974

21. Post MJD, Green BA, Quencer RM, et al: The value of computed tomography in spinal trauma. Spine 7:417–431, 1982

22. Post MJD, Seminer DS, Quencer RM: CT diagnosis of spinal epidural hematoma. AJNR 3:190–192, 1982

23. Pear BL: Spinal epidural hematoma. AJR 115:155–164, 1972

Far-Out Syndrome

13

Leon Wiltse

Signs and symptoms of nerve-root compression are very common in clinical practice. In most cases pain and radiculopathy are caused by disc herniation or degenerative arthropathy. There is one almost totally unknown cause of L5 radiculopathy which presents with specific CT findings on reformatted examinations. This syndrome has been termed the far-out syndrome.

The far-out syndrome (alar transverse process impingement syndrome) occurs in two types of patient: (1) the elderly person with degenerative scoliosis; and (2) a somewhat younger adult with isthmic spondylolisthesis and at least 20% slippage. In both of these groups root compression occurs outside the spinal canal and the neural foramen, as the L5 root descends between the transverse process of L5 and the sacrum.

The 25-degree caudocephalic view (the Ferguson view) is best for visualizing the condition. CT is by far the best diagnostic tool. To show this condition far laterally, the window on the CT scanner must be opened wider than usual. Both coronal and parasagittal views demonstrate the condition, but the coronal view is the more valuable.

Symptoms are those of classic spinal nerve compression. Usually it is the L5–S1 level that is involved, but other levels can be as well. At surgery, it is very important that nerve decompression be carried far enough laterally. This usually means sacrificing the lower one-half of the pedicle and either the lower one-half or all of the transverse process. Part of the body of S1 and of the sacral ala can be removed if the surgeon prefers. Because so much bone is removed, instability is a factor to be seriously considered. How to decompress adequately and still maintain stability often poses a difficult problem.

Compression of the cauda equina and of the spinal nerves as a cause of sciatic pain has been recognized for many years. As early as 1925 Danforth and Wilson[1] described entrapment of the fifth lumbar spinal nerve by peripheral osteophytes at the disc level as a possible cause of sciatica. In 1927 Putti[2] expressed the belief that arthritic changes in the facet joints, as well as the variations of facet joint orientation, including transitional vertebrae, could be responsible for irritating the nerves. He also prescribed facetectomy for the relief of sciatica. Williams,[3] in 1932 wrote that degenerative disc disease at the L5–S1 level could be responsible for pinching of the nerve because of narrowing of the foramen.

Lindbloom,[4] in 1944 showed by anatomic studies that discs could herniate far laterally and compress the spinal nerve. In 1945 Hirsch[5] and Briggs[6] also described cases of patients having nerve entrapment at the foraminal level. Echols and Rehfeldt[8] in 1949 postulated that overhanging facets could be a cause of nerve root irritation. Schlesinger[9] in 1957 presented the idea that entrapment of the S1 spinal nerve in the lateral recess could be a cause of sciatica. Verbiest[10] in 1954 clearly described the syndrome of spinal stenosis, which has been further clarified and a classification formulated by Kirkaldy-Willis, et al.[11] Thus impingement of a spinal nerve anywhere out to the point where it exits from the lateral border of the foramen has been well described and is generally accepted.

This chapter describes nerve compression far laterally, beyond the foramen. Failure to recognize that the nerve can be compressed between the transverse process and the ala of the sacrum accounts for some failures of surgical decompression.

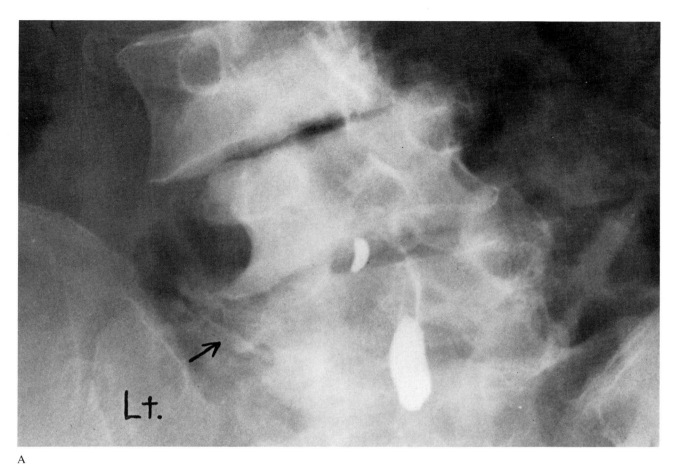

A

FIGURE 13.1 **A.** Typical x-ray showing the left transverse process impinging on the ala. Total decompression with removal of the left (*tvL5*) transverse process will relieve symptoms. (Courtesy of Dr. Marc Asher.) **B.** Coronal view of a CT scan of the left side of the patient whose roentgenogram is shown in **A**. Note that the transverse process of L5 lies against the sacral ala (Sac).

Types of Patient With Far-Out Syndrome

Type I (probably the most common) is the elderly individual with degenerative lumbar scoliosis or asymmetrical disc degeneration at L5, causing tilting of the fifth lumbar vertebra (Fig. 13.1). These patients usually have a primary lumbar curve of no less than 20 degrees and a compensatory lumbosacral curve that causes the transverse process of L5 to dip downward toward the ala. They have usually been unaware of any scoliotic deformity before seeking medical attention. The disc degeneration has often been asymmetrical, with the annular bulges more on the painful side. This bulging displaces the L5 spinal nerve posteriorly so that its course is prolonged in a lateral direction. By being posteriorly displaced, the nerve then proceeds anteriorly so that

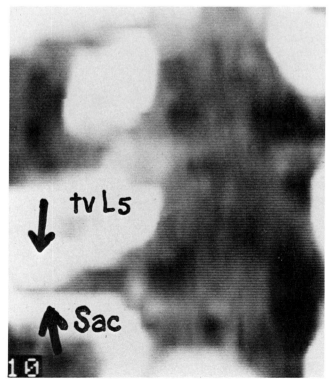

B

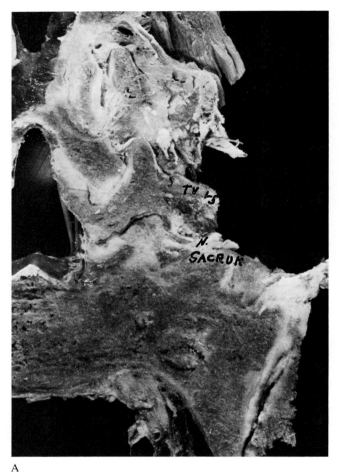

A

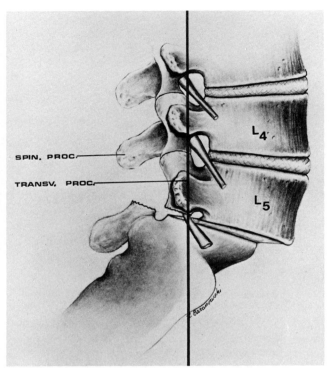

B

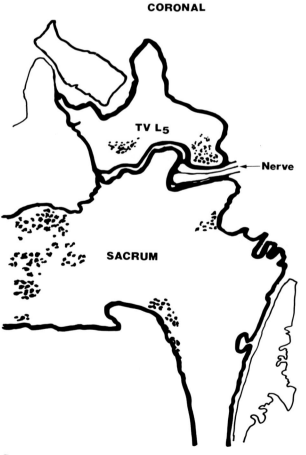

C

FIGURE 13.2 Normal anatomy. **A.** Photograph of a coronal section showing the right transverse process and ala. (*tvL5*) transverse process of the L5 vertebra. (*N*) spinal nerve. **B.** The heavy black line shows the level where the coronal section was taken. **C.** Drawing of the photograph of the pathologic specimen cut in the coronal plane seen in Figure 13.1A. (Reprinted with permission from Wiltse et al. Spine 9, 31-41 1984.)

the base and even the lateral portions of the transverse process compress the nerve against the ala of the sacrum. Some L5 transverse processes often have a rather large accesory process, which compromises the space even more. Very often peripheral osteophytes add to the entrapment.

Previously, radicular pain syndromes in this group of patients had often been explained as being due to foraminal stenosis at the concavity of the major curve. Although there may occasionally be compression around L2–3 at the concavity of the major curve, it is more commonly seen at the concavity of the compensatory lumbosacral curve at the L5 level. The pathology is basically the same, as is the treatment.

Type II is made up of a somewhat younger population group with isthmic spondylolisthesis and at least 20% slippage. The condition can occur bilaterally in these patients, but it usually is unilateral because the forward slippage is most often slightly asymmetrical. Radicular pain in spondylolisthesis patients has traditionally been explained on the basis of fibrous tissue compression or compression of the L5 nerve between the proximal stump of the pars and the body of S1. Stretching the nerves in cases of high-grade olisthesis with progressive slippage has also been incriminated. Twenty percent slippage is the smallest degree of olisthesis we observed to produce far lateral compression. Many people with isthmic spondylolisthesis have somewhat enlarged transverse processes, but not so large as to be considered transitional vertebrae.

As the vertebral body slips forward, the transverse processes move in an anterior, as well as a caudal, direction, allowing them to settle down against the sacrum. We have also seen this type of nerve compression in cases of L4 spondylolisthesis, and there is no reason why it could not occur at higher levels.

In a series of 30 cadaver and fresh autopsy spine specimens, we found one specimen with the anatomic findings that we believed would produce the symptoms described herein. This happened to be a cadaver specimen that demonstrated spondylolisthesis with approximately 25% slippage.

Marked compression of the L5 nerve could be seen between the transverse processes and the sacrum, more severe on the right (Fig. 13.2). Using computerized axial

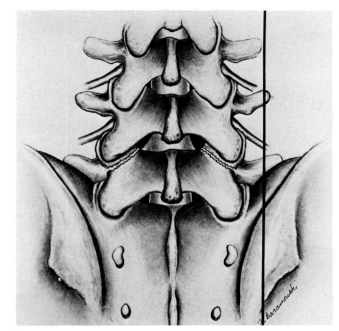

B

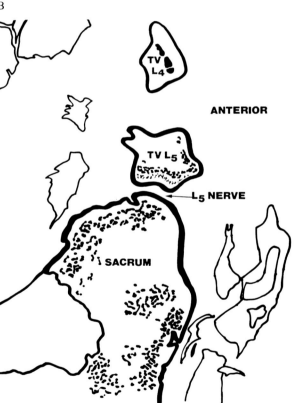

C

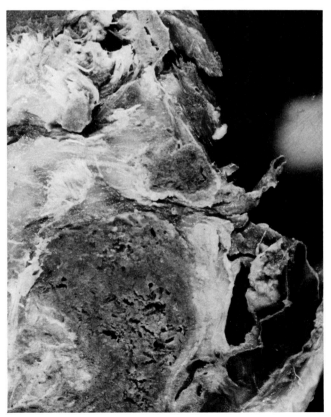

A

FIGURE 13.3 Pathologic specimen. **A.** Photograph of a parasagittal section of a pathologic specimen showing the transverse process down against the ala. **B.** The heavy black line is the point where the saw-cut was made for the specimen in the sagittal view. **C.** Parasagittal section shown in **A** at the point depicted by the heavy black line in **B**. (Reprinted with permission from Wiltse et al. Spine 9, 31-41 1984.)

tomography, both sagittal and coronal sections of this specimen were taken to demonstrate the relationship between the transverse processes and the top of the sacrum, with the nerve exiting between (Fig. 13.3).

When screening patients for the presence of this syndrome, ordinary standing anteroposterior (AP) and lateral views are taken. However, the Ferguson view (20 degrees caudocephalic anterior-posterior x-ray) is the most helpful. When this view is compared with the routine AP view, one can easily see how much better the Ferguson view is for delineating this condition. Myelography is usually done in these patients, and the degenerative type (type I) disorder characteristically shows at least some central canal stenosis. A CT scan is required to show alar transverse process impingement.

On the myelogram, the type II spondylolisthesis case shows a certain amount of canal compromise at the level of olisthesis; but again, computerized axial tomography is by far the procedure of choice to demonstrate far lateral compression.

Technique of Surgical Decompression

For type I, degenerative scoliosis, the patient is placed in the kneeling position, and either a midline or paraspinal approach is used. We much prefer the paraspinal approach if feasible because it makes removal of part of the pedicle and transverse process much easier; however, often there is so much central stenosis both laminae must be removed in the lower levels. In these cases, a midline approach is necessary.

When decompressing the level of far lateral compression, the spinal nerve must be carefully traced out laterally, removing all overlying bone. Usually the caudal one half of the pedicle must be removed along with at least the lower one-half of the transverse process. It may be simpler to remove the entire transverse process. A fusion is not attempted on this decompressed side, but unless the disc at L5 is very narrow and osteoarthritic, a one-level unilateral fusion is done on the other side. Advanced age and poor health may preclude fusion. If possible, total unilateral decompression is limited to one level. Even then, further slippage is a real danger, and fusion would not be done.

Normally, a patient is allowed up when he is able. A corset is seldom used, but if the patient desires he may wear one.

For type II, spondylolisthesis, we also use the paraspinal approach if possible. A unilateral decompression is done unless the pain is severe in both legs. It happens that in spondylolisthesis the pain is usually largely unilateral. It is not necessary to remove the entire lamina of L5 on the painful side. One can simply channel the nerve out through the defective pars and remove the lower portion of the pedi-

cle with the base of the transverse process (or the entire transverse process).[12]

If it is necessary to decompress both sides, we have not done a posterior fusion at the same time. Cloward (personal communication, 1982) recommended his operation in this situation. In a very few cases we have waited a few weeks after total posterior decompression and have then done an anterior interbody fusion using fibula.

The following cases are representative:

Case 1: A 69–year-old white female had low back pain and severe left leg pain, with numbness in the L5 distri-

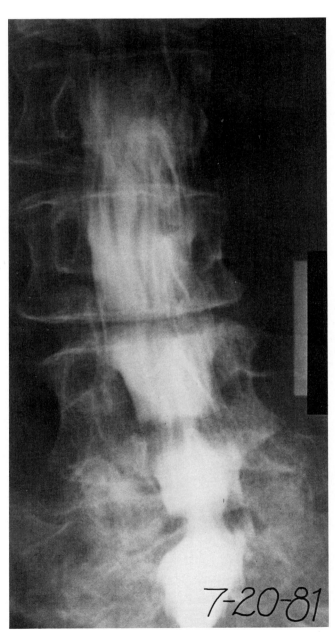

A

bution, for 2 years. She was unable to walk even one block because of back pain and, especially, leg pain. Her plain x-rays revealed that she had degenerative scoliosis and a markedly narrowed disc space at L5. The transverse process of L5 on the painful side was lying against the ala of the sacrum.

On myelography she displayed, in moderate degree, the typical central spinal canal stenosis in the lower lumbar canal. It was the CT scan that was diagnostic. In both sagittal and coronal views, the transverse process on the painful left side was down against the ala of the sacrum (Fig. 13.4).

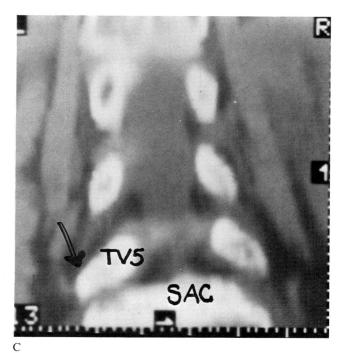

C

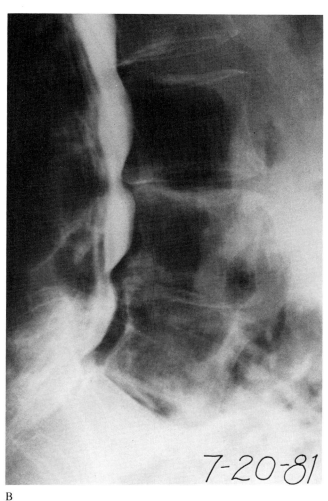

B

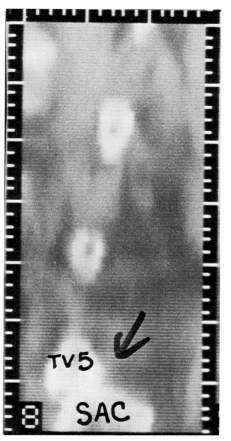

D

FIGURE 13.4 Far-out syndrome. **A.** AP myelogram of 69-year-old woman with very severe left leg pain and some back pain. **B.** Lateral myelogram shows only mild indentations of the metrizamide column. **C.** Coronal view shows marked impingement of the transverse process of L5 (*TV5*) on the sacral ala (*Sac*). **D.** Parasagittal view, cut at the base of the transverse process, again shows marked impingement between TV5 and SAC. (*Figure continued* on page 390.)

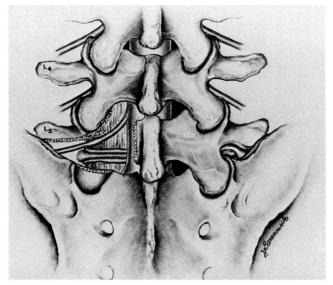

E

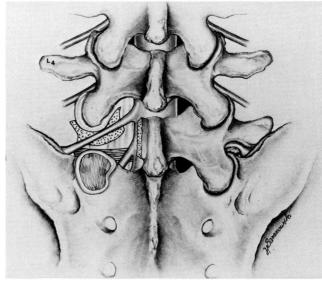

F

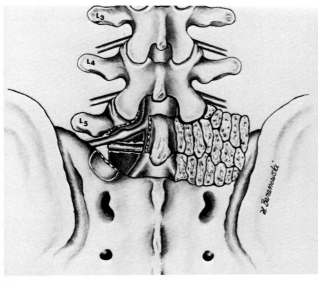

G

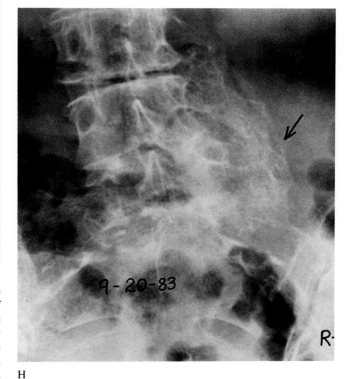

H

FIGURE 13.4 (*cont'd*)   **E.** In order to get the L5 spinal nerve decompressed, it was necessary to take off the lower one half of the pedicle and transverse process. **F.** Sometimes, in order to get the L5 nerve unequivocally decompressed, it is necessary to totally remove the transverse process. **G.** Type of unilateral fusion done on this patient. **H.** AP x-ray taken 30 months after operation shows that the lower one-half of the pedicle and transverse process has been removed on the left. A unilateral fusion has been done on the right from L5 to S1. Because of the narrowing of the L5 disc space, an interbody fusion was not added. The patient obtained a solid fusion. (**E–G:** Reprinted with permission from Wiltse et al. Spine 9, 31-41 1984.)

She underwent surgical decompression of the painful L5 level, with removal of the lower one half of the left pedicle and the entire left transverse process. A unilateral fusion on the right was done. In her case, we believed that

because of the marked narrowing of the fifth interspace no further stabilization beyond the unilateral fusion would be necessary. Approximately 30 months after surgery she is able to walk more than a mile a day. Her one-level unilateral fusion is solid. She does have some residual back pain but no leg pain.

Case 2: A 39–year-old male with isthmic spondylolisthesis and 24% slippage presented with low back pain and right leg pain. On examination, there was decreased sensation in the L5 nerve distribution; sciatic tension tests were markedly positive on the right side only. The CT scan showed approximation of the pedicle, the base of the transverse process, and even the tip of the transverse process to the ala of the sacrum.

At surgery, a complete decompression was done on the painful right side, with removal of the lower one-half of the pedicle. Because of the marked compression of the nerve, the entire transverse process had to be removed. A contralateral one-level posterolateral fusion was done at the same time. Because his L5 disc was fairly wide and we were concerned about further slippage, an L5–S1 interbody fusion of the Crock type was done approximately 10 days after the posterior operation. He was allowed up immediately (Fig. 13.5).

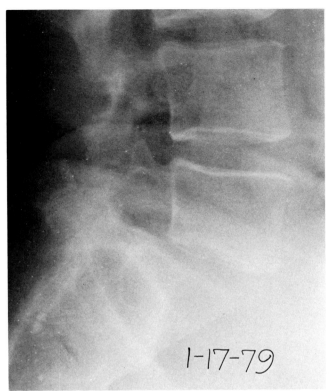

B

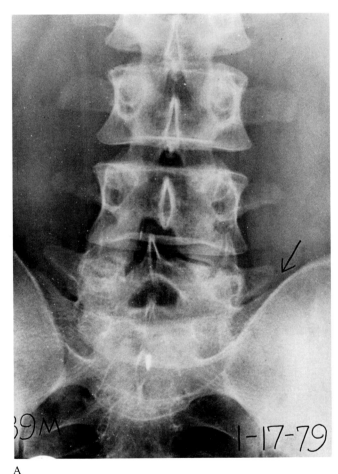

A

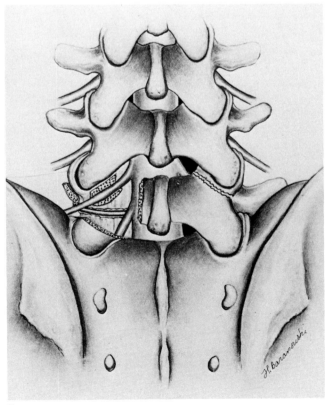

C

FIGURE 13.5 Isthmic spondylolisthesis. **A.** AP x-ray of a 39-year-old male with isthmic spondylolisthesis. Note the close approximation of the right lateral mass and the transverse process of L5 to the ala. At surgery the nerve was seen to be compressed all the way out to the lateral one third of the shaft of the transverse process. **B.** Lateral view, preoperatively. **C.** Type of decompression done in the patient whose x-rays are shown here. The decompression was on the opposite side. (*Figure continued* on page 392.)

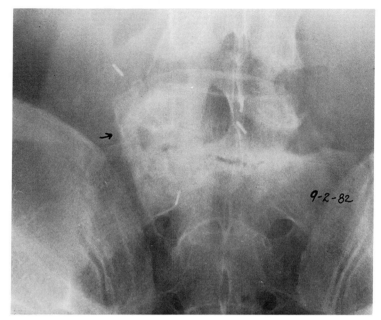

D

FIGURE 13.5 (*cont'd*) **D.** AP view 30 months after operation shows total decompression, with transverse processectomy on the right. Some new bone has formed where the transverse process was removed. The left side shows a unilateral posterolateral fusion. The operation was done through paraspinal approaches, which we believe makes both the decompression and the fusion easier. **E.** Lateral view showing Crock-type interbody fusion 30 months after fusion. (**D, E.**: Reprinted with permission from Wiltse et al. Spine 9, 31-41 1984.)

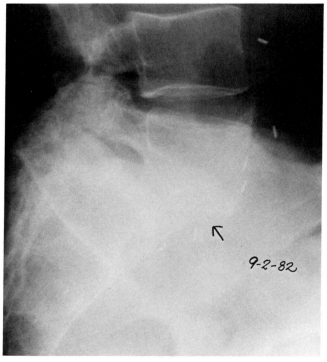

E

slippage in isthmic spondylolisthesis, the condition is also common and probably accounts for many of the failures of the Gill operation. Interestingly, Gill too has recommended that a spinal fusion not be done immediately after his operation, because laying bone over a wide decompression with exposed spinal nerves is likely to produce pain laterally. We also do not recommend fusion across the wide gap between the sacral ala and the L5 transverse process that is inevitable after far lateral decompression.

The question is: Will a unilateral L5/sacrum fusion produce arthrodesis in a high percentage of cases? If there is marked narrowing of the fifth disc space, it probably will; if the fifth disc space is quite normal, it may not. Simple narrowing of a disc space does not increase its stability; severe narrowing with osteoarthritic spurring does. In the patient with type I far-out syndrome, with very marked narrowing of the fifth interspace and osteophytic overgrowth, it is likely that unilateral total decompression can be done, even without fusion, without danger of serious instability.[13]

Summary

The authors have presented a syndrome that occurs in two types of patient: the elderly patient with degenerative lumbar scoliosis, and a somewhat younger adult population with isthmic spondylolisthesis and at least 20% slippage.

The Ferguson view is the best plain-radiographic view for visualizing the condition; however, reformatted CT scanning is also a valuable diagnostic tool. With the CT scan, the approximation of the transverse processes and ala can be visualized well, especially in the coronal view. The

Discussion

The question might be asked: Just how common is this syndrome? In the elderly person who comes to surgery because of lumbar spinal stenosis but who also has degenerative scoliosis of more than 20 degrees, it probably is very common. In the middle-aged adult with more than 30%

descending nerve is usually clearly seen. However, the radiologist must be alerted to reconstruct sagittally all the way out to the tips of the transverse processes or he will miss the lesion.

The symptoms are classic for nerve root compression. This usually occurs at the fifth lumbar nerve, but other levels can be involved, e.g., at the apex of convexity in scoliosis or in cases where there is spondylolisthesis at other than the L5 level.

It is very important that decompression be carried out far laterally, even if it means sacrificing the lower one half of the pedicle and the entire transverse process.

Because so much bone is removed, instability is a factor to be seriously considered. If there is marked joint-space narrowing, with severe osteophytic formation, one may not need to do a fusion. If in doubt, do a unilateral fusion.

References

1. Danforth MD, Wilson PD: The anatomy of the lumbosacral region in relation to sciatic pain. J Bone Joint Surg 7:109–160, 1925
2. Putti V: Pathogenesis of sciatic pain. Lancet July: 54–60, 1927
3. Williams PC: Reduced lumbosacral joint space. JAMA 99–20:1677–1682, 1932
4. Lindblom K: Protrusions of discs and nerve compression in the lumbar region. Acta Radiol (Stockh) 25:195–212, 1944
5. Hirsch C: On lumbar facetectomies. Acta Orthop Scand 17:240–252, 1948
6. Briggs H, Krause J: The intervertebral foraminotomy for relief of sciatic pain. J Bone Joint Surg 27–3:475–478, 1945
7. Wiltse LL, Guyer RD, Spencer CW, Glenn, WV, Porter, IS: Spine 9:31–41, 1984.
8. Echols DH, Rehfeldt FC: Failure to disclose ruptured intervertebral discs in 32 operations for sciatica. J Neurosurg 6:376–382, 1949
9. Schlesinger PT: Low lumbar nerve root compression and adequate operative exposure. J Bone Joint Surg 39A:541–553, 1957
10. Verbiest H: A radicular syndrome from developmental narrowing of the lumbar vertebral canal. J Bone Joint Surg 36B:230–237, 1954
11. Kirkaldy-Willis WH, et al.: Lumbar spinal nerve entrapment. Clin Orthop 169:171–178, 1982
12. Wiltse LL: The paraspinal sacrospinalis splitting approach to the lumbar spine. Clin Orthop 35:116, 1964
13. Hazlett JW, Kinnard P: Lumbar apophyseal process excision and spinal stability. Spine 7:171–176, 1982

Additional Readings

1. Briggs H: Operative aspect of low back pain. J Med Soc NJ 45:404–406, 1948
2. McNab I: Negative disc exploration. J Bone Joint Surg 53A:891–903, July 1971.
3. Mixter WJ, Barr JS: Rupture of the intervertebral disc with involvement of the spinal canal. N Engl J Med 211–5:210–215, August 1934
4. Schlesinger PT: Incarceration of the first sacral nerve in a lateral bony recess of the spinal canal as a cause of sciatica. J Bone Joint Surg 37–A:115–124, January 1955

Cervical and Thoracic Spine

14

Many facilities with confidence and expertise in lumbar CT work have met with considerable disappointment when attempting to extend their diagnostic capabilities to the cervical spine. The authors' experience is no exception, and in retrospect, there are two main reasons: differences in the gross sizes of anatomic structures and in the appropriateness of scanning and filming protocols.

A common mistake is to perform cervical CT examinations with a scanning protocol similar to that used for the lumbar area. In our practice, slice thicknesses of 5 mm were used initially, although were later modified. Slice spacing was decreased from 3 mm to 2.5 mm, and later to 1.5 mm. Formerly, in a typical spine examination, with 5 mm thick images taken every 2.5 mm, five or six cervical interspaces were covered. Gross abnormalities, e.g., severe central-canal stenosis, rotatory scoliosis, subluxations, and large discs, were readily identified. Subtle but important abnormalities, e.g., small, strategically located foraminal spurs and small lateral discs, were not routinely detected.

A significant change of attitude, as reflected in diagnostic confidence and referring physician enthusiasm, occurred when two changes in scanning protocol were instituted. The examination was limited to three or four rather than five or six cervical interspaces, so that, unless otherwise specified, a routine cervical examination covered from mid-C7 body superiorly to mid-C4 body, with additional tilted-axial survey cuts at C2–3, C3–4, and C7–T1. Second, both slice thickness and spacing were reduced to 1.5 mm. This was done to better accommodate the small cervical structures being examined and thereby demonstrate the important subtleties that a coarser scanning protocol simply bypassed.

Perhaps the best way to illustrate the significant improvement in image quality and potential diagnostic accuracy of 1.5 mm thick sections every 1.5 mm over 5 mm thick scans every 2.5 mm is to show the bony detail using each of these techniques. Figure 14.1A illustrates the earlier protocol. This should be compared with the much higher level of bony detail shown in Figure 14.1B. Spondylitic ridges from prominent end-plates and their lateral extension and potential encroachment of foramina represent a good comparative test for bone detail.

The second major reason for early disappointment in cervical work was the incorrect assumption that a single scanning and filming protocol would be as appropriate for cervical examinations as it was for lumbar examinations. Optimal cervical CT diagnosis requires more flexibility in terms of image manipulation and display options.

Disorders of the cervical spine fall into four broad groups: (1) localized lesions of the craniocervical junction; (2) nonarthritic lesions of bone at any cervical level; (3) diseases of the spinal cord, and (4) degenerative diseases of the disc and the vertebral joint. It is very important for the scanning protocol to be tailored to the primary diagnostic category.

Categories (1) and (2) emphasize evaluation of localized osseous lesions, tumors, trauma, and craniocervical junction anomalies. These groups of disorders practically never involve disc spaces. There is adequate low-contrast resolution, even in this type of study, to see cerebellar tonsils and the cervicomedullary junction. For best visualization of bone detail, the examination is performed using thin axial sections with small pixel size and maximal edge enhancement of osseous structures.

394

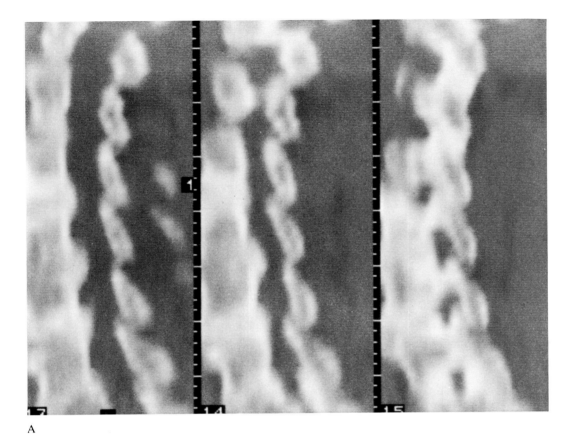

A

B

FIGURE 14.1 Comparison of 5- and 1.5-mm axial slices. **A.** Sagittal reformation of 5 mm thick axial scans performed every 2.5 mm. Note the large degenerative ridges. **B.** Sagittal reformation of 1.5 mm thick axial scans performed every 1.5 mm. Note the small interbody fusion plug between two large central osteophytes. The geometric resolution is much improved when thin axial scans are used.

It is appropriate to trade off low-contrast resolution for bone detail. To achieve this, patients are scanned with a small circle of reconstruction, as in head scanning. The images are targeted to at least life-size (target factor 1.6). On rare occasions, when the lesion in question is very small, obtaining 1.5 mm thick sections every 1 mm increases the proximity of images by 33% (1.5 mm to 1 mm) and may be of diagnostic advantage over 1.5–mm spacing. It is important to properly position the patient's head such that any metallic dental restorations are excluded from the scanning field. This is usually accomplished by hyperextending or markedly flexing the head, depending on what anatomic zones are of primary interest.

When there is a high index of suspicion for disc herniation, the thin-slice technique is preferred. This type of disc examination includes the disc spaces most commonly found to be abnormal: C7, C6, C5. When clinically indicated, T1 and C4 are also included in the reformatted study. It is then desirable, for completeness, to obtain two axial slices at interspaces above and below the reconstruction; this is done with tilted-axial slices for survey purposes. In the unusual instance when evaluation is directed toward the medulla, cerebellar tonsils, or cervical cord for syringomyelia, it is preferable to use a scanning protocol with 5 mm thick images spaced every 2.5 mm, using a soft-tissue reconstruction algorithm. The scan is performed using the smallest possible scanning circle. Studies involving the tonsils and lower medulla extend well into the posterior fossa. When the entire cervical spine must be examined, either because of diffuse disease or syringomyelia, the use of thin sections would be unreasonable. In order to cover such distances, it is necessary to use 5 mm thick scans taken every 2.5–3mm.

To minimize shoulder artifact, the shoulders are passively pulled down to remove the humoral heads from the scanning field whenever possible. This is best accomplished by placing soft, broad armbands on the forearms and attaching these bands to a device that allows gentle but constant shoulder traction (Fig. 14.2). The patient is not told to pull down on the ropes because this nearly always produces cervical motion. Breathing during scanning cannot be avoided, and so patients are instructed to use steady shallow respirations. Swallowing artifacts, however, can be avoided in almost all cases if patients are encouraged to swallow between scans rather than during the data-acquisition phase. The type of artifact caused by swallowing is illustrated in Figure 14.3. One other precaution is to prevent the patients from sliding caudally out of the head holder. When sliding does occur, it is gradual and therefore undetected until the images are later seen with significant distortions.

The choice of size of the scanning field also requires careful consideration. In order to reduce intershoulder artifact, a large scanning field is desirable, although this per-

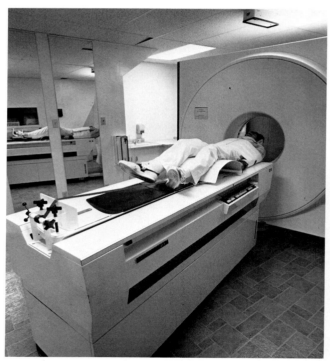

FIGURE 14.2 Patient positioning. A patient properly positioned for a CT scan of the cervical spine. The patient's head is restrained in a plastic head rest, and the arms are pulled down passively by a simple traction device. Note the position of the traction below the plane of the patient's body, which reduces shoulder pain. Traction device (Cat-Trac cervical traction device, CT Innovations, 536 East First Avenue, La Habra, CA 90631).

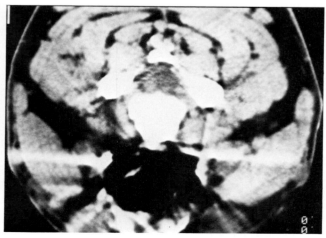

FIGURE 14.3 Artifact produced by motion of the airway caused by swallowing, speaking, or crying. Note that although the bone has not moved, streaks emanate from the airway and cast confusing shadows.

mits only 1.5–mm pixels in the reconstruction. If those scans are then targeted to nearly life-size, an aliasing artifact is produced because of inadequate sampling rate. The artifact is manifest as a fine herringbone pattern in the images (Fig. 14.4). For this reason the scanning circle is made as small as possible and the reformations targeted to nearly life-size. This optimizes the scan for the upper 6 vertebral segments. Supplementary tilted-axial survey slices can be taken at the C7–T1 interspace if shoulder artifact is a problem. As a general rule, it is best to optimize the examination for the majority of the cervical segments being covered and to accept somewhat poorer soft-tissue resolution at the C7–T1 level (due to shoulders). With the tilted-axial supplementary C7–T1 images, considerably more traction on the shoulders can be used over a very short period of time rather than such traction throughout the entire examination.

The standard three-level protocol used by technologists for GE 8800 cervical cases is as follows:

Scouts	AP and lateral
Thickness; spacing	1.5 mm; 1.5 mm
Prospective target	Yes
Calibration file	Infant
Target factor	15 cm F.O.V. (1.6)
Algorithm	1
Raw-data save	No

Survey other levels	Yes
Contrast	No
Process CT/MPR	Yes, life-size
Film	Life-size + bone (12-on-1)

1. Use a passive arm-traction device, preferably with wide arm bands. Provide a leg support to prevent patient sliding, and place the traction bar very low to the table.
2. Use a head holder made of plastic (which does not cause major artifacts) to adequately secure the head; tape the head carefully.
3. Tuck a large flat square sponge under the GE black pad to prevent the patient from sliding.
4. The patient must not swallow during the actual scan.
5. Modify the generator from slow tube cooling to fast tube cooling.
6. Avoid dropping scanner software to the ''R'' level for at least 15 minutes before performing a cervical examination.
7. Apply a dynamic scan for the first 25 slices—using 320 mA and a 15–sec interscan time delay—and complete remainder of scans using 320 mA. For a difficult patient, a second dynamic series can be prescribed using 250 mA.
8. Use a cervical collar to prevent the patient from flexing or extending the head during the scan.

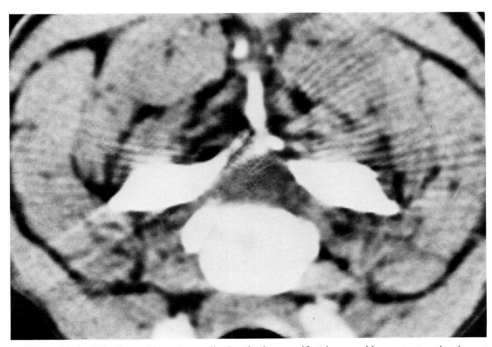

FIGURE 14.4 Aliasing artifact. A peculiar herringbone artifact is caused by reconstruction image pixels that are smaller than the actual sampled volume. For example, in a large-body calibration file, assuming a 5-mm slice thickness, the actual measured volume is 1.5 × 1.5 × 5 mm. Reconstructing this with a target value of 2.8 would produce image pixels of approximately 0.5 mm. A situation has been produced where the display is forced to be more accurate than the measurement of the data, which causes the phenomenon called aliasing.

Craniocervical Junction

Radiologists doing detailed diagnostic work with polytomography of the sella, temporal bones, etc., discovered the cognitive efficiency and convenience associated with the organization of radiographs into highly coned, numbered sequences of images at standardized intervals in multiple perspectives. The filming technique used in CT/MPR examinations encompasses the same approach for the same reasons.

A patient with a normal cranioverterbral articulation is shown in Figure 14.5. Each of the three views is impor-

tant for the evaluation of different anatomic structures. The axial plane is ideal for evaluating the bony neural canal. In the axial plane at the upper cervical levels one must evaluate (1) the bony ring of C1; (2) the relationship of the dens to the anterior arch of C1; (3) the tubercles into which the transverse ligament inserts; (4) the body of C2; and (5) the anterior and posterior rims of the foramen magnum.

The sagittal and coronal planes are best for evaluating the dens, the craniocervical zygapophyseal articulations, and the atlantoaxial joints. Lesions of the dens are best identified on the sagittal view, whereas atlantooccipital joint abnormalities are frequently identified best in the coronal projection. Using thin-section CT with special targeting for bone detail, it is possible to identify all of the minute contours and structures in this region. Even a sclerotic central fusion plane of the two halves of the dens and the C1–2 disc space remnant can be identified (Fig. 14.5C).

This chapter is not meant to be an encyclopedic dissertation on cervical spine disease. The intention is to convince the reader that multiplanar reformatted CT, when properly performed, is in most cases superior, and always at least equivalent, to conventional tomographic examination. In a very substantial portion of cases this type of CT also obviates cervical myelography.

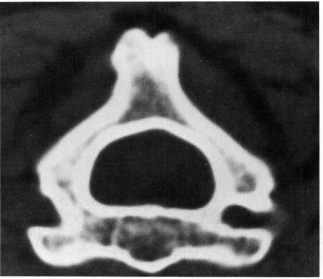

A

FIGURE 14.5 Normal atlantoaxial segment. Axial view of C1 (**A**), axial view of C2 (**B**), sagittal view (**C**), and coronal view (**D**). Reformation of 1.5 mm thick axial scans produced every 1.5 mm. Note the plane of fusion between the two halves of the dens (*arrow*) and the remnant of the C1–2 disc space.

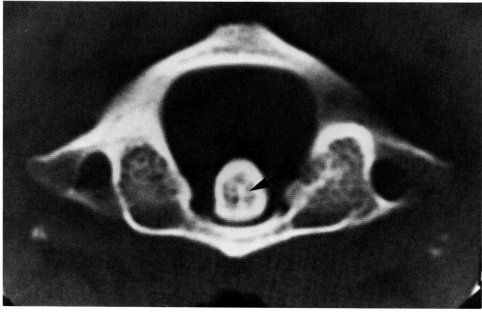

B

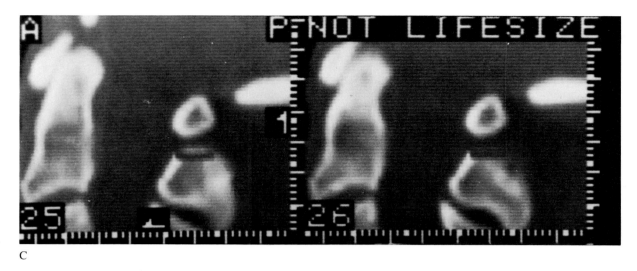

C

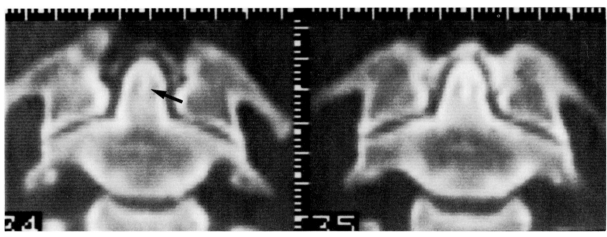

D

Congenital Lesions

Most congenital anomalies of the craniovertebral junction are due to either failure of segmentation or partial vertebral dysplasia. The craniocervical junction develops from the first cervical and fourth occipital somites.[1] The occipital vertebral segment above C1 is called the proatlas. The anterior portion forms the occipital condyles. The posterior portion assimilates with C1 and becomes part of the upper facet surface and the posterior ponticle, forming a bony root over the vertebral artery and the tip of the dens.

Occipital dysplasia is a term used to describe abnormalities of those portions of the craniocervical junction that originate from the occipital vertebral segments.[2] Many patients are asymptomatic. Those who do require medical attention often do so late in life because of pain or signs of myelopathy or lower cranial nerve compression. Assimilation of the atlas is an uncommon anomaly seen in less than 0.3% of patients[3] and is usually associated with other abnormalities.

The patient in Figure 14.6 presented with a myelopathy. Axial CT is difficult to interpret, but no C1 ring is demonstrable. The dens is somewhat peculiar in shape and dramatically dislocated posteriorly. Sagittal reformation confirms assimilation of the atlas with the occipital bone and concomitant upward displacement of the dens through the foramen magnum. The upper cervical spinal cord and medulla, which are surrounded by metrizamide, are displaced posteriorly and compressed between the dens and the posterior rim of the foramen magnum.

Suboccipital dysplasia is a malformation of the C1 and C2 vertebral segments. The most common abnormalities of C1 are vertebral ring clefts and partial aplasia. These occasionally occur in the midline anteriorly or, more commonly, in the center of the posterior arch. Bilateral hypoplasia of the posterior arch is frequently observed, in varying amounts, and must not be confused with fractures. It is important to recognize that if the tomographic axial examination is angled improperly it will produce images that

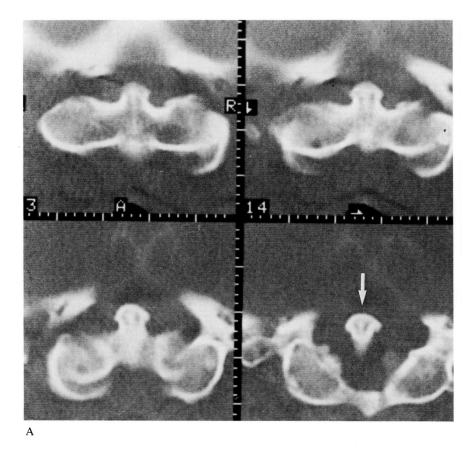

A

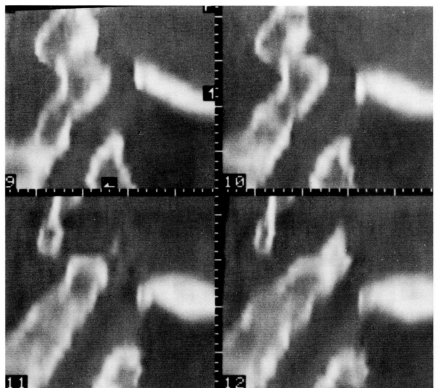

B

FIGURE 14.6 Assimilation of the axis. Axial (**A**) and sagittal (**B**) views computed from 5 mm thick axial scans demonstrate marked posterior dislocation of the dens (*arrow*). The anterior arch of C1 is fused to the anterior lip of the foramen magnum. On sagittal view #12 the dens is seen to be herniated upward into the center of the foramen magnum.

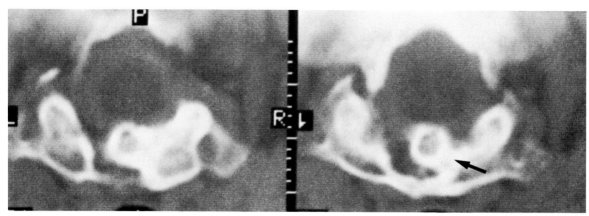

FIGURE 14.7 Fusion of the dens to the arch of C1. Axial scans demonstrate fusion of the dens to the right lateral mass and the tubercle of C1 (*arrow*). The diameter of the spinal canal is not reduced.

cross the plane of the C1 ring obliquely, producing the appearance of bilateral discontinuity. One should be able to deduce this from serial CT scans. Sagittal reformations clearly demonstrate the anatomy of the normal ring.

The axial scans in Figure 14.7 demonstrate unilateral right-sided fusion of the dens to the atlas ring in the area of the tubercle. These lesions are quite rare. They may be associated anomalies of the anterior arch of C1, with varying degrees of dens hypoplasia.

The patient shown in Figure 14.8 has a unique and very complex combination of abnormalities. In the axial plane one can identify a small anterior midline cleft in the anterior arch of C1. This defect should not be mistaken for a fracture because the ends of the defect are normally corticated, which is typical of an anomalous failure of osseous fusion. Likewise, clefts in the posterior vertebral arches have smooth cortical ends. Unfortunately, it was impossible to position the child within the scanner so as to produce axial scans parallel to the plane of C1 because the C1 ring could not be identified on the digital scout radiograph. Hence one might erroneously suspect fractures of the ring laterally.

Sagittal reformations near the midline are most abnormal. They identify an absent or hypoplastic dens. Instead of the normal dens, there is a small soft-tissue mass

with a central zone of ossification. The key image is the coronal reformation (Fig. 14.8C), which represents a plane through the center of the lateral masses of C1 and hence through the abnormal location of the dens. Thoughtful analysis of this one view reveals a lucent cleft between the two halves of a typical hypoplastic dens; there is even continuity of the line with the C1–2 disc space remnant. Above the rounded hypoplastic dens is a pair of tiny ossification centers within the previously noted soft-tissue mass. This patient has an os odontoideum anomaly. It is the only possible explanation for this specific pattern of vertebral maldevelopment. The one problem with the diagnosis is the absence of the bony os. However, this patient also has chondrodysplasia, which accounts for the failure of normal ossification from endochondral bone of the proatlas segment of the tip of the dens. Os odontoideum anomaly is characterized by a normal C2 portion of the axis with bilaterally hypoplastic C1 components. The proatlantal terminal ossicle becomes enlarged and is not normally fused to the dens. The large bony mass may dislocate posteriorly or anteriorly and cause medullary compression. The anterior arch of the atlas is frequently thickened, further compromising the spinal canal (Fig. 14.9).

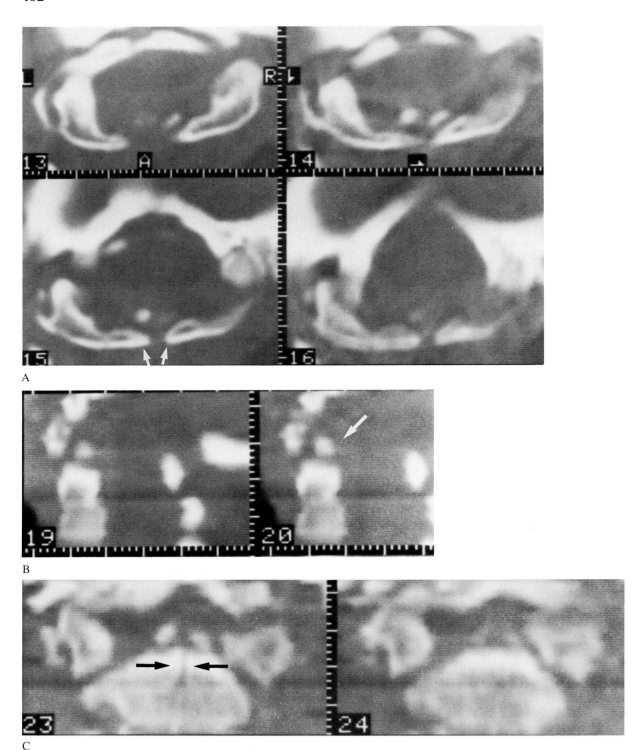

FIGURE 14.8 Unossified os odontoideum. **A.** Axial scans demonstrate a central cleft in the anterior arch of C1. The margins of the defect are covered with cortical bone (*arrow*). There is no normal dens present; in its place is a subtle soft-tissue density (invisible because of the wide window) with two symmetrical calcifications (*arrow*). **B.** Sagittal reformation confirms hypoplasia of the dens. **C.** Coronal reformation defines the problem best. Note hypoplasia of the C2 portion of the body with a central cleft (*arrows*). This represents the fusion plane of the two halves of the malformed dens. The two symmetrical ossification centers are within an os odontoideum that has not ossified.

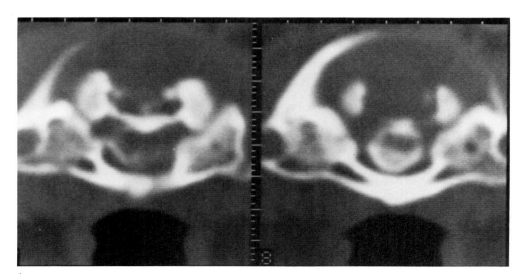

A

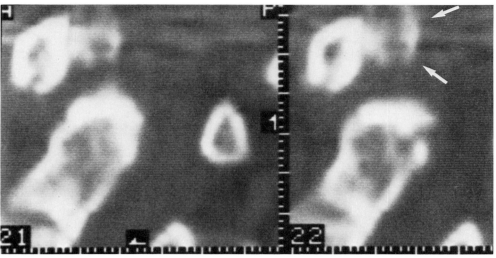

B

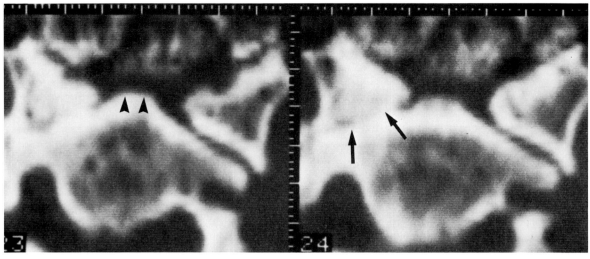

C

FIGURE 14.9 Dislocated os odontoideum. **A, B.** Patient 1. Sagittal reformations demonstrate a large os odontoideum (*arrows*). The os and the entire C1 ring are dislocated anteriorly. The upper spinal cord is compressed between the back of the dens and the posterior arch of C1. **C.** Coronal reformation. Note the rounded hypoplastic dens that is separated from the os (*arrowheads*). There is severe degeneration of the left atlantoaxial joint (*arrow*). (*Figure continued* on page 404.)

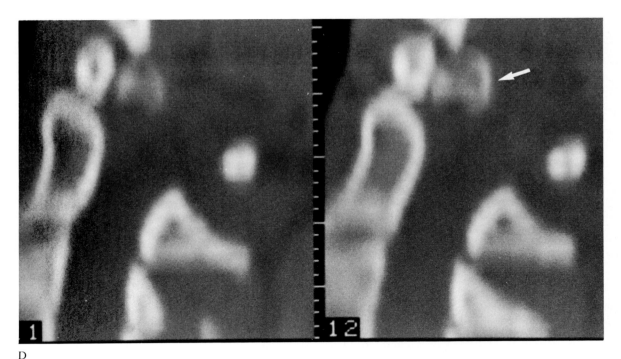

D

FIGURE 14.9 (*cont'd*) **D.** Patient 2. The os odontoideum and the C1 ring are displaced posteriorly. The narrowest diameter of the spinal canal is between the posterior margin of the os and the lamina of C2.

Traumatic Lesions

Conventional radiography defines gross bony spinal integrity and alignment. Major fractures or dislocations are obvious. Ligamentous injury without fracture can be evaluated by very careful flexion/extension films and fluoroscopic examination. However, these procedures frequently underestimate the extent of cervical trauma. Recent advances in thin-section CT and multiplanar reformation have increased the utility of CT so that it has now supplanted conventional tomography in the evaluation of spine trauma.[4–6]

The major advantage of CT is that it is performed in the supine position. No uncomfortable or dangerous manipulation is required to optimize filming. Cervical traction devices can be used without interfering with the scanning procedure. Any required projection can be obtained from the same axial data without significantly increased patient irradiation. Intrathecal metrizamide may be a useful adjunct in acutely traumatized patients with neurologic deficits.

Postoperative scanning of traumatized patients is quite useful for evaluating of abnormalities of alignment as well as spinal canal and neural foraminal compression.

Severe cervical trauma produces symptoms because of neural compression or bony instability. Both can be adequately evaluated by CT. The scans in Figure 14.10 were

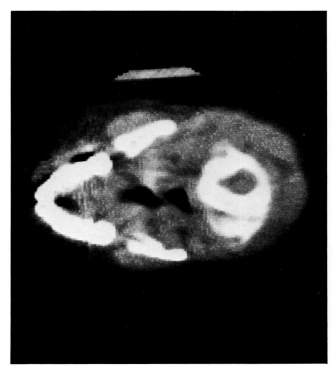

FIGURE 14.10 Rotary dislocation of C1–2. This supine patient's head was rotated 90 degrees to the long axis of his body. The facets are seen to be totally dislocated and the spinal canal is prominently narrowed. (Reprinted with permission from Geehr et al. Comput Tomogr 2:79–97, 1978.)

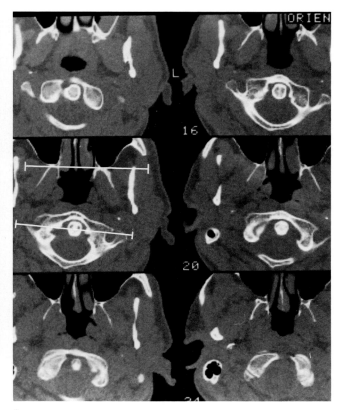

A

performed in 1976 with a first-generation CT scanner. This patient was sleighing down a hill and crashed into a tree. He proceeded to walk back up the hill but suddenly developed severe neck pain. He turned his head to the right, where it became fixed at approximately 90 degrees to the long axis of his body. Routine radiographs and conventional tomograms revealed no fracture and an appropriate relationship of the anterior arch to the dens. However, CT demonstrated total rotatory dislocation of the left C1–2 facets. After appropriate reduction and fixation, the patient made an uneventful recovery. This case is important because it is generally believed that one should see a C1 dens separation in order to make the diagnosis of rotatory subluxation.[4]

Figure 14.11 is a series of axial scans on a patient who was hit by a train. Although he had no major neurologic deficit, he had been complaining of neck pain for 2 years before this scan. Routine radiographs were reported as being normal on several occasions. These axial views are subtly abnormal. Under normal circumstances there is no rotation possible between the occipital condyles and C1. In this patient there is a 13 degree rotation between C1 and the plane of the maxillary sinuses. This should never occur.

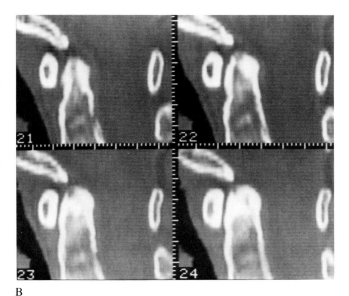

B

FIGURE 14.11 Traumatic cranio-occipital subluxation. **A.** Axial composite, which demonstrates no hint of fracture. The arch of C1 is rotated 13 degrees to the left with respect to the maxilla. This should never occur. **B.** Midline sagittal views are normal. (*Figure continued* on page 406.)

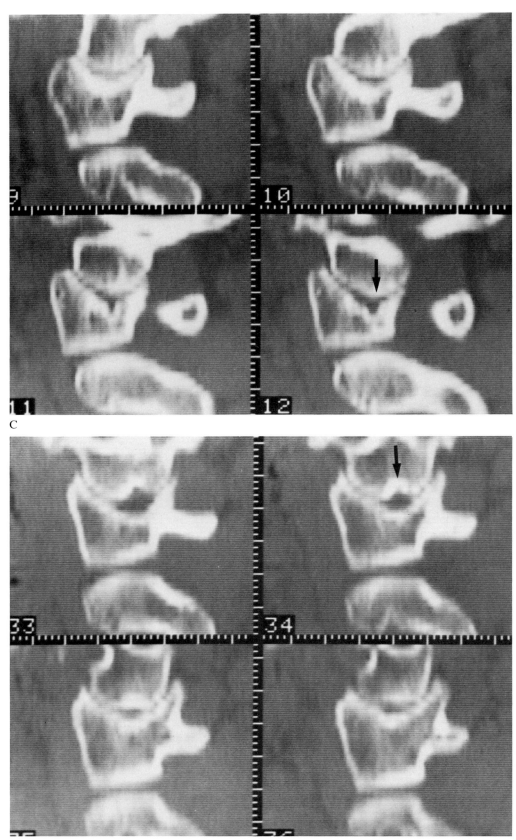

FIGURE 14.11 (*cont'd*) **C, D.** Sagittal views of the left and right atlantooccipital joints, revealing compression fracture of the left lateral mass of C1 and the right occipital condyle (*arrows*).

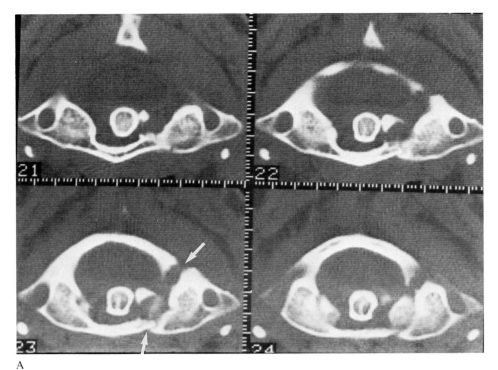

A

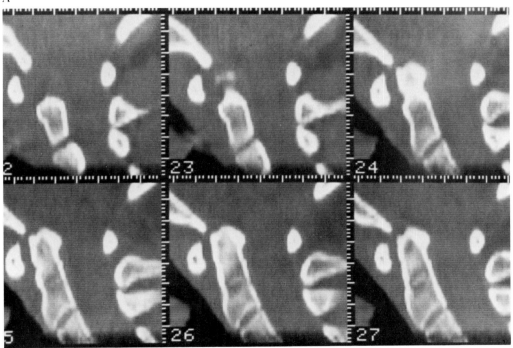

B

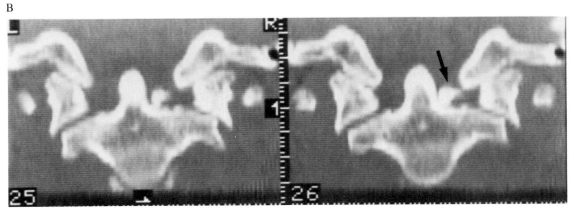

C

FIGURE 14.12 Jefferson fracture. **A.** Axial views demonstrate anterior and posterior fractures of the C1 ring (*arrows*). The dens is subluxed posteriorly. **B.** Sagittal views reveal slight posterior and superior displacement of the dens. **C.** Coronal reformation defines bilateral lateral offset of the C1 facets and a dislocated fragment torn from the right lateral mass (*arrow*).

The relationship of the dens to the anterior arch of C1 is normal. Although the rotation is apparent on these axial scans, the cause is not. On sagittal reformations, however, two occult fractures are noted: On the left there is compression of the occipital condyle; on the right there is compression fracture of the lateral mass of C1. Although this problem does not require surgery, the correct diagnosis was very important because of the medicolegal implications of definable anatomic injury.

The patient shown in Figure 14.12 has a complicated Jefferson fracture. The axial views demonstrate bursting of the arch of C1 on the right. The posterior portion of the fracture occurred in a fairly typical place, adjacent to the lateral mass. The anterior portion of the fracture goes through the anterior arch, but in this case the tubercle is also fractured off. On the sagittal view the dens is shown to be herniated upward toward the foramen magnum. The coronal view demonstrates the bilateral lateral dislocation that is the hallmark of this disorder.

A series of scans on a patient with a hangman's fracture is shown in Figure 14.13. The fracture lines traverse the neural arch at its insertion into the lateral masses. The sagittal view is key here, especially in the evaluation of fracture healing. This is a relatively common motor vehicle injury. Fortunately, by its very nature, it is a self-decompressing lesion, and patients often avoid serious neurologic consequences.

Fractures of the dens are difficult to evaluate in the axial plane. They mostly occur perpendicular to the long axis of the dens and are therefore quite obscure. In Figure 14.14, sagittal reformations demonstrate a displaced fracture through the base of the dens. This amount of displacement was easily diagnosed on routine radiographs. The CT did, however, exclude extradural hematoma or bone fragments.

Nontraumatic destruction of C1 or C2 is usually caused by tumor or infection. Metastases are the most common lesions in this category. Axial scans demonstrate the re-

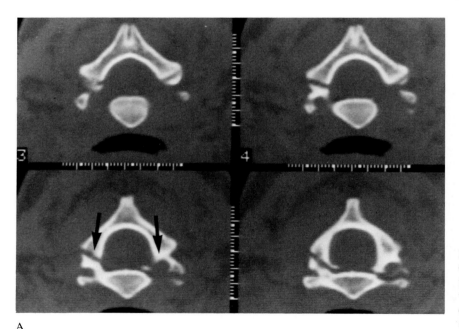

A

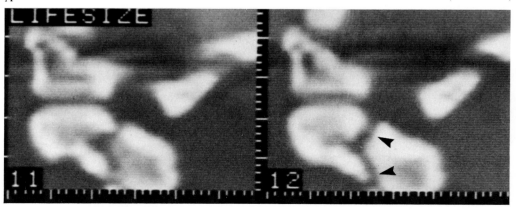

B

FIGURE 14.13 Hangman's fracture of C2. **A.** Axial scans demonstrate bilateral fractures of the neural arch just behind the vertebral body (*arrows*). **B.** Sagittal reformation through the left arch fracture (*arrowheads*).

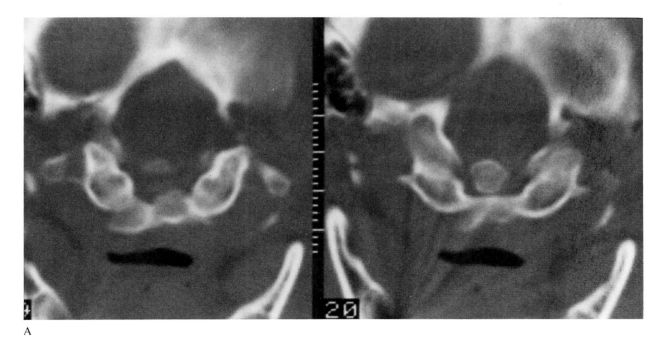

A

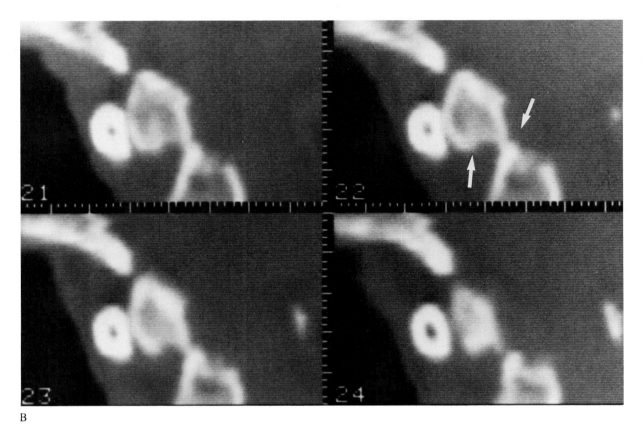

B

FIGURE 14.14 Fracture through the base of the dens. **A.** Axial scans demonstrate malalignment of C1 and C2. The diagnosis of fracture would be difficult without a history. **B.** Sagittal reformation clearly indicates almost total forward dislocation of the fractured dens (*arrows*). The spinal canal is narrowed by more than 50%.

placement of bone by abnormal soft tissue. The differential diagnosis between infection, metastases, and some benign lesions may be quite difficult. Benign processes tend to preserve bony contours, and malignant processes tend to cause more bone destruction. The two unusual patients in Figure 14.15 are quite similar. The first patient had a history of pituitary tumor for many years. A CT scan was performed as part of a routine follow-up because the patient was complaining about difficulty in hearing. Intracranial scans revealed a huge pituitary tumor that eroded the petrous bones. The tumor mass was so extensive it had invaded the ring of C1. The patient in Figure 14.15B had pulmonary coccidiomycosis. He presented with neck pain and a mass in the neck. There is a large lytic, slightly bubbly, destructive lesion of the left articular process that is quite similar to the tumor in Figure 14.15A. One could

not, from the CT appearance alone, exclude the possibility that either lesion is malignant.

Fractures of the midcervical spine can be conveniently divided into categories by the vector of the force producing them. Extension forces tend to cause fracture of the posterior elements with little vertebral body fragmentation. These injuries are especially difficult to evaluate radiographically and are very important clinically because they may produce devastating spinal cord injury with little or no vertebral injury. The axial scan in Figures 14.16A, B demonstrates irregularity of the articular process of C3. Oblique reformation defines a fracture of the superior facet. Fractures of the lateral mass are difficult to diagnose on axial views. This is especially true of compressive fractures (Fig. 14.16C). Oblique, sagittal, or curved coronal reformations eliminate this difficulty.

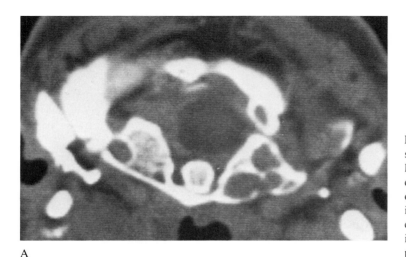

A

FIGURE 14.15 Destructive lesions at C1. **A.** Destruction of the lateral portion of the C1 ring by downward extension of a chromophobe adenoma. **B.** Interosseous infection due to coccidioidomycosis. There is nothing in either instance to allow a specific pathologic diagnosis.

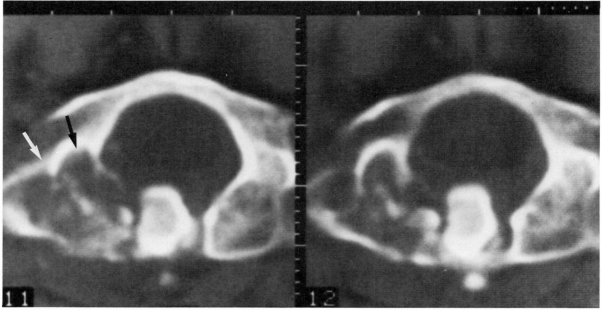

B

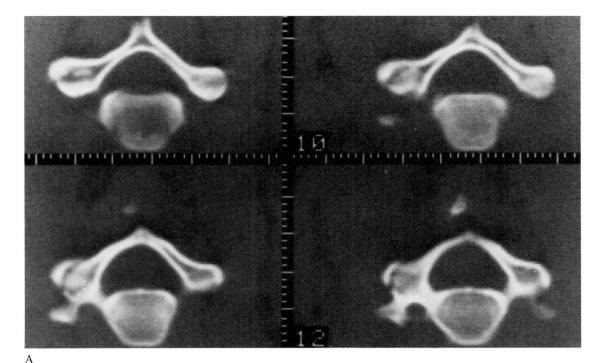

A

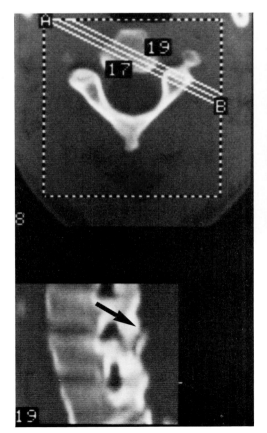

B

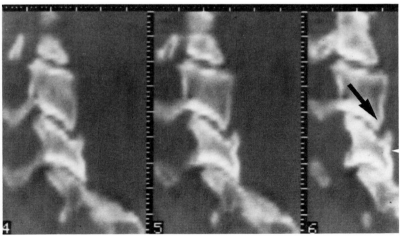

C

FIGURE 14.16 Fracture of the articular process. **A.** Axial scan demonstrates irregularity of the C3 lateral mass. **B.** Oblique reformation defines the flattening and fragmentation of the superior articular process (*arrow*). **C.** Sagital reformation on another patient with compression fracture of the left lateral mass of C6. Note the flattening of the superior articular process and an area of indentation (*arrows*).

An unusual hyperextension fracture is shown in Figure 14.17. This young patient fell from a surf board and was hit on the head. He complained of neck pain, but routine x-rays were reported as normal. During a 2-week follow-up period he developed increasing tingling in the fingers of his left hand. CT scan demonstrates bilateral fractures of the neural arch at the junction with the lateral masses. This, in effect, is the equivalent of a C6 hangman's fracture, which is a self-decompressing injury. The soft-tissue-window sagittal view demonstrates a left-sided disc herniation, which is the most likely cause of his presenting symptom.

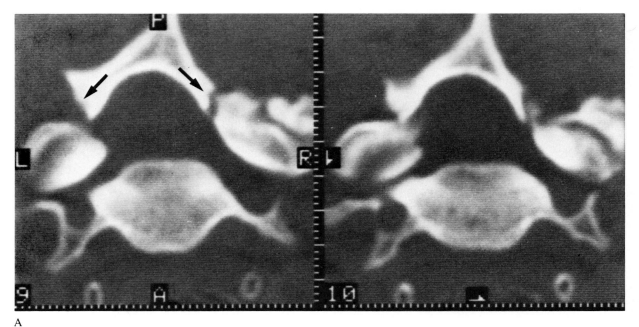

A

FIGURE 14.17   Hangman's fracture of C6. **A–C.** Axial scan (**A**), oblique reformation (**B**), and sagittal reformation (**C**) demonstrate bilateral fractures of the neural arch at the insertion into the lateral mass (*arrows*). There is no fracture of the vertebral body. **D.** Soft-tissue sagittal view reveals a left-sided disc herniation at the level above the fracture (*arrows*) which accounts for the patient's clinical signs. (*Figure continued* on page 413.)

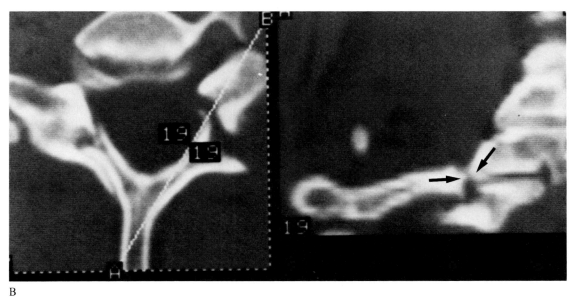

B

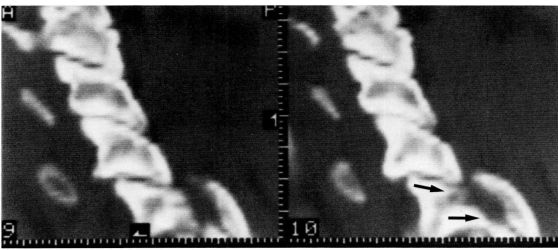

C

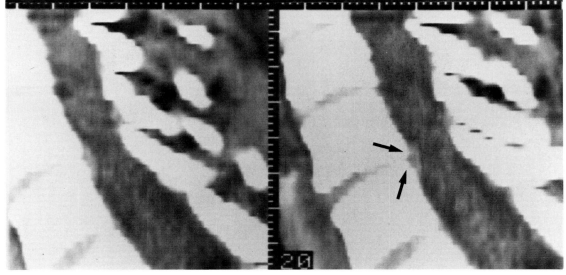

D

Flexion fractures are easier to diagnose because they usually involve some vertebral compression. This is generally diagnosed easily on routine radiographs. The subtleties of the fracture are best seen on CT. Figure 14.18 reveals a compression fracture of C5. Although there is loss of the normal lordotic curve, there is no dislocation. The vertebral body is fractured but not fragmented. The neural arch is intact.

The patient shown in Figure 14.19 has had more severe trauma. On the sagittal reformation one can see a separated bony "teardrop" fracture of C6. The C7 vertebra looks normal. Axial scans demonstrate bursting of the vertebral body with fragmentation. In this case, the neural arch is also fractured, making this an unstable injury. Coronal reformation reveals that the linear central component of the fracture extends in a linear fashion from C6 through C7.

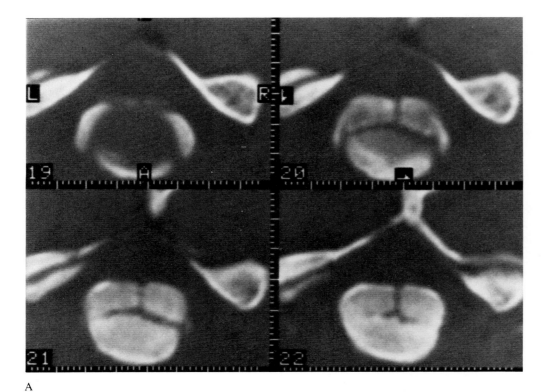

A

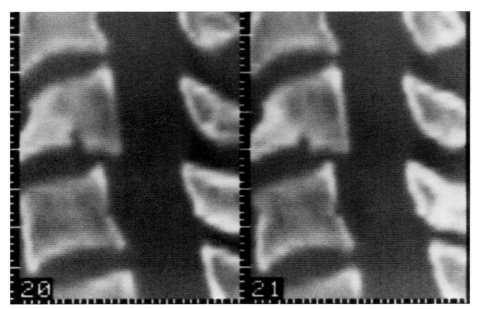

B

FIGURE 14.18 Flexion fracture at C5. **A.** Axial view demonstrates vertebral body fracture with normal neural arch. **B.** Sagittal views show the vertebral compression to advantage.

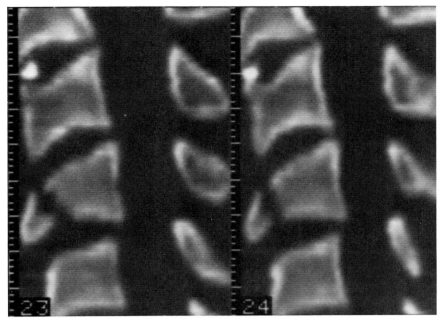

A

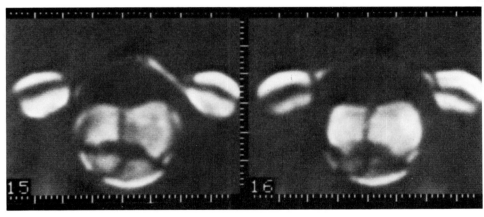

B

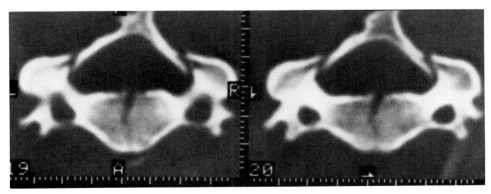

C

FIGURE 14.19 Compression fracture at C6 and C5. **A.** Sagittal views demonstrate a compression "teardrop" fracture of C6. The C5 vertebra looks normal. There is loss of the normal lordosis, but no bone is subluxated into the canal. **B, C.** Axial scans reveal fracture of the body and neural arches of C6 and C5. (*Figure continued* on page 416.)

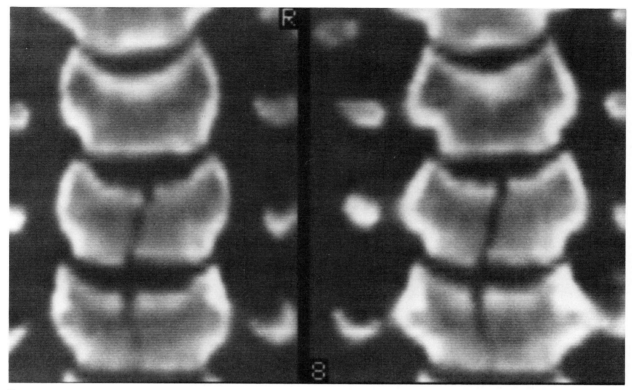

D

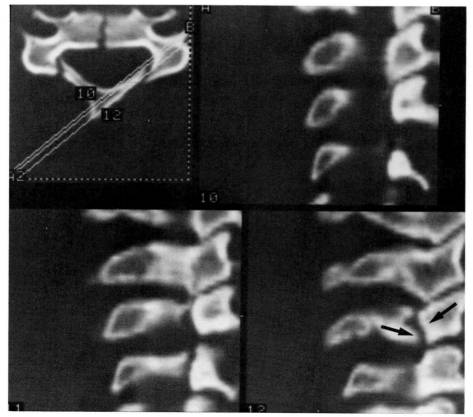

E

FIGURE 14.19 (*cont'd*) **D.** Coronal views show that the fracture line is continuous from C5 through C6. **E.** Oblique reformation depicts fracture at the insertion of the posterior arch (*arrows*).

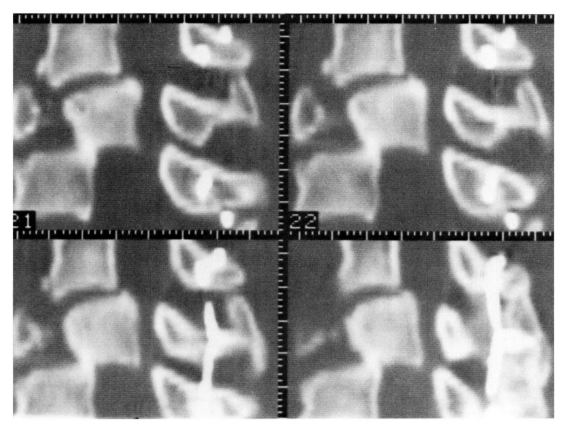

FIGURE 14.20   Burst fracture of C5. Sagittal reformation performed after spinal fusion demonstrates marked spinal stenosis due to retropulsion of the posterior portion of the fractured vertebral body.

The patient shown in Figure 14.20 was evaluated because of increased myelopathy after decompression and fusion for a bursting fracture of C5. He demonstrates the most severe end of the spectrum. Scans with sagittal reformations demonstrate that the fusion is intact but that there is very severe bony encroachment on the spinal canal. The vertebral body has broken into two fragments—one propelled forward and the other propelled posteriorly into the spinal canal. The sagittal diameter is severely reduced.

Soft-Tissue Abnormalities

Visualization of intraspinal soft-tissue structures without intravenous or intrathecal contrast enhancement requires excellent low-contrast resolution and careful soft-tissue photographic technique. Extramedullary tumors or cyst formation can frequently be detected on nonenhanced scans, especially when the spinal canal is normal in size and when there is a normal amount of cerebrospinal fluid (CSF) acting as a contrast medium. Figure 14.21 shows excellent definition of the cervical cord edges at C3–4. The four axial views are also convincing for a large low-density cystic area within the cord shadow; this was a large cervical syrinx that extended inferiorly over several levels. Many patients with Arnold-Chiari malformation and syringomyelia have cystic lesions large enough to be evaluated without metrizamide. Also, downward tonsillar herniation is easily seen on sagittal reformations. In normal patients there is always a triangle of CSF at the cervicomedullary junction behind the cord shadow. When tonsils herniate downward, this space becomes filled with brain-density material (Figs. 14.21C, D). It is very important when looking for tonsilar displacement to be sure that the patient's head is flexed so that the teeth are away from the plane of interest.

Intrathecal contrast medium is usually required when attempting to diagnose posttraumatic syrinx because the cavities tend to be somewhat smaller and localized. Figure 14.22 is a metrizamide-enhanced example of a syrinx shown after diffusion of metrizamide across the cord into the syrinx. It is not known exactly how metrizamide enters the cord. Some think it is due to transependymal or transpial diffusion, but others believe that pores are formed that con-

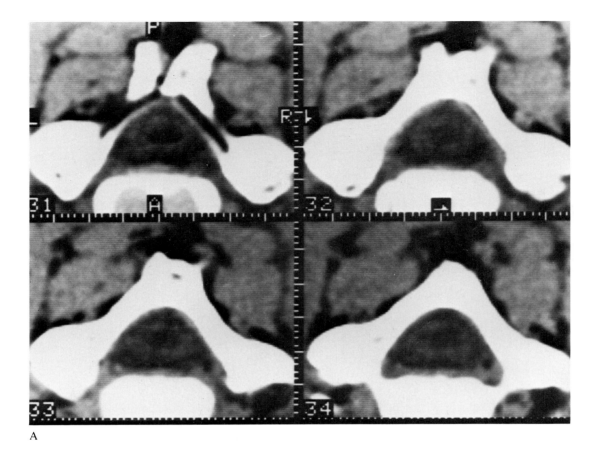

A

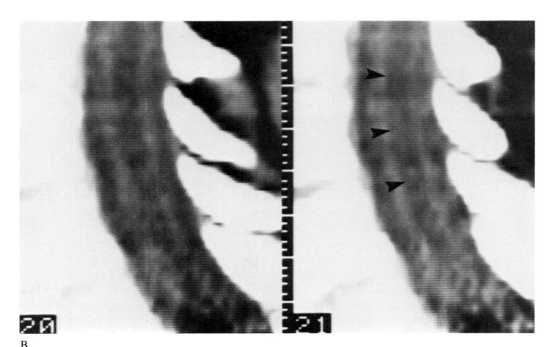

B

FIGURE 14.21 Syringomyelia. Axial (**A**) and sagittal (**B**) views demonstrate a large water-density collection in the center of the cervical spinal cord (*arrowheads*). **C.** Another patient with Arnold-Chiari malformation and syrinx. The top of the cystic space is seen at the level of C2 (*arrows*). The space behind the cervicomedullary junction is filled with soft tissue rather than CSF. **D.** Normal craniocervical junction, for comparison. Note the posterior triangle of CSF.

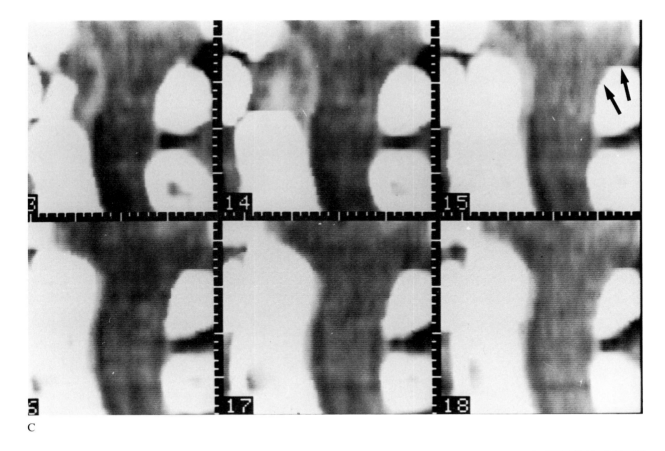

C

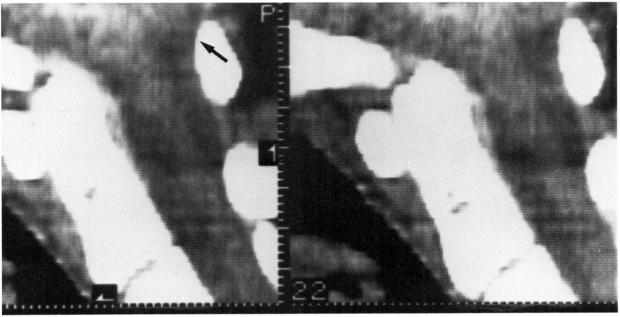

D

nect the central canal to the subarachnoid space. It is important for surgeons who contemplate external shunting of syrinx cavities to know the caudal extent. It is usually preferable to place the shunt tubing as low in the cyst as possible. Axial images should always be carried inferiorly until there is no trace of the syrinx.

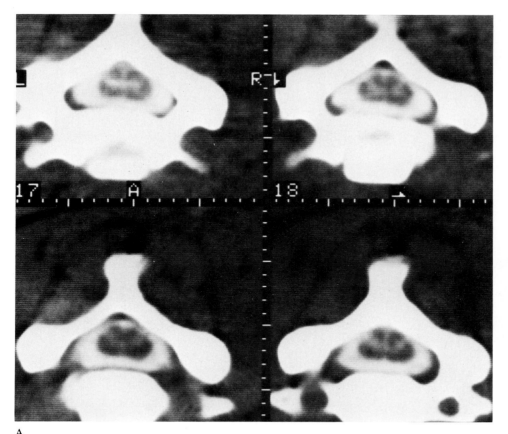

A

FIGURE 14.22 Syringomyelia—metrizamide CT. **A.** Axial scans through the midcervical spine reveal a somewhat flattened cervical cord filled with metrizamide. **B.** Sagittal reformation of the craniocervical junction confirms tonsilar herniation (*arrow*). **C.** Axial scan through the midthoracic area shows the bottom of this extensive cavity.

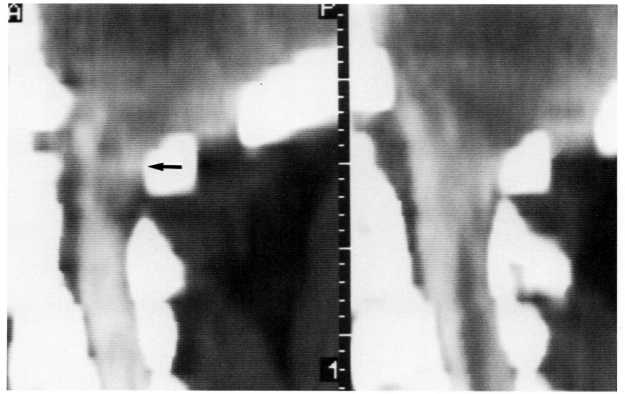

B

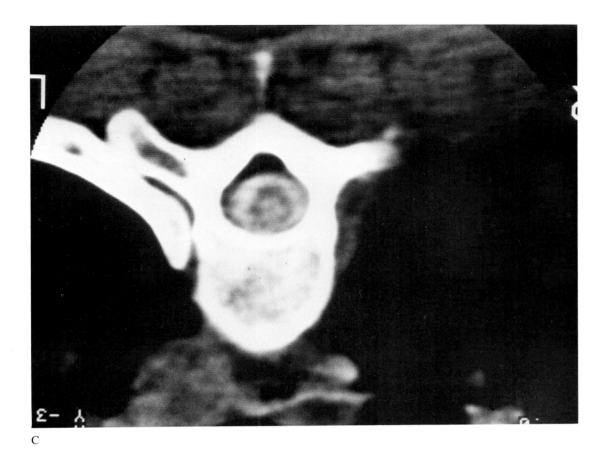

C

Tumors

Most extradural tumors are easily evaluated even without intravenous contrast injection or intrathecal metrizamide. Primary bone lesions are the easiest category to diagnose. They produce either hyperostosis or bone destruction.

An "ivory vertebra" at the thoracocervical junction is shown in Figure 14.23. This is difficult to fully evaluate in the axial perspective alone. There is obvious sclerosis of a vertebra, but whether this is limited to one segment is difficult to establish from the axial views. There is clear

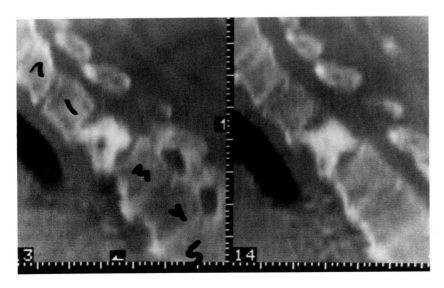

FIGURE 14.23 Ivory vertebrae. Sagittal view demonstrates ivory vertebrae due to metastatic carcinoma.

evidence for bone destruction and widening of the left T1–2 foramen. This is optimally demonstrated on the sagittal plane.

The patient in Figure 14.24 has a carcinoid tumor metastatic to his thoracic spine. A conventional myelogram was thought to be normal, but because of signs of severe cord compression, a scan was ordered the same day. Axial scans and sagittal reformations demonstrate significant cervical cord compression caused by the expansile hyperostotic metastasis. In fact, the same information could have been obtained without the use of intrathecal metrizamide, saving the patient a lumbar puncture. Bony metastasis from carcinoid is relatively uncommon. When it occurs, however, it tends to produce prominent hyperostosis. This patient had several markedly expanded ribs from other metastatic deposits.

The case in Figure 14.25 represents a curious calcified abnormality occupying approximately one-third of the lateral aspect of the central canal in this Japanese man with radiculopathy and myelopathy. There is no pathologic proof of what this represents, but the possibility of a burned-out, calcified meningioma should certainly be considered in the differential diagnosis. It is interesting to note a complete lucent halo around the lesion, suggesting a dural or ligamentous origin rather than an unusual lesion arising from the bone. In any case, the important diagnostic points of this scan are that: (1) the lesion producing the symptoms is not a disc herniation or ridge that would be operated from anteriorly; (2) it is a benign process; and (3) it is very unlikely to grow.

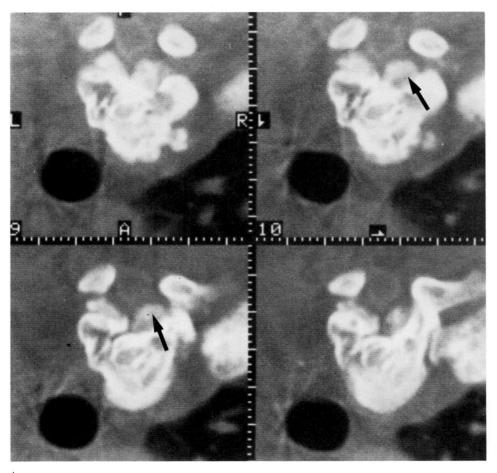

A

FIGURE 14.24 Metastatic carcinoid tumor. **A.** Axial scans displayed for bone detail reveal evidence of previous interbody spine fusion. There is a large bony tumor extending posteriorly into the canal (*arrow*). **B.** Sagittal reformation showing posterior displacement of the metrizamide-filled theca by a large bony tumor (*arrows*). **C.** Coronal reformation defines lateral canal compression by the mass (*arrows*). The theca and the cord are displaced to the left.

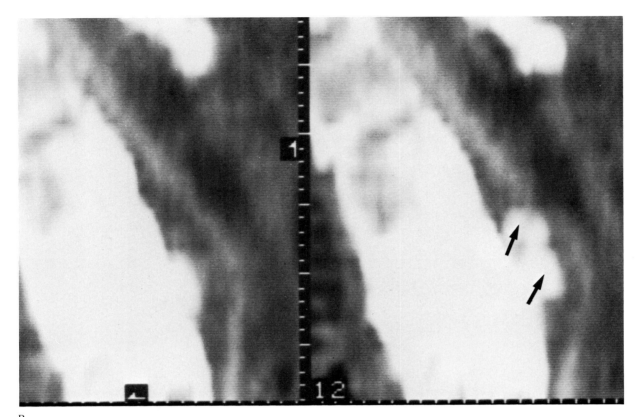

B

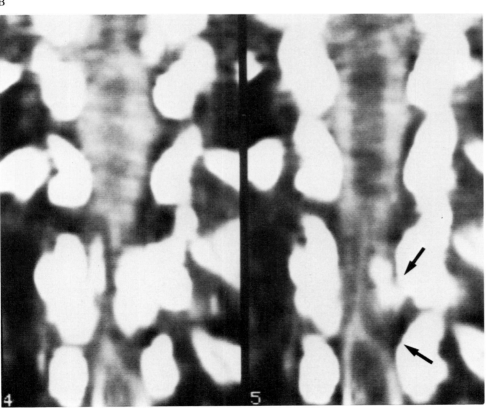

C

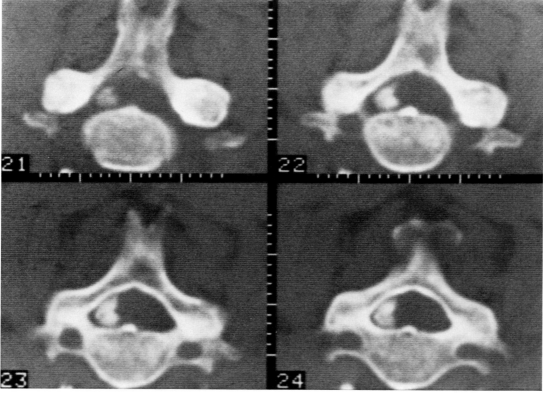

FIGURE 14.25   Benign intraspinal calcification. There is a dense well-defined bony mass that is completely separable from the vertebral ring. This most likely arises from the dura.

Intravenous infusion causes tumor enhancement relative to the thecal contents.[7] This is most useful for the evaluation of meningiomas, neurofibromas, and the other extradural soft-tissue tumors. Figure 14.26 is a sagittal reformation on a patient who many years before had resection of a meningioma. The study was performed after intrave-

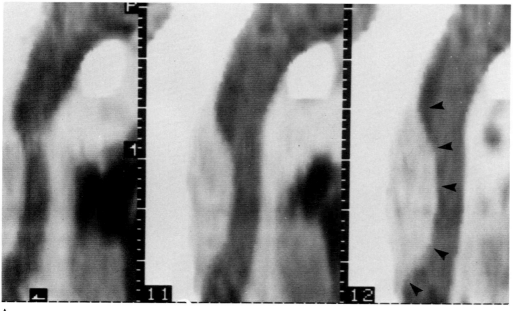

A

FIGURE 14.26   Recurrent meningioma. **A.** Sagittal view after intravenous contrast enhancement. The full extent of the mass is clearly visible (*arrowheads*). The spinal cord is displaced posteriorly (*arrows*). **B.** Axial views demonstrate a large anterior zone of enhancement. The anatomy of the tumor is much easier to conceptualize on the sagittal views.

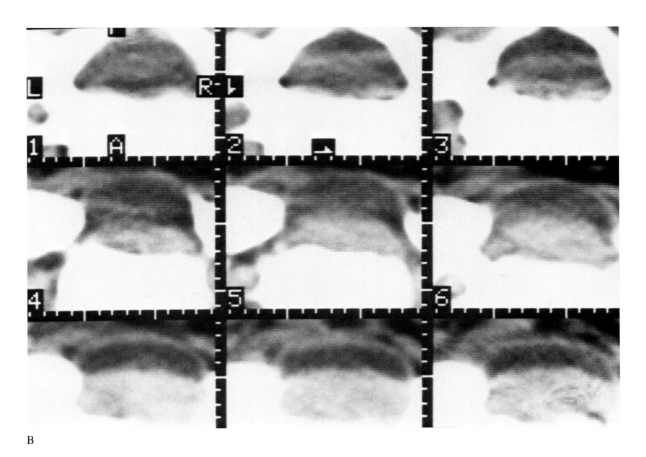

B

nous contrast infusion and with 5 mm thick axial slices taken every 2.5 mm. The meningioma enhances relative to the thecal contents and is seen on all three views.

Meningiomas represent 25–45% of primary spinal tumors; approximately 20% of meningiomas occur in the cervical region. They tend to be intradural masses, but they may extend beyond the neural foramina in a dumbbell fashion, making them indistinguishable from schwannomas. Because they enhance prominently, they should be evaluated with intravenous enhancement.[8] The lesion would be diagnosable even without enhancement because of its mass effect, which is unmistakable on sagittal views.

Neurinomas (schwannomas) account for approximately 25% of intradural extramedullary tumors.[9] They are frequently dumbbell-shaped and caused by extension through

the neural foramina. Because they are slow-growing, they cause smooth remodeling of bone and enlargement of a neural foramen rather than true bony destruction. These tumors are enhanced after intravenous contrast injection and are usually distinguishable from the spinal cord.[10] The scan in Figure 14.27 was performed many years after partial surgical removal of a neurofibroma. The tumor enhances prominently when compared to the spinal cord, which is displaced posteriorly and to the left. The large low-attenuation fluid collection represents a pseudomeningocele. As in the previous case, a myelogram would add little objective information to that found on CT. CT is ideal for demonstrating both intradural and extradural components of dumbbell tumors.

The upper cervical spinal canal on a patient with a previously treated cerebellar medulloblastoma is shown in Figure 14.28. The scan reveals lateral dural or epidural lesions in the lateral gutters, extending over several vertebral segments. The patient presented at the time of the scan with neck pain and tingling in the fingers. She underwent radiation therapy, with dramatic relief of symptoms. A metrizamide myelogram was performed and was thought to be normal. Repeat CT still demonstrated epidural masses but with shrinkage and concavity where before radiotherapy there had been medially convex tumoral lesions. Identical CT findings were seen in a second patient who proved to have cervical lymphoma. Dural or epidural tumors generally enhance relative to the thecal contents. They are especially well seen where there is a moderate amount of CSF. There are no specific radiographic features that allow the differentiation of downstream "drop metastasis" from blood-borne metastatic tumors.

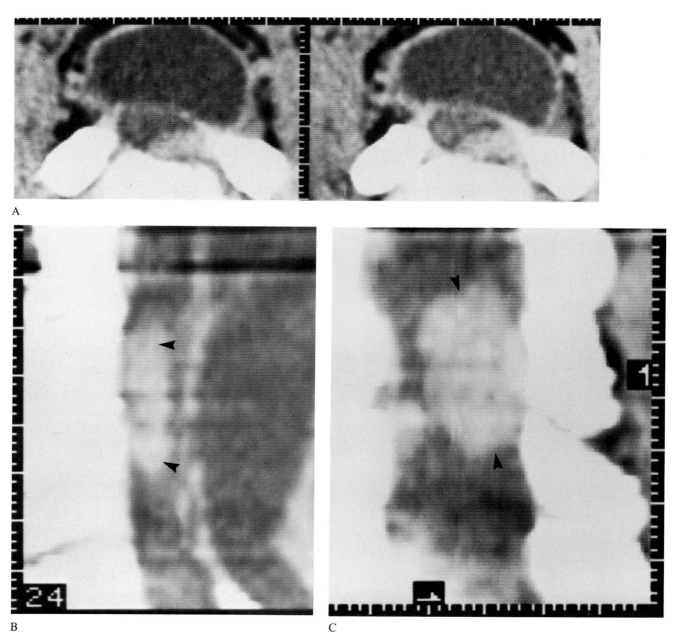

A

B   C

FIGURE 14.27   Schwannoma. **A.** Axial scans performed after intravenous contrast injection reveal prominent enhancement in the tumor mass (*arrows*) relative to the spinal cord. It is difficult to identify the cord with certainty from this view alone. There is a large posterior fluid collection. **B.** Sagittal view allows one to see the entire height of the tumor (*arrowheads*), and its relationship to the vertebral disc spaces. **C.** Coronal reformation demonstrates the side-to-side diameter of the mass (*arrowheads*), completing the three-dimensional picture.

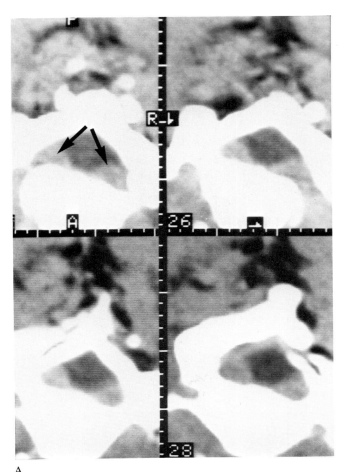

A

Cervical Disc Disease

The difficulty in seeing cervical disc herniation on CT scans is inversely related to the size of the disc abnormality. The axial and sagittal planes are more important than the coronal planes in most cases. Disc herniation appears as an area of high soft-tissue attenuation, extending posteriorly or posterolaterally from a disc space. The contours are almost always smooth, as seen on all CT projections. Lateral disc herniation may be best viewed on oblique reformations. This allows optimal visualization of the exiting root and its relationship to the disc. Figure 14.29 demonstrates two patients with central disc herniation noted on the axial views. The disc herniation in Figures 14.29A, B would probably cause a moderate central myelographic defect. The sagittal view is much more convincing with regard to amount of protrusion and likely myelographic defect. The patient in Figures 14.29C, D, however, has two extremely large central disc herniations which are severely compromising the spinal cord.

FIGURE 14.28 Metastatic medulloblastoma. **A.** Axial scan before local radiation therapy reveals prominent soft-tissue masses impressing the thecal sac (*arrows*). **B.** Axial scans during a course of radiation therapy, after a "normal" myelogram. Note that the masses are now concave and the thecal compression is reduced.

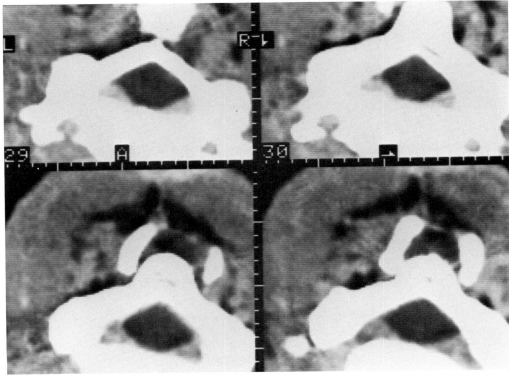

B

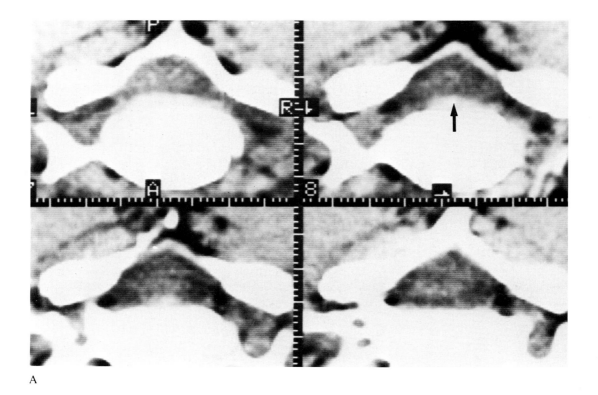

A

B

FIGURE 14.29 Central disc herniation. Axial (**A**) and sagittal (**B**) views demonstrate a high-density anterior extradural defect emanating from the disc space (*arrows*). The lesion is much more obvious in the sagittal view. Note that the normal exiting nerves within the foramina are surrounded by fat, which serves as a good contrast agent for distinguishing foraminal disc herniation. Axial (**C**) and sagittal (**D**) views of patient 2 reveal marked disc herniation, with severe canal compromise. Two herniations are seen on the sagittal images (*arrows*).

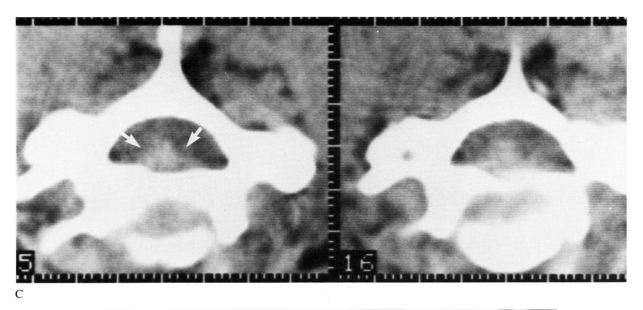

C

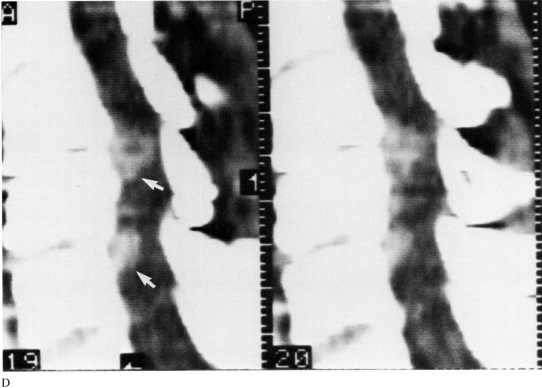

D

The combination of the two right-angle projections removes all doubt about the presence of an extradural soft-tissue defect.

The next case involves a diagnostic/therapeutic dilemma. This patient sustained a football injury, with significant tingling and numbness in the distribution of the left C6 nerve root. Figure 14.30 represents a scan performed 2 weeks after the injury. It leaves little doubt as to the presence of *both* a left-sided ridge causing foraminal narrowing plus a coexisting soft-tissue disc herniation. On a previous study immediately after injury, (2 weeks earlier), the coarser scanning protocol (5 mm thick images every 2.5 mm) resulted in a good-quality study (not shown) that definitely demonstrated a left-sided ridge. However, that examination left two radiologists differing as to the actual presence of a soft-tissue component. The second, more detailed and more restricted examination clearly established the presence of both conditions to the satisfaction of both radiologists. This influenced the surgeon's decision to proceed with surgery for the soft-tissue disc component.

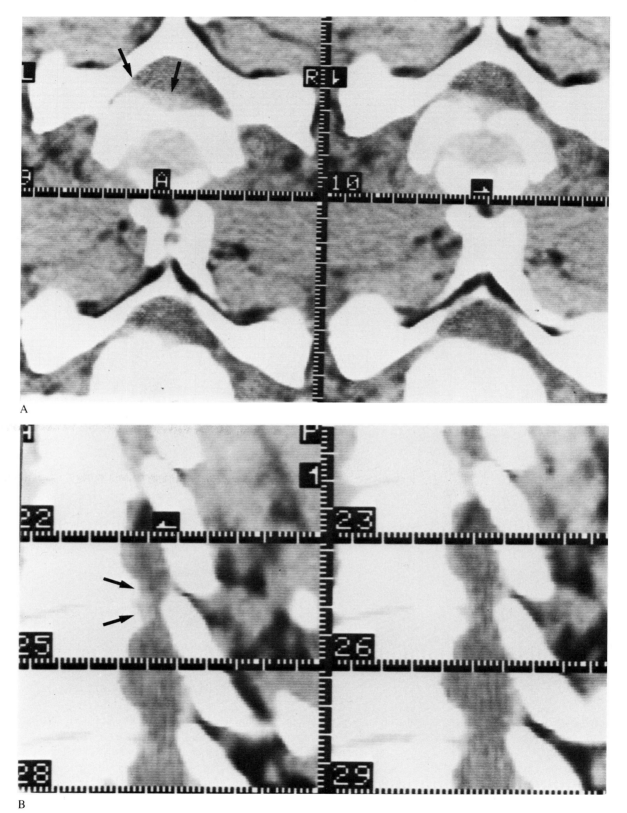

FIGURE 14.30 Lateral cervical disc. Axial (**A**) and sagittal (**B**) views define a prominent lateral extradural defect (*arrows*) that extends across the disc space and into the lateral gutter and the medial end of the foramen.

The disc case shown in Figure 14.31 is not at all subtle owing to the presence of calcification in the posterior margin of the disc fragment. The differential diagnosis of postoperative scar from recurrent disc herniation is less commonly a problem in the cervical spine. The rules for making this differentiation are the same. Scar is high in density but diffuse and infiltrating. It replaces epidural fat along the distribution of the involved neural segment. It is not a smooth, localized mass with borders (Fig. 14.32).

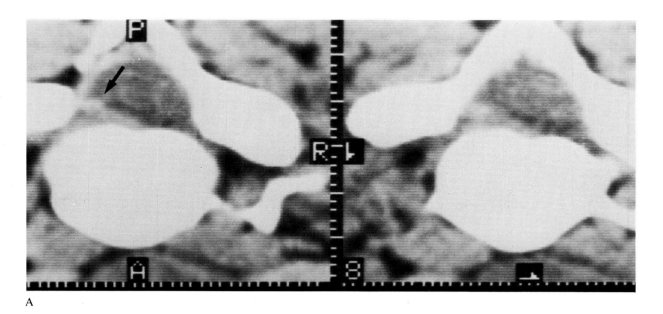

A

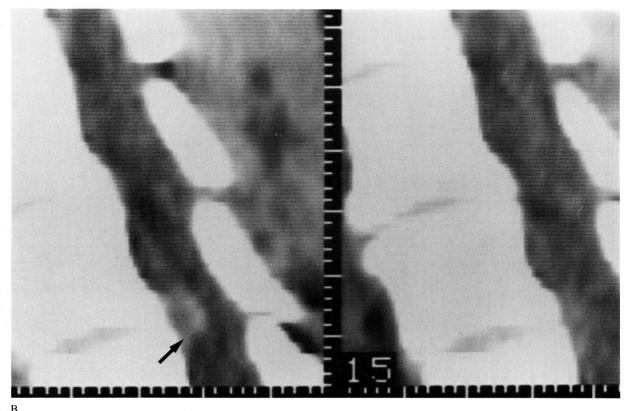

B

FIGURE 14.31 Herniated disc with calcification. Axial (**A**) and sagittal (**B**) views show a lateral disc herniation with a small peripheral calcification (*arrows*).

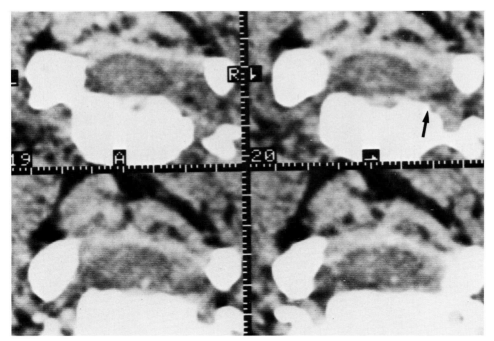

A

FIGURE 14.32 Postoperative scar. Axial (**A**) and sagittal (**B**) views demonstrate a homogeneous, ill-defined soft-tissue density (*arrow*) extending into the neural foramen at the site of surgery. This is the hallmark of postoperative fibrosis.

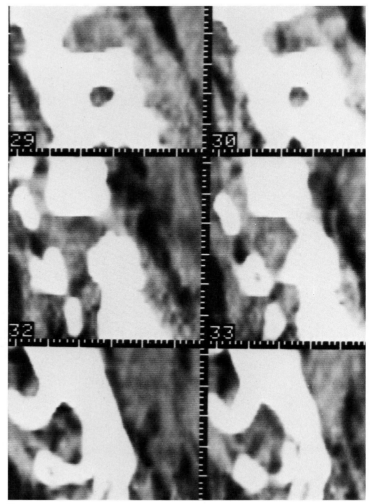

B

Spondylosis, Spurs, Ridges, and Foraminal Stenosis

To a very large extent, spondylosis, spurs, ridges and foraminal stenosis fall under the broad category of degenerative disc lesions and are frequently found in association with abnormalities of the disc. Using thin-section CT, it is now possible to evaluate osteophytic ridging and spurring and to judge the effects these bony overgrowths have on the central canal and the neural foramina. The disc spaces become narrow as the nuclear material loses its ability to remain adequately hydrated. This narrowing can strip the annular fibers from their bony attachment, producing spurs and ridges. With further reduction in disc space height, the uncinate processes that ride high above the vertebral end-plates become increasingly abnormal.

The uncinate processes are smooth, shoulder-like curved ridges along the superior posterolateral surfaces of the vertebral bodies that are capped with cartilage medially. Normally, 1–2 mm of radiographic lucency is seen between the upper cortical margin of the uncinate process and the adjacent inferior vertebral end-plate (Fig. 14.33). As the disc space narrows, the uncinate processes lie closer to, and finally come into direct contact with, the adjacent end-plates.

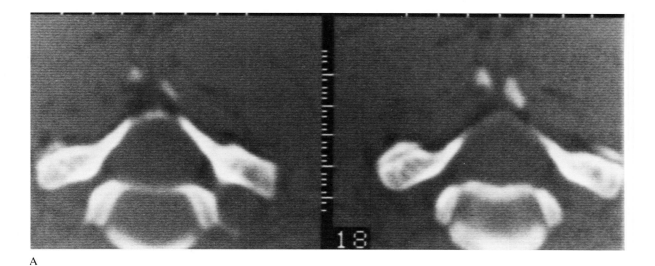

A

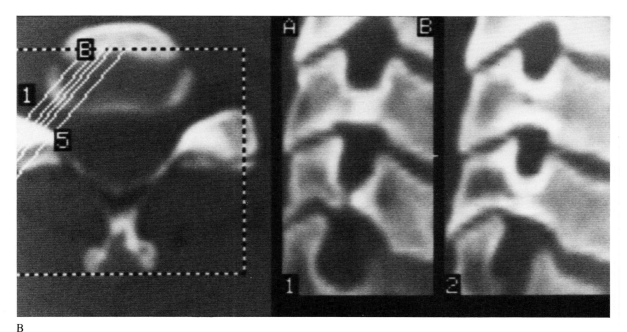

B

FIGURE 14.33 Normal uncinate processes. Axial (**A**) and oblique (**B**) projections. Between the uncinate process and the inferior end-plate of the upper vertebra there normally is 1–2 mm of cartilage.

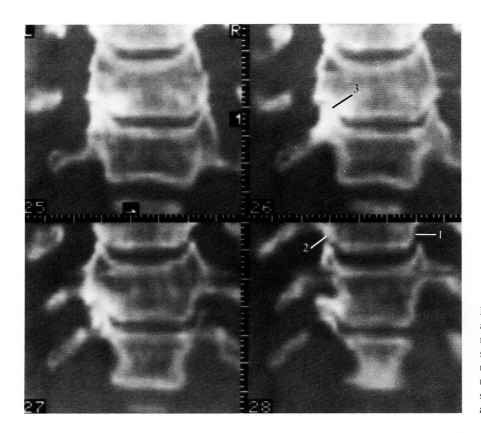

FIGURE 14.34 Uncinate spur formation. Coronal reformation demonstrating a normal uncovertebral joint (*1*), mild uncinate narrowing (*2*), and severe uncinate narrowing and spurring (*3*).

Hyperostotic ridging and spurring become more prominent once contact occurs. These ridges may extend posteriorly to compress the lateral portion of the spinal canal, posterolaterally to compress the exiting nerve roots, or laterally to compress the vertebral artery. Figure 14.34 is a series of reformations from 1.5 mm thick axial CT data that demonstrate the normal and progressively abnormal uncinate processes. The normal cortex of the process and its cartilaginous cap are clearly identifiable. Lateral extension of uncinate spurs is also clearly definable at the most abnormal level.

The normal neural foramina are shown in Figure 14.35 in multiple projections. One should, in most cases, be able to identify the exiting roots surrounded by fat. The optimal

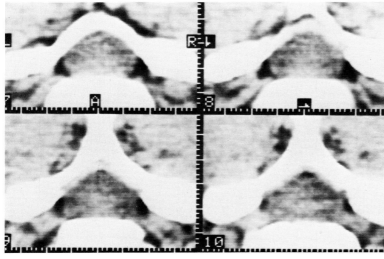

A

FIGURE 14.35 Normal cervical neural foramina. Note that the exiting roots are surrounded by fat. Axial (**A**), sagittal (**B**), and coronal (**C**) views. (*Figure continued on pages 435, 436.*)

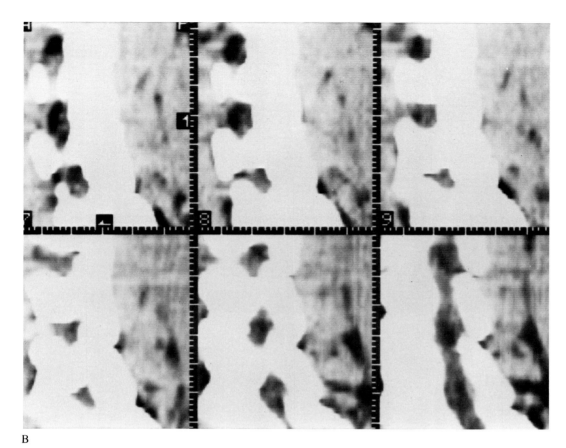

B

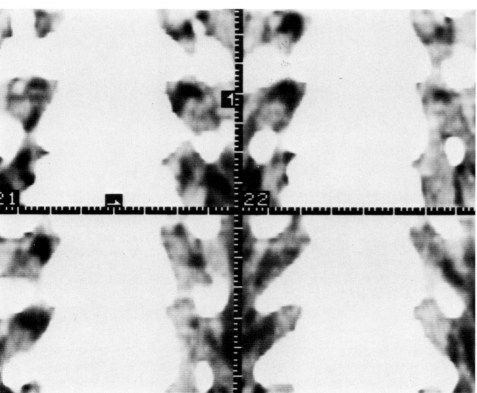

C

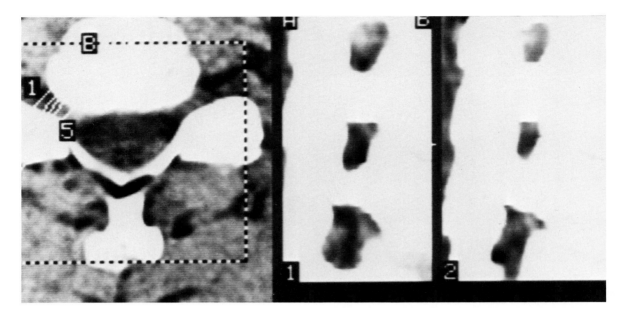

D

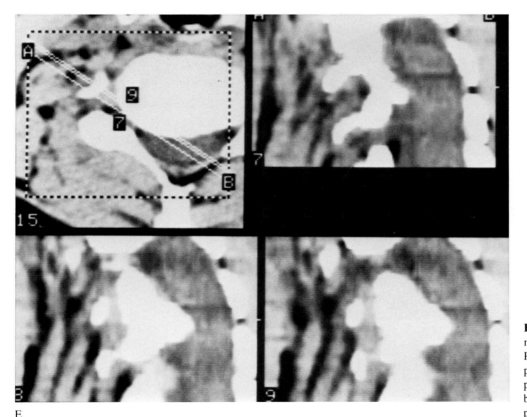

E

FIGURE 14.35 (*cont'd*) Normal cervical neural foramina. Perpendicular oblique (**D**), and parallel oblique (**E**) views. On the parallel oblique view it is possible to see the roots of the brachial plexus forming.

projection is much more oblique than in the lumbar spine, where the view would be closer to a true lateral or sagittal projection. The difference is subtle. Evaluation of foramina using both bone-window and soft-tissue-window photography of the identical image is important and necessary because the bone-windowed images tend to underestimate foraminal encroachments, whereas the soft-tissue photographs tend to overestimate the encroachments.

The abnormal scan in Figure 14.36 illustrates severe lateral canal and foraminal compression caused by a large

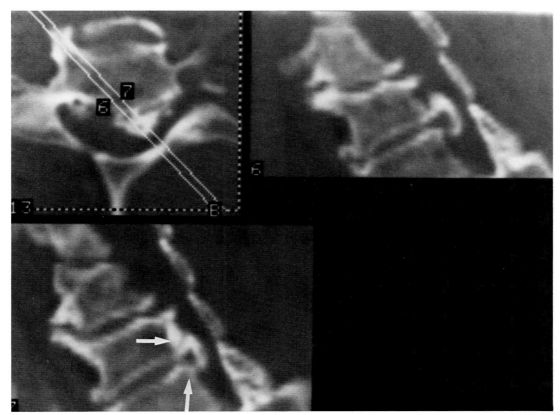

FIGURE 14.36 Uncinate spurs. Oblique reformation on a patient with a large pair of degenerative ridges (*arrows*)—one from the uncinate process and another from its parallel mate on the undersurface of the vertebral end-plate.

pair of spurs—one from the uncinate process and a parallel mate from the inferior end-plate above. The medial two thirds of the neural foramen is narrowed, an extremely important observation. Most surgeons perform anterior cervical osteophyte removal and interbody fusions. Using this interdiscal approach it may be difficult or impossible to visualize the lateral extent of the uncinate ridge. We have seen a number of cases where even major central decompression was inadequate for relieving radiculopathy from a far-lateral-extending uncinate ridge.

The series of views in Figure 14.37 shows a patient with more extensive disease at multiple levels. Large degenerative ridges arising from the vertebral end-plate significantly encroach on both the central canal and the foramina at more than one level.

Gas is frequently noted in severely degenerated lumbar discs, and this "vacuum" effect is well documented on CT. Similarly, gas is frequently noted in the cervical area when thin CT sections are performed (Fig. 14.38). It is interesting that this gas is noted far more often on the CT scans than on conventional films or on the scanner's digital ScoutView.

Narrowing and degeneration of a cervical disc space may rarely be associated with intrabody disc herniation.

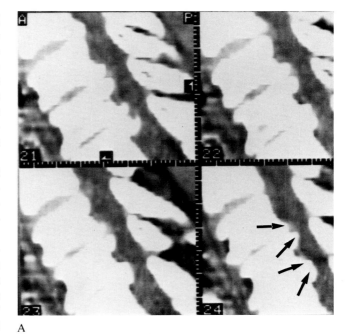

A

FIGURE 14.37 Multiple degenerative ridges. **A.** Sagittal views demonstrate large end-plate and uncinate ridges (*arrows*), which narrow the spinal canal severely. (*Figure continued* on page 438.)

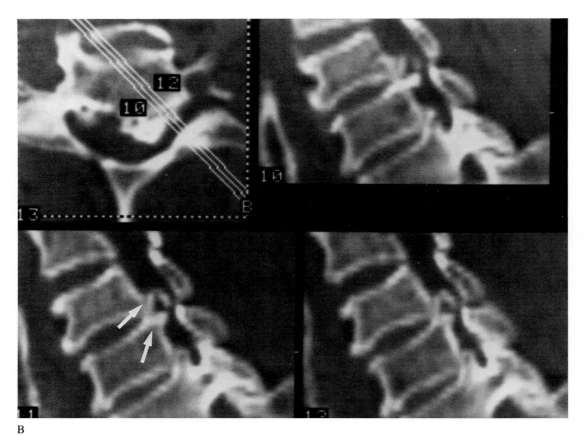

B

FIGURE 14.37 (*cont'd*) **B.** Oblique views demonstrate large end-plate and uncinate ridges (*arrows*), which narrow the spinal cord severely.

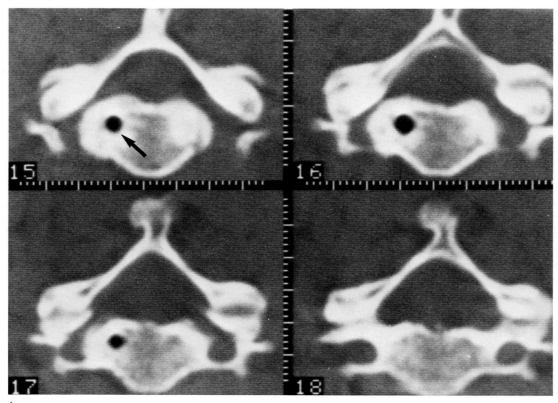

A

FIGURE 14.38 Vacuum disc effect. Axial (**A**), sagittal (**B**), and coronal (**C**) views demonstrate a degenerative uncinate ridge with a bubble of gas (*arrow*) within the disc space, extending into a cystic cavity in the end-plate.

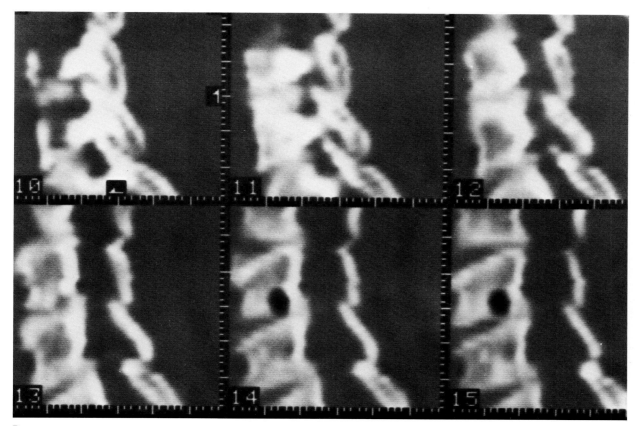

B

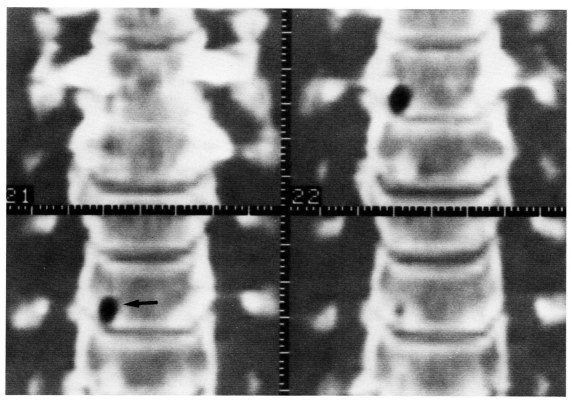

C

This is much less common in the neck than in the lumbar spine. The radiographic appearance of cervical Schmorl's node is identical to that in the lumbar spine (Fig. 14.39). The lucent defects involve the vertebral end-plate and are surrounded by a dense rim of sclerosis.

Obviously not all abnormal disc spaces are due to degenerating discs. The child in Figure 14.40 has a slightly widened but markedly irregular disc space. The most striking finding was a very large retropharyngeal soft-tissue mass anterior to the abnormal C2–3 disc space (not shown). This

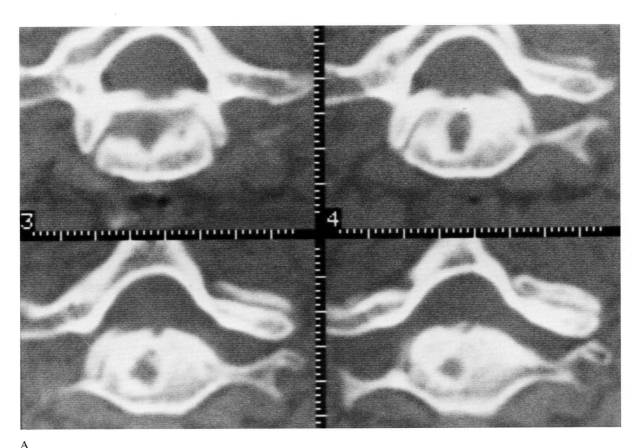

A

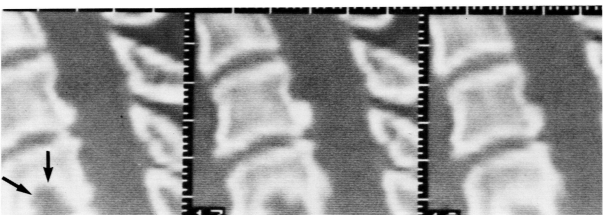

B

FIGURE 14.39 Cervical Schmorl's node. Axial (**A**) and sagittal (**B**) views demonstrate an unusually large lucent vertebral defect (*arrows*) with a sclerotic rim characteristic of interbody herniation.

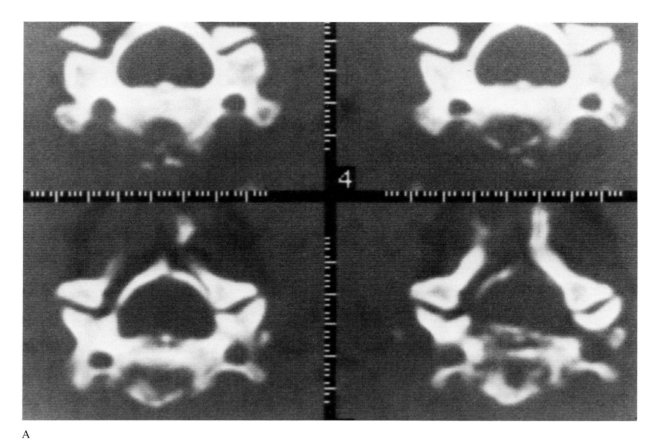

A

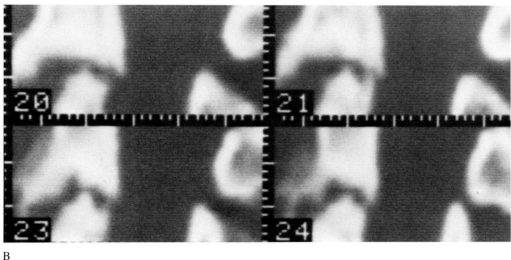

B

FIGURE 14.40 Tuberculous discitis. Axial (**A**) and sagittal (**B**) views on a child with tuberculous adenitis with extension into the C2–3 disc space. The interspace and the vertebral end-plates are irregular and eroded.

almost always signifies some type of infection. Tuberculosis was proved in this patient.

A C3–4 subluxation is shown in Figure 14.41 in bone-windowed sagittal composite views. The sagittal view is much more accurate than the axial view in identifying precisely where and to what extent critical central-canal stenosis exists in the presence of subluxation. Axial views generally overestimate the amount of central-canal space available for the spinal cord. The reason is that the critical

stenosis is usually between the upper posterior margin of a superior end-plate of the lower vertebra and the ventral surface of the lamina of the subluxated vertebral body. This critical stenosis often exists at a very steep angle and cannot be adequately assessed in axial views alone unless the gantry could be tilted to approximately 60 degrees. (See Chapter 15.)

Forestier's, or "DISH," syndrome, is characterized by prominent bony ridging and anterior hyperostotic bars

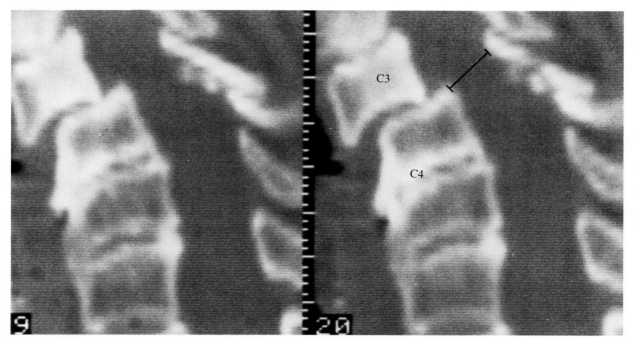

FIGURE 14.41 Rheumatoid subluxation. Sagittal reformation demonstrates narrowing and degeneration of the C4 disc space with more than 5 mm of subluxation. The narrowest diameter of the canal is between the body of C4 and the lamina of C3.

which may be large enough to cause dysphagia due to esophageal compression. Large osteophytic ridges may also extend into the spinal canal, causing a severe myelopathy (Fig. 14.42). Another cause of myelopathy from cervical cord compression is the unusual syndrome of ossification of the posterior longitudinal ligament. This syndrome is most commonly seen in people of Japanese extraction, but it is occasionally encountered in other population groups as well. CT scans distinguish between ligamentous ossification and more common osteophytic bony spinal stenosis (Fig. 14.43). In any case of cervical spinal stenosis due to bony compression, it is crucial that the entire stenotic area be evaluated, all associated foraminal compressive lesions be identified, and a clear anatomic picture of the surgical field be available preoperatively.

Degenerative arthritis of the facets may cause localized pain and, when associated with hypertrophic spurring, may compress nerves within the neural foramina. Because of the sloping orientation of the cervical facets, the joints are better viewed in the sagittal projection than in the axial view. The patient in Figures 14.44A–C has severe destructive arthritis of both facets. Note the irregularity of the articular processes, the bone sclerosis, and the cystic degeneration. The neural foramen is compressed by osteophytes descending from the apex of the joint, as well as by uncinate spurs.

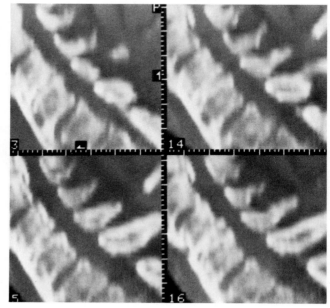

FIGURE 14.42 "DISH" syndrome. Sagittal reformation demonstrates prominent anterior osseous bony fusion of the vertebral bodies characteristic of Forestier's syndrome. Posterior intercanalicular ridges tend to be smaller than anterior prevertebral ridges.

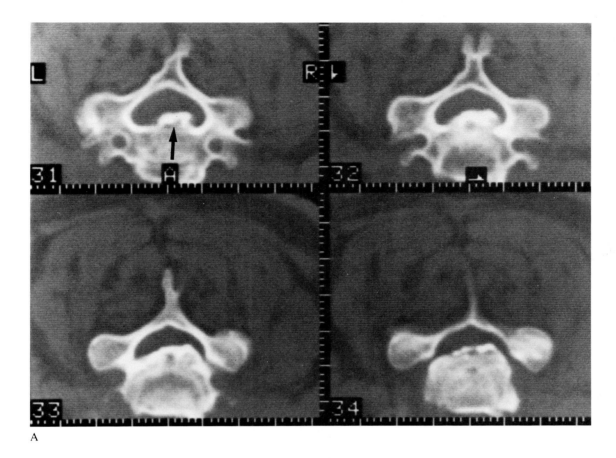

A

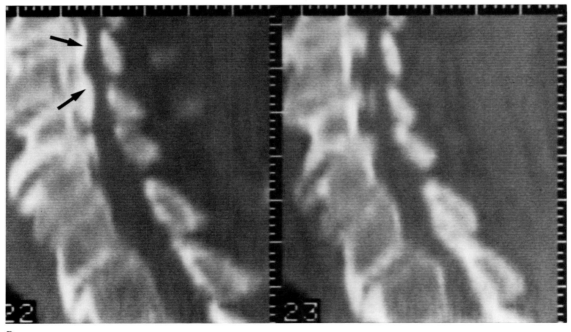

B

FIGURE 14.43 Calcification of the posterior longitudinal ligament. Axial (**A**) and sagittal (**B**) views reveal large irregular ossification of the posterior longitudinal ligament (*arrow*). On the sagittal view one can easily distinguish this from degenerative osteophytes.

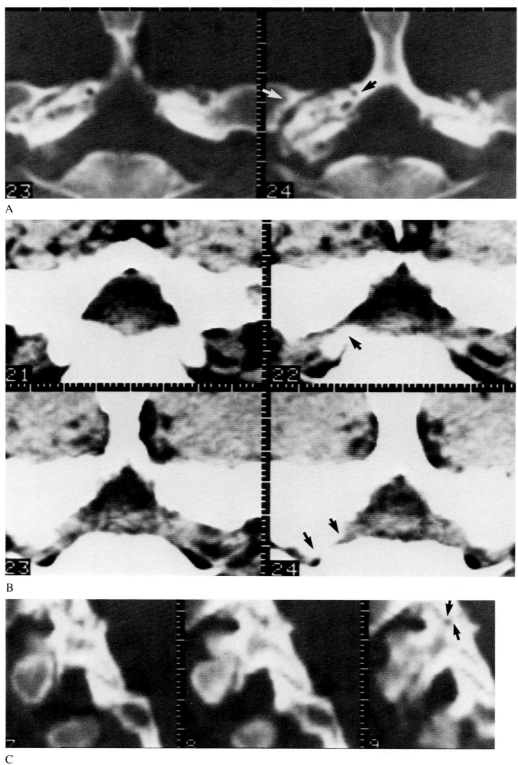

FIGURE 14.44   Degenerative arthritis of the facets. Axial bone (**A**) and soft-tissue (**B**) views demonstrate degenerative arthritis of the facets, worse on the left than on the right. The exiting nerves are compressed by bony spurs from the joints and uncinate processes. Sagittal view (**C**) demonstrates downward-projecting facet spurs. Axial (**D**) and sagittal (**E**) views on a second patient who had a fracture of C7 reveal localized posttraumatic arthritis of the left articulation. Note gas within a degenerative cyst.

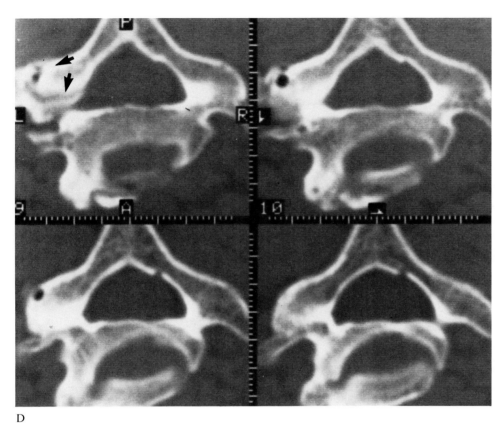

D

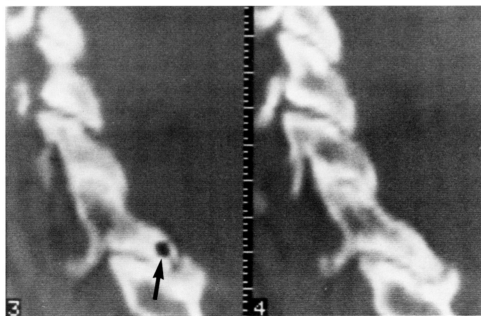

E

A second patient (Figs. 14.44D, E) had a compression fracture at C7. This scan, showing severe localized degenerative arthritis, was perfomed because of subsequent neck pain. It is not clear why some people develop severe articular arthritis and some are spared. What is clear, however, is that these changes may cause clinical symptoms and therefore must be described by CT.

Cervical Interbody Fusions

The anterior approach to the cervical disc space, as described by Southwick and Robinson[12] and Cloward,[13] has become one of the most important surgical procedures for the treatment of degenerative disc disease and spondylosis. It is therefore important to describe the anatomy of this type of surgery, as seen by CT, as well as the common postoperative complications.

After identification of the involved disc, the disc space is excised from the front and the disc material removed. An attempt is made to remove all or most of the cartilaginous end-plate without removing too much subchondral bone. A bone graft is inserted into the widely retracted disc space to increase disc space height,[14] open the foramina, and fuse the interspace. During the immediate postoperative period (Fig. 14.45) it is possible to clearly identify the cortical margins of the bone graft. On sagittal and curved coronal reformations the bone plug is seen wedged tightly in the enlarged disc space. The interface plane becomes less distinct as new bone grows into the graft from the adjacent vertebrae. It may take up to 6 months to form a contiguous solid fusion (Fig. 14.46).

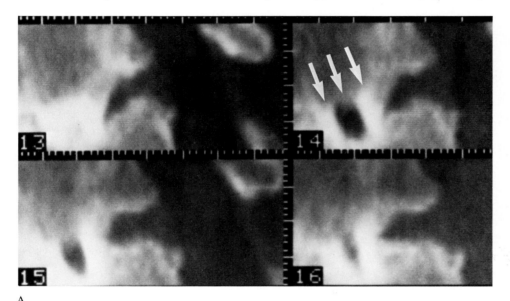

A

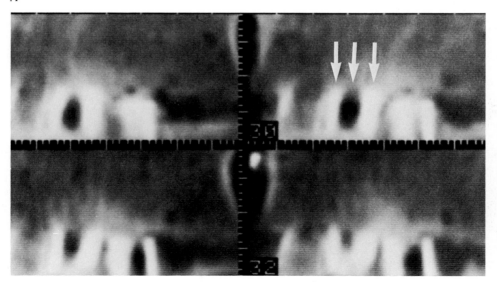

B

FIGURE 14.45 Interbody spine fusion. Sagittal (**A**) and coronal (**B**) views on a patient scanned within 2 weeks of interbody spine fusion. During this phase, one is able to identify the cortical and medullary portions of the graft. A cleavage plane is seen between the graft and the vertebral end-plate (*arrows*). Note that during the acute phase of healing the medullary cavity of the graft is lucent.

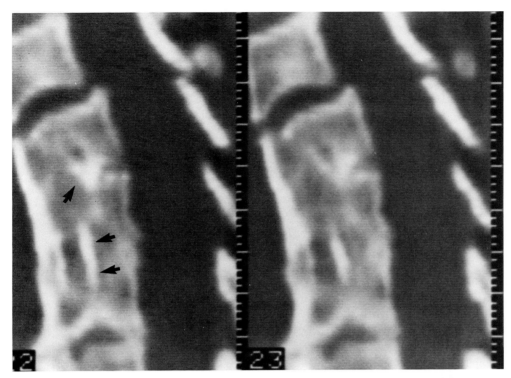

FIGURE 14.46 Interbody spine fusion. Sagittal scan on a patient with healed interbody fusions. There is bone trabeculation traversing the operated disc spaces (*arrows*).

The earliest change in the failing interbody fusion is lucency or "haloing" at one or both ends of the graft. When dissolution of the graft occurs, the disc space height decreases, becomes lucent, and may sublux. Failure of osseous fusion is best identified on sagittal and curved coronal reformations.

Occasionally a patient with failure of fusion develops an abnormal angulation at the pseudarthrosis (Fig. 14.47). This may be associated with radiculopathy or neck pain.

Some patients with successful anterior decompression and interbody fusion continue to have symptoms, which may be due to residual unrelieved foraminal or spinal cord

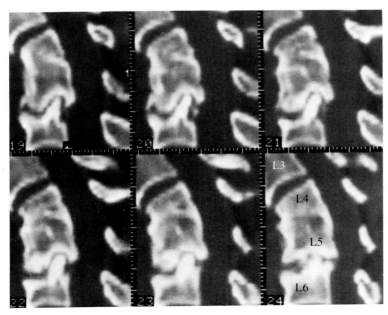

A

FIGURE 14.47 Failed interbody fusion. **A.** Sagittal reformations on a patient with a solid interbody fusion between C4 and C5 and a failed interbody fusion between C5 and C6. There is a halo of lucency between the superior end-plate and the top of the bone plug. C5 is posteriorly subluxed on C6. (*Figure continued on page 447.*)

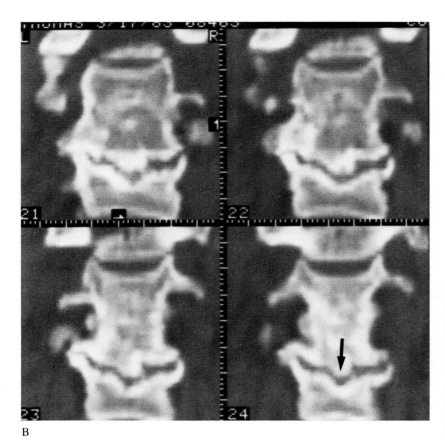

FIGURE 14.47 (*cont'd*) **B.** Coronal reformations on a patient with a solid interbody fusion between C4 and C5 and a failed interbody fusion between C5 and C6. There is a halo of lucency between the superior endplate and the top of the bone plug. C5 is posteriorly subluxed on C6.

compression by osteophytes or ridges. Because of the nature of the surgery, recurrent or residual disc herniation is not a serious consideration. Another cause of pain during the immediate postoperative period is dislocation of the bone plug. This is a rare but potentially disastrous complication (Fig. 14.48).

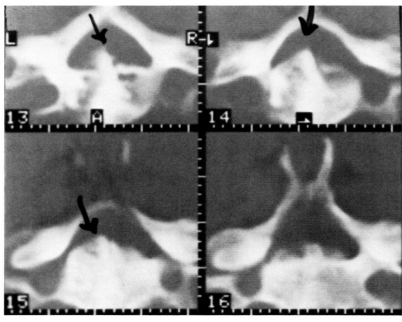

FIGURE 14.48 Dislocated interbody fusion. Axial (**A**) and sagittal (**B**) scans on a patient with a fused interbody fusion. There is dislocation of the bone plug (*arrows*), with severe cervical spinal stenosis.

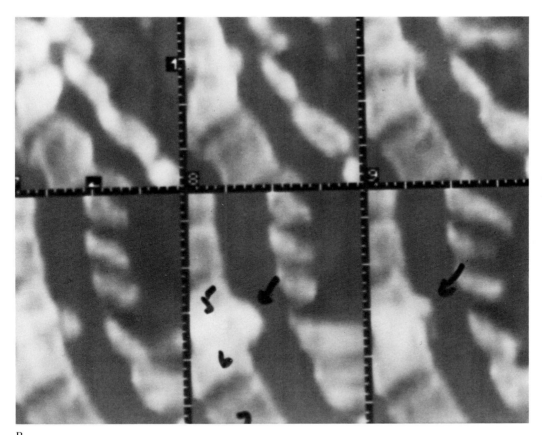

B
FIGURE 14.48 (*cont'd*) **B.**

It is not uncommon for patients to present for evaluation many years after successful interbody fusion because of another radiculopathy or neck pain. One of the common causes of the syndrome is degeneration of the disc above the surgical fusion. A solid low or midcervical fusion places added stress on the next highest disc space, and degenerative changes occur in the disc space and the zygapophyseal joints (Fig. 14.49).

True disc herniation may also occur above such a fusion. This is exactly analogous to the degenerative disease that occurs above and below areas of congenital fusion. Figure 14.50 shows a patient with congenital fusion be-

tween C4 and C5. It is difficult to distinguish this from a small surgical fusion. Sagittal reformations reveal a common fused lateral mass attesting to the congenital nature of the disorder.

Less commonly, an entire cervical vertebral body must be removed. This typically occurs in patients with tumoral replacement of bone or with severe cervical trauma. A multilevel graft is usually used when this type of surgery is performed. Figure 14.51 shows a bone plug that has replaced two cervical vertebral segments. Axial sections represent the caudal and cranial ends of this graft. In neither set of axial images does the graft appear solid. The extent

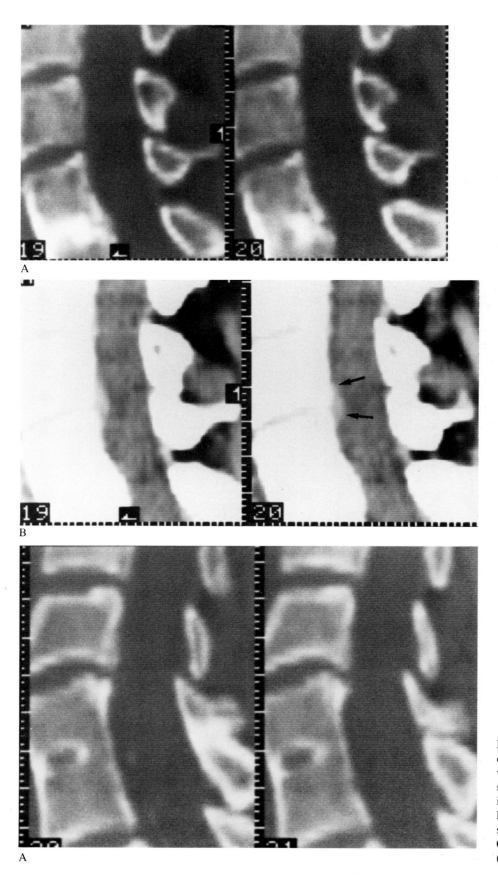

A

B

A

FIGURE 14.49 Degenerative disc disease above a successful spinal fusion. Bone-window (**A**) and soft-tissue-window (**B**) sagittal reformation demonstrates narrowing of the intervertebral disc space, with disc herniation at the level above the spine fusion (*arrows*).

FIGURE 14.50 Congenital cervical fusion. **A.** Midsagittal scans reveal solid fusion across a narrow disc space. Note the degenerative disease in the interspace above the fusion. **B.** Lateral sagittal views demonstrate a common facet for C6 and C5. Note the two neural foramina (*arrows*).

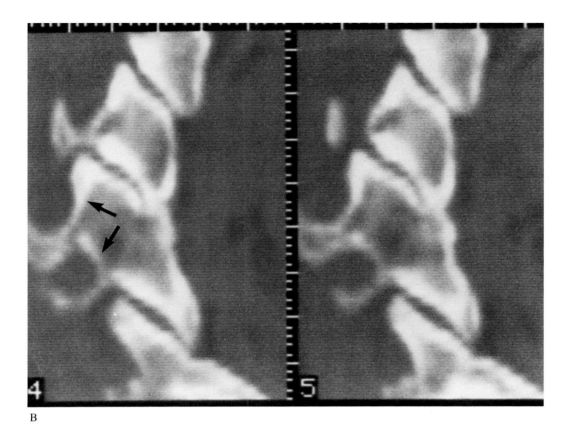

B

to which this axial perspective is misleading, with regard to fusion stability, is readily seen in the reformatted bone-window sagittal image. There is trabecular bone at both ends of this graft, which appears to be completely solid.

References

1. Sarwar M, Kier EL, Virapongse C: Development of the spine and spinal cord. In Newton TH, Potts DG (eds): Modern Neurology, Vol. 1: Computed Tomography of the Spine and Spinal cord. Clavadel Press, San Anselmo, California, 1983, pp. 15–30
2. Naidich TP, McLone DG, Harwood-Nash DC: Malformations of the craniocervical junction. In Newton TH, Potts DG (eds): Modern Neurology, Vol. 1: Computed Tomography of the Spine and Spinal Cord. Clavadel Press, San Anselmo, California, 1983, pp. 355–366
3. Von Torklus D, Gehle W: The Upper Cervical Spine: Regional Anatomy, Pathology, and Traumatology: A Systematic Radiological Atlas and Textbook. Grune & Stratton, New York, 1972
4. Shapiro R, Youngberg AS, Rothman SLG: The differential diagnosis of traumatic lesions of the occipito-atlanto-axial segment. Radiol Clin North Am 9:505–526, 1973
5. Brant-Zawadzki M, Minagi H: CT in the evaluation of spine trauma. In Federle MP, Brant-Zawadzki M (eds): Computed Tomography in the Evaluation of Trauma. Williams & Wilkins, Baltimore, 1982
6. Martilla KR, Cooper PR, Sklar FH: The influence of thin section tomography on the treatment of cervical spine injuries. Radiology 127:131, 1978
7. Handel SF, Lee Y: Computed tomography of spinal fractures. Radiol Clin North Am 19:69, 1981
8. Aubin M-L, Jardin C, Bar D, Vignaud J: Computerized tomography in 32 cases of intraspinal tumor. J Neuroradiol 6:81–92, 1979
9. Dorwart RH, LaMasters DL, Watanabe TJ: Tumors. In Newton TH, Potts DG (eds): Modern Neurology, Vol. 1: Computed Tomography of the Spine and Spinal Cord. Clavadel Press, San Anselmo, California, 1983, pp. 115–147
10. Rubinstein CJ: Tumors of the central nervous system. In Atlas of Tumor Pathology, Series 2, fasc. 6. United States Armed Forces Institute of Pathology, Washington, DC, 1972
11. Baleriaux-Waha D, Terwinghe G, Jeanmart L: The value of computed tomography for the diagnosis of hourglass tumors of the spine. Neuroradiology 14:31–32, 1977
12. Southwick WO, Robinson RA: Surgical approaches to the vertebral bodies in the cervical and lumbar regions. J Bone Joint surg 39A:631–644, 1957
13. Cloward RB: The anterior approach for removal of ruptured disks. J Neurosurg 15:602–617, 1958
14. Bohlman HH, Robinson RA: Anterior approaches to the cervical spine. In Ruge D, and Wiltse LL (eds): Spinal Disorders: Diagnosis and Treatment. Lea & Febiger, Philadelphia, 1977, pp. 125–131

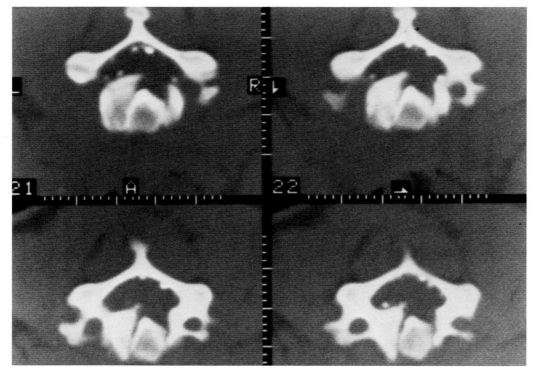

A

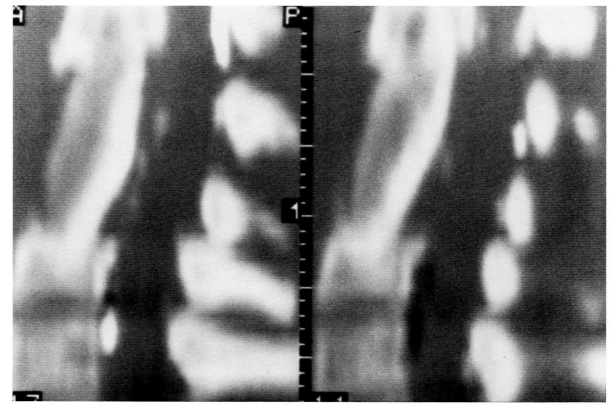

B

FIGURE 14.51   Cervical vertebrectomy. Axial (**A**) and sagittal (**B**) views reveal a graft traversing two vertebral interspaces. The sagittal view is necessary to prove successful fusion.

Advanced Cervical Rheumatoid Arthritis

15

Ronald L. Kaufman

Rheumatoid arthritis is a systemic rheumatic disease that can involve most synovial-lined diarthrodial articulations. Cervical involvement in this patient group varies from 3% to 85% of the population reviewed, depending on the severity and chronicity of involvement. When all admissions to Rancho Los Amigos Hospital Arthritis Service (a tertiary care combined orthopedic rheumatologic arthritis rehabilitation center) were prospectively evaluated for rheumatoid cervical spine involvement during calendar year 1980, we found a 72% incidence. This included inflammatory changes of cervical subluxation at atlantoaxial or subaxial levels and nonsclerotic disc and apophyseal joint narrowing. The average age of this patient group was 58 years, and the average disease duration was 19 years. The female:male ratio was 3.8. The most common levels of involvement were atlantoaxial, followed by C3–4 and C4–5; multiple levels were involved in 20% of these patients.

During this time period, 7 of the 166 hospitalized patients with rheumatoid arthritis had frank cervical myelopathy, an incidence of 4% of all patients and 6% of those with cervical spine radiographic changes. The demographic characteristics of this myelopathic subgroup of rheumatoid patients did not differ from those of our general population. The most common clues of myelopathy were nonspecific, generalized functional decrease and weakness.[1] In addition to the higher incidence of subluxation at every level, over 70% had multiple levels of subluxation.

Clinical and Radiographic Evaluation

Clinical evaluation of patients with severe rheumatoid arthritis is difficult because of the concomitant peripheral and entrapment neuropathies, severe deformities, and aberrant or lacking articular function. Because neurologic signs can be misleading and symptomatology is usually nonspecific, a confirmatory test is often necessary to document the presence of structural compression and all levels of abnormality. The standard for evaluation of myelopathy is radiographic myelography. This procedure has many drawbacks, e.g., the discomfort of dye instillation, headaches after the procedure, and dye-specific side effects such as arachnoiditis or confusion. Additionally, many alternative positions are required to define the lesion in question. Patients with severe rheumatoid arthritis find these alternative positions difficult to maintain because of severe shoulder and lower-extremity abnormalities, nodules, and dermal sensitivity. Consequently, although myelography is recommended, it is rarely done in the preoperative evaluation of these patients.

Computerized tomography with multiplanar reconstruction (CT/MPR) has totally replaced myelography in our evaluation of patients with suspected myelopathy secondary to rheumatoid arthritis or other types of inflammatory systemic rheumatic disease, i.e., psoriatic arthritis[2] and ankylosing spondylitis. This technology has many advantages over myelography and routine CT. CT/MPR allows complete visualization in an orthogonal representation and, additionally, can generate oblique and curved sections in any plane. Dural structures can usually be visualized without contrast introduction. Also, in the cervical structures there is an osseous network of foramina transversaria that lead the vertebral arteries from the level of C6 through C1 and ultimately to the basilar artery. Whereas the foramina transversaria exist at C7, the vertebral artery usually courses anteriorly to them. The single drawback to CT/MPR, as compared to myelography, is that it is a static study, whereas routine radiographs and standard myelograms can be done with flexion and extension views.

CT/MPR Compared with Plain Radiographs

The review of radiographs with CT/MPR against the background of the patient's clinical presentation has validated the usefulness of this method compared with using historic controls. This protocol has replaced the myelogram since 1979, and several observations are clear:

1. Neurologic abnormalities can be correlated with structural lesions as defined by CT/MPR; they range from spinal cord to nerve root to vertebral artery involvement.
2. All levels of skeletal involvement are revealed by CT/MPR, although frequently in the absence of radiographic abnormalities. This is usually explained by the presence of unsuspected subaxial rotary subluxation or overlapping structures, i.e., shoulders or head-on cervical structures.
3. Rotary atlantoaxial and subaxial subluxation can cause vertebrobasilar artery symptomatology.
4. CT/MPR is essential for the preoperative planning of the appropriate levels for cervical fusion, obviating the need for reoperation for subsequent subluxation of previously minimally abnormal/unsuspected lesions.

At this point a caveat is appropriate. All evaluations must, in concert, validate the presence of myelopathy in order to suggest that surgical fusion is appropriate. Clinical findings in the absence of confirmatory radiographic and CT/MPR abnormalities do not justify surgery any more than does subluxation in the absence of clinical findings. It must also be remembered that the cord in the midsagittal diameter is 10 mm at the atlantoaxial level and 7 mm in the subaxial levels (Table 15.1). Inflammatory changes can resorb osseous spinal canal structures and allow major degrees of subluxation to occur in the presence of a canal with the capacity to accommodate the spinal cord.

Table 15.1 Spinal Canal and Cord Normal Measurements

Vertebra	Spinal canal radiographic mean (range) (mm)	Spinal cord by metrizamide CT (mm)
C1	21.3 (16–30)	7.2 ± 1.6
C2	19.2 (16–18)	6.5 ± 2.0
C3	19.1 (14–25)	6.2 ± 2.2
C4		6.0 ± 1.5
C5	18.5 (14–25)	6.2 ± 2.3
C6		6.4 ± 2.7
C7	17.5 (13–24)	6.8 ± 2.5

Characteristic Alterations of Inflammatory Cervical Spine Involvement

Examples of characteristic findings in rheumatoid cervical spine disease follow at this point. They can be grouped into atlantoaxial and subaxial changes. Figure 15.1 demonstrates the normal C1–C2 anatomic relationships. The most common abnormality at the atlantoaxial level is horizontal

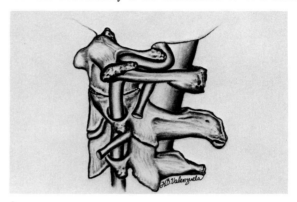

A

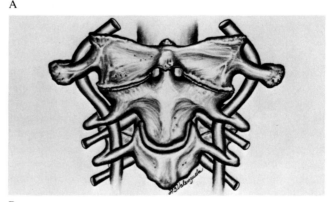

B

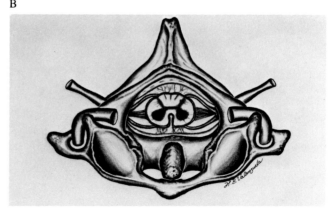

C

FIGURE 15.1 C1–C3, showing normal relationships of vertebrae, vertebral arteries, spinal nerve roots, and dural structures. **A.** Viewed laterally. **B.** Viewed anteriorly. **C.** Viewed axially, with the dens shown.

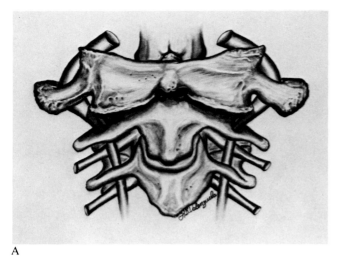

A

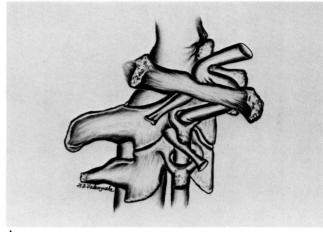

A

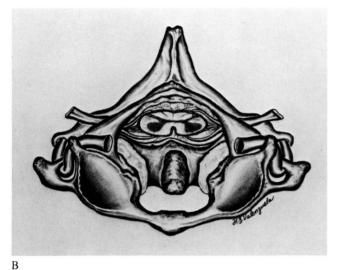

B

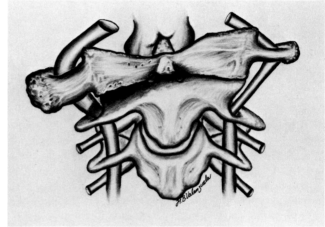

B

FIGURE 15.2 Symmetrical anterior subluxation of C1 on C2. **A.** Anterior view. **B.** Axial view, with encroachment at the spinal cord and vertebral arteries.

symmetrical subluxation (Fig. 15.2). The other characteristic change is vertical penetration, which occurs because of resorption at the atlantoaxial articulation. These types of subluxation can occur separately or in combination. Horizontal anterior atlantoaxial subluxation is present if the distance between the posterior aspect of the anterior ring of C1 is more than 2.5 mm in a woman or 3 mm in a man from the anterior aspect of the odontoid. Vertical penetration has occurred if the line joining the hard palate to the outer table of the occiput is more than 4.5 mm caudad to the tip of the dens on a lateral radiograph.

The progression of atlantoaxial synovitis can be asymmetrical, yielding to a tilt of the ring of C1 on C2, and it is usually associated with some rotation of C1 on C2 (Fig. 15.3). Any of these atlantoaxial alterations can occur

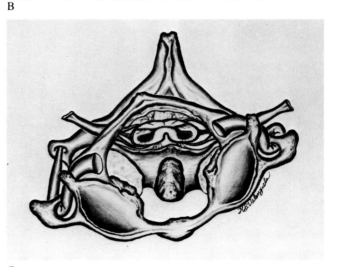

C

FIGURE 15.3 Asymmetrical rotary subluxation of C1 on C2. **A.** Lateral view. Note tortuous course of the vertebral artery. **B.** Anterior view. Note rotation, with associated contralateral head tilt. **C.** Axial view, showing concomitant spinal cord and vertebral artery encroachment.

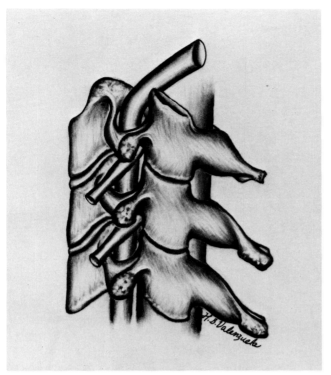

FIGURE 15.4 Lateral view of C3–C5, showing the normal relationship of the vertebral bodies, vertebral artery, apophyseal joints, and dural contents.

in isolation or in combination. The final type of subluxation at the atlantoaxial level is true lateral subluxation. In our experience, symmetrical severe vertical penetration, lateral subluxation, and rotary subluxation have been associated with vertebrobasilar artery signs and symptoms. Posterior subluxation of C1–C2 has been reported in traumatic C-spine disease, but it has not been seen by us in inflammatory disease.

Subaxial subluxation occurs at all levels from C2 through the C7–T1 articulation, but most commonly at C3–C4 and C4–C5 (Fig. 15.4). Subaxial subluxation is less well quantitated; however, White et al. has suggested that a measurement greater than 3.5 mm is greater than is normally physiological.[3] The significant measurements are the remaining diameter in the spinal canal. As in the atlantoaxial involvement, horizontal anterior subluxation is the most common and reflects involvement at the apophyseal and neurocentral joints (Fig. 15.5). Also similar to the atlantoaxial level, subaxial involvement can be asymmetrical and can result in rotary subluxation (Fig. 15.6). This has not been previously reported, and it is difficult to visualize on routine lateral or anteroposterior radiographs. However, after appreciation of this type of subluxation on CT, review of radiographs shows some consistent alteration. With rotary subluxation viewed on lateral radiographs, it is seen that apophyseal joints do not overlap one side on the other

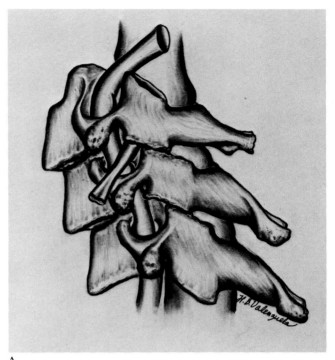

A

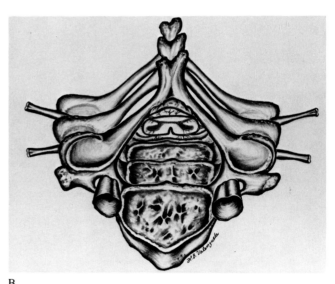

B

FIGURE 15.5 Staircase subluxation of C3,4,5. **A.** Lateral view. **B.** Axial view (also review Figure 15.11).

but are translated anterior or posterior (with the anterior overlying the vertebral body), and/or the neural foramen at the involved level is visualized when not normally seen on true lateral views. These changes do not hold at the C2–3 level or at the C6–7 level: The neural foramina are usually seen at these levels on lateral radiographs, whereas the others are visualized only with oblique views.

The normal osseous relationships between the first cervical vertebra (C1) and the dens of the second cervical vertebra (C2) are seen in Figure 15.7. The C1 ring is visu-

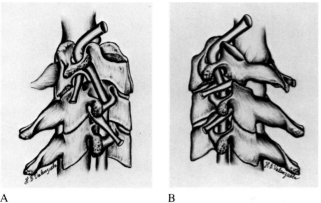

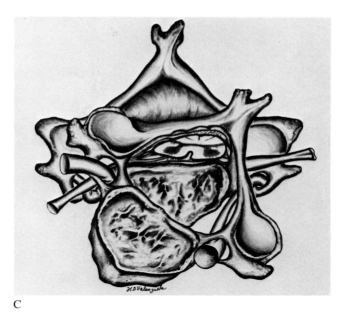

FIGURE 15.6 Rotary subluxation of C3 on C4. **A.** Lateral view. Note the visualization of the neural foramen on a true lateral view. **B.** Lateral view showing the anterior displacement of the apophyseal articulation. **C.** Axial view of an extreme rotary subluxation of C3 on C4. Note the vertebral artery embarrassment.

alized symmetrically in the identical axial sections, with the plane of the sagittal section on the right signified in the upper image by a midsagittal line. The measurement shown is from the transverse ligament (posterior to the dens) to the posterior ring; it demonstrates adequate capacity for the average 10-mm spinal cord. The level of the axial section is shown on the right superior margin of the sagittal section by a tick mark.

The complex deformity shown in Figure 15.8 is at the atlantoaxial complex, with anterior subluxation, vertical penetration, and asymmetrical lateral mass erosion; this resulted in a rightward facial rotation and a rightward head

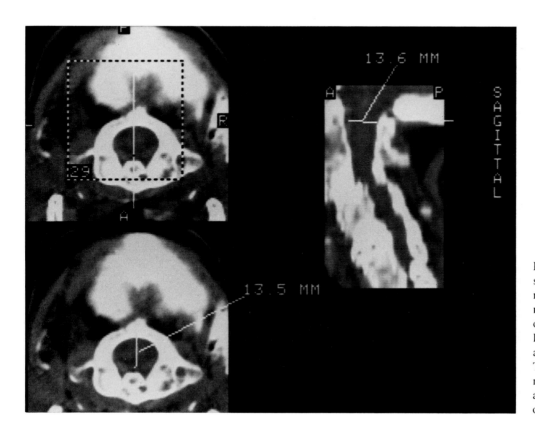

FIGURE 15.7 Axial and sagittal views in a patient with rheumatoid arthritis, showing normal relationship at the level of C1. The dens, transverse ligament, and dural structures are seen on the axial view. There is adequate measurement from the transverse ligament to the posterior ring of C1.

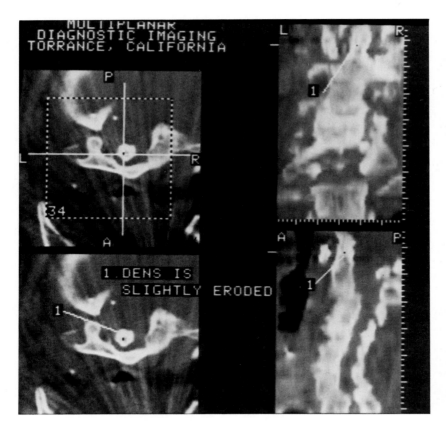

FIGURE 15.8 Axial, coronal, and sagittal views in a patient with rheumatoid arthritis and asymmetrical subluxation of C1 on C2. C1 and cranium are rotated to the patient's right and are also subluxated to the right, as seen on the coronal view. The sagittal view verifies the anterior subluxation and reveals vertical penetration.

tilt because of subluxation to the right at the atlantoaxial articulation on the right. Usually the rotation is contralateral to the head tilt unless lateral subluxation also occurs. The axial image clearly shows space between the dens and the anterior ring of C1, and this is confirmed on the sagittal image. In addition, the degree of vertical penetration over the superior margin of C1 can be seen in the sagittal image, and the degree of penetration into the foramen magnum can be seen in the coronal image.

Another example of vertical penetration at the atlantoaxial level can be seen in Figure 15.9. The axial section shows the body of C2 inside the ring of C1 to the extent that a single 3 mm thick section allows visualization of the right and left foramina transversaria of both C1 and C2. The sagittal section shows the dens protruding 12 mm above the superior margin of C1 and 8.4 mm above the foramen magnum.

Sequential C1–2 axial sections, slices 13–28, are demonstrated in Figure 15.10A. C1 is anterior to C2 and is rotated approximately 65 degrees to the axis of C2. The left lateral mass of C1 is anterior to the midportion of the body of C2, as shown on slices 23–27. The path of the vertebral artery on the left can be estimated by locating the foramen transversarium of C2 on slice 22, and of C1 on slice 27. Figure 15.10B helps to explain this deformity by demonstrating complete resorption of the dens. Figure 15.10C shows inadequate space for dural structures at the level of C1–2: 8.1 mm in an area where the cord measures 10 mm.

The curved coronal reconstructions Nos. 1–14 are shown in Figure 10.15D. These further define the severe head tilt to the right, with rotation to the right. Section 9 shows the

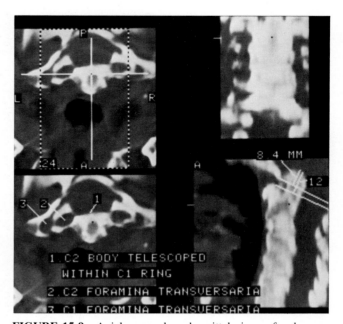

1. C2 BODY TELESCOPED
   WITHIN C1 RING
2. C2 FORAMINA TRANSVERSARIA
3. C1 FORAMINA TRANSVERSARIA

FIGURE 15.9 Axial, coronal, and sagittal views of a rheumatoid arthritis patient with vertical penetration of 8.4 mm above the foramen magnum and 12 mm above the ring of C1.

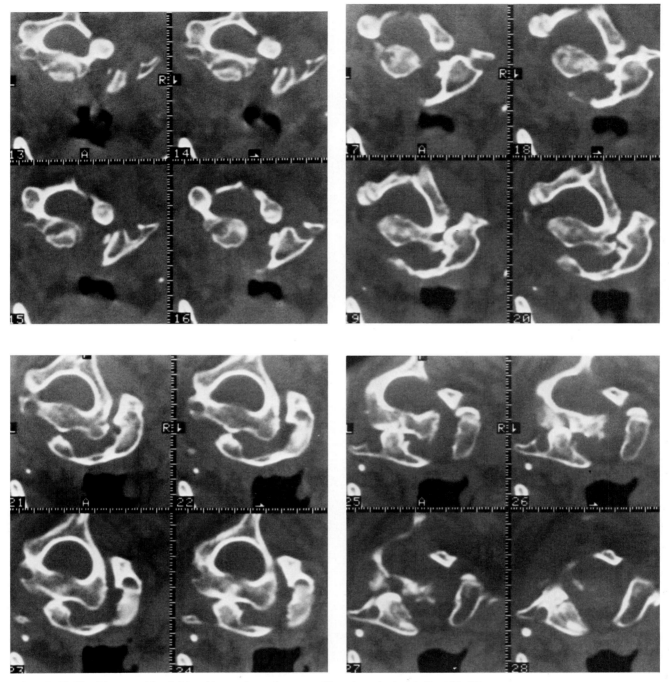

FIGURE 15.10 Rheumatoid arthritis with anterior and rotary subluxation. **A.** Axial slices 13–28. Sequential views of the C1–C2 articulation. **B.** Axial and midsagittal views through the body of C2, showing complete dens resorption. **C.** Axial and midsagittal views through the ring of C1, showing the degree of anterior subluxation and the decrease in the spinal canal. **D.** Sequential curved coronal views clearly show the severely altered anatomy of the lateral masses of C1 on C2, with rightward subluxation and head rotation. (*Figure continued* on pages 460, 461, 462.)

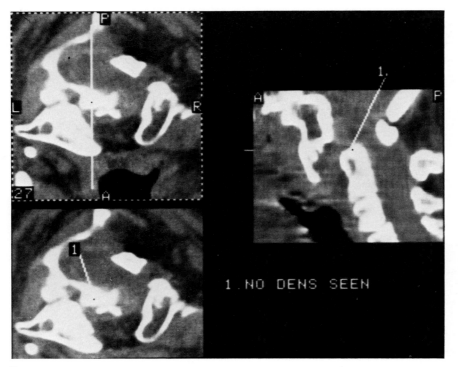

B

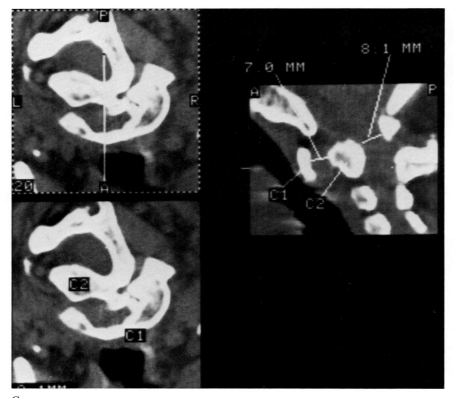

C

FIGURE 15.10 (*cont'd*)

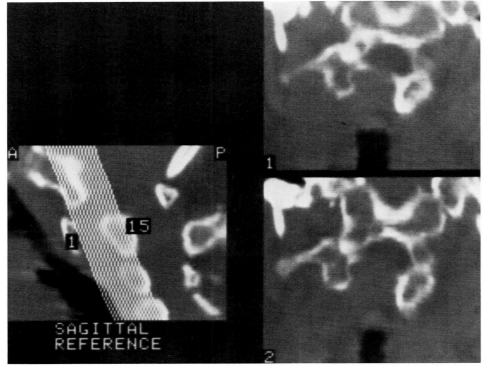

D1

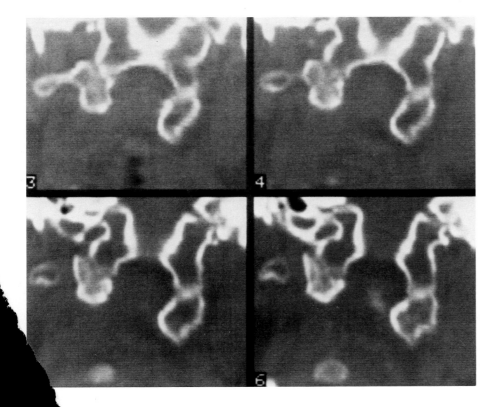

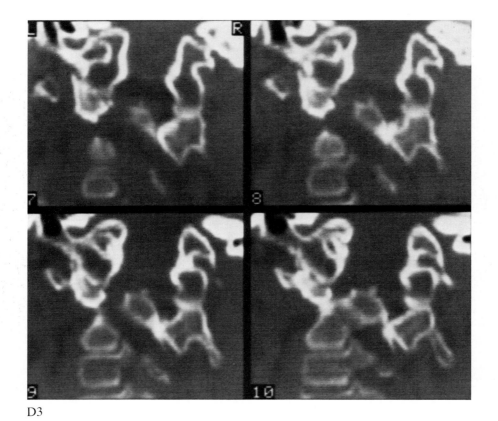

D3

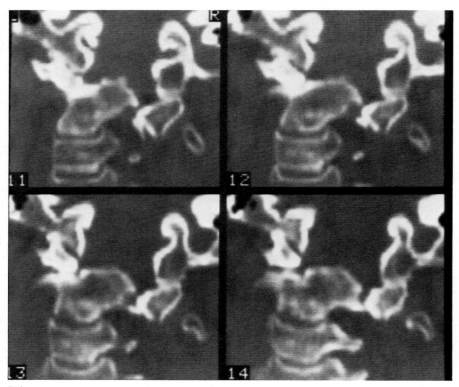

D4

FIGURE 15.10 (*cont'd*)

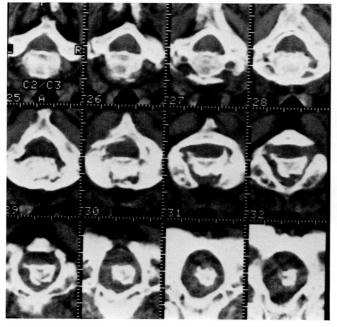

A

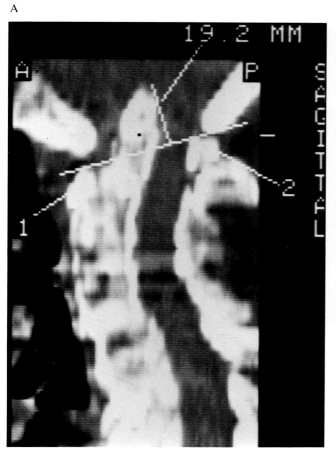

B

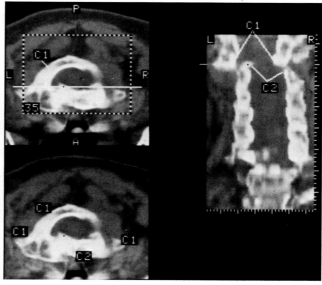

C

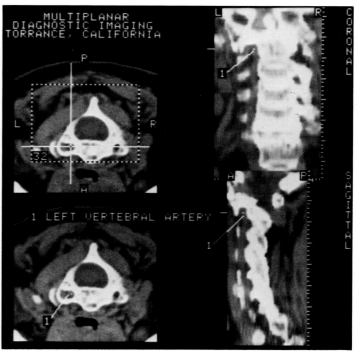

D

FIGURE 15.11 Rheumatoid arthritis with vertical penetration (**A, B**) and later subluxation (**C, D**). **A.** Sequential axial sections 25–36 (foramen magnum 34–36). **B.** Axial and midsagittal view detailing 19.2 mm vertical penetration above the ring of C1. **C.** Axial and coronal views of lateral subluxation of C1 on C2. **D.** The course of the left vertebral artery from the patient in **C**, with the intersection of sagittal and coronal planes at the pixel (*1*).

lateral mass of C1, with its transverse process barely articulating with C2, also again confirming the absence of the dens.

Sequential axial sections of vertical symmetrical subluxation of C1–C2 is shown in Figure 15.11A (slices 25–36). Figure 15.11B demonstrates how essential the reconstructed alternative views are to the interpretation of axial sections. The dens is shown by a black dot on both the axial and the sagittal sections, and the severity of vertical penetration is shown on the sagittal view. Figure 15.11C shows pure lateral subluxation of C1 on C2, and the vertebral artery is visualized in Figure 15.11D.

Subaxial subluxation in inflammatory arthritis can be at a single level, or it can be in staircase fashion as in Figure 15.12. This case serves to prove an important point with regard to the controversy between reconstructions and tilt-

ing-gantry perpendicular sections. The single 3 mm thick axial section cuts through portions of the vertebral bodies of C2–C5. The spinal canal is shown in the midsagittal reconstruction to be at 65 degrees to the long axis of the spinal canal, an angulation uncorrectable by tilting-gantry techniques.

As previously mentioned, subaxial subluxations can occur with a rotational component (Fig. 15.13). Figure 15.13A shows sequential axial sections 16–30, with section 30 at the level of C2 and section 16 at C6. Of particular interest is the axis of C3 in slice 25 compared with slices 16 and 30. Further clarification is seen in Figure 15.13B, which shows the rotation on the axial plane as well as the inaccuracy of the above axial measurements. The axial section shows a 13.5-mm diameter, which is actually 3.5 mm on the midsagittal oblique measurement, a critical narrowing.

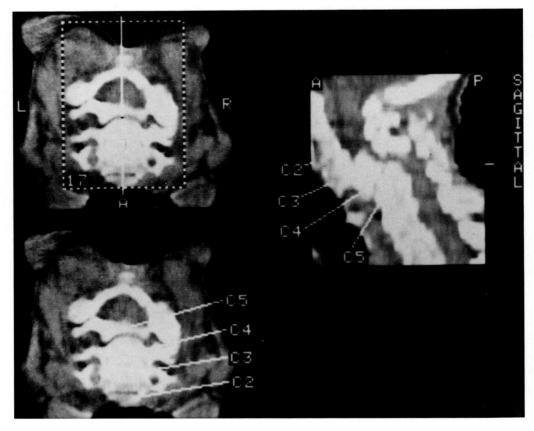

FIGURE 15.12 Axial and sagittal views of subaxial staircase subluxation; the spinal canal dimension at its narrowest level was 1.5 mm.

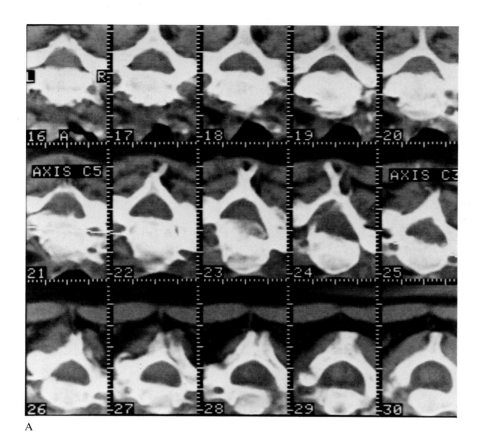

A

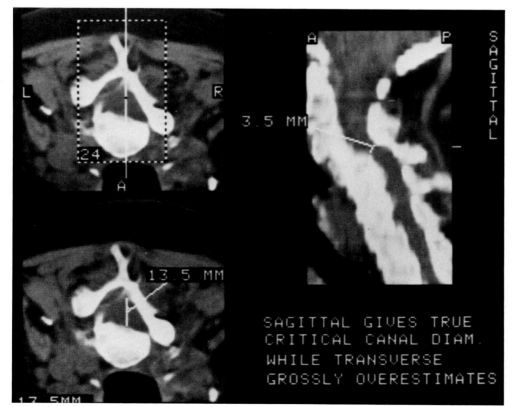

B

FIGURE 15.13 Rheumatoid arthritis, with rotary subluxation at C3. **A.** Axial slices 16–30. **B.** Axial slice 24 shows the adequate axial canal but a severely stenotic midsagittal oblique measurement of 3.5 mm.

Further demonstration of the requirement for rapidly generated alternative-view reconstructions is shown in Figure 15.14. The sequential axial sections in Figure 15.14A (sections 13–24) show that the spinal canal is only encroached on in slice 19. Figure 15.14B illustrates that the severity is more fully appreciated when this is viewed in the midsagittal section, reflecting an oblique measurement of 3.5 mm in an area where the spinal cord averages 7 mm.

CT/MPR can also evaluate the status of all the neural foramina; in fact, it is probably best shown on oblique reconstructions through this area. Figure 15.15A shows the area of interest and the intersection of the sagittal and coronal planes on the axial section at the left neural foramen at the C4–5 level. The neural foramen is shown to be patent on all three views. Figure 15.15B shows another neural foramen to be severely stenotic.

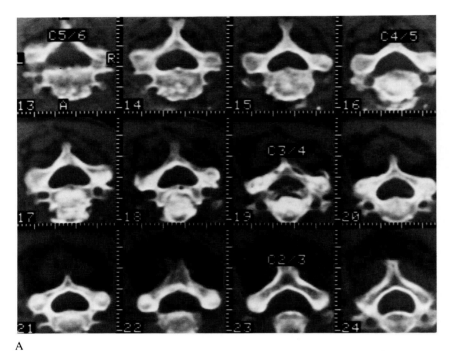

A

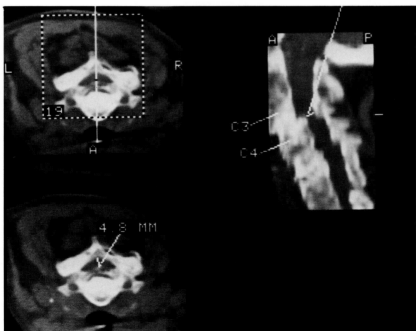

B

FIGURE 15.14 Rheumatoid arthritis, with C3–4 subluxation. **A.** Sequential axial sections 13–24. **B.** Axial slice 19, with the midsagittal reconstruction showing the oblique measurement to be 3.5 mm.

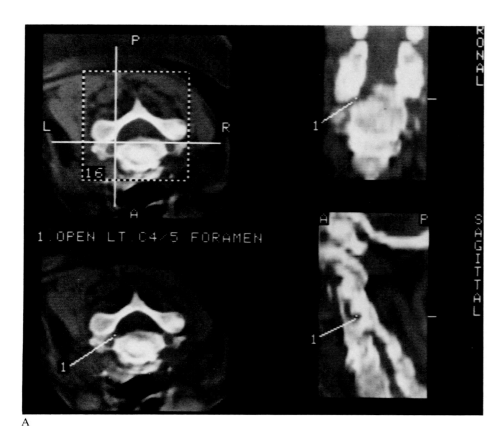

A

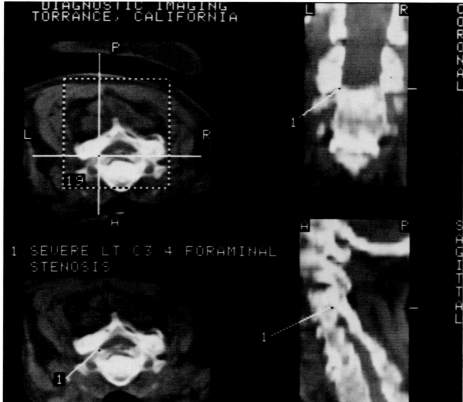

B

FIGURE 15.15 Foraminal stenosis. **A.** Axial, coronal, and sagittal views of the left neural foramen of C4–5. **B.** Axial, coronal, and sagittal views of a severely stenotic C3–4 foramen.

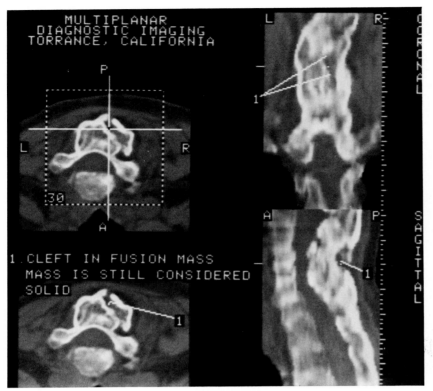

FIGURE 15.16   Axial, coronal, and sagittal views of a mature posterior cervical fusion in a patient with rheumatoid cervical myelopathy after an extensive multilevel procedure.

Finally, Figure 15.16 evaluates a posterior cervical fusion mass and shows it to be intact and fused to the cervical structures. Although a cleft is pointed out, a review of sections sequentially in sagittal and/or coronal orientations shows the fusion to be solid.

In conclusion, CT/MPR is essential in the preoperative evaluation of patients with cervical myelopathy secondary to rheumatoid arthritis and other forms of inflammatory polyarthritis. It is also an effective aid in the workup of a patient with unusual clinical findings that are unexplained by routine radiographs. CT/MPR can largely replace myelography in the evaluation of these patients and thereby reduce both cost and morbidity. Cervical structures can be detailed to evaluate osseous integrity and relationships as well as encroachment at the spinal cord, nerve roots, or vertebral arteries.

References

1. Kaufman RL, Glenn WV: Rheumatoid cervical myelopathy: evaluation by computerized tomography with multiplanar reconstruction. J Rheumatol 10:42–54, 1983
2. Blau R, Kaufman RL: Erosive subluxing cervical spine disease in psoriatic arthritis. In preparation
3. White AA, Johnson RM, Panjabi MM, et al: Biomechanical analysis of clinical stability in the cervical spine. Clin Orthop 109:55–96, 1975

CT Image Processing Using Digital Networks

Michael L. Rhodes

16

Several digital image transmission networks have been proposed, studied, and measured for local-area medical applications. Cox and co-workers[1] used an axiomatic, structured approach to their network design, whereas Meyer-Ebrecht[2] designed an architecture using a hierarchical approach.

Characteristics for an interdepartmental radiology system outlined by Dwyer et al.[3] with components later implemented by Anderson and colleagues.[4] Performance measures were reported by Rasmussen[5] and Gayler[6] and their co-workers. In all cases, networks were designed with special hardware to link a variety of image display devices at high transmission rates.

Local image communication (e.g., within a hospital) emphasizes fast response and format compatibility between several medical imaging modalities. In this setting, where digital images from CT, ultrasound, angiography, and common x-ray devices are accessed by several widely distributed work stations,[1-6] wide-bandwidth ($\sim$56,000 characters/sec or faster) communication channels are essential. Other software issues of file format conversions and communication protocol standards have plagued such systems.

The image processing service described here uses a commercial digital network to connect the computers of CT scanners. The network service shares image processing tasks with remote sites during the times that the scanners are otherwise idle. The network is nationwide, emphasizes resource sharing, uses moderate-bandwidth (4800 or 9600 baud, i.e., 480 or 960 characters/sec) dedicated leased telephone lines, and is restricted at this time to only a few types of CT scanner. Furthermore, because it offers services that are not interactive, it is able to optimize computer resources without routine interruption from users.

Discussion begins by a brief overview of classic computer network topologies, with an emphasis on their application to CT, magnetic resonance imaging (MRI), and other medical imaging modalities. This somewhat technical introduction to networks demonstrates the unique characteristics of medical image communication as opposed to the more common applications of computer communication in the banking, retail, and management information industries. In the sections that follow, a more selective focus is made on the topology, hardware, image-processing, and operational characteristics of a network that is now composed of over 50 CT scanner systems throughout the United States. The chapter concludes by summarizing the network performance during its first 35 months of operation.

Evolution of Computer Networking

Data and image communication is emerging as one of the most strategically important sectors within the information processing industry.[7,8] A driving technology in the medical component of this industry is CT and, more recently, magnetic resonance imaging. The key reason for this trend is that data communication, especially image communication, allows a wide distribution of information. Information exchange in medicine means cost-effective medical care. Communication systems minimize the duplication of equipment and film, the volume of information archived, and manual transmission of reports.

An important aspect of networks and their application to medical imaging is simply the ability to communicate easily with these image-generation systems. Because they can be accomplished without travel to each connected system, program updates, system repairs, and system diagnostics are becoming key benefits of network approaches to the distribution and maintenance of medical technology. These are important side effects of medical imaging networks, whose initial value and perceived merit was limited to resource sharing and information distribution alone. Ultimately, as a major element in today's expanding role for medical data and medical image processing, computer communication provides a cost-effective way to deliver the highest-quality medicine possible on a global scale. There are no remaining technical barriers to international computer communication.

To understand the current and emerging capabilities in today's computer communication networks, we need to put in perspective the network evolution that has occurred during the past two decades. The first networks, during the 1960s, connected a terminal operator directly to a host computer. All facilities were dedicated. The terminal, the communication processor, and the host computer were all assigned to a single task. As a result, only large applications, e.g., airline reservation systems, could justify and afford to use communications. The American Airlines STAR system was one of the early successful applications of that technology. Figure 16.1 illustrates a typical computer configuration during the 1960s. One can think of these early configurations as really no different from a modern multiuser computer system, with the exception of having terminals geographically distant from the host—terminals connected by telephone leased lines directly to the computer.

During this initial phase there was little real networking activity as we know it today. Terminals had wires connected directly, point to point, to the single central computer system (one can understand how the STAR system got its name). There was no interaction between multiple computer systems at this early date. In addition, limitations were imposed by the "hard-wire" implementation of such

systems, because all of the controllers and multiplexors (equipment that allows multiple dialogues over a single wire) were incapable of switching to other applications.

During the 1970s progress was made in nearly every area of computer communication to increase the ease and flexibility of networking. Progress made during this decade allowed the widespread use of networks that was later realized in the 1980s. An outline of these contributions introduces key concepts of computer communication that are now commonplace.

First of all, communication was provided between multiple host computer centers. Basically, this is the first genuine networking function that took place. The next development was to attach remote processors to provide some other form of sharing or concentration. These first steps included a form of concentration within the networking capability, trunking, line switching, and support for multiple host processors. In other words, we had implementations that began to optimize the way in which physical connections are made efficient; genuine network issues were now addressed.

The concept of trunking, which concentrated lines between network nodes, was introduced during the 1970s. This capability is desirable for many reasons. With multiple circuits, there is a limit to the number of characters that can be transmitted per second between two network nodes. This volume of characters per second, or bandwidth, is limited by economics—the larger the bandwidth, the more expensive the rental of the line. Such lines are rented from the local or, in cases of long distance, regional telephone utility companies (also known as the "common carriers"). However, if multiple circuits or a large bandwidth are needed between multiple locations, the user is left with no other choice than to install multiple links.

The first concept of trunking was to combine the multiple links between nodes and consolidate them as a trunk. The resulting combined bandwidth would allow the addition

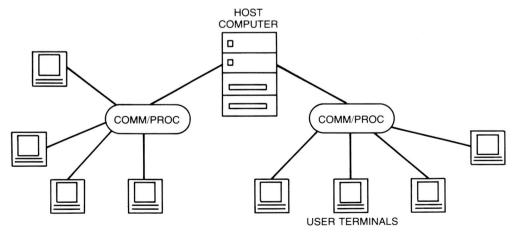

FIGURE 16.1   The topology of a limited network approach to computer communications of the 1960s. (*COMM/PROC*) communications processor.

of the individual line capacities and, on occasion, would provide a basic link between two nodes that could then be treated as a single line of very large bandwidth. Data now could flow on multiple links between the nodes without being dedicated to one physical line.

In addition to increased bandwidth, trunking provided some reliability and a measure of protection by means of link backup. If a line was getting a high error rate, for example, or was put out of service, there would be an automatic fallback to the remaining circuits on that trunk, with no disruption in service other than, possibly, diminished response time. A logical connection between nodes, in any case, was maintained. Because the error sensing and backup was automated, no apparent interruption of the link was sensed between the connected nodes.

The concept of alternate routing was introduced as the second major capability. In a multiple-node network, alternate routing allowed the designer, by means of a software option, to choose an alternate path through some other nodes in the network. It provided for a backup method to enable continued communication in spite of a major catastrophe. For example, should a snow storm in Denver sever the physical line connection between Los Angeles and Chicago, trunks established with an alternate route between these cities are able to avoid the service disruption.

The majority of network dialogues now, and especially for the early applications of digital networks, consisted of short bursts of characters, which can be understood in the light of airline reservations where only a few key words are needed for most transactions. This type of traffic sends so many short bursts of data surrounded by control characters that lines of moderate bandwidth (4800 or 9600 baud) are effectively underutilized. This traffic characteristic justifies the next major advance in networking—concentration. The principle here is simply to avoid the loading of the network with unnecessary traffic, and in this way a given bandwidth is better utilized. Essentially, more processing is delegated to the remote processor to "concentrate" only the key components of the user's dialogue into a compact form to be sent to the host computer. This type of concentration became especially important to reduce long-haul connection charges for computer links.

For a variety of reasons—many in response to a growing concern for reliability—the concept of multiple host processors became more attractive. Increasingly large data bases also encouraged the development of multiple host communication and the data-base management system to support their access. Now networks began to change their topology from star to ring and skeletal configurations. In these distributed topologies a "central" data base was only a conceptual location having no single physical position in a real sense; it was actually distributed among several host computers within the network. The result emphasized resource sharing and allowed more applications to become network options. Figure 16.2 illustrates this more flexible and further distributed network topology.

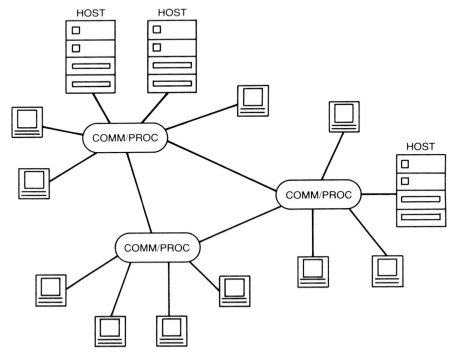

FIGURE 16.2 A distributed network topology for resource sharing typical of computer communications of the 1970s. Distributed data base, services, and multicomputer interconnections begin to be commonplace.

During the 1980s computer communication continues to be more diverse. Embedded within networks are regional data centers that are themselves networks. Each of these regional centers utilizes all forms of common carriers and local facilities. Regional networks, depending on their size, can be called local area networks, similar to those commonly proposed for large hospital medical centers.

At this time there are many competing technologies for local area networks, with no clear leader. CT, MRI, and digital radiographic computer systems can be connected to share image information by twisted-pair wire, coaxial cable, fiberoptics, or in some instances microwave links. Their relative merit and current problems are beyond the scope of this outline. The generic issues in networking during the 1980s are discussed here: packet switching (also called message switching), session and circuit switching, the standardization of transmission protocols, the commercial introduction of satellites, gateways, and the attachment of local area networks.

Circuit switching is familiar to most of us: Common voice-grade dial-up telephone connections are circuit switched. This means that a physical connection between the telephone receiver in your hand and the receiver in the hand of the person you speak with is made electrically. Telephone companies have electronic "switching stations" that actually cause a continuous wire connection between telephone users.

Packet switching is not so simple. Instead of an actual connection, as in circuit-switched links, a "virtual" connection is made. Between points A and B, messages forming the dialogue are split into standard-size packets. Because dialogue in the environment of computer communication usually means file transfers, packets then are simply groups of characters forming part of a file. Even if the dialogue represents English sentences exchanged between distant users, we can think of the individual sentences as files also.

Packets travel independent paths across the network to reach their destinations. For example, packets coming from point A to point B are assembled at point B to rebuild the original message transmitted from point A. This process of disassembly and packet transmission followed by reassembly at a destination node delivers important benefits to the network user.

First, because each packet is individually addressed and is able to find its own way across the network, reliability is improved. Links in the network that become disabled cause packets to reroute to another node along an alternate path of links to the ultimate destination. This is done by logic resident at packet processors at each node. Message integrity is also improved. As packets arrive they are verified against a copy held at the sending node. If it is without error, the packet is accepted, the copy at the sending node is deleted, and the packet is forwarded to the next available node in the path toward its destination. This

"store-and-forward" protocol ensures that packets migrating through the network are error-free—no packet is accepted from a node unless it is identical to the copy at the sending node.

Another advantage of packet switching is found in the design of node processors. No processor is dedicated to a particular connection, so their design is standard and expandable. This also allows bandwidth to be dynamically allocated; load-sharing is then easily accommodated. As a node becomes congested and slows response time, selection of alternate paths to maintain acceptable response is inherent to the strategy.

Network options are becoming integral to computer operating systems. Network packages are now sold as standard software to computer system buyers, just as programming languages (BASIC, FORTRAN, PL/I, PASCAL, etc.) were offered in the past. This trend has important consequences that further encourage network proliferation. One consequence is session switching. Now, as a side effect of the network's integration with a computer's operating system, multiple network dialogues can take place simultaneously through one or several terminals. This is an inherent feature of multiuser operating systems, which have evolved independently of network issues. Such operating systems are able to keep track of several users simultaneously, without burden to system users.

Session switching is the capability to use a single line for several concurrent dialogues. It takes several forms. At one level a session is a logical link or process of an operating system; at another level it may simply be the multiplexing of several conversations over a single link. The key aspect of either form is flexibility. Several conversations can take place regardless of the number of lines or terminals a computer system may have connected to a network. In practical terms, this means a user at one terminal can easily switch environments from one dialogue to the next. He may start a file transfer between one remote computer and the host, switch to a new environment where a second file transfer is begun with a different remote computer, and continue such session switching until the early file transfer is complete. This feature is used to great advantage by the medical image-processing network discussed later in this chapter.

In spite of all the progress made by computer communication during the past two decades, none has been as helpful to the commercial success and general public use of networks as has the international standardization of communication protocols. This was a necessary step to successfully interconnect computer systems from different manufacturers. For packet-switched networks, X.25 has been the most widely accepted protocol. Using this and other similar protocols, commercial network service providers can lower service charges to all of their customers because no special ad hoc protocols need their support. Network service providers can also concentrate and trunk traffic themselves

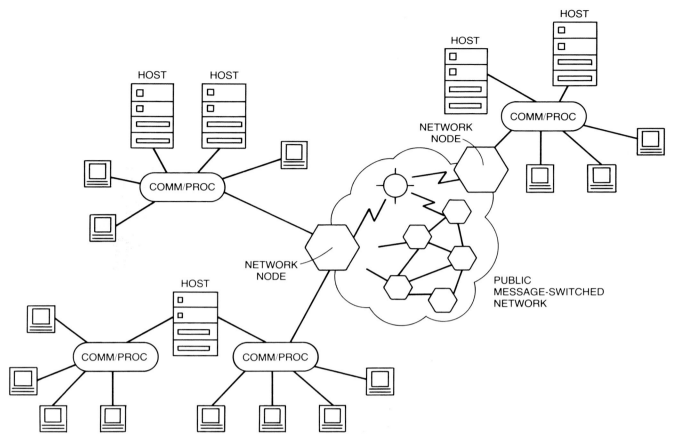

FIGURE 16.3 Local-area and single-computer systems connected to a public data communications network. Public networks allow any computer system to communicate with any other system by enforcing a standard communications protocol—X.25.

using a protocol that is optimal for higher-bandwidth traffic (e.g., X.75).

A typical interconnection of three computer systems to a public message-switched network is illustrated in Figure 16.3. Once subscriber packets enter the public network, issues of the actual transmission of packets are left to the public network. It is solely the concern of the public network whether satellite, microwave, fiberoptic, terrestial line, or radio is used to transmit packets.

When network traffic is voluminous, satellite transponder channels are leased by network service providers to trunk their customers' packet-switched computer dialogues between nodes having concentrated long-haul traffic. For the network that is discussed later in this chapter, traffic is sent routinely on satellite channels for cross-country dialogues. Exactly when and how often this is used is left to the network provider. The overall effect is a more reliable, widely distributed, and less expensive service for the network subscriber.

A description of network gateways provides a logical final block to the pyramid of increasing sophistication outlined in the preceding text. Numerous industrial, military, academic, governmental, and commercial message-switched networks are now in service. Gateways are network nodes that allow interconnection of networks. In practical terms, this means that a commercial message-switched network, e.g., GTE Telenet, is able to provide its customers with global access. Any network, anywhere, that uses X.25 as a protocol can interconnect to Telenet via a gateway.

Gateways were introduced above as the top of the evolutionary hierarchy of network developments spanning digital computer communication over the past two decades. This can be understood in terms of the types of interconnections that have taken place in computer networks: terminals-to-computers, computers-to-computers, computers-to-networks, and now gateways (networks-to-networks). In the sections that follow, attention is refocused to characteristics of the only network that is currently connected to CT scanners distributed nationwide in the United States.

Network Hardware

In August 1981, using GTE Telenet's X.25 public network service, two CT scanners separated by 3000 miles were connected. This connection allowed routine CT image processing for a CT scanner at Massachusetts General Hospital to be shared between several computers in Torrance, California. The network provides an image-processing service (it does not include radiologic interpretation). High-volume CT image processing that would be economically impractical for the remote site to perform alone is shared between the network computers. The economies delivered by this approach are genuine, regardless of the type of scanner connected. Circuit-board and standard wire connections that allow a CT scanner to be network-connected, whether it be one X.25 network or another, are briefly outlined here.

Currently, the network is not able to connect to all scanner systems. For compatible scanners, no changes to the scanner's computer are necessary beyond the addition of a single-line synchronous-interface circuit card, which fits directly into the computer chassis. Figure 16.4 illustrates this configuration for a GE system. A cable from the synchronous-interface card extends to the 4800- to 9600-baud modem that is supplied by the commercial telecommunication provider.

This level of integration with the scanner's computer allows all network communication instructions to be issued by software alone. Users need not dial a telephone for computer communication or use any specialized equipment; all the communication capability of the network is available at the CT scanner's keyboard and videoscreen.

Network Operation

From an operational standpoint, network services require little effort. The CT technologist at a remote site triggers network processing by initiating the "CTNET" program just before leaving at night. The CTNET program requests the identity of cases to be network-processed and then simply enters a wait state until signaled by the host computer in California. The CT technologist in California then executes an instruction to connect the host computer with the remote system. The remote CT scanner's computer and the large central host computer then conduct a dialogue involving extensive compression of the data transmitted to the host computer.

Incoming files are screen presentations that represent a survey of each case. That is, for each case submitted, a composite picture is formed and then sent to the host computer. This survey view includes the first, middle, and last axial slices of the case, plus lateral and anteroposterior digital plain views that may have been taken to locate the axial slices.

This survey presentation is used by CT technologists in California to select processing options for the case. Among other tasks, they position and adjust the region of interest (within which a complete set of sagittal and coronal planes are generated), clip the digital plain views for their inclusion in later composite pictures, select the curvature for network-generated curved image planes (curved coronals), and direct the order in which remote sites are processed.

Once processing options are chosen for all cases submitted, a dialogue takes place between the remote CT scanner's computer and the host system. This automated correspondence generates the formatted set of pictures that is selected for each of the cases submitted.

Images generated by the host computer are written over the disk storage locations that were previously occupied by the axial picture files generated by the scanner. As many cases as can be loaded on a scanner's storage system can be submitted to the network.

A common misconception regarding the network service is that all of the CT image data are transmitted to

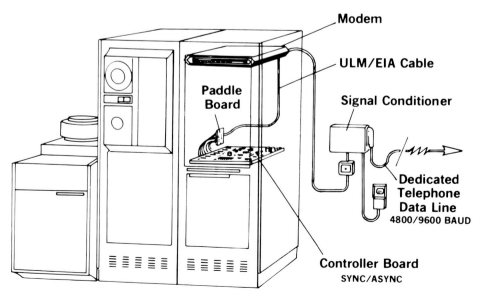

FIGURE 16.4 Electronics and telecommunications gear attached to a CT scanner system to allow network communications.

the host computer in California and processed there, and then resultant pictures are transmitted back. This is not the case. What and how much image data are transmitted between a remote site and the host computer depends on: (1) the type of study requested; (2) network traffic congestion; and (3) the software revision in effect. Some (not all) of the image data for every case are transmitted between the remote computer and the host computer. When submitted cases arrive in California, each case is examined by a certified CT technologist at the host system to determine processing options.

The network shares processing with the remote users. Some processing for every case is done at the host site, and several system utilities take place solely at the remote site: file allocation, disk space recovery, and file deletions. The result is an image-processing service that shares resources—image processing takes place at both facilities.

Full-Case Transmission

On occasion, full cases (32–35 CT slices) are transmitted between sites via the network. This situation is rare and currently is not encouraged due to the length of time a leased line is occupied. The time required to transmit each case without any data compression is determined quite simply: (32 slices/case) × (160,768 bytes/slice) × (8 bits/byte)/(4800 bits/sec)(60 sec/min) = 142.9 min.

The assumption here is that full bandwidth of the line is achieved. We have experienced an effective line speed of only 87% of that rated. The loss, we suspect, is caused by protocol overhead introduced by the telecommunication provider. Depending on the image quality and resolution, compression routines can reduce the time required to transmit (142.9 min) to less than 1 hr. Even under these circumstances, the network cannot presently sustain more than 50 such requests per day. For the routine image processing service there is never a need to transmit full cases; only regions of interest require transmission.

SUMMARY

Nearly every working day an exchange of files takes place between the host and each remote computer connected to the network. In the flurry of this digital communication where now, over 50,000 CT exams have been processed, software maintenance emerges as a key advantage to the distributed approach to network image processing. Several examples illustrate this point. More than 32 software revisions were distributed to remote users during the first 35 months of operation. Files are routinely replaced, substituted, deleted, and created by the host system. In addition, system configuration (in terms of available memory, disk space utilization, and current revision of remote software) is all automatically reported to the host system and its operator at the time of connection for each site.

The ease with which the host computer communicates with remote systems translates to network reliability. On no occasion has a technologist had to travel to a remote site to resurrect a system that has crashed. All software residing at a remote site can be reinstalled directly from the host computer using a simple network connect program. Downtime from remote sites has therefore been very rare.

Computer communications have revolutionized the world we live in. Though limited to special applications in the past (airline reservations systems), computer communications have now reached us all via our bank (automatic teller systems) and more recently by introduction to our living rooms via personnel computers. Benefits of simple communication between medical computer systems are numerous and too valuable to ignore.

References

1. Cox JR, Blaine GJ, Hill RL, Jost RG: Study of a distributed picture archiving and communication system for radiology. SPIE Vol. 318 (Part I), Picture Archiving and Communication Systems (PACS) for Medical Applications, SPIE, Bellingham, Washington, pp. 133–140, January 1982
2. Meyer-Ebrecht D: The management and processing of medical pictures: an architecture for systems and processing devices. In: Proceedings of the Workshop on Picture Data Description and Management, IEEE, pp. 202–206, 1980
3. Dwyer SJ, Templeton AW, Anderson WH, et al: Salient characteristics of a distributed diagnostic imaging management system for a radiology department. SPIE Vol. 318 (Part I), Picture Archiving and Communication Systems (PACS) for Medical Applications, SPIE, Bellingham, Washington, pp. 194–204, January 1982
4. Anderson WH, Tarlton MA, Hensley KS, et al: Implementation of a diagnostic display and image manipulation mode. SPIE Vol. 418, PACS II for Medical Applications, SPIE, Bellingham, Washington, p. 225, May 1983
5. Rasmussen WT, Stevens I, Hayes PD, et al: Remote Medical Diagnosis System (RMDS) Advanced Development Model (ADM) Radiology Performance Results. NOSC TR 683, Naval Ocean Systems Center, San Diego, California, November 1981
6. Gayler B, Gitlin J, Rappaport W, et al: Teleradiology — An evaluation of a microcomputer-based system. Vol. 147, Number 8, Radiology, 1981
7. Groenke RM: Network evolution: putting it in perspective. Computerworld 18:SR/3–SR/6, 1984
8. Harper WL, Pollard RC: Data Communications Desk Book: A Systems Analysis Approach. Prentice-Hall, Englewood Cliffs, New Jersey, 1982

CT Applications of Medical Computer Graphics

17

Michael L. Rhodes

Few applications of computer graphics show as much promise and early success as that for CT. Unlike electron microscopy, ultrasound, business, military, and animation applications, CT image data are inherently digital. CT pictures can be processed directly by programs well established in the fields of computer graphics and digital image processing. Methods for reformatting digital pictures, enhancing structure shape, reducing image noise, and rendering three-dimensional (3D) scenes of anatomic structures have all become routine at many CT centers. In this chapter we provide a brief introduction to computer graphics terms and techniques commonly applied to CT pictures and, when appropriate, to those showing promise for magnetic resonance images. Topics discussed here are image-processing options that are applied to digital images already reconstructed. Image reconstruction topics—those concerning the formation of digital images from raw projection data—are not considered.

Methods of special interest here are those already proved in other applications that may become important diagnostic aids in a clinical environment. After a brief introduction to the components forming a typical clinical image workstation, we review image enhancement techniques, digital filters, image operators, edge detection, object isolation, and methods for viewing anatomy using orthogonal, oblique, and curved surfaces. These topics represent the expanding role that computer graphics is taking in clinical medicine. For example, in many 3D imaging applications, random-shaped objects reconstructed from serial sections are isolated to display their overall structure in a single view. Image data from magnetic resonance is particularly well suited to structure isolation techniques because of its volume scanning capability. It is anticipated that clinical interest in such views will gather strength as magnetic resonance imaging (MRI) becomes more commonplace. Here methods are presented for locating all contours of random-shaped objects intersected by a series of digital image planes. Characteristics most favorable to clinical CT applications are discussed. Phantom and clinical CT data are used to illustrate the performance of each technique.

The goal of structure isolation helps to introduce many common image-processing topics. The sequence of their discussion here reflects their historic development, their increasing sophistication, and the evolution from their application to two-dimensional (2D) image data to efficient program execution using image data that are 3D. Algorithms that were sufficiently fast in two dimensions are not necessarily best suited for data that are 3D. This can be illustrated by edge detection.

In the final portion of this chapter techniques for "slicing" CT image data are presented, and geometric principles that describe the specification of oblique and curved images are outlined. Clinical examples are included.

Workstation Components and Terminology

Three types of display systems comprise more than 95% of all terminals connected to computers. The most common (terminals restricted to the presentation of modest amounts of text at high speed) are ignored here; their operation is straightforward. The two remaining classes of computer display system are calligraphic displays and raster displays. Calligraphic displays "draw" the parts forming a picture in any sequence given by the computer. The electron beam in a calligraphic display is positioned and swept across the screen in a pattern that traces discrete lines and characters to make a picture. Raster displays make pictures in the same way that television (TV) sets do; they paint a picture row by row across the screen from top to bottom. Deflection amplifiers, deflection yokes, and other electronic circuitry for raster systems are now mass produced and are ideally suited for CT, MRI, and other digital radiographic gray-scale images. Calligraphic systems, on the other hand, are not well suited for gray-scale digital pictures but are the preferred presentation technology for line drawing and wire-frame pictures.

The TV commercials we see showing car and plane bodies having surfaces modeled by chicken-wire frames are examples of the ideal application for calligraphic display systems. Computer-aided design and other drafting applications use calligraphic systems almost exclusively. A key difference between the two systems is that calligraphic systems display information in any order, whereas raster systems display information that must be ordered top to bottom, left to right. Components forming either system are

similar, but raster technology is emphasized here because of its integral role in CT diagnosis.

Components forming a typical CT image workstation are shown in Figure 17.1. In its most simple form, the console acts as an image memory device. Digital images (e.g., 512 × 512 pixels in size) can be stored for temporary viewing. New images selected for viewing write over the image previously resident in the console's image memory. The term ''frame buffer'' has gained popular acceptance for referring to this volatile memory component of the display system.

CT images are viewed in detail using several presentation options to clearly illustrate anatomic structure. These adjustments are necessary because of the limited gray-scale differentiation of human vision. They allow the viewer to spread his gray-scale visibility spectrum to selective ranges of pixel values. Electronic circuitry that allows this was already in place on standard raster systems long before the proliferation of CT scanners. Image generation systems based on infrared, x-ray, magnetic resonance, and optical sensory scanners can all produce digital information that exceeds

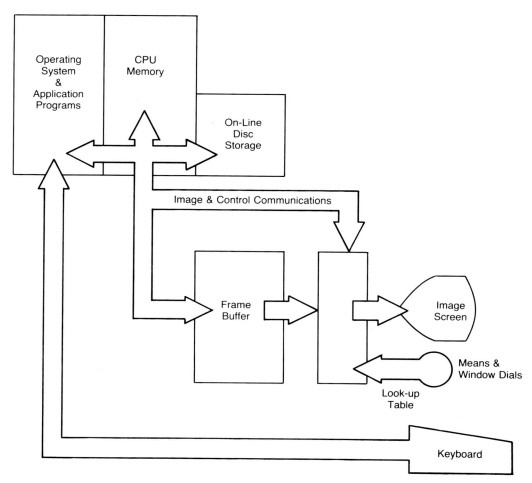

FIGURE 17.1 Components forming a raster display workstation that is typical for CT and MRI applications.

the gray-scale capabilities of human vision. From this background, "lookup" tables were designed to allow flexible viewing of digital (raster-organized) pictures.

The role played by a lookup table in a raster workstation is illustrated in Figure 17.1. It provides a gray-scale brightness value for each of the possible values stored in the frame buffer. Pictures are displayed by a frequent (typically 30/sec) scan of the frame buffer. As each pixel is read from the buffer, its brightness value is looked up in a table. If pixels have values from -500 to $+500$, a lookup table will have 1000 entries. The entry found in the table position equal to the pixel's value is a number that determines its brightness (the strength of the electron beam is modulated at the pixels location by this relative value).

This frame buffer to lookup table to screen scanning process is continuous—if it were done once, the screen would flash and fade to a blank as the screen phosphor gradually lost its charge. By continually scanning, an image persists on the screen as a stable picture. Screens having short-persistence phosphor allow new pictures (new frame buffer contents) to be swept onto the screen quickly without leaving a ghost of the previous display. Quick switch to new pictures is not the only reason for this approach; new presentations of the same picture require the same short persistence. Changes to the content of the lookup table, between screen refreshes, results in new presentations of the same image information.

Note in Figure 17.1 that the lookup table is directly accessed by the console or by program control. The lookup table itself sends output to only the display screen. Under program control or by devices attached directly to the lookup table, image presentations can be adjusted instantaneously by mean and window values.

The frame buffer receives digital image data from the computer systems. Although recent computer system architectures allow direct transfer of image data from the computer system's disk to the frame buffer, the most common path for image data is via the computer's address space. That is, under software (program) control, a digital picture is transferred from the computer system's disk through the computer system's memory onto the frame buffer in a sequence of subpicture components. This transfer—disk to memory to frame buffer—is typically the slowest component of any interactive workstation. This slow transmission of image data is ultimately due to disk access and transfer rates that are typically 10 times slower than memory-to-memory transfers within the computer system.

Recently several technologic advances to reduce image data transmission delays have begun to appear in workstations. Because of the continuing cost reduction in semiconductor memory, large frame buffers are becoming more commonplace. Now, several full pictures (eventually, all the slices for a given case) can be stored at the workstation's frame buffer. Workstations for some MRI scanners are to have frame buffers for up to 16 slices.

Thresholding and Operator Methods for CT Image Enhancement

Thresholding

Digital images from CT systems are composed of picture elements (pixels) located by coordinate pairs (x,y). Each pixel has a value, f(x,y), typically between 0 and 4095 (corresponding to the positive integer values for 12 bits). A reduction in range corresponds to a lower number of bits for some imaging modalities, e.g., 8 bits (0–255) for many ultrasound devices. Although 256 or more shades of gray can be presented, simple black/white presentation is sometimes preferred to illustrate a single density range that highlights anatomic structure. For example, contrast injections are often viewed with window and level settings adjusted to show contrast medium alone as white against a black field. This is done at the display console, interactively, by dial adjustments to the lookup table. The display processor changes its presentation of the underlying image data at screen refresh rates. Changes appear to the user instantaneously. Entries in the lookup table for each f(x,y) are reassigned to brighten one range of values and suppress (make darker) the values of f(x,y) outside the selected range. Carefully adjusted settings can cause the presentation of soft tissue [below some $f'(x,y)$] to be black, whereas pixels having values above f'(x,y) can be displayed white. This interactive technique is useful for tracking the extent of contrast medium or to acquire a simple, segmented view for a range of pixel values, $f'(x,y) < (f(x,y) < f''(x,y)$.

Thresholding is a useful image presentation technique for quickly and interactively viewing structures that have near-homogeneous values of f(x,y) and that are different from surrounding tissue. Using the lookup table, an image is presented that effectively isolates such a structure from its surroundings. Because no change to the underlying image data is made, however, a logical segmentation of the image is not available. There is no computer-readable, logical entity, or data structure, unique to a single anatomic structure that a computer program can access. What is needed is a data structure that represents those pixels [g(x,y), a subset of f(x,y)], that form the volume, area, or surface of a single anatomic entity. Once this is done, subsequent steps may be taken to show the isolated structure to better advantage.

Images segmented by thresholding are the result of a pixel-by-pixel selection process that is indiscriminate in terms of spatial features. Any pixel that satisfies a value criterion for f(x,y) is accepted; others are rejected. Binary images are the customary results of thresholding, but band-passed gray-level images are also possible. Later in this chapter there are illustrations of several realistic 3D synthetic views of anatomic structures that use thresholding as a key preprocessing step to their scene-rendering technique.

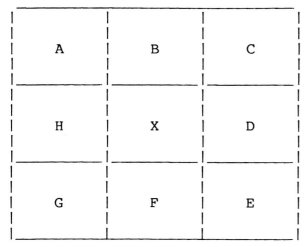

FIGURE 17.2 The 3 x 3 pixel pattern for image operations.

Operator Methods

Operator methods are common edge-detection techniques using spatial filters for satellite, radar, geologic, and other 2D image applications. These digital operators report sharp changes in image gray-level values. Fourier frequency filters are the classic linear operators for such 2D image processing because high spatial frequencies correspond to sharp changes in intensity. Other digital operators introduced[1-5] have varying success for specific applications (see Frei and Chen[6] for general description). These operators are said to be "blind" by their indiscriminate application to all image points: Edges of interest (forming a discrete structure) and those of structural insignificance are treated alike. No structure-dependent information is utilized.

Seven operators are described here and applied to CT image data. In addition to their application for edge detection, methods for simple thresholding, low- and high-pass filtering, and detection of gray-level "step" edges to indicate boundaries are included. In all cases the 3 × 3 pattern of pixels shown in Figure 17.2 is used as reference. Low- and high-pass filters, Kirsch and Sobel operators are presented as described by Bullock.[5] The pseudo-Laplacian operator is described using similar notation.[7] Edge operators can be implemented on CT systems as user options that allow preprocessing of images as an aid to diagnosis. Their addition would complement the image thresholding options already present on most CT display consoles.

Low-Pass Filters

The most simple low-pass filter assigns pixel point X the average $(A + B + C + D + E + F + G + H)/8$. Variants of the simple low-pass filter give added weight to the original value of pixel X. Low-pass filters are commonly used to smooth images that suffer from noise or sharp intensity discontinuities. This is demonstrated by comparing the original CT image in Figure 17.3A with the result of a low-pass filter in Figure 17.3B.

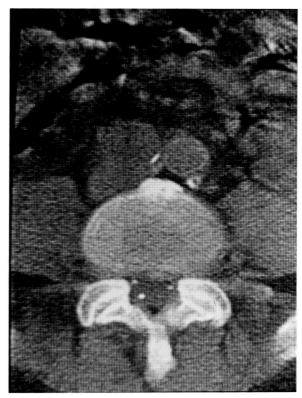

A

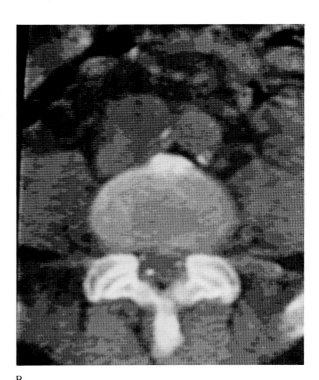

B

FIGURE 17.3 Effects of low-pass filtering a CT image of the spine. **A.** High-frequency image noise originally present. **B.** Image after the low-pass filter operator is applied.

High-Pass Filters

Two related derivative operators are presented here: the gradient

$$[(df/dx)^2 + (df/dy)^2]^{1/2}$$

and the Laplacian

$$(d^2f/dx^2) + (d^2f/dy^2)$$

For digital images, finite differences (instead of derivatives) are used, giving

$$D_x(f) = f(x+1,y) - f(x,y) \text{ for } df/dx$$

$$D_x^2(f) = f(x+1,y) + f(x-1,y) - 2f(x,y) \text{ for } d^2f/dx^2$$

with similar terms for y-derivatives. Finite differences are preferred in those cases where preprocessing time is critical to system response. Other factors influencing this choice is availability of hardware support for floating point and square-root operations.

Gradient

Variations of the gradient avoid computational costs by using the simple sum or maximum (MAX) of $|D_xf|$ and $|D_yf|$ instead of the square root of the sum of the squares. Using points arranged as shown in Figure 17.2 we can define

$$\text{GRAD-MAX (X)} = \text{MAX} (|D-X|,|F-X|)$$

(x − y origin at A, positive y A − G, positive x A − C). An alternative pseudogradient can be defined using addition of terms:

$$\text{GRAD-SUM (X)} = |D-X| + |F+X|$$

Laplacian Operator

Variations of the Laplacian at a point examine only the orthogonal neighbors[7] and those that use all eight neighbors.[5] Both forms are discussed.

For the *orthogonal Laplacian operator*, four 4-neighbor Laplacian operators were examined by Schacter and Rosenfeld.[7] One, the absolute pseudo-Laplacian, is defined as:

$$\text{ABSOLUTE PSEUDO-LAPLACIAN (X)} = \text{MAX} (H+D-2X, B+F-2X)$$

An *8-neighbor Laplacian operator* is implemented by averaging over an image window and subtracting this value from a weighted center pixel value[5]

$$\text{8–N LAP (X)} = 8X - (A+B+C+D+E+F+G+H)$$

Roberts Operator

The Roberts operator is one of the most commonly used operators, having both historic and practical interest. Roberts operator assigns pixel values using the following

$$\text{ROBERTS (X)} = [(X-E)^2 + (F-D)^2]^{1/2}$$

which is often simplified[8]

$$\text{SIMPLIFIED ROBERTS (X)} = |X-E| + |F-D|$$

Sobel Operator

The Sobel operator uses an estimation of x and y partial derivatives with weightings based on the proximity of points to the center pixel X. The partial derivatives are

$$\text{Sobel x-derivative} = SD_x$$
$$= (C+2D+E) - (G+2H+A)$$
$$\text{Sobel y-derivative} = SD_y$$
$$= (C+2B+A) - (E+2F+G)$$

Using these

$$\text{SOBEL GRADIENT(X)} = [(SD_x)^2 + (SD_y)^2]^{1/2}$$

which can be approximated

$$\text{SIMPLIFIED SOBEL (X)} = |SD_x| + |SD_y|$$

Ofthe seven operators, the Sobel operator was the most successful for edge enhancement of CT images.[9] Note the transition from the original CT image in Figure 17.4A to the edge-enhanced result of a Sobel operator[8] shown in Figure 17.4B. No special significance is attached to edges forming one structure as opposed to any other. Images having a strong bimodal distribution of intensity—one characteristic distribution for objects of interest and another for background—are ideal subjects for edge operators. Under these conditions, all edges found are significant. Several research domains process image data with typically bimodal distributions. The Roberts operator,[10] for example, is a common gradient-like operator used for outlining clouds in satellite images, large thermal currents and patches illustrated in infrared pictures, or vegetation patterns in satellite photos. The Roberts operator is also used to reduce gray-level images to line-drawing representations.[11] Operator methods have a long history in medical image processing.

Hall et al.[12] used an operator method to detect and locate the cardiac outline. A threshold is obtained from the first-order gray-level distribution in the cardiac rectangle. Thresholding the gray level there produces a one-bit representation of gradients in the cardiac area. The performance of this method is sensitive to the overlap of gray levels in the lung and heart areas and suffers from spurious and disconnected edges despite postprocess smoothing to encourage connection.

Chow and Kaneka[1] used a method similar to that used by Hall et al.[12] but first segmented the entire picture into small overlapping areas. A gray-level histogram is taken for each area. Each local region of the image containing a portion of a boundary is characterized by a mixture of two normal distributions of gray levels (one histogram hill represents background, and the other represents the object). A

regions that contain several edges the technique is unable to distinguish between the true and erroneous edge. Two difficulties are inherent to their approach: (1) for many classes of pictures the histogram is not bimodal; and (2) differing thresholds between picture segments do not encourage edge connection. This method is unsuitable for 3D interactive applications because of extensive preprocessing: Images are segmented, local distributions are found, thresholds determined, and local binary decision applied—a time-consuming process.

Another technique, suggested by Weszka et al.,[13] requires preprocessing of the entire picture to obtain a bimodal distribution using a Laplacian operator. A threshold is then selected from a strongly bimodal resultant gray-level histogram. This technique, however, suffers the same shortcomings as does that of Chow and Kaneka[1]: True and erroneous edges are not discriminated, and no constraints encourage connection of boundary points.

Contour-Following Methods for Edge Detection

There are numerous edge-detection algorithms published for 2D digital images,[1-7,9-19] but fewer for processing 3D data.[20-25] Because of their accuracy and interaction, 2D techniques have been appropriate for most applications, including even those that involve 3D data. For example, in microscopy, computer-calibrated tracing pens are used to locate structure contours for computer graphics display. Tracings are made for each digitized photograph prepared from microscopes focused at regular levels within a transparent specimen. For opaque specimens, image planes that show a specimen's newly exposed surface are digitized after slices are cut at regularly spaced intervals. Dramatic views of the human brain,[26] neural tissue of the vertebrate retina,[27] and more recently muscle and skeletal structures of the arm and hand[28] have been produced using such contour-tracing techniques.

The complete 3D scene-building process is illustrated in Figure 17.5, from manual tracings of structures reported by CT images (Fig. 17.5A) to "tiled" surfaces (Fig. 17.5B) to shaded views of the skull, ventricles, and lesion (Fig. 17.5C). Figure 17.6 gives us a 3D presentation of cadaver contours of the arm and hand made by manual digitization of cross sections cut at regular intervals.

Edge detection for slow image generation systems can use 2D methods applied manually or interactively without extensive additional cost in computing time. Data generated are off-line, and except for a few image-processing research facilities, automatic photograph to scanner to digital file creation is so protracted that manual 2D edge-finding methods are best suited. A few of the early and successful applications of 2D contour-following techniques for edge detection are outlined here.

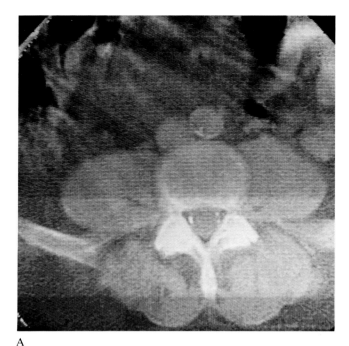

A

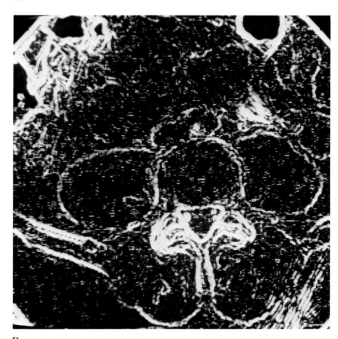

B

FIGURE 17.4 Sobel operator applied to CT image of the spine. **A.** CT image of the spine before Sobel operation. **B.** Edge-enhanced image using Sobel operator.

threshold is found for each region using a maximum likelihood analysis of the two distributions and local area thresholds. A binary decision is then performed for each region.

This technique was found to be effective for detecting edges in pictures that contain very few objects, but for

Contour-following methods are designed to ensure boundary point connection and to emphasize structure-dependent information to find edges. These techniques are sequential algorithms that apply a decision function to each candidate boundary point. Contour following is typically faster than full-field thresholding methods, because the number of candidate edge points is limited to only connected neighbors.

Techniques suggested by Ausherman et al.[14] and Sezaki and Ukena[18] are based on the value of the gradient of the possible boundary point and its spatial relationship with the previously detected edge points. Gradient values are used to detect edges at a local level, and the spatial relationship is used to ensure connectivity of the contour and to detect the edge at a global level. For both algorithms, global information is based on previously detected edge points: Once an error in an edge point has been made, subsequent errors are more likely to occur. No provision is available to evaluate an edge to avoid error propagation. Initialization is another difficulty with contour following: "Good" initial point and global heuristics are required to begin boundary detection.

To avoid erroneous edge points and subsequent error propagation that troubled techniques by Ausherman et al.[14] and Sezaki and Ukena,[18] combined threshold and contour-following techniques were proposed.[15,16]

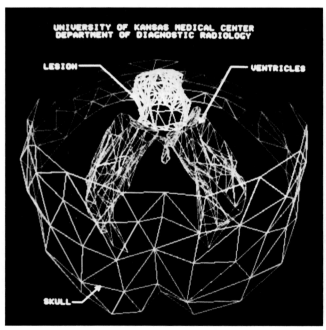

A

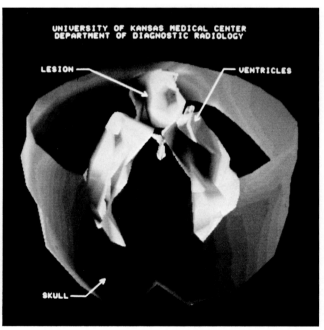

B   C

FIGURE 17.5 Shaded view of human skull, ventricle, and lesion, outlined manually, tiled, then shaded with semitransparency. (Courtesy of SJ Dwyer III, PhD, Department of Diagnostic Radiology, University of Kansas Medical Center.) **A.** Contour-data-illustrated CT cross section of structures isolated. **B.** Add cues to the overall shape are given the view when polygonal tiles are added to approximate the surface. **C.** A semitransparent, shaded graphic view adds a sense of realism to the isolated structures.

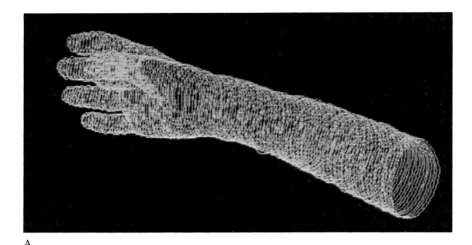

A

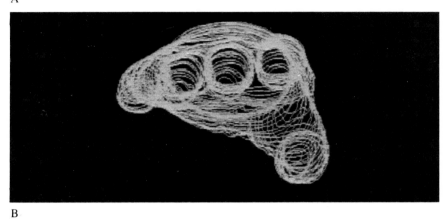

B

C

FIGURE 17.6 Cadaver contours of the arm and hand made by manual digitization of cross sections cut at regular intervals along the arm. **A.** Axial view. (Courtesy of M Kabo, PhD, UCLA Division of Orthopaedic Surgery and the Veterans Administration, Los Angeles, CA.) **B.** Contours rotated for coaxial view. **C.** Skin, bone, nerve, and muscle structures highlighted to illustrate their relative size and anatomic position.

Ballard and Sklansky[15] used a dynamic programming technique to obtain the optimal set of points that maximize a ''figure of merit'' defined by the equation

$$\text{MAX}_{Z(1),Z(2),\ldots,Z(N)}$$

$$\left\{ \sum_{k=1}^{N} G[Z(k)] + Q \sum_{k=1}^{N-2} g[Z(k), Z(k+1), Z(k+2)] \right\}$$

where $G[Z(k)]$ = the gradient value at point $Z(k) = (x,y)$

Q = a negative weighting factor

$g[Z(k),Z(k+1),Z(k+2)]$ = a low curvature

with the constraint $|Z(i) - Z(j)| \leq 2^{1/2}$

This technique used a complex search technique unsuitable for processing pictures with many elements, and the decision function is awkward for general application; terms in the equation above would require adjustment for each object to be outlined. In spite of these difficulties, notable success in image enhancement of digitized chest films has been demonstrated by Ballard and Sklansky.[15] Its broad application is promising in light of future picture archiving and communications systems, where storage, transmission, and presentation of chest films would be digital.

To avoid the difficulties found in Ausherman and Dwyer[14] and Sezaki and Ukena,[18] Chien and Fu[16] proposed a backtracking-lookahead algorithm. They included backtracking capability to avoid erroneous edges and proposed a strategy for general applications. Local and global measures used by their evaluation function are determined by preprocessing that reduces the search space and forms a set of candidate edge points. From this set of points a final boundary set is obtained by applying curvature (global) constraints that are estimated to best fit the boundary to be extracted.

Their technique successfully outlined the cardiac and lung boundary in chest x-ray pictures using curvature constraints represented by a fourth-order polynomial with positive second-order derivative. Their edge detection method is dependent on boundary estimates used as a priori information for the decision function. However, for application to clinical CT data, curvature and surface estimation should be the result of edge detection, not a required parameter for boundary detection to begin. In addition, processing 3D data introduces new problems not yet considered in terms of computer memory and logical connection between CT slices.

3D Methods for Structure Isolation

Whenever digital image generation is slow, or when only a few parallel planes are available for 3D applications, there is no need for fast or automatic algorithms to find structure cross-section contours. However, once a large volume of image data (comprising several planes) is produced quickly,

and when fast object isolation is desired, an automatic 3D method is needed. Such characteristics describe the environment for clinical analysis of data from CT scanners, ultrasound, and MRI devices.

Like many image-processing operations, edge detection for clinical image analysis should be on-line, need little user interaction, and execute with speed close to the rate at which images are generated. Methods described here are directed to those applications where fast automatic results are desired for 3D image analysis. Using edge detection as an example, our goal is to illustrate algorithms and hardware systems that isolate a single structure quickly, with as little user interaction as possible. Using such systems, a radiologist may start the isolation process, resume other duties, then return to a display with the object's contours isolated.

Structure boundaries can be so complex or obscure in 2D and 3D image data that no automatic method can locate structure edges successfully. For example, tumors may appear so subtle in CT brain scans that careful image examination may not disclose their presence. In cases such as these, patient history, symptoms, and physician experience are essential ingredients to the human edge-detection process. In other cases scanned by CT, no clear edge may in fact be present. For example, a destructive process may be widespread but make no substantive changes to the x-ray absorption characteristics of the invaded tissue.

Acceptable accuracy of automatic boundary detection depends on the type of images examined, the image quality, and the algorithm chosen. In repetitive examination of similar images, benefits can be derived from using a priori knowledge or global information gained from earlier images; for example, edges can be postulated when local information is inconclusive or low in quality. In the case of chest-film screening applications, automatic pattern recognition, edge detection, and classification techniques can rely heavily on a priori information. As already discussed, this was shown by Ballard and Sklansky[15] to be a useful approach. In such screening applications, computational techniques are not likely to change from one patient's chest film to that of the next patient.

The natural cognitive process that identifies an object and determines its surface is not well understood. Any modeling of such cognition by digital computers is a poor imitation of a human capability that can recognize objects in some way by the use of several senses. Objects embedded in a series of digital images can be isolated from surrounding pixels only by a methodical, sequential selection task that ultimately examines image data at the level of individual pixels. Routine digital techniques have no global information regarding the membership of a pixel in the class of those representing one object's cross section from another. The task is reduced to a classification process—an examination of spatial and sensory features attached to each pixel. The sensory features, in the case of CT images, corresponds to a relative density, or x-ray attenuation coefficient, for each picture element. Spatial features correspond to adjacency relationships that each pixel may share with its 3D neighbors.

As in any digital representation, the real object is being approximated by discrete samples that record characteristics of voxels that may partially intersect, be located within, or be located entirely outside the object of interest. The discrete representation introduces approximations to the actual cross section of the object. An object surface, then, is also an estimate. As image resolution becomes more fine, in all three axes, errors introduced by partial-volume estimates are reduced. Given the image data defined by any digital sample, what remains is to define rules for the computer, so that by using these rules it can isolate the extent of single objects and segment them from their surroundings. In what follows, we briefly define rules for object and surface isolation.

We can define the notion of digital connectivity by using the natural concepts of connectedness defined somewhat rigorously by Rosenfeld[29] and adapted to our CT application here.

Let I denote the set of all integer triples (i,j,k), which are picture elements in 3–space. Let $A = (i_1,j_1,k_1),...,(i_q,j_q,k_q)$ be any q-tuple of (i,j,k)'s, $q \leq 1$. We call A a right-path in space if for each p, where $1 \leq p < q$, we have $|i_p - i_{p+1}| + |j_p - j_{p+1}| + |k_p - k_{p+1}| < 1$: The condition allows $(i_{p+1},j_{p+1},k_{p+1})$ to be the same as (i_p,j_p,k_p) or any of its six orthogonal neighbors. Similarly, we call A an angle-path in space if for each p, $MAX(|i_p - i_{p+1}|,|j_p - j_{p+1}|,|k_p-k_{p+1}|) \leq 1$; this condition also allows $(i_{p+1},j_{p+1},k_{p+1})$ to be the same as (i_p,j_p,k_p), its eight horizontal, vertical, diagonal neighbors on plane k_p, or any of the nine neighbors on either plane $k_p + 1$ or $k_p - 1$. The set of 26 angle neighbors of (i,j,k) is denoted by AN(i,j,k) and the set of six right neighbors by RN(i,j,k), (a proper subset of AN). Similar definitions are found in Herman and Liu,[23] Liu,[21] and Artzy et al.,[24] where right neighbors and angle neighbors have corresponding terms to designate classes of connectivity.

Boundary detection for a variety of images requires a flexible algorithm—one that does not rely on strong gradients or complex global figures of merit to find an edge. For instance, an edge gradient surrounding a structure may not always determine boundaries. The gradient for a brain tumor may be strong on its border with cerebrospinal fluid (CSF) but very weak near healthy brain tissue. Edges found using connection of picture elements known to be within the boundary are less sensitive to gradient variations along the edge.

Methodology to detect the surface of embedded volumes in 3D is presented here. The two methods outlined—region growing and cubic surface detection—are different from preceding edge-detection techniques that are guided by measures and estimates of the edge to be detected. Instead, a sequential decision approach, e.g., contour following, is combined with spatial and gray-level measures of the picture elements within a region to determine boundaries. Key 3D aspects of both isolation algorithms lie in their ability to provide connection between planes automatically, to enter new ones, or to reenter image planes when necessary to find complete object boundaries. Both algorithms illustrate attention that is due the control of search strategies using 3D image data: Without careful design, such programs can easily overwhelm a computer system and deliver results too slowly for any clinical utility. This 3D control of edge detection is given after presentation of 2D aspects of one algorithm and its data structures.

Region Growing

The region-growing algorithm introduced below is 2D and based on an image-segmentation algorithm developed by Yakimovsky and Cunningham.[19] The algorithm's 2D nature is maintained in a 3D data environment. Although 2D region growing can be extended to "volume" growing, we have limited the search for structure edges to planar data first. By processing as much as possible per plane, the planar arrangement of image data is exploited and the frequency with which image planes are read from auxiliary storage is reduced: I/O delays are short and infrequent. Additional execution speed is made possible by using large I/O buffers. Because of the memory savings made possible by the algorithm's data structures, larger portions of each image can be core resident during execution.

A scenario of computer-issued prompts and user replies determines three inputs interactively: an image array (usually a subsection of a CT picture defining the region of interest); a region acceptance criterion that is used to determine region membership (this usually takes the form of a simple threshold, band-pass requirement); and a set of seed pixels, which are pixels chosen by the user and known to be part of the structure to be isolated. Seed pixels are the first to be tested for region membership.

The algorithm produces two results: an area image containing all pixels found to be in the region on plane k = CK and an edge image containing only the structure's surface intersection with the plane. The algorithm is a simple ordered search process that examines perimeter pixels of a growing region:

> Every seed pixel tested by the algorithm, and found to be a region member, generates eight (or fewer) candidate pixels to be tested for membership. Only the eight neighboring pixels are possible candidates, and of these only pixels not already region members are chosen. Pixels chosen as candidates are placed in a queue to be tested for membership. Those that fail acceptance are discarded and do not generate candidate pixels; those that pass are entered as region members and generate candidate pixels themselves. Terminate when the candidate queue is empty and no additional seeds are provided for the plane.

The algorithm is a breadth-first search that examines all eight same-plane neighbors of each pixel already found to be a region member. The algorithm is said to be breadth-first (as opposed to depth-first) by the fact that all nearest-neighbor pixels are tested for membership before the examination of pixels that are neighbors of neighbors. This breadth-first strategy influences key dynamic characteristics of the program's data structures, memory utilization, and speed (see Rhodes[9] for details).

If we add the restriction that only one candidate can be accepted for membership (for each pixel already chosen), we form an algorithm that constructs paths of one pixel width. Added provisions for ordering the eight candidates for selection, backtracking on dead-end edges, and end-point/start-point identity forms a contour-following algorithm that can use the organization and data structures of region growing for implementation.

Because typically far fewer pixels are tested for contour membership than for region membership, the contour follower has a clear advantage in execution speed but complicates the connection strategy as the planar algorithm advances from one image plane to the next. For example, "bubble" surfaces within an object are difficult to detect automatically using contour following as the planar algorithm. Such surfaces are detected as a matter of course using region growing, and because of this we have used region growing for our clinical implementation.

In the material that follows we confine planar aspects of edge finding to region growing and use terminology from digital connectivity defined earlier to form an automatic plane-connection strategy for a region-growing algorithm. (The corresponding strategy for a contour-following algorithm requires similar pixel testing with added provisions to detect "bubble" surfaces.)

Plane Connection

As region growing proceeds from plane k to plane k + 1, at least one seed pixel is needed for each area in k + 1 that is a structure cross-section angle connected to a region member on plane k. For some structures one seed pixel is sufficient on each plane (consider a sphere intersected by parallel image planes), whereas other structures require multiple seeds (consider a fork intersected by planes normal to its axis). For complete isolation of random objects, all pixels angle-connected to region members need examination for region membership, a requirement that may exhaust core memory.

A solution is required to eliminate the need for extensive computer memory. One is provided by a data communication strategy to transmit seeds generated from plane k to region-growing software operating in either neighboring plane. Two concurrent subroutines interact: One transmits seeds generated from the area image of plane k to another receiving routine that tests seeds for acceptance and initiates region growing. This method, described below, uses I/O buffer space to read the plane k area image from auxiliary storage; no large candidate queue is needed.

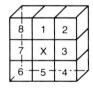

8 2-D Neighbors

Volume Pixels found
in plane k

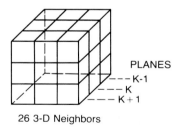

PLANES
--- K-1
--- K
--- K+1

26 3-D Neighbors

Candidate Volume Pixels
to check on planes
k + 1 and k-1

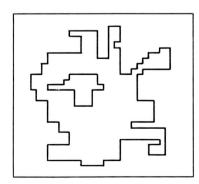

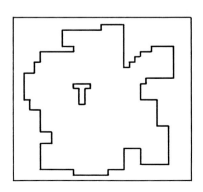

FIGURE 17.7 Digital connectivity for volume elements.

Each pixel in the area image of plane k + 1 or k − 1, depending on direction of advance, generates nine seed pixels (the angle neighbors on plane k + 1). In effect, this action creates the set of candidate pixels shown in the lower right of Figure 17.7 from the region members shown in the lower left. Seeds angle connected to area members on the neighboring plane (candidate records) are transmitted until all pixels in the area image are exhausted.

When a seed is accepted for region membership in the new plane, transmission of seeds to the region grower is suspended and region growing begins about the accepted seed. During region expansion all pixels examined in plane k + 1 have their right neighbors in plane k eliminated. This action eliminates seeds already tested for membership from the pool of potential region members. (Figure 17.8 illustrates the strategy.)

Reentering Image Planes

The S-shaped structure in Figure 17.9, intersected by five parallel image planes, illustrates the need for image-plane reentrance to isolate complete structure contours. Table 17.1 shows five cases where region growing is applied to locate

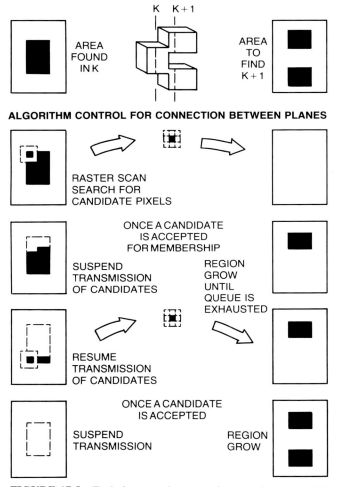

FIGURE 17.8 Technique to advance region growing in one CT slice to continued search in the next CT slice.

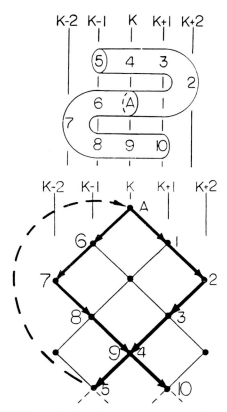

FIGURE 17.9 An S-shaped structure intersected by five planes to illustrate the need to reenter image planes to detect all structure contours when only one cross section is initially identified.

Table 17.1 Contours Found Using Five Seed Placements

Case No.	Grow region from initial seed in area[a]	Sequence of planes examined	Sequence of contours found	Contours missed
1	4 (5,3)	k,k + 1,k + 2,k − 1,k − 2	4,3,2,5	1,A,6,7,8,9,10
2	A (6,1)	k,k + 1,k + 2,k − 1,k − 2	A,1,2,6,7	3,4,5,8,9,10
3	9 (8,10)	k,k + 1,k + 2,k − 1,k − 2	9,10,8.7	1,2,3,4,5,6,A
4	2	k + 2,k + 1,k,k − 1,k − 2	2,3,1,4,A,5,6,7	8,9,10
5	7	k − 2,k − 1,k,k + 1,k + 2	7,6,8,A,9,1,10,2	5,4,3

[a]For seeds in parentheses, the same planes are examined and the same contours are found, but in different order.

structure surface intersecting these planes. If control of the planar algorithm is limited to one examination of each plane, an incomplete set of cross-sectional contours for the structure will be detected. Note that in every case some contours are not discovered.

Complete contours for many simple structures can be found using a single initial seed and one examination per plane. However, for objects of random or unknown shape, well placed seeds cannot always be provided. Regardless, a 3D region growing should find all angle-connected volume members, given any single pixel as seed. This is possible by reentering image planes that may have more region members than previously determined. For the "S" structure (case 4, Table 17.1) this would mean "turning the corner" at plane k − 2, reentering plane k − 1, k, and k + 1 to locate contours 8, 9, and 10.

When a graph is used to represent states of a process and the nodes of the graph are labeled by state descriptors, the nodes and arcs form a directed graph indicating a sequence of state changes. Intuition suggests that such a directed graph can be used to represent image plane access by the isolation algorithm (the lower portion of Figure 17.9 illustrates such a graph). The problem of controlling entry to planes for complete object isolation can now be treated as controlling the creation of a directed graph.

The plane reentrance algorithm is simple: The algorithm searches in one direction from plane to plane, finding object cross sections in each. Whenever a new cross section can be found in the immediately preceding plane, the algorithm interrupts its current plane-to-plane advance, remembers where it is, and turns around to advance in the opposite direction. The algorithm "remembers" where it

"turned" by placing the identity of the current plane in a turnpoint stack. A stack is a computer structure that behaves similar to a spring-aided stack of dishes, like those seen in cafeterias. The first dish placed in the stack is the last dish removed; in other words, a first in last out (FILO) list.

The process continues in the new direction, always "looking over its shoulder" as it proceeds. Advance in one direction ends when no pixels in the next plane are accepted as part of the target object's volume, or when the limit of z-axis planes has been reached. This condition returns control to the last turnpoint to be resumed (the stack is "popped"), until advance is again halted.

The algorithm terminates when plane-to-plane advance is halted and there are no nodes in the turnpoint stack that can be used to resume processing. The algorithm is a depth-first search because turnpoint nodes (planes) are stored in a FILO stack. The most recently interrupted plane-to-plane advance is resumed next.

Note that image planes are entered if, and only if, a new set of area pixels are found, and all possible areas are found when each plane is entered. Thus image planes are entered the least number of times to find all contour cross sections for a structure.

Phantom and Patient Results for Region Growing

The phantom test demonstrates the ability of the algorithm to reenter image planes using actual CT data. Figure 17.10 shows two phantoms scanned to test region growing. On the right in Figure 17.10, the phantom block was scanned to test the algorithm to locate forked structure contours; on

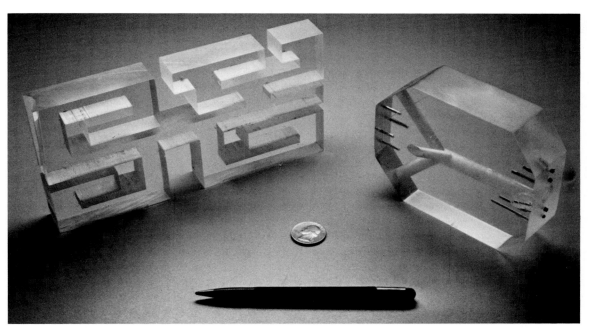

FIGURE 17.10   Phantom Plexiglas blocks used to test region growing.

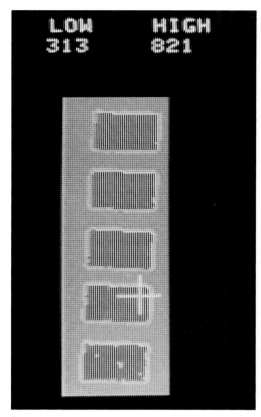
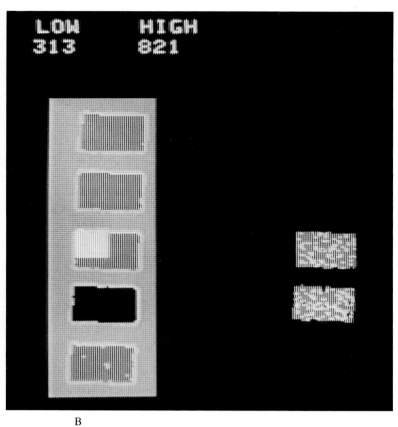

A   B

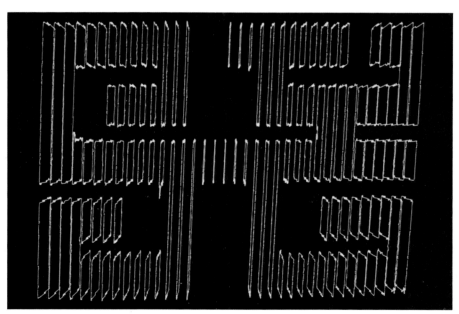

C

FIGURE 17.11 Region growing to find contours of the Plexiglas phantom. **A.** One seed on one CT slice provided to the algorithm to isolate the entire structure. **B.** Intermediate results of region growing. On the right, areas of a neighboring plane are shown. The white square within the Plexiglas cross section is region expanding to the structure's limits. **C.** Contours found by the technique, matching these end-on cross sections with the photograph in Figure 17.10, demonstrate that all cross sections have been found. (*Figure continued* on page 490.)

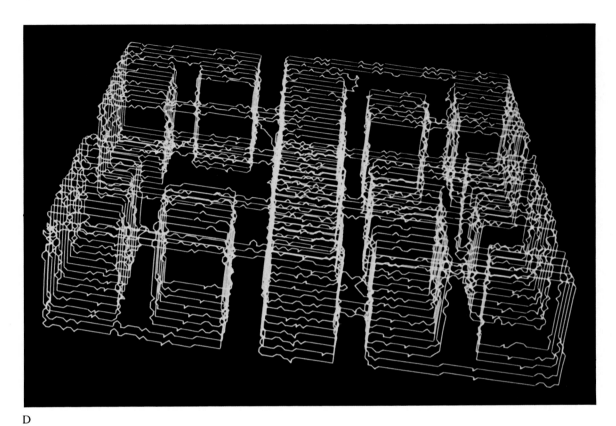

D

FIGURE 17.11 (*cont'd*)   **D.** Oblique view of the cross sections.

the left, a test phantom is shown that was CT scanned to form a file of 35 parallel image planes. Each plane is centered 4 mm apart and normal to the long (left to right) axis of the phantom. The phantom is Plexiglas and was cut to form a complex maze pattern so areas on one plane are disconnected, but connected from plane to plane. The left half of the phantom forms an S-shaped structure similar to that used earlier to introduce the problem of image plane reentrance. The right half of the phantom, connected by a single path, further complicates the algorithm's task.

Figure 17.11A shows only one seed provided to the algorithm to isolate the entire phantom. Note that five disconnected areas are part of the phantom—only one seed is given to the algorithm. (Multiple seeds can be user supplied, but only one is given here for our test.)

The status of one plane during algorithm execution is shown in Figure 17.11B. One disconnected area is "blacked out" (because pixels there have been found earlier) and a new area is about to be discovered (using seeds from a neighboring plane shown on the right side of Figure 17.11B).

A composite view of contours from all planes is shown in Figure 17.11C,D. Matching lines with the photograph in Figure 17.10 shows the entire phantom structure isolated. The algorithm determined the phantom contours in less than 20 min using a GE 8800 S/140 computer. Using five initial seeds, execution time was reduced to less than 14 min.

The composite photograph in Figure 17.11 shows an-

atomic structures isolated by reentrant region growing. Execution times for each structure depends on structure size, frequency of plane reentrance (shape complexity), number of seeds first provided, and whether filtering operations were chosen to preprocess image data.

Few computers have sufficient core memory to store complete 3D image data for typical CT, ultrasound, or microscopic applications. A virtual memory organization is a practical and common solution for such large core memory requirements. In methods described in this chapter, as in Liu,[21] a virtual memory is implemented to access the cube of image data searched for structure edges. Such techniques emulate a core memory of "virtually" infinite size similar to that used in operating systems.[30] Virtual memories implement a "sleight of hand" memory-replacement operation using only the actual core memory available. When requested data is not core-memory-resident, a "page fault" condition is raised. This condition causes replacement of data in the core with that requested. The switch occurs transparent to the requesting program so a virtually large core memory is apparent. Frequent page faults, however, slow algorithm execution because each fault initiates a data transfer from disk to memory.

A key feature of the region-growing method as described here lies in its ability to reduce I/O costs by finding automatically all structure contours possible per plane and entering planes less frequently than methods that do not restrict processing to planes-at-a-time. Additionally, the plane-connection strategy used here can be used to automatically tally contour connections for surface building programs[27,31] that operate on multiple discrete objects. Contours for several structures isolated from CT data are illustrated in Figure 17.12.

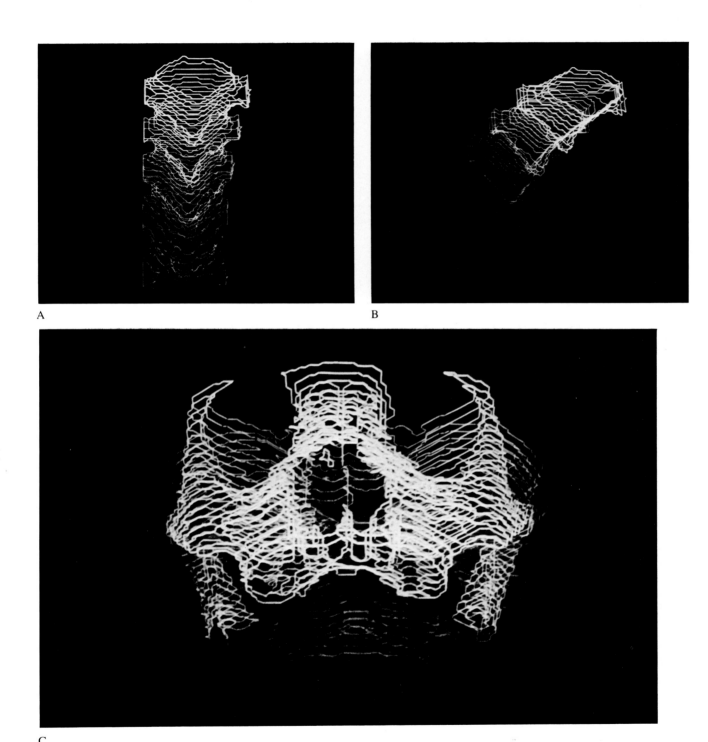

A

B

C

FIGURE 17.12 Contours found by region growing. **A.** Lumbar spinal canal tilted slightly toward the viewer. **B.** Oblique view of the spinal canal. **C.** Midfacial portion of the skull. (*Figure con-tinued* on page 492.)

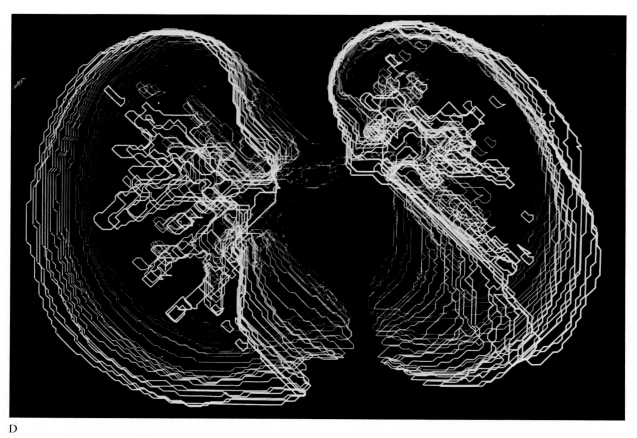

D

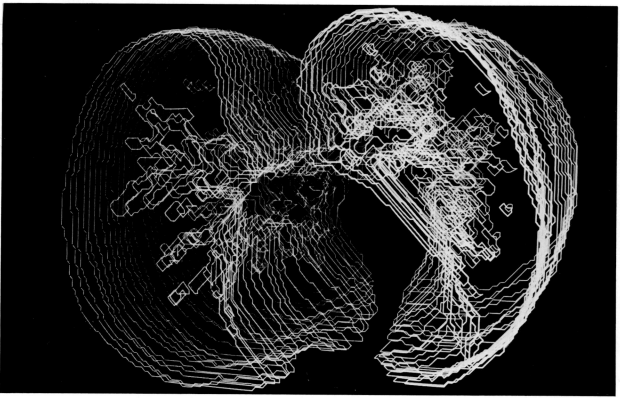

E

FIGURE 17.12 (*cont'd*)   **D.** Bottom-to-top view of lung, extracted from CT image data. **E.** Oblique view of the lung.

Once contours are found for an object, subsequent steps taken to render its 3D presentation use techniques and algorithms well founded in computer graphics. The first step is to create a surface covering the object's contours. This can be done several ways. (See Fuchs et al.,[31] Christiansen and Sederberg,[32] Keppel,[33] Schantz and McCann,[27] and Cook et al.[34] for a useful overview.) The goal in each method is to generate a logical representation of the surface. Patches, triangles, or polygons are commonly used to represent the "chicken-wire" mesh that defines such surfaces. Figure 17.13 illustrates this step. Difficulties during this step are in the area of surface building between planes. Contours at two levels that represent a forking structure usually require human intervention. For example, it is difficult to determine the transition surface automatically from the single contours marking the palm and knuckle portion of a hand through the multiple contours forming the fingers.

Ultimately, by tiling techniques, an object's surface is represented by a single file of polygons. Typically, each polygon contains vertices that are points forming the contours at two adjacent sections. Shaded synthetic 3D views of the structure are made by a series of operations that are applied to each polygon:

1. Each polygon is *transformed* to the desired location for viewing. This includes transformation caused by translation, rotation, and perspective polygon shape deformation.
2. Each polygon is then *clipped*, if necessary, so that only that portion of the structure which is visible through a virtual window, or viewport, is considered for subsequent steps.
3. *Hidden surface sorting.* The polygons that remain are sorted so that only polygons that are visible (not obstructed by others for a given viewer location) are considered for shading.
4. *Shading.* A vector is determined for each of the remaining polygons to determine its orientation relative to both the viewer and to one or more simulated light sources and their reflections. For polygons having a light ray incidence equal to and opposite to the viewpoint incidence, the shaded color is brightest. For polygons with more oblique and unequal light and viewer incidence rays, the shaded color tends to be dim.

Described above is one of several ways to render a synthetic computer graphic view of a 3D object. Figures 17.14 and 17.15 illustrate the results of this approach. Other techniques, using polygon files, include ray tracing[35] and more integrated approaches of the stepwise technique outlined here.[27,36–41] A comprehensive review of this approach to shaded-raster image synthesis appears in Sutherland et al.[42] Yet another technique for viewing 3D views of structures isolated from CT data is briefly reviewed in the following section.

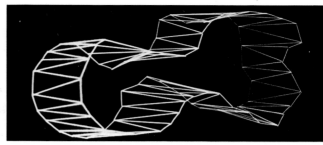

A

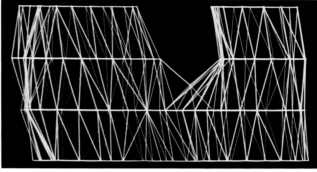

B

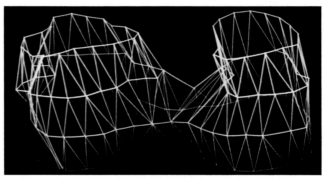

C

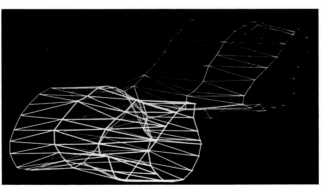

D

FIGURE 17.13 Contours. **A.** Two contours tiled by polygonal patches. **B.** Tiled from four planes. The bifurcation requires a user-added intersection point between the second and third planes (counting from the bottom). **C.** Rotated view. **D.** Rotated view with vectors dimmed furthest from the viewer.

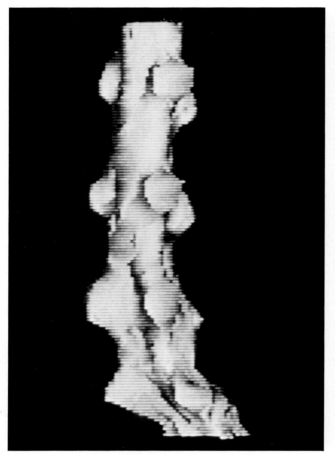

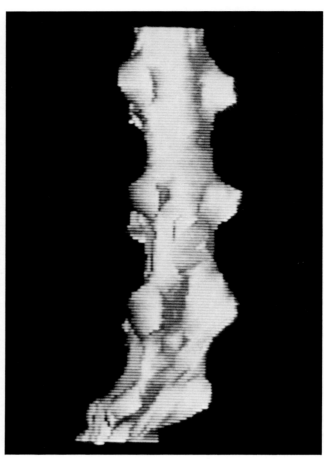

A B

FIGURE 17.14 Lumbar spinal canal. **A.** Shaded view based on contours shown in Figure 17.12. **B.** Rotated alternative view.

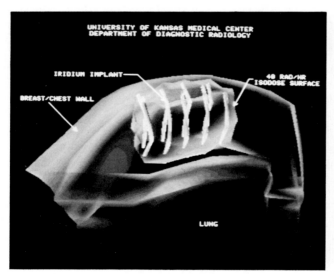

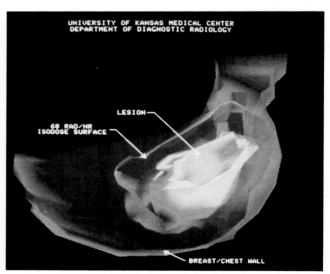

A B

FIGURE 17.15 Semitransparent 3D views of the breast show radiation implant position and an isodose surface of radiation. **A.** Lateral prone view of the breast illustrating the radiation implants and an isodose surface. **B.** An alternate view of the breast that illustrates the lesion and a semitransparent isodose radiation surface. (Courtesy of SJ Dwyer III, PhD, Department of Diagnostic Radiology, University of Kansas Medical Center.)

Cuberille Approach to Surface Detection

Of all the properties that one may use to compare the two structure-isolation techniques, accuracy and speed are clear assets for the cuberille approach. This is not to say that region growing or any approach that uses contour representations of structures is inaccurate, but less approximation is introduced in the cuberille method. Results of this method show surfaces composed of unit volume elements (voxels) that are either axial CT voxels or voxels interpolated between CT slices. Essentially, the structure seen is made at the time of interpolation, where a solid cubic interpolated volume is generated and thresholded. Subsequent surface detection is the process that exposes the embedded object's surface to view.

As shown earlier, contour representation of structures requires "tiling" of surface patches or polygons between contours at various levels. Because there are many criteria for finding an acceptable set of tiles that connect two contours, an element of approximation is necessarily introduced. The only approximation introduced by the cuberille method is during the interpolation step. Interpolation, one could argue, is an arithmetic pure form of approximation where no heuristics need be introduced.

Cuberille surface detection was first introduced for clinical applications of CT diagnosis by Liu,[21] modified somewhat by Herman and Liu[23] to use local gradients to aid thresholding, and later optimized by a clever spatial sorting technique by Artzy et al.[24] This approach uses an image volume in 3-space composed of unit cubes. Notions of connectivity between cubes is more restricted than that outlined earlier in this chapter. For example, objects isolated by the cuberille approach disallow digital connectivity to be angle-connected. In terms of geometry, this means that objects which touch by the corners of two voxel cubes are considered disjoint.

The process (much simplified here) takes five steps. The first step is subregioning, where a region of interest is selected from each of the regularly spaced CT slices comprising a CT examination (usually an orthogonal polyhedron is selected but parallelepipeds are also possible). Within this area, the second step interpolates voxels to form a block of unit voxel cubes. The third step thresholds the block to create a binary representation where voxels failing the threshold condition are marked 0 and those that pass are marked 1. The fourth step is the unique and definitive aspect of the cuberille process. It is the task that efficiently traverses the binary 3-space to locate an object surface given the identity of a single voxel (or face of one cubic voxel) known to be part of the object's surface. Details of the algorithm are given by Herman and Liu[23,43] and Artzy et al.[24] The fifth and final step is a shading process similar to that outlined in earlier sections. Interesting efficiencies and unique problems regarding cuberille shading are outlined by Chen et al.[44] The views of the right neuroforamina, C4–T1 (Fig. 17.16), and the pre- and postoperative views

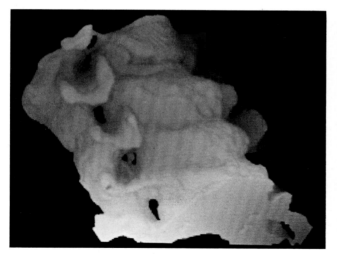 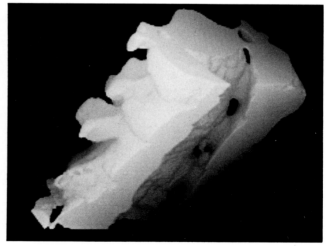

A   B

FIGURE 17.16 3D images, based on CT slices, of right neural foramina, C4–T1. The lamina and spinous processes have been removed from the reconstructed images. Anterior oblique view (**A**) and posterior oblique view (**B**) demonstrate a nodular bony bridge that crosses and constricts medial aspect of the C6–7 foramen. This lesion was not defined on cervical spine films or a myelogram. Although the scan revealed small osseous densities at the C6–7 neural foramina, the degree of foraminal narrowing could not be appreciated on either the routine axial images or the multiple oblique longitudinal reformatted images of this region. The anatomic detail provided by 3D display led to successful surgery. (Reprinted with permission from Goldberg et al: J Neurosurg, in press.)

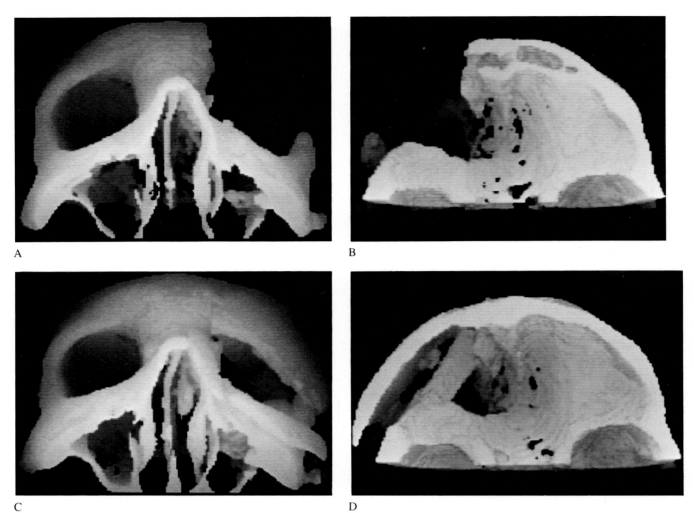

A

B

C

D

FIGURE 17.17   3D images, based on CT slices, of the preoperative (**A, B**) and postoperative (**C, D**) skull of a patient involved in a motorcycle accident. (Reprinted with permission from Morales et al: Volume Assessments Using Three-Dimensional Imaging. 1983 ASPRS*PSEF*ASMS Annual Meeting, Dallas, Texas, October–November 1983.)

of the skull (Fig. 17.17) demonstrate the dramatic 3D clues to shape that are delivered to the user by the cuberille approach.

A comparison of the cuberille method with contour-tiling approaches for clinical 3D imaging illustrates key differences that some researchers find controversial. Issues first outlined by Herman[43] are extended here:

1. *Slice-to-slice connection*. Any structure of modest complexity has cross sections in a series of regularly spaced slices with disconnected components. Although the complete set of contours can be found for these structures, tiling such a set of contours (having one or more bifurcations) is nontrivial. Usually human intervention is needed for even relatively simple structural shapes (e.g., palm-to-finger cross sections). The cuberille approach is not confronted by this problem.

2. *Surface approximations*. Tiling techniques determine an optimal, nearly optimal, or simply acceptable approximation of the surface of a structure by arbitrary measures (i.e., minimal surface area, minimal enclosed volume, speed to surface). As pointed out earlier, no such heuristic approximation is introduced by the simple interpolation of the cuberille method. There has been and continues to be, however, some dispute as to whether the tiling approximation is any worse than the arithmetic approximation of interpolation.

3. *Clinical response*. Although shaded graphics views based on polygons are rendered with increasing speed, the cuberille method enjoys a decided advantage. This is further reinforced by the fact that those systems that are able to generate views quickly based on the tiling approach are special-purpose and represent an added barrier to its

clinical utility. Cuberille methods use the standard CT workstation. Special-purpose hardware built for the cuberille method has further sped this technique (e.g., Contour Medical Systems, Inc., Mountain View, CA).

4. *Realism.* The tiling technique can rely on nearly 20 years of computer graphics contributions that have brought synthetic 3D imaging to a level of realism difficult to match by the straightforward cuberille method. The question of course is whether what appears realistic is actually the most accurate presentation of the "true" surface of the object. The cuberille method is under further development to begin to tap many of the classic contributions to realistic scene generation in order to improve its surface presentations. Improvements can be seen in efforts reported by Chen et al.[44]

Extracting Oblique Planes from Serial Sections

Several researchers have reported definite diagnostic advantages of CT views oriented off the axial plane commonly provided by CT scanners. Byrd and co-workers[45,46] pointed out practical advantages to coronal views for diagnosis of brain and intraorbital disorders in children. Sagittal CT views have been used by Osborn and Anderson,[47] Anderson and Koehler,[48] and Mondello and Savin,[49] in the evaluation of lesions of the nasopharynx and paranasal sinuses. Oblique views also have been found useful for demonstrating orbital masses[50] and, more recently, subtle meningioma in the optic sheath.[51] The acceptance of off-axis views is further endorsed by early researchers in MRI. The apparent unrestricted orientation of views in MRI is widely acknowledged as a key asset to its potential routine clinical utility.

In all of the CT cases cited above, gantry-direct off-axial views were used primarily, although not exclusively, for accurate review. Standard image formats provide an important reference to visualize anatomic position and shape. Indeed, thorough examinations for subtle diagnostic evidence are best made with unlimited image orientations and registration between all formats. Byrd et al.[45] pointed out early that "scanning in the coronal plane is still only an adjunct to the axial view, since at present the disadvantages of increased artifacts and the uncomfortable position make coronal CT inadvisable as the only study."

During the past several years gantry-direct oblique views have been facilitated by CT manufacturers using tilted-gantry scanners. When correctly positioned, oblique views of unsurpassed resolution result. However, precise patient-scanner alignment for such views is still difficult to realize. Automated aids have been introduced (e.g., CT-generated digital plain-film views), but views are limited to those the gantry provides, and no registration or limited registration is available with the more familiar axial transverse, sagittal, and coronal formats.

A technique for constructing general views—image planes oblique to one or more orthogonal axes—is outlined here. Using these methods, tilted-gantry CT is not required, yet unlimited image orientations with registration to standard image formats are made possible. In what follows, principles of oblique plane extraction from a raster-organized, regularly spaced image data set are outlined.

Specification of Oblique Planes

Orientation of an oblique plane is an interactive process where analog dials and multiple images are displayed to help users specify their request. There are as many ways to specify oblique planes as there are programs to do so; each CT manufacturer uses a technique unique to itself. We use here a general approach, unrestricted by any single image orientation. Here images displayed are planes in a cube of image data viewed from three mutually orthogonal directions. The gantry-direct z-axis series provides image information to construct the two additional sets of views: sagittal planes normal to the x-axis and coronal images normal to the y-axis. Pixels in the sagittal and coronal sets are interpolated from the regularly spaced axial transverse images. Further details can be found in Rhodes et al.[521]

Para-axial Oblique Planes

Paraaxial oblique planes are specified using an axial transverse image and two analog dials to position and pitch an axial oblique plane intersection line. Endpoints of the intersection line are positioned around the dashed box marking the limits for sagittal-coronal reconstruction. Once endpoints are located, the oblique plane is extracted, then rotated for display. Figure 17.18 illustrates a multiplanar format

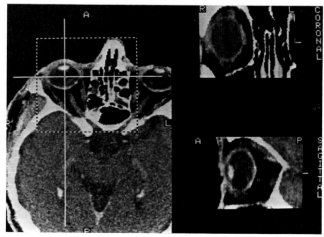

FIGURE 17.18 A multiplanar display of CT orbit anatomy. On the left is an axial picture that is the middle of a series of regularly spaced slices. At top right is a reformatted coronal view passing through the midorbit. Similarly, at bottom right, the sagittal view passes through the central portion of the orbit. Superimposed registration lines over the axial picture locate the alternative views.

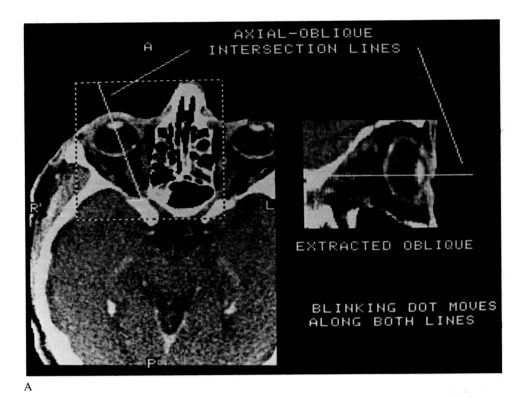

A

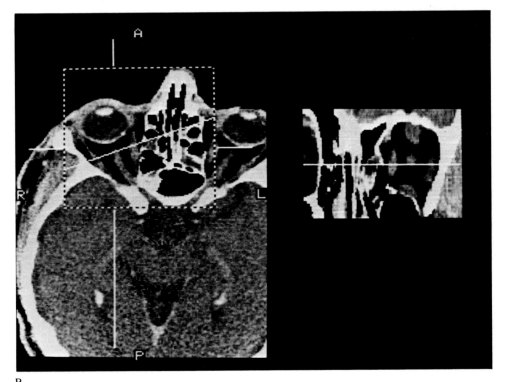

B

FIGURE 17.19 Para-axial views of the orbit. **A.** The paraaxial image on the right is coincident with the optic nerve. Note the registration line superimposed over the axial picture; the same line of pixels appears on the right, superimposed on the paraaxial plane. **B.** A second paraaxial image, on the right, is perpendicular to the optic nerve. As in **A,** registration lines help users to orient the two pictures.

for analysis of orbit anatomy. Two paraaxial obliques of the same case are shown in Figure 17.19. Figure 17.19A represents an oblique oriented along the optic nerve, and in Figure 17.19B an oblique perpendicular to the optic nerve is shown. The process for locating pixels in the oblique plane and that for providing transformation graphics for its display are identical to the general case for extracting obliques, as described in the following section.

General Oblique Planes

As for paraaxials, general oblique planes are selected by showing their intersection with standard image formats. However, unlike paraaxials, these planes can be truly oblique: Resultant views are perpendicular to no reference axis. Sagittal and coronal intersections of the desired oblique are determined using either analog dials to provide parameters or subprograms that locate and display the oblique plane.

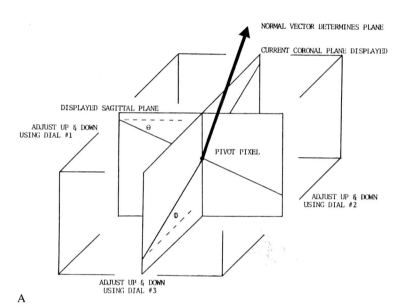

FIGURE 17.20 Geometry of oblique planes as compared to sagittal and coronal images. **A.** Geometry illustrating the selection of true oblique planes from sagittal and coronal views. **B.** The oblique plane selected by intersection lines illustrated in **A.**

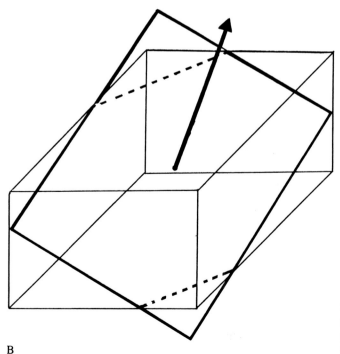

Figure 17.20A illustrates these geometric parameters using a new coordinate system defined by sagittal planes. A pivot pixel common to sagittal and coronal images is used to register intersection lines on both planes. Angles θ in the sagittal image and ϕ in the coronal image determine orientation angles of the oblique. Using three pixels selected on lines user-specified, an equation for the plane is determined:

$$Ai + Bj + Ck + D = 0 \qquad (1)$$

Figure 17.20B shows the oblique plane specified by the intersection lines of Figure 17.20A. The plane equation defines the normal vector shown. The oblique presentation of the orbit on the left in Figure 17.21 is perpendicular to no standard axes. Oblique intersection with the sagittal and coronal views on the right in Figure 17.21 are shown as superimposed lines. The oblique image corresponds to tilting the axial plane slightly downward (see the oblique-sagittal intersection line). Note that the extracted oblique allows the vestibule to be more clearly visualized, due in part to an added pitch relative to the coronal planes.

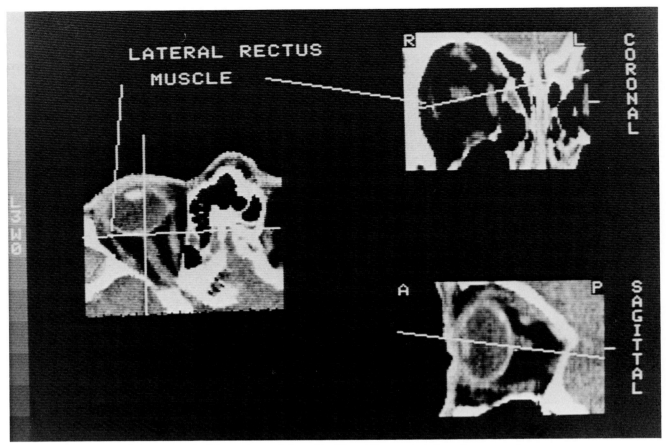

FIGURE 17.21   At left is a general oblique plane of the orbit. The oblique orientation allows the vestibule to be more clearly visualized without losing visibility of the optic nerve. Intersection lines on the right show that the extracted image is oblique to both sagittal and coronal planes.

Image Extraction

Earlier work[53] transformed the entire cube of pixels, transected by the oblique plane, to position the oblique plane viewer perpendicularly. Pixels were then eliminated in front of and behind the plane of interest. The method here selects for transformation only those pixels forming the oblique plane. The pixel location algorithm is described here, and the transformation necessary to reorient oblique planes or display is introduced briefly.

All sagittal images intersected by the oblique plane are examined for pixels coincident to both planes. Because the domain of our search is limited to the image cube of sagittal planes, we can sometimes reduce the range of one or more coordinates. Only a subset of the image data [pixels(i,j,k), where IMIN≤i≤IMAX, YMIN≤j≤YMAX, KMIN≤ k≤KMAX] need be examined. For each sagittal plane (k = constant), pixels intersecting the oblique plane describe a line:

$$Ai + Bj = -(Ck + D) = \text{constant} \qquad (2)$$

Knowing the intersection line equation, we then extract

from image data the pixel value for each (i,j,k) satisfying Eq. (2), then reassign each (i,j,k) to a new position (i′,j′,k′) for viewing. A composite transformation of three rotations is made to orient the plane for screen viewing.

Digital Aliasing

Close inspection of any gray-level digital image shows inherent problems in rendition of detail. Crow[54] listed these difficulties as characteristic to situations in which edge, small object, and fine texture are rendered on digital displays. For example, along edges on the silhouette of an object or a crease on an object's surface, edges appear ragged or "staircased." Polyhedral-shaped oblique planes, as on the left side of Figure 17.22, invariably demonstrate this effect. In situations in which small objects or minute texture are processed for display, picture elements can overlap one another, causing gaps or Moire patterns of holes to appear throughout the resulting view. Software-generated oblique CT images also fall prey to this type of aliasing. For example, some pixels forming the oblique plane in

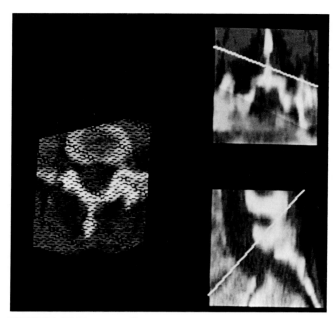

FIGURE 17.22 The effect of digital aliasing is illustrated by the oblique image shown on the left. Note that the orientation of the oblique is perpendicular to the lordic curvature (see sagittal intersection line) but is tilted to view the lateral bone process on one side and the foraminal canal on the opposite side (see coronal intersection line).

Figure 17.22 are written over their neighbors, causing holes to appear.

Aliasing degrades detail of software-extracted obliques in two similar ways. The first is related to the sampling of Eq. (2) to locate oblique plane pixels and the second to raster console resolution.

High-frequency information along an oblique intersection line of Eq. (2) can be missed because of a low sampling frequency. For example, Figure 17.23A shows a digital approximation for a straight line with only three samples taken, one for each row. The approximation is degraded to three disconnected pixels. If pixels along the line were colored periodically red, white, and blue, our sample could lead us to believe the line is solid and entirely red when viewed from point 1 or similar perspectives. However, other viewpoints uncover the discontinuity in our digital sample. When the lines of Figure 17.23A are viewed from point 2, gaps in the line are evident. Analogous image degradation occurs with clinical data. The digital holes appearing in Figure 17.22 are due in part to a low sampling frequency for selecting pixels forming the oblique plane.

Figure 17.23A demonstrates that image orientation may obscure the effects caused by a low sampling frequency. However, all digital holes appear when lines or planes are oriented perpendicular to the viewer's line of

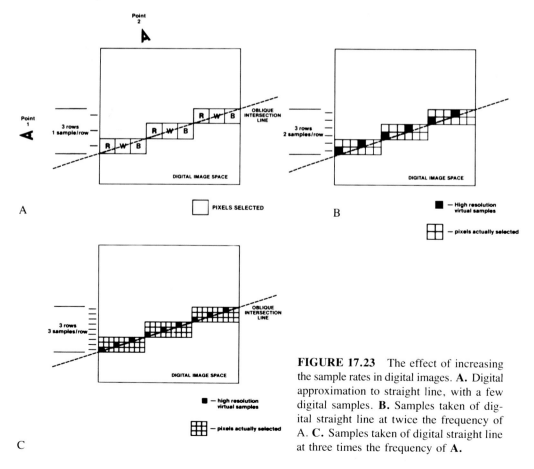

FIGURE 17.23 The effect of increasing the sample rates in digital images. **A.** Digital approximation to straight line, with a few digital samples. **B.** Samples taken of digital straight line at twice the frequency of A. **C.** Samples taken of digital straight line at three times the frequency of **A.**

sight. Because perpendicular orientations are desired for CT diagnosis, all holes must be eliminated.

Oblique views can be improved by increasing image data resolution. Unfortunately, this is not a practical alternative for CT applications, and aliasing problems can persist even at high resolution. In Figure 17.23B, gaps still appear in the digital line, although the resolution is twice that of Figure 17.23A. However, regardless of holes that persist in Figure 17.23B, a solution is suggested. Using higher sampling rates along rows intersected by the oblique plane, the size of holes have been reduced. If samples are taken at higher frequency, we can simulate an image resolution sufficient to eliminate image holes. In this implementation, the sampling frequency has been increased to simulate pixel selection in high-resolution data.

An oblique sagittal intersection line is taken from each sagittal image. The number of samples to take in the interval of sagittal rows should exceed twice the number of columns intersected by the oblique plane. This technique delivers enough pixels to eliminate holes, as shown in Figure 17.23C, but they are again subject to aliasing when transformed to the digital display.

Oblique planes are specified at a precision determined by the available word size. If N bits of precision are used, the plane is defined to a resolution of 2^N virtual pixels (R_v). However, to form the plane, pixels are chosen at the image cube resolution (R_i). Because typically $R_i << R_v$, pixels selected sometimes form a rough surface. Although no holes appear because of high sampling rates, some pixels are above or below their neighbors, sharing only an edge rather than a pixel surface to maintain surface continuity (Fig. 17.24). A digital surface transecting an integer 3–space is illustrated in Figure 17.24. Pixels that share only an edge for surface continuity are seen to be edge-connected and can be described in terms of digital connectivity.[29]

Holes can appear for digital planes when transformed for viewing. Sample pixels that form an oblique surface can be sufficiently coarse (highly edge-connected) to cause some pixels to be written over their neighbors when transformed to screen positions. The result is the same as that occurring for low sampling rate: Digital holes appear in the final view.

In order to reduce the effects of aliasing, select pixels along oblique sagittal intersection lines at twice data resolution and then convolve the selection with a function T to "thicken" the selected oblique plane to two pixels. By ordering image-building routines, oblique planes thus generated have the quality that all pixels selected on the oblique are visible; pixels filling holes are from the adjacent plane behind the oblique. Two key advantages make this method desirable for extracting oblique planes: (1) resultant views are fast—oblique planes are extracted at speeds bound by disk access time; and (2) no additional interpolation from gantry data is required—pixels are selected from a precomputed data cube.

Extracting Pictures of Curved Surfaces

As diagnostic viewing flexibility improves for CT and MRI data, image orientations are suggested that are unrestricted by orthogonal picture storage and addressing structures common to these digital imaging technologies. For example, images generated by most techniques are planar and most often are perpendicular to some reference axes. This section reviews the technique to specify, locate, and display a type of digital image that is 3D in its description but flat in its presentation, an image that follows the structural shape of anatomy. More simply, the technique to generate pictures like "curved coronal" views is discussed here. Because details of this technique were already outlined in Chapter 2, only a brief recapitulation is provided here.

A set of regularly spaced axial CT images is required to generate a curved coronal reformation. As an example, a series of 24 scans of a lumbar spine is obtained using 5-mm thick CT sections every 3 mm. From this series, a midsagittal image is generated to act as reference for choosing a curved coronal reformation (see Chapter 2). It is specified by selecting several pixels (approximately 15) along the desired curvature. A mathematic expression to represent the smooth curve formed by joining these points is then automatically determined. The expression is an 8-term polynomial of the form:

$$f(x) = a_0x^7 + a_1x^6 + a_2x^5 + a_3x^4 + a_5x^2 + a_6x^1 + a_7$$

Terms (a_nx^k) are determined using a polynomial interpolation approach similar to that found in Gerald.[55] The polynomial is then interpreted as an addressing mechanism. It is used to extract pixels from axial CT data to form the coronal image curved along the polynomial.

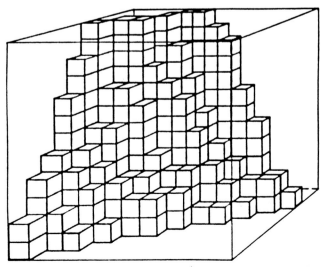

FIGURE 17.24 An oblique surface transecting a digital cube.

It is also possible to generate a family of curved co-ronals that matches exactly the polynomial in curvature but that is separated by a standard distance between curved sections. The format for such a family of curved coronals includes use of the midsagittal section as a reference, where each curved coronal is numbered as a registration aid. (Chapter 2 illustrates several clinical examples of this format.)

One can generalize the curved-surface extraction technique to surfaces that are perpendicular to no axis. In the general case, curved surfaces can be represented by nonlinear parametric polynomial equations (e.g., B-splines, Bezier curves, and patches). Early work by Coons[56,57] and Bezier[58] and more recently by Riesenfeld[59] and Schoenburg,[60] as well as an evaluation of several methods by Barsky,[61] have demonstrated their power and flexibility in spite of a general reluctance to use them because of their complexity of formulation and computational expense. Those medical applications where a generalized curved-surface description is needed (e.g., the surface containing foraminal nerve roots for a patient with spondylolysis and/or scoliosis) require a much simplified spline model over the area of interest. Even under these unusual circumstances, spline techniques for specification of such twisted surfaces can be easily generated. Once determined, curved-surface image extraction is straightforward, because of its inherent parametric form. At this writing no such surfaces have yet been generated for such a medical application.

References

1. Chow CK, Kaneka T: Boundary Detection of Radiographic Images by a Thresholding Method. IBM Report RG3203, December 1970
2. Carton E, Weszka J, Mohr J, Rosenfeld A: Some Basic Edge Detection Techniques. University of Maryland Technical Report TR-277, December 1973
3. Hueckel MH: An operator which locates edges in digitized pictures. J ACM 18:1:113–125, 1971
4. Peli, T, Malah, D: A study of edge detection algorithms. Comput. Graphics Image Processing, vol. 20, pp. 113–125, 1971
5. Bullock B: The Performance of Edge Operators in Images with Texture. Hughes Air Company Technical Report, Malibu, California, October 1974
6. Frei W, Chen CC: Fast boundary detection: A generalization and a new algorithm. IEEE Trans Computers, C-26:988–998
7. Schacter EJ, Rosenfeld A: Some New Methods of Detecting Step Edges. University of Maryland Technical Report TR-461, September 1976
8. Duda RC, Hart PE: Pattern Classification and Scene Analysis. Wiley-Interscience, New York, 1973
9. Rhodes ML: An algorithmic approach to controlling search in three-dimensional image data. In: ACM Siggraph '79 Proceedings, Chicago, 1979, pp. 134–142
10. Roberts IG: Machine perception of three-dimensional solids. In Tippett J (ed): Optical and Electro-optical Infor Proc. MIT Press, Cambridge, Massachusetts, 1963, pp. 159–197
11. Ramer EU: The transformation of photographic images into stroke arrays. IEEE Trans Cir Sys CAS-22:363–373, 1975
12. Hall EL, Lodwick GS, Kruger SJ, et al: Direct Computer Diagnosis of Rheumatic Heart Disease. Technical Report, Department of Electrical Engineering, University of Missouri, Columbia, June 1971
13. Weszka JS, Nagel RN, Rosenfeld A: A Technique Facilitating Threshold Selection for Object Extraction from Digital Pictures. Technical Report 243, University of Maryland, May 1973
14. Ausherman DA, Dwyer SJ, Lodwick GS: Extraction of connected edges from radiographs. IEEE Trans Comput C-21:753–758, 1972
15. Ballard D, Sklansky J: Tumor detection in radiographs. Comput Biomed Res 6:299–321, 1973
16. Chien YP, Fu KS: A decision function method for boundary detection. Comp Graphics Image Proc 3:125–140, 1974
17. Rosenfeld A, Thurston M: Edge and curvature detection for visual scene analysis. IEEE Comp C-28, 1971
18. Sezaki N, Ukena K: Automatic computation of cardiothoracic ratio with application to mass screening. IEEE Trans Biomed Engin BME-20, July 1973
19. Yakimovsky Y, Cunningham R: On the Problem of Embedding Picture Elements in Regions. Jet Propulsion Laboratory Technical Report No. 33–774, Pasadena, California, June 1976
20. Mazziotta JC, Huang HK: THREAD (three-dimensional reconstruction and display) with biomedical applications in neuron ultrastructure and computed tomography. Proc Natl Comp Conf AFIPS 45:241–250, 1976 (AFIPS Press, Montvale, New Jersey)
21. Liu HK: Two- and three-dimensional boundary detection. Comp Graphics Image Proc 6:123–134, 1977
22. Rhodes ML, Glenn WV, Klinger A: Interactive volume and surface isolation using computer tomographic data. In: Proc San Diego Biom Symp February 1–3, 1978, pp. 403–411
23. Herman GT, Liu HK: Dynamic boundary surface detection. Comput Graphics Image Proc 7:130–138, 1978
24. Artzy E, Frieder G, Herman GT: The theory, design, implementation and evaluation of a three-dimensional surface detection algorithm. Comput Graphics Image Proc 15:1–24, 1981
25. Herman GT, Webster D: Surfaces of organs in discrete three-dimensional space. In Herman GT, Natterer F (eds): Mathematical Aspects of Computerized Tomography. Springer-Verlag, Berlin, 1980, pp. 204–224
26. Cohen P, Livingston R, Sumners R: Application Programs for Computer Graphics, "Dynamic Viewing of CT Image Data," 16-mm film, Roche Laboratories Inc. and the Neuroscience Department, University of California San Diego, La Jolla, California, 1978
27. Shantz MJ, McCann GD: Computational morphology: three-dimensional computer graphics for electron microscopy. IEEE Trans Biomed Eng BME-25:99–102, 1978
28. Kabo JM, Meals R: Personal correspondence. UCLA, Division of Orthopaedic Surgery, Biomechanics Research Section, Rehabilitation Center 21–65, 1000 Veteran Avenue, Los Angeles, California 90024

29. Rosenfeld A: Connectivity in digital pictures. J ACM 17:146–160, 1970

30. Denning PJ: Virtual memory. Comput Surv 2:153–189, 1970

31. Fuchs H, Kedem ZM, Uselton SP: Optimal surface reconstruction from planar contours. Comm ACM 20:693–702, 1977

32. Christiansen HN, Sederberg TW: Conversion of complex contour line definitions into polygonal element mosaics. Comput Graphics 12:187–192, 1978

33. Keppel E: Approximating complex surfaces by triangulation of contour lines. IBM J Res Dev 19:2–11, 1969

34. Cook LT, Cook PN, Lee KR, et al: An algorithm for volume estimation based on polyhedral approximation. IEEE Trans Biomed Engin, BME-27, 1980

35. Whitted T: An improved illumination model for shaded display. Commun ACM 23:343–349, 1980

36. Schumacker R, Brand B, Gilliland M, Sharp W: Study for Applying Computer Generated Images to Visual Simulation. AFHRL-TR-69–14, US Air Force Human Resources Laboratory, 1969

37. Newell J, Newell R, Sancha T: A solution to the hidden surface problem. Proc ACM Natl Conf 1972, pp. 443–450

38. Warnock JE: A Hidden Surface Algorithm for Computer Generated Halftone Picture Representation. Technical Report 4–15, University of Utah, Salt Lake City, June 1969

39. Watkins GS: A real-time visible surface algorithm. PhD dissertation and Technical Report UTECH-CSC-70–101, University of Utah, Salt Lake City, June 1970

40. Weiler K, Atherton P: Hidden surface removal using polygon area sorting. Comput Graphics 11:214–222, 1977

41. Sechrest S, Greenberg DP: A visible polygon reconstruction algorithm. Comput Graphics 15:17–27, 1981

42. Sutherland IE, Sproull RF, Schumacker RA: A characterization of ten hidden-surface algorithms. Comput Surv 6:1–55, 1974

43. Herman GT: Three-Dimensional Imaging from Tomograms. Medical Image Processing Group, TR No. M1PG58, Department of Computer Science, SUNY, Buffalo, New York, June 1981

44. Chen LS, Herman GT, Reynolds RA, Udupa JK: Surface Rendering in the Cuberille Environment. TR No. M1PG87, Department of Radiology, University of Pennsylvania, Philadelphia, January 1984

45. Byrd SE, Harwood-Nash DC, Barry JF, et al: Coronal computed tomography of the skull and brain in infants and children. Radiology 124:710–714, 1977

46. Byrd SE, Harwood-Nash DC, Fitz CR, et al: Computed tomography of intraorbital optic nerve gliomas in children. Radiology 129:73–78, 1978

47. Osborne AG, Anderson RE: Direct sagittal computed tomographic scans of the face and paranasal sinuses. Radiology 129:81–87, 1978

48. Anderson RE, Koehler PR: An accessory patient table for multidirectional CT scanning. Radiology 130:802–803, 1979

49. Mondello E, Savin A: Direct sagittal computed tomography of the brain. J Comput Assist Tomogr 3:706–708, 1979

50. Komaki S, Baba H, Matsuura K: Oblique computed tomography for orbital mass lesions. Radiology 129:79–80, 1978

51. Fox AJ, Debrun G, Vinuela F, et al: Intrathecal metrizamide enhancement of the optic nerve sheath. J Comput Assist Tomogr 3:653–656, 1979

52. Rhodes ML, Glenn WV, Azzawi YM: Extracting oblique planes from serial CT sections. J Comput Assist Tomogr 4:649–657, 1980

53. Klinger A, Rhodes ML, Kostanick CV, Glenn WV: General view imagery from parallel image planes. In: Proceedings of the San Diego Biomedical Symposium, 1–3 February 1978, pp. 387–391

54. Crow FC: The aliasing problem in computer-generated shaded images. Commun ACM 20:799–805, 1977

55. Gerald CG: Applied Numerical Analysis, ed. 2. Addison-Wesley, Reading, Massachusetts, 1980, pp. 174–182

56. Coons SA: Surfaces for Computer-Aided Design of Space Forms. Technical Report No. MAC-TR-41, Project MAC, MIT, Cambridge, Massachusetts, June 1967. Available as AD-663 504 from NTIS, Springfield, Virginia

57. Forrest AR: On Coons' and other methods for the representation of curved surfaces. Comput Graphics Image Processing 1:341–359, 1972

58. Bezier PE: Mathematical and practical possibilities of UNISURF. In Barnhill RE, Riesenfeld RF (eds): Computer Aided Geometric Design. Wiley, London, 1972

59. Riesenfeld RF: Applications of B-Spline Approximation to Geometric Problems of Computer-Aided Design. PhD thesis, Syracuse University, Syracuse, New York, May 1973. Available as Technical Report No. UTEC-CSc-73–126, Department of Computer Science, University of Utah

60. Schoenberg IJ: On spline functions (with supplement by TNE Greville. In Shisha O (ed): Inequalities. Academic Press, New York, 1967

61. Barsky BA: A description and evaluation of various 3–D models. IEEE Comput Graphics Applications 4:38–52, 1984

Index